COMMUNITY-BASED
PARTICIPATORY
RESEARCH
FOR HEALTH

COMMUNITY-BASED PARTICIPATORY RESEARCH FOR HEALTH

From Process to Outcomes

second edition

MEREDITH MINKLER
NINA WALLERSTEIN

Editors

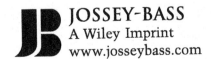

JOSSEY-BASS
A Wiley Imprint
www.josseybass.com

Published by Jossey-Bass
A Wiley Imprint
989 Market Street, San Francisco, CA 94103-1741—www.josseybass.com

Jossey-Bass books and products are available through most bookstores. To contact Jossey-Bass directly call our Customer Care Department within the U.S. at 800-956-7739, outside the U.S. at 317-572-3986, or fax 317-572-4002.

Jossey-Bass also publishes its books in a variety of electronic formats. Some content that appears in print may not be available in electronic books.

Library of Congress Cataloging-in-Publication Data has been applied for.

ISBN 13: 978-0-470-26043-2

SECOND EDITION

10 9 8 7 6 5 4

CONTENTS

PART ONE: INTRODUCTION TO COMMUNITY-BASED PARTICIPATORY RESEARCH

PART FOUR: METHODOLOGICAL AND ETHICAL CONSIDERATIONS IN PLANNING AND CONDUCTING CBPR

PART FIVE: USING CBPR TO PROMOTE SOCIAL CHANGE AND HEALTHY PUBLIC POLICY

SEVENTEEN: THE ROLE OF CBPR IN POLICY ADVOCACY — 307

Makani Themba-Nixon, Meredith Minkler, & Nicholas Freudenberg

EIGHTEEN: USING CBPR TO PROMOTE ENVIRONMENTAL JUSTICE POLICY: A CASE STUDY FROM HARLEM, NEW YORK — 323

Peggy Shepard, Victoria Breckwich Vásquez, & Meredith Minkler

PART SIX: NEXT STEPS AND STRATEGIES FOR THE FUTURE OF CBPR

APPENDIXES

TABLES, FIGURES, AND EXHIBITS

TABLES

FIGURES

EXHIBITS

THE EDITORS

MEREDITH MINKLER, DrPH, MPH, is professor and chair of health and social behavior at the School of Public Health, University of California (UC), Berkeley, where she was also founding director of the UC Center on Aging. She has more than thirty years' experience in working with underserved communities on community-identified issues through community building, community organizing, and community-based participatory research (CBPR). Her current research interests include documenting the impacts of CBPR on public policy, partnering with local community groups in CBPR efforts, and national studies of racial and ethnic disparities in disability among older adults. Minkler is coauthor or editor of seven books and more than one hundred and fifty articles and book chapters in community-based participatory research, community health education, health promotion, community organizing, and critical gerontology. Her books including *Forgotten Caregivers: Grandmothers Raising Children of the Crack Cocaine Epidemic* (with Kathleen M. Roe, 1993), *Critical Perspectives on Aging* (with Carroll L. Estes, 1991), and the edited volume *Community Organizing and Community Building for Health* (2nd edition, 2005).

NINA WALLERSTEIN, DrPH, MPH, is professor in the Department of Family and Community Medicine (DFCM) and was the founding director of the MPH Program at the University of New Mexico. She currently directs the Center for Participatory Research in the DFCM's and vice president's Office of Community Health's Institute for Public Health, and is co-director of the developing Community Engagement Research unit of the Clinical Translational Science Center. For over thirty years she has been involved in empowerment and popular education and in participatory research with youths, women, tribes, and underserved communities in the United States and in Latin America. She is author, coauthor, or editor of six health and adult education books, including *Problem-Posing at Work: Popular Educator's Guide* (with Elsa Auerbach, 2004); an empowerment curriculum for the Americas (in Spanish and Portuguese); and over 100 articles and book chapters on intervention research, adolescent health, alcohol prevention, healthy communities, and empowerment, including materials for the WHO health evidence network (http://www.euro.who.int/HEN/Syntheses/empowerment/20060119_10). Her current research focuses on community capacity development in tribal communities, culturally centered translational research, and the study of participation and partnership processes in creating effective community-based participatory research outcomes.

To the memory of three remarkable human beings
who inspired us
and gave without measure:
Michael Wallerstein, Roy Minkler, and Donald H. Minkler

THE CONTRIBUTORS

JO MARIE AGRIESTI is a leading representative with UNITE HERE in Chicago. She has over thirty-five years of experience in the labor movement and was instrumental in initiating national work and health initiatives focusing on room cleaners.

ALEX J. ALLEN III is vice president of community planning and research at Isles, Inc. He provides leadership for Isles' community-based participatory neighborhood planning, facilitating neighborhood planning processes that involve community stakeholders in collectively addressing land use, transportation, service delivery, and other vital community issues. He also provides direction for community-based participatory research that supports, evaluates, gains a better understanding of communities, and measures the impact of Isles' work.

ROBERT E. ARONSON, DrPH, MPH, is associate professor in the Department of Public Health Education at the University of North Carolina at Greensboro. He currently serves as vice chair of the Greensboro Health Disparities Collaborative.

JENNIFER AVERILL, RN, PhD, is associate professor of nursing at the University of New Mexico. Her clinical and research interests include health care issues and access for multicultural elders (especially in isolated rural areas), community partnership models for making change in the health care system, and critical ethnographic research aimed at engaging community members in the problem-solving process.

MAGDALENA M. AVILA, DrPH, is assistant professor in the Department of Health, Exercise and Sports Science, University of New Mexico College of Education. Her work and research are focused on social justice, community health and health equities, and social determinants of health. She is a coauthor of the landmark principles of environmental justice, developed in 1991 during the Summit on Environmental Racism.

ARI MAX BACHRACH has been doing public health, harm reduction, and HIV research work with marginalized communities in San Francisco since 1996. He is currently studying in the City College of San Francisco Nursing Program and will soon receive his RN degree.

ANDREA CORAGE BADEN, MPH, is a consultant with Community-Campus Partnerships for Health, assisting schools and programs of public health to enhance their capacity to collaborate with communities around reducing racial and ethnic health disparities. She is currently completing her doctorate in medical sociology at University of California, San Francisco, with a research focus on environmental justice, health inequities, and community-academic collaboration.

QUINTON E. BAKER is principal consultant with QE Baker Associates, providing consulting services to community-based organizations and other agencies and organizations in the public and nonprofit sectors. He also serves as associate investigator with the Division of Public Health and the Center for the Advancement of Collaborative Strategies in Health of the New York Academy of Medicine.

ROBIN BAKER, MPH, is a health educator with more than thirty years' experience in the occupational health field. She is director of the Labor Occupational Health Program at the University of California, Berkeley, Center for Occupational and Environmental Health, in the School of Public Health. She is an advocate for effective, action-oriented worker education and leadership.

BEVERLY BECENTI-PIGMAN is the current chair of the Navajo Nation Human Research Review Board (NNHRRB) (www.nnhrrb.navajo.org). She is a wife, a mother, a grandmother, and a respected member of the Chinle, Arizona, local Chapter House, the local unit of governance on the Navajo Nation. She was formally a tribal judge and deeply understands and treasures Native sovereignty and self-governance of tribal research.

ADAM B. BECKER, PhD, MPH, received his PhD degree from the University of Michigan School of Public Health. He has used community-based participatory research to examine and address the impact of stressful community conditions on the health of women raising children, youth violence prevention, and the impact of the social and physical environment on physical activity. He is currently executive director of the Consortium to Lower Obesity in Chicago Children (CLOCC).

LORENDA BELONE, MPH, is a member of the Navajo Nation and currently a PhD candidate in the University of New Mexico (UNM) Department of Communication and Journalism, with a health communication concentration. She is a Robert Wood Johnson Fellow and also a research scientist with the UNM MPH program. She has worked on several National Institutes of Health and Centers for Disease Control and Prevention capacity research projects with Native American communities of the Southwest.

BEA BOWMAN is administrator of the Navajo Nation Human Research Review Board. She has worked with the NNHRRB for over five years and is responsible for organizing the NNHRRB agenda and meetings.

HILARY BRADBURY, PhD, is a writer, researcher, business consultant, educator, and journal editor. Her work focuses on the human and organizational dimensions of sustainable development. She is research associate professor and director of Sustainable Business Programs at the University of Southern California's Center for Sustainable Cities. She can be reached at Hilary.Bradbury@usc.edu.

VICTORIA BRECKWICH VÁSQUEZ, MPH, MA, DrPH, is a graduate of the University of California, Berkeley, and currently works as chief of the Community Health Action

& Assessment Section in the City of Berkeley Public Health Division. Her academic and practice interests are in Latino health issues, international community development, and community engagement and strategic partnerships to eliminate health inequities.

LELAND BROWN, MPH, was founder and director of the Global Bridges Group, which assists public agencies and private corporations in improving community and customer services and internal processes and relationships. He worked internationally on relief efforts and health improvement in Thailand and Nicaragua, and consulted widely in the United States on change processes, the business case for diversity, and community health initiatives. He received his graduate degree in health planning and policy from the University of California, Berkeley, and was credentialed as a project management professional. His untimely death in early 2008 was deeply felt by his large circle of family, friends, and admirers around the world.

MARIANNE P. BROWN, MPH, was director of the University of California at Los Angeles (UCLA) Labor Occupational Safety and Health Program for twenty years and has twenty-nine years of experience in workplace health and safety. She has written many workplace health and safety articles published in journals, books, and the popular press.

MARGARET CARGO, PhD, is senior lecturer in health promotion, School of Health Sciences, University of South Australia. She has been doing participatory research with vulnerable populations for fifteen years. Her research focuses on assessing the governance of participatory partnerships and accounting for context and implementation in the evaluation of participatory interventions.

SUZANNE B. CASHMAN, ScD, is associate professor and director of community health in the Department of Family Medicine and Community Health at the University of Massachusetts Medical School. Formally trained in health services research, evaluation, and administration, she has spent thirty years conducting evaluation research, teaching graduate courses in public health, and developing partnerships aimed at helping communities improve their health status. Prior to her faculty appointment, she spent a decade in community-oriented primary care at the Carney Hospital and the Center for Community Responsive Care, both in Boston.

VIVIAN CHÁVEZ, DrPH, MPH, is associate professor in the Department of Health Education at San Francisco State University. Her scholarship is partially informed by her standpoint as a woman of color and concerns the mind-body divide, community organizing, and global health. She is a coeditor of *Prevention Is Primary: Strategies for Community Well-Being* (Jossey-Bass, 2007).

ANN CHEATHAM-ROJAS, PhD, is a consultant who works with social justice organizations and was formerly research coordinator at Asians and Pacific Islanders for Reproductive Health (APIRH). Cheatham has worked on social change issues using popular education, participatory action research, epidemiology, and organizing with Southeast

Asian girls in California, with farmworkers and day laborers in Ohio and California, and with other communities in California.

KRISTEN CLEMENTS-NOLLE, PhD, MPH, is associate research professor at the University of Nevada, Reno Department of Health Ecology. She received her master of public health degree in behavioral sciences and her PhD degree in epidemiology from the University of California, Berkeley. She formerly worked as an epidemiologist for the San Francisco Department of Public Health, conducting HIV research with hard-to-reach populations, and she emphasizes participatory research approaches to epidemiological and evaluation studies.

NETTIE COAD is executive director of the Partnership Project in North Carolina. She is also a resource trainer for the People's Institute for Survival and Beyond and serves on a broad array of community boards. Coad has been a leader and organizer in her Greensboro neighborhood for over twenty-eight years, serving eight terms as president of the board for her neighborhood association.

JASON CORBURN, PhD, is assistant professor in the Department of City and Regional Planning and a member of the Global Metropolitan Studies initiative at the University of California, Berkeley. His research focuses on the links between environmental health and social justice in cities, notions of expertise in science-based policy making, and the role of local knowledge in addressing community-based environmental and public health problems. Corburn's book *Street Science: Community Knowledge and Environmental Health Justice* (MIT Press, 2005) won the 2007 Paul Davidoff Best Book Award from the Association of Collegiate Schools of Planning.

MARK DANIEL, PhD, is professor and Research Chair for Social Epidemiology in the School of Health Sciences, University of South Australia, Adelaide. He has engaged in participatory research with First Nations in Canada and Aboriginal Australians to develop community-directed initiatives for prevention of cardiometabolic diseases. His research focuses on the role of social and built-environment factors in chronic disease, and how to intervene on these issues.

BONNIE DURAN, DrPH, MPH, is associate professor in the Department of Health Services, University of Washington School of Public Health and Community Medicine, and is also a director at the Indigenous Wellness Research Institute. Her research is focused on alcohol, drug, and mental disorder services and prevention, on social determinants such as historical trauma and violence, and also on cultural and spiritual protective factors. She has worked in public health practice, research, and education for over thirty years.

EUGENIA ENG, DrPH, MPH, is professor of health behavior and health education at the University of North Carolina (UNC) and director of the Kellogg Health Scholars Postdoctoral Program at UNC. She has extensive experience in community-based participatory research and is the principal investigator for the Cancer Care and Racial Equity Study (CCARES).

SHELLEY FACENTE, MPH, received her graduate degree from University of California, Berkeley, and now works as coordinator of evaluation and quality assurance for HIV Counseling, Testing, and Linkage for the City of San Francisco. Her past research projects have included community-based research in Amsterdam, the Dominican Republic, and San Francisco.

STEPHANIE ANN FARQUHAR, PhD, is associate professor in the School of Community Health at Portland State University. She works with community organizations and local agencies to address the environmental and structural determinants of health in Oregon.

STEPHEN FAWCETT, PhD, is Kansas Health Foundation Distinguished Professor of Applied Behavioral Science at the University of Kansas. He is also director of the KU Work Group for Community Health and Development, a World Health Organization Collaborating Centre. In his work he uses behavioral science and community development methods to help understand and improve conditions that affect community health and development.

SARAH FLICKER, PhD, is assistant professor with the faculty of environmental studies at York University in Toronto and an Ontario HIV Treatment Network Scholar. Her research interests are in the areas of youth health promotion, HIV, and community-based participatory research. Flicker sits on a number of community boards and believes strongly in community partnerships for research and action.

SHELLEY FRAZIER, MPH, (Navajo), is Dziltl'ahnii, born for Kinlichíi'nii. Her maternal grandparents are Tsin sikaadnii, and her paternal grandparents are Táchii'nii. Frazier is the national Just Move It campaign coordinator for the Indian Health Service Shiprock Health Promotion Program and National Prevention Initiative. She is a key partner in the Healthy Native Communities Fellowship and coordinates a wide variety of activities aimed at building and strengthening healthy families and communities from the local to the national level.

NICHOLAS FREUDENBERG is Distinguished Professor of Public Health at Hunter College, City University of New York, and has worked with community and advocacy organizations in New York City for more than twenty years. His most recent work focuses on public health advocacy campaigns to change corporate practices that harm health.

CHARLES GOETCHIUS is a field director with the California School Employees Association (CSEA). He has spent over thirty years in the labor movement. Prior to joining CSEA, he was a staff director for UNITE HERE, representing room cleaners employed in hotels.

LAWRENCE W. GREEN, DrPH, is adjunct professor in the Department of Epidemiology and Biostatistics at the University of California, San Francisco (UCSF), and leader of the Society, Diversity and Disparities Program at UCSF's Comprehensive Cancer Center. He was lead author of the original participatory research guidelines while at the University of British Columbia, and he directed the Centers for Disease Control and Prevention Office of Science and Extramural Research, where the reliability testing of the guidelines included in this volume was conducted.

ADRIAN GUTA is undertaking PhD studies in the Department of Public Health Sciences at the University of Toronto. His research interests are in the areas of youth, sexual diversity, HIV, research ethics, and community-based participatory research.

J. RICARDO GUZMAN, MSW, MPH, has been CEO for the Community Health & Social Services Center (CHASS) in Detroit for the past twenty-six years. During this period he has increased funding and expanded primary health care services to the uninsured residents of Detroit by increasing the number of federally qualified health centers, and he has received numerous national and local awards for his role in expanding access to culturally and linguistically appropriate health services for the African American and Hispanic communities.

HELEN ANN HALPIN, PhD, MSPH, is professor of health policy and director of the Center for Health and Public Policy Studies at the School of Public Health, University of California, Berkeley. She is also a senior health policy adviser to presidential candidate Barack Obama. Dr. Halpin's research interests are in increasing access to health insurance, consumer experiences in managed care, and the integration of health promotion and disease prevention services in the U.S. health care system.

TREVOR HANCOCK, MD, is a public health physician and health promotion consultant who has worked for local communities; municipal, provincial, and national governments; health care organizations; and the World Health Organization. The main focus of his work has been in the area of healthy cities and communities, an area he helped to pioneer.

SUSANA HENNESSEY LAVERY, MPH, is a health educator with the San Francisco Department of Public Health, Community Health Promotion and Prevention Branch, working on tobacco control, food systems, and community health worker (*promotores de salud*) efforts. Previously she served as the community health education coordinator at La Clinica de la Raza in Oakland, California.

BARBARA A. ISRAEL, DrPH, MPH, is professor in the Department of Health Behavior and Health Education at the University of Michigan School of Public Health. She has extensive experience conducting community-based participatory research projects in Detroit, Michigan, examining and addressing the social and physical environmental determinants of health inequities.

LORETTA JONES, MA, is founder and executive director of Healthy African American Families (HAAF) II and a community gatekeeper. She has dedicated her entire life to the healing of community and society at large. Her career as a civil rights activist, health policy advocate, and social architect has spanned more than thirty years. In an effort to level the playing field for all people, she continues her unyielding commitment as a change agent against disparities in human health, development, and opportunity.

MARITA JONES, MPH, is field coordinator with the National Prevention Initiative and director of the Healthy Native Communities Fellowship, and also helps to coordinate the Community Wellness Champion Forums with the Indian Health Service. Her passion for learning and connecting with people has led her to work with several communities throughout Indian country and across cultural boundaries. Marita received her MPH degree in community health education and health promotion from Loma Linda University.

NORA JONES is a retired Guilford County secondary school teacher. She is chair of the Partnership Project and a member of the Guilford County Enrichment Board.

PAUL KOEGEL, PhD, is an anthropologist and mental health services researcher, a senior behavioral scientist at the RAND Corporation, and associate director, RAND Health. His research focuses on improving the lives of underserved individuals, with an emphasis on using participatory methods toward that end.

NIKLAS KRAUSE, MD, PhD, MPH, is associate professor of medicine at the University of California, San Francisco, and an occupational epidemiologist with a research focus on the prevention of work-related injury, disability, and chronic musculoskeletal and cardiovascular diseases among ethnically diverse and vulnerable populations.

DANA LANZA, MA, is executive director of the Environmental Grantmakers Association. Earlier, she founded Literacy for Environmental Justice, which brought free urban environmental education projects to more than 10,000 public school students in Bayview Hunters Point and surrounding neighborhoods in San Francisco. Lanza has taught at New College of California and has been a fellow with the Donnella Meadows Leaders Program and with the California Women's Foundation Policy Institute.

PAM TAU LEE is a health educator with twenty years of experience working with unions, worker centers, joint labor-management committees, and community based organizations. She is a practitioner of popular education and community-based participatory research whose work has made major contributions to improving the working conditions of immigrants and women.

SEAN MCDONALD is a master's degree candidate at the University of Toronto, currently studying in the Faculty of Information and the Knowledge Media Design Institute. Previously, he was coordinator of communications and knowledge exchange at the Wellesley Institute in Toronto.

KRISTINE MALTRUD, MPH, works with communities and groups as an evaluator and planner. She is committed to the practice of participatory evaluation and research, encouraging the wisdom and expertise that resides in every community. She currently works with American Indian and Alaska Native communities throughout the United States in the areas of leadership development and increasing community capacity. She received her MPH degree from University of California, Berkeley.

AILEEN MEAGHER is a champion for consumer involvement in health care initiatives involving research, programming, and policy development. Her leadership has been instrumental in advancing the inclusion of consumers in community-based research partnerships across a number of urban health issues, including homelessness, mental health, and research ethics. She currently chairs the Community Advisory Panel on Mental Health at St. Michael's Hospital in Toronto.

SHAWNA L. MERCER, PhD, MSc, is director of the Guide to Community Preventive Services (Community Guide), at the Centers for Disease Control and Prevention (CDC). The Community Guide uses participatory approaches to engage with its intended users in conducting systematic reviews of the effectiveness of community, environmental, population, and health care system interventions in public health. Previously, Mercer was a senior scientist and deputy director of the CDC Office of Science and Extramural Research, where she codeveloped and oversaw a $12 million grant program for community-based participatory prevention research and conducted research and evaluation assessing the value of participatory research for bridging gaps between research and practice.

JAIME MONTAÑO is a Latino community health educator with extensive experience in the development and implementation of individual-level and small-group structural and policy interventions designed to improve sexual outcomes, reduce high-risk drinking, and prevent domestic violence among Latino immigrants. He is particularly experienced in the application of natural helper and lay health approaches using existing social structures, such as soccer leagues. Born in Mexico City, Montaño has worked in community-based participatory health promotion and disease prevention for over ten years.

ANGELA NI is completing her BA degree in political economies of industrialized society at the University of California, Berkeley. She is a research assistant in the School of Public Health as well as a peer adviser in the International and Area Studies department. Ni has studied in China and Taiwan as well as the United States and plans a career that will combine her interests in political science, international studies, and health policy.

R. SCOTT OLDS, PhD, is professor of health promotion at Kent State University. His primary research interests are adolescent and college student substance use prevention. His work employs community-based approaches that coalesce varied groups to marshal resources necessary to effectively respond to this significant public health challenge.

JOHN OETZEL, PhD, is professor and chair in the Department of Communication and Journalism at the University of New Mexico, where he studies the impact of culture on problematic communication in work groups, organizations, and health settings. He is author of over fifty articles and book chapters and author, coauthor, or coeditor of three books: *Intercultural Communication: A Layered Approach* (in press), *Managing Intercultural Communication Effectively* (with Stella Ting-Toomey, 2001), and *The Sage Handbook of Conflict Communication: Integrating Theory, Research, and Practice* (co-edited with Stella Ting-Toomey, 2006).

NANCY "LYNN" PALMANTEER-HOLDER, MEd, (Colville), has over twenty-five years of professional experience in education, community development, and administration in education, health, and human service programs on American Indian reservations. She currently is a doctoral student and National Institute of Mental Health (NIMH) Prevention Research Trainee working with the Center for Indigenous Health Research at the University of Washington's Indigenous Wellness Research Institute. Her interests include using community-based participatory research to develop social welfare Indian health policy as a tool for health promotion, and ethical approaches to health research on American Indian reservations.

EDITH A. PARKER, DrPH, MPH, is associate professor in the Department of Health Behavior and Health Education at the University of Michigan School of Public Health. Her work focuses on the development, implementation, and evaluation of community-based participatory public health interventions, including the Community Action Against Asthma project and the Detroit Community-Academic Urban Research Center, both focused on Detroit, Michigan.

CHRIS PERCY, MD, is a family practice physician with Northern Navajo Medical Center in Shiprock, New Mexico. He serves multiple roles as director of Community Health Services and as chair of the Indian Health Service Health Promotion Task Force. He has been a champion of communities being in the driver's seat and of using Navajo traditional philosophies to guide the work of the health promotion program.

CHERI PIES, MSW, DrPH, is director of the Family, Maternal, and Child Health Programs for Contra Costa Health Services. She is also on the faculty of the School of Public Health at the University of California, Berkeley, as lecturer in the Maternal and Child Health Program and community codirector of the Doctor of Public Health program. Her professional work and interests include implementing a life course perspective in maternal and child health practice, education and training, community capacity building, development of longitudinal data systems for planning and evaluation, photovoice, women's health and reproductive health issues, women and HIV, and parenting support for nontraditional families.

MARGARET A. POTTER, JD, MS, is associate dean at Pittsburgh University School of Public Health, and director of a center focused on issues of practice-based research and scholarship. She spent a sabbatical year in the Office of Science and Extramural Research at the Centers for Disease Control and Prevention.

REBECCA RAE, MCRP, MWR, is Jicarilla Apache from Dulce, New Mexico. She has a dual MA degree in community and regional planning and in water resources from the University of New Mexico (UNM). Currently, she is a graduate research assistant in the MPH program of the Department of Family and Community Medicine at UNM.

PETER REASON is professor of action research/practice and director of the Centre for Action Research in Professional Practice in the School of Management at the University of Bath. His major academic work has been to contribute to the development of a participatory worldview and associated approaches to inquiry, and in particular to the theory and practice of cooperative inquiry. He is coeditor (with Hilary Bradbury) of *The Handbook of Action Research: Participative Inquiry and Practice* (2001 and 2008, 2nd edition).

ERIKA REED-GROSS, MHS, is a Senior Study Director at Westat where she is responsible for managing public health research projects with the Centers for Disease Control and Prevention and other agencies in public health and health promotion.

SCOTT D. RHODES, PhD, MPH, CHES, is a public health scientist whose research focuses on the development, implementation, and evaluation of interventions designed to improve the health and well-being of vulnerable communities and using community-based participatory research approaches. His research explores sexual health, HIV and sexually transmitted disease (STD) prevention, and health disparities among vulnerable communities, including disparities involving substance use and obesity. Rhodes has extensive experience working in partnership with Latino communities, urban African American adolescents, persons living with HIV and AIDS, men of color, self-identified gay and bisexual men, and men who have sex with men.

CASSANDRA RITAS earned her BA degree from Hunter College and her MPP degree from the Kennedy School of Government at Harvard. She works in New York City with communities defined by geography and experience to achieve individual and collective well-being through collaboration, research, and action.

JERRY SCHULTZ, PhD, is codirector of the Work Group for Community Health and Development at the University of Kansas and directs content development for the Community Tool Box (CTB), a global online resource for community building. In 2007, he received the Society for Community Research and Action Award for Distinguished Contribution to the Practice of Community Psychology.

AMY J. SCHULZ, PhD, MPH, is associate director of the University of Michigan's Center for Research on Ethnicity, Culture and Health, and associate professor in the Department of Health Behavior and Health Education at the School of Public Health. She has a long-standing commitment and research record focused on the contributions of social factors (racial, ethnic, and socioeconomic) to disparities in health. Her current research focuses on community-based participatory approaches to understanding social inequalities as they influence health disparities, with a particular focus on the health of urban residents.

SARENA D. SEIFER, MD, is founding executive director of Community-Campus Partnerships for Health and research associate professor of public health at the University of Washington in Seattle. She currently resides in Toronto, where she serves on the steering committee of the Toronto Community-Based Research Network.

EVELINE SHEN, MPH, has worked for over eighteen years in reproductive justice, environmental justice, and community development, using core strategies of community organizing and youth organizing with communities of color to promote self-determination. She is currently executive director of Asian Communities for Reproductive Justice and holds an MPH degree from University of California, Berkeley, in community health education.

PEGGY SHEPARD is executive director and co-founder of WE ACT for Environmental Justice (also known as West Harlem Environmental Action), founded in 1988. Based in Harlem, WE ACT works to build community power to improve environmental health, policy, and protection in communities of color. Shepard is a recipient of the 10th Annual Heinz Award for the Environment and the Dean's Distinguished Service Award from Columbia University's Mailman School of Public Health in 2004.

JANE SPRINGETT, PhD, is professor of health promotion and public health at Liverpool John Moores University, England, where she is director of the Institute for Health. She also is a visiting professor at Kristianstad University in Sweden. Springett has a doctorate in urban geography and a long-standing research interest in healthy cities and communities. Her main research interests are joint work and organizational change, participatory evaluation, and action research in a variety of settings.

RANDY STOECKER, is associate professor in the Department of Rural Sociology at the University of Wisconsin, with a joint appointment in the University of Wisconsin-Extension Center for Community and Economic Development. He moderates and edits COMM-ORG: The On-Line Conference on Community Organizing and Development (http://comm-org. wisc.edu), and writes, conducts trainings, and speaks frequently on community organizing participatory research and evaluation and on community information technology.

JEFFREY L. STOWELL, JD, is president of Community Systems Group and an alumnus of the University of Kansas and the University of Kansas School of Law. He has worked to help communities across the nation use technology as a tool in their efforts to improve health, wellness, and social justice and in their evaluations of those efforts.

SAMARA F. SWANSTON has practiced environmental law for more than twenty years and is a former Superfund attorney with the Environmental Protection Agency, where she was awarded the EPA's highest honor for her work in environmental justice. A former manager of the Department of Environmental Conservation's Superfund program and executive director and general counsel of the Watchperson Project of Greenpoint-Williamsburg, Swanston currently serves as counsel to the Environmental Protection Committee of the New York City Council, a part-time administrative law judge, and a visiting professor at the Pratt Institute Graduate School for Urban Planning and the Environment.

GREG TAFOYA is a degree candidate in the University of New Mexico MPH program, with a concentration in community health interventions. He is a member of Santa Clara Pueblo, NM, where he was raised, and is also of Sauk and Fox descent. Greg is committed to serving communities through participatory approaches and public health research that benefits all partners involved.

MAKANI THEMBA-NIXON is executive director of the Praxis Project, a nonprofit organization dedicated to supporting community-based media and policy advocacy to advance equity and justice. She is author of *Making Policy, Making Change* (1999). Her latest book, coauthored with Hunter Cutting, is *Talking the Walk: Communications Guide for Racial Justice* (2006).

ROSANNA TRAN, MPH, is a program officer with the California HealthCare Foundation and received her graduate training at the University of California, Berkeley. Her community-based public health experience includes work on program evaluation, HIV prevention and care, language access and cultural competence, and problem gambling with a focus on Asian and Pacific Islander American Communities.

ROBB TRAVERS, PhD, is a scientist and director of community-based research (CBR) at the Ontario HIV Treatment Network. He is also an associate research scientist at the Centre for Research on Inner City Health at St. Michael's Hospital, Toronto. He received his PhD degree in public health sciences from the University of Toronto, and subsequently codeveloped (with Sarah Flicker) and taught Canada's first undergraduate course in CBR in the Health Studies Program there.

WILLIAM A. VEGA, DCrim, is currently professor in the Department of Family Medicine at the David Geffen School of Medicine at the University of California, Los Angeles. He formerly served as professor of public health at University of California, Berkeley, and professor of psychiatry at the Robert Wood Johnson Medical School of New Jersey. Vega's research projects on health, mental health, and substance abuse in the United States and Mexico have resulted in several books and over 160 articles and book chapters.

CAROLINE C. WANG, DrPH, MPH, is adjunct faculty member in the Department of Health Behavior and Health Education at the University of Michigan's School of Public Health. A creator of the photovoice methodology, she consults on photovoice projects nationally and internationally. She is a coeditor of the book *Visual Voices: 100 Photographs of Village China by the Women of Yunnan Province,* and a coeditor of *Strength to Be: Community Visions and Voices.*

KENNETH B. WELLS, MD, is a psychiatrist and director of the Health Services Research Center at University of California, Los Angeles (UCLA). He is also professor in the UCLA Geffen School of Medicine in Psychiatry as well as professor in the UCLA School of Public Health and senior scientist at RAND Corporation, Santa Monica.

KALVIN WHITE, PhD, received his doctorate in counseling psychology from the University of Utah. He is currently program director for the Office of Dine Science, Math, and Technology for the Department of Dine Education, Navajo Nation. White is one of the Navajo Nation Council Education Committee's three appointees to the Navajo Nation Human Research Review Board (NNHRRB). He is an active participant on the board and has assisted with the organization and implementation of the NNHRRB research conference.

STEVE WING teaches epidemiology at the University of North Carolina School of Public Health and conducts research on occupational and environmental health. His recent work has focused on the health impacts of ionizing radiation, industrial animal production, and environmental injustice. He is a founding member of the North Carolina Environmental Justice Network.

MICHAEL A. YONAS, DrPH, is assistant professor in the Department of Family Medicine at the University of Pittsburgh School of Medicine and has completed a Community Health Scholars postdoctoral fellowship, with specialized training in community-based participatory research, at the University of North Carolina. He is the founder and director of the Visual Voices project, a participatory approach to working with young people and communities to learn about and collaboratively address issues of health and wellness through the arts.

ACKNOWLEDGMENTS

Many people helped us to make this book a reality, and we are especially grateful to the many coauthors whose hard work and belief in the power and potential of community-based participatory research (CBPR) are reflected in the pages that follow. Each of them writes with commitment and passion for this alternative research paradigm, whether as a community partner, academic researcher, or professional in the field for whom facilitating and conducting participatory action-oriented research with, rather than on, communities is a continuing goal.

The second edition of a volume like this one is also a gift from the publisher, and we are particularly indebted to Andy Pasternak, Seth Schwartz, and the staff at Jossey-Bass for believing in this book enough to make this second edition possible. Editorial staff Kelsey McGee, Elspeth MacHattie, and Sarah Miller also were of great help with their expert copyediting and advice.

Beyond those listed as contributors to this volume are the countless community partners, academic colleagues, research assistants, and practitioners who have shared with us and our fellow authors through their own writings and their more personal stories, theoretical frameworks, illuminating case studies, ethical dilemmas faced in practice, and other insights that have enriched this book, and our understanding, immeasurably. Although too numerous to mention here by name, their contributions are cited throughout the book, and they are deserving of special thanks and recognition.

We also would be remiss in not mentioning by name some of the many friends, colleagues, and community partners who have contributed so richly to our own understanding of empowerment, community participation, and public health as social justice. In addition to the contributors to this edition, they include public health leaders Joyce Lashof, H. Jack Geiger, Victor Sidel, Ruth Sidel, Ronald Labonté, Richard Jackson, John Frank, David Williams, and Margarita Alegría.

Each of us also is supported and inspired by our colleagues at the University of California, Berkeley, and the University of New Mexico (UNM), Albuquerque, respectively. We acknowledge in particular, Emily Ozer, Denise Herd, Cheri Pies, S. Leonard Syme, Linda Neuhauser, Rachel Morello-Frosch, Amani Nuru Jeter, Brenda Eskenazi, Pam Tau Lee, Robin Baker, and William Satariano at Berkeley; and at UNM, Jennifer Averill, Magdalena Avila, Lisa Cacari-Stone, Celia Iriart, Arthur Kaufman, Julie Lucero, Tassy Parker, Veronica Plaza, Victoria Sanchez, Lily Velarde, William Wiese, and Robert Williams, who helped create the UNM Center for Participatory Research.

We also owe great thanks to the scholars, former scholars, staff, and advisory board of the Kellogg Health Scholars program, from whom we also have learned a great deal about community-based participatory research and its deep roots in community building. The W. K. Kellogg Foundation, The California Endowment, Community-Campus Partnerships for Health, and the Community-Based Public Health Caucus of the American

Public Health Association also are thanked for their trailblazing work in and support of CBPR on multiple levels.

Our colleagues at PolicyLink, and especially Angela Glover Blackwell, Judith Bell, Mildred Thompson, and Victor Rubin, with their commitment to using the lessons of community building on the ground to inform and shape healthy public policy, also have been a source of real inspiration as we have worked to focus this new edition more heavily on the potential for affecting change on the policy level through CBPR.

Our graduate students at Berkeley and UNM have been a source of tremendous learning and inspiration, and we thank them for continuing to ask the hard questions and stretch the boundaries of conventional paradigms, stretching our own thinking in the process. At the same time, we also must individually thank our teachers in the communities with which we have worked and our families and friends, since the second edition of this book, like the first, came to fruition thanks in part to their stimulation and support.

For Meredith, community teachers include the residents of San Francisco's Tenderloin hotels, the Oakland grandmothers raising grandchildren, the staff and members of the Chinese Progressive Association, the community of Bay Area people with disabilities, and the participants in the Youth Empowerment Strategies Program in West Contra Costa County. I am also deeply indebted to the men and women of Concerned Citizens of Tillery, North Carolina, and to their visionary leaders Gary Grant and Naeema Muhammad, who exemplify a standard of community organizing and true collaborative research to which I can only aspire.

Among my family and friends my late father, Roy Minkler, was my inspiration, guide, and shining light, even in his last days, and the greatest teacher I have ever known, both in his decades of work with and for the children of San Francisco and more personally with his own five children. My mother, Frances Minkler, has shown in her long struggle with Alzheimer's the same gifts of love, concern for others, and optimism that characterized the whole of her life. My late uncle and dear colleague, Donald H. Minkler, was also a tremendous source of pride and love, whose own courageous battle with Alzheimer's, like his lifelong giving as a physician, teacher, and international family planning leader, touched so many lives. My siblings, Donna, Jason, Chris, and Joan, are each among my closest friends, and a source of pride in the separate paths they have taken and the values they share. Together with my extended family members they have, each in their own way, contributed to this project. I am very grateful as well to the support provided by close friends, including Kathleen M. Roe, Rena Pasick, Marty Martinson, Esme Fuller Thomson, Claire Murphy, Larry Wallack, Nance Wilson, Martha Holstein, and Rusty Springer. The sheer mechanics of a project like this one can be overwhelming, and I owe a special debt to my friend and tireless research assistant, Angela Ni, without whose caring and commitment, organizational skills, and unfailing sense of humor this project never could have been completed, much less done on schedule. My husband, Jerry Peters, and our son, Jason, have been the source of much support, love, and humor, and I owe them special thanks for sticking with me through the long hours this project entailed.

From Nina, great appreciation goes to the advisory committees and local research teams from the tribes I have had the honor of working with, including the elders, social service and health providers, youths and other community members from Jemez, Sandia, and San Felipe Pueblos, the Band of Ramah Navajo, and the Navajo Nation, my colleagues at the Albuquerque Area Indian Health Board, in particular Marianna Kennedy and Rita Kie, and from the New Mexico Department of Health and Health Councils, who have pioneered healthy communities and local health decision making. On the national level, I have deep gratitude to the members of the national advisory committee for the pilot CBPR process-to-outcomes grant, who have provided guidance and gentle, but persistent, redirections to the ongoing work of myself and my colleague Bonnie Duran. Internationally, I owe a debt to my Latin American colleagues who have opened my eyes to new visions of empowerment, equity, and health promotion: Marcia Faria Westphal, Rosilda Mendes, Claudia Bogus, Marco Akerman, Vera Lucía Pereira Lima, Mario González Sobera, Marta Lucia Gutiérrez, and Maria Theresa Carqueira. My research team has been extraordinary in its support: first and foremost Bonnie Duran, who has informed so much of my CBPR thinking, and at UNM, Lorenda Belone, Greg Tafoya, Rebecca Rae, Scott Atole, Julie Lucero, Lisbeth Rios, Isis Serna, Jennifer Sandoval, and John Oetzel.

Among my family and friends, my late brother, Michael Wallerstein, was a source of inspiration in his ground-breaking work on inequality and political and economic systems, as well as being a personal support for each new direction that I have attempted in my life. I am grateful to my father, Robert Wallerstein, who has provided professional and personal guidance, most recently an introduction to his psychological capacity scales, which my colleagues and I are exploring to adapt to community partnerships. I owe to my mother, Judith Wallerstein, a belief in strong independent women, which she carried from her mother who fled as a young child from Russia and which she passed on to me and my sister, Amy, whom I have also always admired and tried to emulate in her capable and independent choices. My close family of this generation, Glenn, Liz, and the kids, Jonah, Hannah, Benjamin, and Nikki, give me faith in this world, as do special friends who have helped me this year to keep my work and my transitions in context: Eda, Suzanne, Michele, Barbara, Robin, and the POCA Sangha. I couldn't do this work without the love, debates, and helping hours from my lifelong partner, David Dunaway, and our son, Alexei, whom I have had the pleasure of watching grow, as he moves out to his own separate, but connected, life.

PART

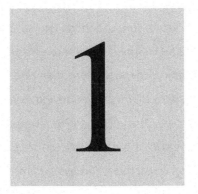

1

INTRODUCTION TO COMMUNITY-BASED PARTICIPATORY RESEARCH

In the six years since the first edition of this book went to press, community-based partici-patory research (CBPR) has achieved growing attention as a collaborative approach to research that offers new hope for studying and addressing some of our most intractable health and social problems. In contrast to more traditional investigator-driven research, CBPR begins with an issue selected by, or of real importance to, the community, and involves community members and other stakeholders throughout the research process, including its culmination in education and action for social change. An overarching term for a wide variety of approaches such as action research, participatory action research, mutual inquiry, and feminist participatory research, CBPR is not a method but an orientation to research (Cornwall & Jewkes, 1995) that emphasizes mutual respect and co-learning between partners, individual and community capacity building, systems change, and balancing research and action (Israel, Schulz, Parker, & Becker, 1998). As Lawrence Green and Shawna Mercer (2001) suggest, CBPR thus effected a change in the balance of power by which "research subjects became more than research objects. They gave more than informed consent; they gave their knowledge and experience to the formulation of research questions" (pp. 1926–1927) and to many other aspects of the research process.

We begin in Chapter One with a broad overview of CBPR, including the reasons for its growing popularity among researchers, funders, and community and other partners. We briefly describe the notion of CBPR as a continuum of approaches and highlight its special relevance for addressing issues of health disparities and inequities. We also provide in this first chapter the goals and purposes of this book, which include in particular a desire to provide both newcomers to the field and more advanced scholars and practitioners a highly accessible text that will offer historical, conceptual, and practical grounding, as well as a variety of tools and techniques that can be used in applying this approach to action-oriented research with a wide range of community and other partners to address an equally wide range of health concerns and disparities. In Chapter One we also introduce several new issues and emphases that are a special focus of this second edition. These include greater attention to external validity, practice-based evidence, and implementation contexts (Fixsen, Naoom, Blasé, Friedman, & Wallace, 2005; Green, 2006) and to the evolution of the field of CBPR from a primary focus on process to an equally strong emphasis on the study of CBPR outcomes, particularly on the policy level. The book's increased use of case studies is described as providing professionally trained researchers and their community partners with useful examples of the integration of theoretical and practice-based concepts, situating the latter in real-world CBPR settings.

Chapter One also introduces the book's increased accent on diverse venues for CBPR, including nursing and academic and clinical medicine (Macaulay & Nutting, 2006; Wells &

Norris, 2006) and a closer look at CBPR in tribal communities. We highlight as well the book's increased attention to involving community partners in data analysis and interpretation and on moving into action, particularly policy-level action, through CBPR.

In Chapter Two, Nina Wallerstein and Bonnie Duran offer a deeper look at CBPR and other participatory research approaches, situating this tradition historically, conceptually, and in practice. The authors provide a more in-depth look at the notion of CBPR as a continuum of approaches ranging from the "Northern tradition" of action research rooted in the work of German social psychologist Kurt Lewin (1946) in the 1940s to the more revolutionary "Southern tradition" grounded in the popular education work of Brazilian educator Paulo Freire (1970, 1982), along with other critical theory, feminist, postmodern, and postcolonial contributors to the field.

In Chapter Three, Barbara A. Israel and her academic and community partners share the core set of principles they developed through their work at the University of Michigan Urban Research Center. These principles, including conceptualizations of CBPR as a participatory, empowering, and co-learning process that accents systems development and balances research with action, are widely used as touchstones in the field. Yet as the chapter authors also point out, every partnership is unique, and each CBPR initiative should therefore create its own set of guidelines for practice.

We conclude Part One with a case study that does just that, while also demonstrating the immense potential of CBPR in fields like clinical and community medicine. In Chapter Four, Loretta Jones and her colleagues discuss the new form of CBPR known as community-partnered participatory research (CPPR) and its principles and core beliefs. Jones and her colleagues also describe how a CPPR partnership involving the University of California, Los Angeles (UCLA), Medical School and the RAND Corporation has used this approach in the planning of a large experimental design study to test CPPR as an implementation strategy for evidence-based depression care interventions.

We hope the first part of this book will give readers a solid understanding of the conceptual and practical base of CBPR and its utility in diverse settings with a range of community-based partnerships. We also hope Part One will encourage readers to explore these challenges further and discover how versatile this orientation is for varied settings, using varied methodologies.

REFERENCES

Cornwall, A., & Jewkes, R. (1995). What is participatory research? *Social Science & Medicine, 41*, 1667–1676.

Fixsen, D. L., Naoom, S. F., Blasé, K. A., Friedman, R. M., & Wallace, F. (2005). *Implementation research: A synthesis of the literature* (FMHI pub. no. 231). Tampa, FL.: University of South Florida, Louis de la Parte Florida Mental Health Institute, National Implementation Research Network.

Freire, P. (1970). *Pedagogy of the oppressed*. New York: Seabury Press.

Freire, P. (1982). Creating alternative research methods: Learning to do it by doing it. In B. L. Hall, A. Gillette, & R. Tandon (Eds.), *Creating knowledge: A monopoly? Participatory research in development* (pp. 29–38). New Delhi: Society for Participatory Research in Asia.

Green, L. W. (2006). Public health asks of systems science: To advance our evidence-based practice, can you help us get more practice-based evidence? *American Journal of Public Health, 96*(3), 406–409.

Green, L. W., & Mercer, S. L. (2001). Can public health researchers and agencies reconcile the push from funding bodies and the pull from communities? *American Journal of Public Health, 91*, 1926–1929.

Israel, B. A., Schulz, A. J., Parker, E. A., & Becker, A. B. (1998). Review of community-based research: Assessing partnership approaches to improve public health. *Annual Review of Public Health, 19*, 173–202.

Lewin, K. (1946). Action research and minority problems. *Journal of Social Issues, 2*, 34–46.

Macaulay, A. C., & Nutting, P. A. (2006). Moving the frontiers forward: Incorporating community-based participatory research into practice-based research networks. *Annals of Family Medicine, 4*, 4–7.

Wells, K., & Norris, K. C. (Eds.). (2006). The Community Health Improvement Collaboration: Building community-academic partnerships to reduce disparities [entire issue]. *Ethnicity & Disease, 16*(1, Suppl. 1).

CHAPTER

1

INTRODUCTION TO COMMUNITY-BASED PARTICIPATORY RESEARCH

NEW ISSUES AND EMPHASES

MEREDITH MINKLER & NINA WALLERSTEIN

GROWING INTEREST among health professionals and academics in finding new ways to study and address complex health and social problems has intersected in recent years with increasing community demands for research that is *community-based,* rather than merely *community placed.* The new focus on translational research to improve intervention outcomes within diverse cultures and contexts (Bammer, 2005; Fixsen, Naoom, Blasé, Friedman, & Wallace, 2005; Neuhauser, Richardson, MacKenzie, & Minkler, 2007) has also shone a spotlight on the potential of action-oriented and community-partnered approaches to health and health disparities research.

In the United States, *community-based participatory research* (CBPR) is increasingly being used as an overarching term for this alternative research paradigm. Building on the work of Barbara Israel, Amy Schulz, Edith Parker, and Adam Becker (1998) in Michigan and of Lawrence W. Green and his Canadian colleagues (1995), the W. K. Kellogg Foundation's Community Health Scholars Program (2001) defined *community-based participatory research* in the health field as "a collaborative approach to research that equitably involves all partners in the research process and recognizes the unique strengths that each brings. CBPR begins with a research topic of importance to the community with the aim of combining knowledge and action for social change to improve community health and eliminate health disparities" (p. 2).

Together with many related action research and participatory research traditions, CBPR turns upside down the more traditional applied research paradigm, in which the outside researcher largely determines the questions asked, the tools employed, the interventions developed, and the kinds of results and outcomes documented and valued (Gaventa, 1993). For, in the words of Budd Hall (1992), "participatory research fundamentally is about who has the right to speak, to analyze and to act" (p. 22). Although often and erroneously referred to as *research methods,* CBPR and other participatory approaches are not methods at all but *orientations to research.* As Andrea Cornwall and Rachel Jewkes (1995), have pointed out, what is distinctive about such approaches "is not the methods but the methodological contexts of their application"; what is new is "the attitudes of researchers, which in turn determine how, by and for whom research is conceptualized and conducted" and "the corresponding location of power at every stage of the research process" (p. 1667). Central to CBPR and related approaches is a commitment to consciously muting the distinction between who does the studying and who gets studied (or decides what gets studied). Similarly, enhancing community members' awareness of the assets they bring as researchers and agents of change is a hallmark of CBPR (Israel, Eng, Schulz, & Parker, 2005). As Cargo and Mercer (2008) suggest, "A key strength of [participatory research] is the integration of researchers' theoretical and methodological expertise with nonacademic participants' real-world knowledge and experiences into a mutually reinforcing partnership" (p. 327).

In epidemiology, often described as the *basic science* of public health, movement toward a more participatory and action-oriented approach has also been increasingly advocated and demonstrated (Krieger, 2000; Lantz, Israel, Schulz, & Reyes, 2005; Leung, Yen, & Minkler, 2004; Wing, 1998). Michael Schwab and S. Leonard Syme (1997) are among those pointing up the potential of such an approach, which embraces "the experience and partnership of those we are normally content simply to measure" (p. 2050).

Such perspectives, of course, are not without critics. Although participatory research is gaining legitimacy in academic circles (see Appendix B), much of the academy remains skeptical of participatory and action-oriented approaches to scholarship (Buchanan, Miller, & Wallerstein, 2007; Coghlan, 2004; Northridge et al., 2000). This book addresses these concerns regarding scientific rigor in later chapters and also includes numerous case studies that demonstrate that CBPR can be both community driven and scientifically sound. In the process we underscore the message of environmental epidemiologist Steve Wing (1998) when he notes that if this nation is to transform society to eliminate health disparities and promote social justice, "a more democratic and ecological approach to scientific study is necessary," one in which "education between scientists and the public must take place in both directions" (p. 250). It is with this *orientation to research,* with its heavy accent on issues of trust, power, dialogue, community capacity building, and collaborative inquiry toward the goal of social change to improve community health outcomes and eliminate health disparities, that this book is concerned.

THE GROWING SUPPORT FOR CBPR

Community-based participatory research has received increasing recognition in public health, as evidenced in its being named by the Institute of Medicine (IOM) as one of eight new content areas in which all schools of public health should offer training (Gebbie, Rosenstock, & Hernandez, 2003). The IOM described CBPR-enhanced public health as "epidemiology enriched by contemporary social and behavioral science because it incorporates what we have learned about community processes and engagement, and the complex nature of interventions with epidemiology, in order to understand how the multiple determinants of health interact to influence health in a particular community" (p. 7).

Beyond public health, a solid tradition of participatory research exists in nursing (see, for example, Anderson & McFarlane, 2004; Falk-Rafael, 2004; Averill, 2005; see also Appendix F), and growing interest in the participatory research potential for medicine also is evident. In North America, practice-based research networks (PBRNs), which initially stressed collaborative research with physicians, are broadening their reach to include patients, family members, and communities (Green, 2007; Macaulay & Nutting, 2006; Westfall, VanVorst, Main, & Herbert, 2006). Special issues of such peer-reviewed publications as the *Journal of General Internal Medicine* (Felix-Aaron & O'Toole, 2003) and *Ethnicity & Disease* (Wells & Norris, 2006) have been published. In both the United States and the United Kingdom, new journals devoted to participatory research (that is, *Progress in Community Health Partnerships* and *Action Research*) have been successfully launched, and a book devoted to methods in CBPR for health (Israel et al., 2005) is widely used and cited. Nationally and internationally, a plethora of academic and community centers and also broad networks supporting participatory research may now be found (see Appendix L).

Federal and philanthropic support for CBPR in the health field has also grown substantially in recent years (Minkler, Blackwell, Thompson, & Tamir, 2003; see also Appendix B), albeit still lagging far behind that available for more traditional approaches to health research. As described in Appendix B, following the early lead of the National Institute of Environmental Health Sciences (NIEHS) and the Centers for Disease Control and Prevention (CDC), many divisions in the National Institutes of Health (NIH) have increasingly called for proposals mandating the use of CBPR to study and address health disparities. New, NIH-funded Clinical and Translational Science Centers (CTSCs) also represent a major opportunity to bring CBPR into health sciences research through required community engagement components, which seek community involvement in defining research priorities to transform the academic research enterprise.

Large and small philanthropic organizations, prominently including the W. K. Kellogg Foundation in the United States (wkkf.org) and the Wellesley Institute in Canada (www.wellesleyinstitute.com), are supporting both participatory research and its use to help effect health-promoting changes in programs, policies, and practices. Through the Community Track of its Kellogg Health Scholars Program, the W. K. Kellogg Foundation (2008) further supports postdoctoral training of a new cadre of researchers with experience in CBPR and a commitment to scholarly and pedagogical use of this approach in their future careers.

New tools and approaches have also been developed, making possible more rigorous and relevant assessment of CBPR, with special attention to its effectiveness in attending to both CBPR principles and the ethical and methodological challenges often inherent in this work (see Chapter Twelve and Appendixes C and G).

Finally, and most important, CBPR and related approaches increasingly have been identified as promising strategies for research aimed at studying and reducing health disparities (Israel et al., 2005; Wallerstein & Duran, 2006; Wells & Norris, 2006). As Paula Lantz and her colleagues (2005) point out, "even if research is purely descriptive (for example, it is attempting to identify patterns and differentials in some phenomenon by race, ethnicity or social class), a participatory approach can help to reframe or refocus the research questions in ways that improve the research" (p. 245).

Building on these developments, this book's aim is to excite students, practitioners, and scholars in public health, medicine, nursing, social work, community psychology, and other disciplines about the potentials of CBPR as a potent alternative to outside expert–driven research approaches to studying health and social problems. We hope that both those with substantial experience in CBPR and newcomers to this paradigm will find themselves challenged by the theoretical frameworks offered, the ethical and methodological dilemmas explored, and the theory-driven case studies used throughout to illuminate this approach. The intent of this new edition is to continue to ground the field through relevant theoretical frameworks and case studies while also offering some new directions. As discussed later in this chapter, key among these new directions is more emphasis on outcomes of CBPR, including policy-related outcomes, indicators of sustainability, and factors that predict outcomes. Additionally, this book explores new applications of CBPR (for example, in the data analysis phase of research) and new settings for this endeavor, including clinical and other organizational settings. We begin here, however, by taking a step back to look more closely at the processes, goals, and principles that lie at the heart of this orientation to research.

SEMANTICS AND CORE PRINCIPLES

Since the publication of the first edition of this volume in 2003, the term *community-based participatory research* has achieved growing popularity, particularly in the United States. Numerous variations of the term exist, however; key among them are *action research* (widely used in the U.K., Australia, and New Zealand); *community-based research*—often the preferred term in Canada (Flicker & Savan, 2006); *participatory action research* and *participatory research* (widely used in many developing countries);

mutual inquiry; feminist participatory research; and most recently perhaps, *community-partnered participatory research* (Jones & Wells, 2007; see also Chapters Two and Four). Adherents to these different terms continue to engage in lively debate over which one—and which corresponding approach—best captures the principles and ideological commitments espoused. We argue, however, that although these different approaches often vary in goals and in change theories, they also share a set of core principles and characteristics (Wallerstein, 1999; Wallerstein & Duran, 2006), summarized by Israel and her colleagues (1998, 2005; see also Chapter Three), who say of CBPR that

- It is participatory.
- It is cooperative, engaging community members and researchers in a joint process in which both contribute equally.
- It is a co-learning process.
- It involves systems development and local community capacity building.
- It is an empowering process through which participants can increase control over their lives.
- It achieves a balance between research and action.

Building on the work of scholars of color and feminist participatory researchers, such as Patricia Hill Collins (2000), bell hooks (1989), Patricia Maguire (2006), M. Brinton Lykes (1997), and Ella Edmonson Bell (2006), we add to these principles that attention to issues of gender, race, class, and culture should also be central to CBPR, as these issues interlock and influence every aspect of the research enterprise. Especially in the health field, in the United States, where the four-decade Tuskegee study of untreated syphilis in black males remains an indelible reminder of the human costs of unethical scientific research (Thomas & Quinn, 2001), issues of race and ethnicity and of racism must not be overlooked. As discussed in Chapter Five, such realities underscore the need to acknowledge, through "cultural humility," that although no one can ever be "competent" in another's culture, individuals can demonstrate an openness to critical reflection and learning about each other's cultures while also examining the biases they bring to the table and being open to genuine partnership (Tervalon & Murray-Garcia, 1998).

The contributors to this volume each bring their own values and assumptions to CBPR, and their different but complementary views provide alternative perspectives on the processes of and forces shaping respectful engagement with communities in combining research with education and action for change. CBPR is used in this book as an overarching name for this orientation to research and praxis, which stresses the principles and values just outlined and explored in greater detail in subsequent chapters.

Although there has been a growing convergence of principles and values, the majority of participatory and action-oriented approaches to research stem from two separate traditions that fall on opposite ends of a continuum (this topic is discussed in depth in Chapter Two). At one end of the continuum is action research in the tradition of Kurt Lewin (1946) and his followers (Coghlan, 2004; Greenwood & Levin, 1998), for whom the accent is on involving people affected by a problem in practical problem solving through a cyclical process of fact finding, action, and evaluation. As illustrated in Chapter Thirteen, the term *action research* has more recently been used, particularly in the U.K.

and Australia, to reflect an overarching family of "participatory inquiry and practice" approaches (Reason & Bradbury, 2008; Stringer & Genat, 2004; Stringer, 2007). In the United States, however, the term *action research* continues most commonly to reflect the narrower and often more conservative approaches used in industrial psychology and related fields. In this tradition there is some, but not necessarily extensive, involvement of affected individuals and typically little commitment to broader social change objectives (Brown & Tandon, 1983; Coghlan, 2004).

At the other end of this continuum is the more emancipatory focus of the *participatory research* (PR), *collaborative action research,* and *participatory action research* (PAR) traditions, which have their roots in popular education and related work in the 1970s with and by oppressed peoples in Africa, Asia, and Latin America (Hall, Gillette, & Tandon, 1982). Such approaches often developed as a direct counter to the often "colonizing" nature of the research to which these peoples were subjected (Fals-Borda & Rahman, 1991; Freire, 1982; Swantz, Ndedya, & Masaiganah, 2006). As Budd Hall (1999) has suggested, "participatory research was very largely theorized and disseminated from a social movement or civil society base: (p. 35). Among the original premises were the importance of 'breaking' what Hall referred to as the 'monopoly over knowledge production' by universities . . . [with] recognition that the academic mode of production was, and remains, in some fundamental way, linked to different sets of interests and power relations than [those held by] women and men in various social movement settings or located in more autonomous community-based, nongovernmental structures" (p. 35).

As discussed in Chapter Two, feminist participatory research approaches, postmodern research, and postcolonial research are among the important contributors to PR and PAR in this tradition. The accent placed by feminist scholars on the importance of *voice*—of having women speak of their own experience and reality, in part as a means of understanding power relations—has thus heavily shaped the work of many participatory researchers (including Cornwall & Jewkes, 1995; Lykes, 1997; Maguire, 2006). Feminists and postcolonial research traditions have similarly reinforced structural transformation as the ultimate goal of an integrated activity combining "social investigation, educational work, and action" (Hall, 1981, p. 7; Maguire, 2006). Finally, and in an interesting alternative to discussions that most often take place from the perspective of academically trained research partners, the new term *street science* is used by Jay Corburn (2005) to describe an approach to environmental health justice that "joins local insights with professional techniques." As Corburn suggests, street science "does not devalue science, but rather revalues forms of knowledge that professional science has excluded and democratizes the inquiry and decision-making processes" (p. 3; see also Ansley & Gaventa, 1997).

As the contributors to this volume well demonstrate, CBPR can and does occur at many places along the continuum from Lewinian action research through participatory (action) research. Yet for all involved to really live up to the definition and espoused principles of CBPR for health—principles accenting having true partnerships between outside researchers and communities and achieving a balance between research and action toward the goal of ending health disparities—it is the emancipatory end of the continuum that ideally should serve as a gold standard for CBPR practice. Particularly for professionals in fields like public health and social welfare, with their roots in concerns for social justice, CBPR in this latter sense provides an important goal for which to strive in their collaborative work with communities.

CBPR AND THE FIGHT TO ELIMINATE HEALTH DISPARITIES

In August 2005, the tragedy of Hurricane Katrina and its bitter aftermath starkly revealed the depth of the race and class disparities in health and life chances in the United States generally and epitomized in New Orlean's Ninth Ward. Through the images seen around the world on television screens and the Internet, many people came to grips with the extent to which there is a "Third World" within the "First World" that is the United States (Omi, 2000) and that in this Third World, mini-Katrinas happen on a daily basis (see Chapter Five). As PolicyLink founder and chief executive officer Angela Glover Blackwell is fond of pointing out, perhaps the only silver lining to Katrina was that it forced Americans to confront head on the dramatic race and class-based inequities that continue to exist in this country and in the process brought about the most sustained dialogue on race and poverty in America since the civil rights movement. It is a goal of this book to contribute to that dialogue, in part as the contributors explore through multiple case studies the continued profound health and social inequities based on race, ethnicity, class, gender, age, disability, sexual orientation, and gender identity and well documented in the literature (Krieger, Rowley, Herman, Avery, & Phillips, 1993; Marmot & Wilkinson, 2006; Schulz & Mullings, 2006; Williams, Neighbors, & Jackson, 2003). But readers also will see how involving communities of color and other stigmatized groups as equal partners in a strengths-based and action-oriented research process, beginning with community definition of the problem to be explored, can improve the quality and outcomes of the research.

The need for new approaches in the efforts to study and address health disparities and inequities cannot be overstressed. Despite some recent progress, racial and ethnic disparities in health and health care access and quality remain profound and have been associated with sociostructural factors such as poverty, racism, minimal public infrastructure, lack of employment opportunities, and neighborhood characteristics (Berkman & Kawachi, 2003; Gee, Spencer, Chen, & Takeuchi, 2007; Krieger et al., 1993; Smedley, Stith, & Nelson, 2003; Williams et al., 2003). Environmental factors, such as outdoor air quality and the prevalence of mite allergens or mold in low-income homes, often exacerbate asthma and other conditions in communities of color, which are disproportionately located in poor neighborhoods (Krieger, Allen, Roberts, Ross, & Takaro, 2005; LaVeist, 2005). Finally, when social capital, which is measured in terms of social networks and feelings of reciprocity and trust (Szreter & Woolcock, 2004; Kawachi, Kennedy, Lochner, & Prothrow-Stith, 1997), is low, it has been shown to bear a relationship to poverty and health disparities (James, Schulz, & van Olphen, 2001). New research showing low social capital in neighborhoods characterized by racial or ethnic heterogeneity (Putnam, 2007) is particularly disturbing, underscoring as it does how far this nation has to go in developing cross-cultural understanding and trust (see Chapter Five).

The fight against disparities can be won only if the most oppressed communities can be fully engaged as partners in exploring and in taking action to address the health and social problems about which they—not experts as outsiders—care most deeply (Minkler, 2005; Wells & Norris, 2006).

GOALS OF THIS BOOK: CONTINUING CONCERNS AND NEW EMPHASES

Our primary goal in this book is to provide a highly accessible text that will stimulate practitioners, students, academics in health and related fields, and their community partners as they engage—intellectually and in practice—in community-based participatory research as an alternative approach to collaborative inquiry for action to eliminate health disparities. Further, and although much cutting-edge participatory research continues outside the United States (see, for example, Mosavel, Simon, van Stade, & Buchbinder, 2005; Reason & Bradbury, 2006; Rice, 2007; Stringer, 2007), our purpose is to focus primarily on CBPR in the contemporary United States, in part so that we can more carefully attend to the geopolitical and sociohistorical contexts that are so central to this work. We frequently draw on the wisdom of leading PR, AR, and PAR scholars and practitioners in developing nations, the U.K., Canada, Australia, and elsewhere (De Koning & Martin, 1996), and believe that many of the skills and conceptual and ethical issues raised will have relevance beyond the United States. We also acknowledge our deep indebtedness to earlier landmark participatory research in North America, to which we cannot do justice here (see Park, Brydon-Miller, Hall, & Jackson, 1993). These classic studies address, for example, popular epidemiology in occupational and environmental health in Appalachia conducted over two decades ago by and with the Highlander Research and Education Center in Tennessee (Couto, 1987; Lewis, 2006; Merrifield, 1993).

As we build on this rich history, our central concern is with helping students, scholars, community members, and practitioners in fields such as health, social welfare, and city and regional planning become more inspired by, comfortable with, and proficient in applying CBPR approaches in their community-based work. Within this context the contributors to this volume explore such issues as cross-cultural and power dynamics in the CBPR process, with particular attention to race and racism; methods and techniques for helping communities identify their strengths and concerns; issues of rigor and validity in CBPR; and special considerations in conducting CBPR with hidden populations, youths, and other diverse groups.

Alongside these continuing concerns, however, this new volume introduces—and considers in more depth—several new emphases. The first of these grows out of an increased call across public health, medicine, and related disciplines for evidence-based practice and outcomes-based research (Green, 2006; Green & Glasgow, 2006). A recognition that evidence in one setting is no longer sufficient for translating interventions to diverse settings has led to calls for greater attention to external validity, *practice-based evidence,* and implementation contexts (Hall, 2001; Fixsen et al., 2005; Miller & Shinn, 2005; Green, 2006). Examining the added value of CBPR and the pathways through which CBPR may improve health has become increasingly important with the growing attention to translational research (Bammer, 2005; Best, Hiatt, & Norman, 2005; Neuhauser et al., 2007; see also Chapter Twenty-One). Consistent with these concerns, the focus of the field of CBPR is evolving from an initial and continued interest in *process* (that is, in how to form authentic partnerships or involve community members in the research) to an interest in the study of *outcomes,* whether these are systems change CBPR outcomes (that is, health-promoting policies or practices) or outcomes related to health and the reduction of health disparities. In this second edition we study CBPR processes leading to outcomes within a translational context, as a potential key to better understanding implementation and sustainability within interventions research. In addition to new chapters presenting case studies selected in part because they feature demonstrated effectiveness in getting to outcomes, we have included updated chapters from the first edition that now discuss documented, longer-term outcomes. Our strengthened emphasis on case studies provides professionals with valuable examples of integrating theoretical and practice-based concepts, as these case studies situate and apply these concepts in real-world CBPR settings.

We also provide in this new edition a final chapter that explores the contributions of CBPR to outcomes and the potential pathways to both intermediate system change outcomes and more distal health changes. Reporting on the first-year results of a two-year pilot study to identify these core processes and pathways, the chapter offers a unifying conceptual model to guide researchers' and practitioners' thinking in this area and inform future intervention research. The chapter also offers a series of hypotheses that could profitably be tested for their ability to move the field forward. Although we present this work as an integrative chapter at the end of the book, readers who are familiar with CBPR may wish to read it early on, using its discussion of the state of the science of CBPR and the challenges in the field to provide context as they explore the various case studies and theoretical, ethical, and methodological issues discussed in other chapters.

A second new focus of this book involves the growing interest in academic and clinical medicine in incorporating CBPR in work with patients, providers, and health and other social service agencies (Felix-Aaron & O'Toole, 2003; Macaulay & Nutting, 2006; Wells & Norris, 2006). As Loretta Jones and Ken Wells point out (2007), "community-based participatory research has been used more as a paradigm for public health than for clinical or health services research," and "many features of CBPR, such as spending time in the community, power sharing, and action research methods, might challenge physicians given their clinical training" and the demands and expectations of their work (p. 407). Yet as Jones and Wells go on to note, in medicine too, new collaborations and NIH funding opportunities (see Appendix B) are encouraging physicians and other clinicians to employ CBPR in innovative ways (Macaulay & Nutting, 2006; Wells & Norris, 2006). Although this book remains focused primarily on the use of CBPR in community settings and within the context of public health, we have broadened our gaze in this second volume to increase its utility to physicians, nurses, social workers, and other clinicians who are exploring the use of CBPR within health care and provider contexts (see Chapter Four and Appendix F).

As discussed in Chapters Three and Sixteen, although CBPR frequently involves community partners in issue selection, study design, and data collection and dissemination, data analysis is typically left up to the academic or other outside research partners. The third new area of emphasis in this volume concerns actively involving community partners in data analysis and understanding both the advantages and the challenges of doing so (see Chapter Sixteen). We further have devoted more attention to participatory evaluation with community partners, both in the expanded and updated chapter on that theme (see Chapter Twelve) and in case studies, such as the study of the Healthy Native Community Fellowship (see Chapter Ten).

A final expanded area of emphasis involves the use of CBPR to help bring about policy changes. Several seminal works in this area have been produced, key among them the user-friendly monograph *Speaking Truth, Creating Power,* by Cassandra Ritas (2003), available through Community-Campus Partnerships for Health. Yet efforts to document the impacts of CBPR on policy have been slower in coming. Of the sixty CBPR case studies identified through the comprehensive literature review commissioned by the Agency for Healthcare Research and Quality (Viswanathan et al., 2004), just thirteen were seen as having a strong policy focus. With support from funders including the W. K. Kellogg Foundation and The California Endowment, several efforts to chronicle the impacts of CBPR on policy have since gotten under way and are building the evidence base in this area (see, for example, Morello-Frosch, Pastor, Sadd, Porras, & Prichard, 2005; Petersen, Minkler, Breckwich Vásquez, & Baden, 2006; Minkler et al., 2008; Minkler, Breckwich Vásquez, Tajik, and Petersen, 2008). In this second edition we contribute an expanded overview chapter on CBPR and policy and three case studies designed to show the breadth and diversity of work in this area (see Chapters Seventeen through Twenty).

In sum this second edition offers the reader several new and expanded areas of emphasis that reflect some of the exciting developments in the theory and practice of community-based participatory research. The chapter authors have in common a belief in the power of CBPR, tempered with an awareness of the very real ethical and practical dilemmas that arise in the course of CBPR application. Speaking from both personal experience in the field and a broad understanding of underlying theoretical, methodological, and ethical and value issues, they help the reader to grapple with some of the steps and considerations that underlie ethical and effective community engagement. The contributors share as well the formal and informal theories guiding their work, because, in the words of social epidemiologist Nancy Krieger (2000), "by clarifying our theories we are likely to enhance our understanding of what kinds of questions we need to ask, and with whom it is we need to think and work, to generate knowledge and action useful in rectifying social inequalities in health" (p. 27).

Finally, the book's contributors provide, through both case studies and an appendix of concrete tools, a host of techniques and methods that may be useful in working collaboratively with communities in different phases of the CBPR process.

ORGANIZATION OF THIS BOOK

In Chapter Two, Nina Wallerstein and Bonnie Duran situate CBPR and other participatory research approaches historically, conceptually, and in practice, identifying a far-reaching sweep of historical and theoretical underpinnings, including the popular education work of Brazilian educator Paulo Freire (1970, 1973, 1982) and other critical theory, feminist, postmodern, and postcolonial contributions to the field.

In Chapter Three, Barbara Israel and her academic and community partners share the core set of principles they developed through their work at the University of Michigan Urban Research Center, and discuss ethical considerations for the field, including a recommendation that each CBPR initiative come up with its own set of guidelines. Loretta Jones and her colleagues conclude Part One with an introduction, in Chapter Four, to the new form of CBPR known as *community-partnered participatory research* (CPPR) and its principles and core beliefs. Jones and her colleagues also describe how a CPPR partnership involving the University of California, Los Angeles (UCLA) Medical School and the RAND Corporation used this approach in the planning of a major experimental design study to test CPPR as an implementation strategy for evidence-based depression care interventions.

In Part Two we grapple further with issues of trust, power, dialogue, and race or ethnicity and racism as we focus on the challenges of building relationships with community members, clinical providers, and policymakers in multiple settings. In Chapter Five, Vivian Chávez and colleagues examine the multiple dimensions of race and privilege, historical trauma and internalized oppression, and conversely, the existence of strong social movements in communities. The context these factors create for understanding cross-cultural CBPR is also examined.

Although this book is premised on the assumption that concerned outside researchers can make useful contributions to community-driven research, Randy Stoecker, in Chapter Six, takes a step back to examine that assumption, asking whether outside academics do have a legitimate role to play in participatory research and then offering "guideposts" for effective and ethical engagement. Further exploring many of these issues, Ann Cheatham-Rojas and Eveline Chen then analyze in Chapter Seven a CBPR project involving Cambodian girls studying sexual harassment in their school. They illustrate in the process the powerful contributions youths can make as genuine partners in CBPR efforts. Issues of trust, dialogue, and problem solving when working with youths and also outcomes, such as new school and district policies to prevent sexual harassment and the birth of a new nonprofit organization of and by young Cambodian women, are among the topics discussed.

Conducting research with "hidden populations" presents special challenges to trust building and effective cross-cultural partnerships. In Chapter Eight, the final chapter in Part Two, Kristen Clements-Nolle and Ari Bachrach describe and analyze the CBPR approach employed in the first major epidemiological study of and with transgender people, including the multiple roles of community partners in gaining access to this hidden and stigmatized population. A ten-year retrospective look at this project and its many subsequent program, policy, and practice outcomes is provided, along with lessons learned.

Part Three focuses on one of the most important but often neglected processes in CBPR—creating a setting in which community members, rather than outsiders, truly drive the decisions around issue selection and actively participate in project and partnership evaluation.

In Chapter Nine, Meredith Minkler and Trevor Hancock discuss three core principles that lie at the heart of ensuring community-driven issue selection: starting where the people are, building on community strengths, and fostering authentic dialogue. They then present a variety of collaborative strategies for identifying strengths and issues, such as windshield tours, town hall meetings, community asset and risk mapping, a modified Delphi technique, and neighborhood indicator development.

Next, in Chapter Ten, Marita Jones, Shelley Frazier, and their colleagues explore the successes and challenges encountered in using Internet-based tools in a CBPR partnership to build local capacity, cross-community sharing, leadership, and knowledge creation in geographically dispersed urban and rural communities. The national Healthy Native Community Fellowship and the Just Move It physical activity program, which serve tribes and tribal agencies across the nation, are used to illustrate the utility of the Internet in such capacity-focused collaborations.

In Chapter Eleven, Caroline Wang and Cheri Pies explore the potency and challenges of the *photovoice* method, which integrates "community participation, health concerns, and the visual image" for collective action for change (Wang & Burris, 1994, p. 177). Using as a case study the experiences of a local health department working on maternal child health issues with low-income residents, they illustrate the strengths of photovoice in broadening and deepening academics' and practitioners' understandings of local concerns and strengths, and how these understandings may in turn help a community to effect change.

In Chapter Twelve, the final chapter in Part Three, Jane Springett and Nina Wallerstein critically examine participatory evaluation, consider its relationship to participatory research, explore the multiple and sometimes conflicting roles of the evaluator, and contrast participatory and traditional evaluation. They end with a brief case study of a statewide youth policy project in New Mexico, which shows how collaborative development of youth and policy change indicators facilitated program effectiveness.

Part Four turns a spotlight on some of the knottiest issues in CBPR: the validity and quality of the research and the many difficult ethical and practical issues involved in the implementation of research findings. We begin, in Chapter Thirteen, with Hilary Bradbury and Peter Reason's thoughtful examination of these issues, such as how to identify "choice points" for improving the quality of action research, and how to "broaden the bandwidth of validity" to include how well a program is grounded experientially and whether it builds infrastructure so that the work may endure over time.

In the following chapter, Chapter Fourteen, Meredith Minkler and Andrea Corage Baden draw on both reviews of the literature and in-depth interviews from a cross-site case study analysis (Minkler et al., 2008a, 2008b) to explore the impacts of CBPR on the outside researchers, the research quality and methodology, and the way in which CBPR addresses power differentials between community and academic partners.

To further illustrate a number of the methodological and ethical issues faced in CBPR, Part Four also presents several in-depth case studies. In Chapter Fifteen, Stephanie Farquhar and Steve Wing discuss two unique community-academic partnerships designed to document and expose health problems and potential social and environmental racism in rural North Carolina. They pay particular attention to how academic and community partners handled the controversies generated when findings had political fallout, such as charges of bias and "unscientific" research, and demands to disclose confidential data sources. In Chapter Sixteen, the last chapter of this section, Suzanne Cashman and her colleagues use brief case studies (involving surveys, geographic information system [GIS] mapping, focus groups, and mixed methods) to highlight the involvement of community partners in data analysis and interpretation. Illustrated is the value of authentic partnerships in producing far richer understandings of a problem area than outsiders could achieve working on their own, and in leaving behind a community of people better able to systematically study and act on their issues in the future.

One of the defining features of CBPR that sets it apart from more traditional research approaches is its commitment to action (Israel et al., 1998; Minkler, 2005). Part Five takes an in-depth look at the action component of CBPR, giving particular attention to how CBPR can foster health-promoting policy changes in the public and private sectors. Makani Themba-Nixon, Meredith Minkler, and Nicholas Freudenberg begin this examination, in Chapter Seventeen, by summarizing two conceptual frameworks for understanding the public policymaking process in the United States and also a third framework more directly tailored to policy advocacy through CBPR. Drawing on case examples they then illustrate the roles and entry points for CBPR partners interested in influencing policy. In Chapter Eighteen, Peggy Shepard and her colleagues describe one of the most frequently cited examples of a successful effort to study and address the disproportionate exposure to environmental insults in low-income communities of color. Although the original CBPR collaboration between West Harlem Environmental Action (WE ACT) and its academic partners took place well over a decade ago, its successes in helping to bring about policy change and the continuing collaborative work it has helped to spawn are useful reminders of the need to look at CBPR efforts over the long haul.

Although policy is most often thought of in broad public policy terms, the potential for improving health through changes in private sector arenas should not be forgotten. In Chapter Nineteen, Pam Tau Lee and her colleagues examine two union-supported CBPR projects, undertaken by university partners and hotel room cleaners in San Francisco and Las Vegas. These authors document the key role of the room cleaners in the research—including their high-level participation at the bargaining table—and in bringing about contract changes to improve workload and other working conditions.

In Chapter Twenty, Victoria Breckwich Vásquez and her colleagues explore the efforts of a partnership between a youth-focused environmental justice organization and a local health department to promote policy changes to address lack of access to fresh fruits and vegetables in a low-income neighborhood in San Francisco. The chapter chronicles the partnership's innovative data collection, its work with city policymakers to mount a major new program incentivizing local stores to become "Good Neighbors," and the impacts of this work on fresh food access locally as well as on broader state policy efforts.

In this book's final chapter Nina Wallerstein and Bonnie Duran and their research team return to a central theme of this volume while also offering a bridge to future efforts to understand the pathways through which CBPR processes lead both to intermediate capacity and systems level outcomes and to more distal health changes. These authors present a logic model that captures the core participatory characteristics and mediating or moderating processes that may matter most in getting to outcomes in CBPR. Enhanced partnerships, culturally based interventions, institutional practice changes, and policy changes are among the core factors identified.

The book concludes with twelve appendixes designed to provide a variety of tools and applications to outsider researchers and their community partners so that they can put some of the messages central to this volume into practice in their own CBPR efforts. Among the instruments included are sample protocols for community–outside researcher collaboration in CBPR; tools for communities to use in conducting their own asset and risk mapping; a brief historical look at federal support for participatory research in the United States; and new, reliability-tested guidelines for assessing participatory research in health promotion. The appendixes include as well a glimpse of CBPR in the field of nursing; recommendations for modified institutional review board (IRB) questions when reviewing CBPR proposals; insights into the use of "undoing racism" training in the context of CBPR; recommendations and resources that academic CBPR partners can use for strengthening their case for promotion and tenure; and contact information for many key CBPR centers and networks based in North America.

SUMMARY

Growing disillusionment with the limitations of traditional, "outside expert" approaches to understanding and addressing some of our most complex health and social problems have helped shine a spotlight on the potential of the alternative paradigm, which in the United States increasingly goes under the heading of community-based participatory research. An orientation to action-oriented inquiry, rather than a particular methodological approach, CBPR is time consuming and filled with challenges as local communities and their outside research collaborators navigate difficult ethical and methodological terrain, addressing issues of power and trust; race, ethnicity, and racism; research rigor; and, often, conflicting agendas (Maguire, 2006; Minkler, 2005; Stringer, 2007). Leveraging sufficient funding for CBPR also is a challenge, and although increasing substantially over the past decade, such financial support lags far behind the level of funding available for more traditional research approaches. Yet as the contributors to this volume demonstrate, CBPR also holds immense promise for insuring that research focuses on topics of deep concern to communities and is conducted in ways that can enhance validity, build community capacity, promote systems change, and work to reduce health disparities. At the same time, CBPR can foster the conditions in which professionally trained researchers adopt the role of co-learner, rather than outside expert, and communities better recognize and build on their strengths and become full partners in gaining and creating knowledge and mobilizing for change. As CBPR continues to evolve as a field of practice and an orientation to research, a new emphasis is being placed on the pathways linking processes to outcomes and on applications across a wide range of disciplines, settings, and populations. By introducing the reader to such issues using a broad brush, this first chapter has attempted to set the stage for the more in-depth coverage of each issue in the pages that follow.

QUESTIONS FOR DISCUSSION

1. Cornwall and Jewkes are cited in this chapter as arguing that community-based participatory research is not a research method per se but rather an "orientation to research" that reflects a very different stance from that taken by traditional research approaches in relation to communities and community members. How would you

describe this alternative research paradigm to a friend or colleague who's never heard of CBPR? Also, what other elements, if any, would you add to the definition, cited earlier, of CBPR used by the Kellogg Community Health Scholars Program (2001, p. 2): "a collaborative approach to research that equitably involves all partners in the research process and recognizes the unique strengths that each brings. CBPR begins with a research topic of importance to the community with the aim of combining knowledge and action for social change to improve community health and eliminate health disparities"?

2. CBPR is described in this chapter as a particularly promising approach for health disparities research. What characteristics of this orientation to research might especially lend themselves to the study of health and social problems that adversely affect people from underserved communities?

3. The authors describe CBPR as existing on a continuum running from action research (in the tradition of Kurt Lewin) on one end to the more "emancipatory" approaches (such as participatory research or participatory action research [PAR]) on the other. They go on to suggest that the more emancipatory forms of CBPR represent a "gold standard" for which professionals might strive. Do you agree with this characterization? Why or why not?

KEY TERMS

Action research   Participatory action research   Health disparities

REFERENCES

Anderson, E. T., & McFarlane, J. M. (2004). *Community as partner: Theory and practice in nursing* (4th ed.). Philadelphia: Lippincott Williams & Wilkins.

Ansley, F., & Gaventa, J. (1997, Jan.–Feb.). Researching for democracy and democratizing research. *Change,* pp. 46–53.

Averill, J. B. (2005). Merging critical ethnography with community-based action research in studies of rural elders. *Journal of Gerontological Nursing, 31*(12), 11–18.

Bammer, G. (2005). Integration and implementation sciences: Building a new specialization. *Ecology and Society, 10*(2). Retrieved Mar. 19, 2007, from http://www.ecologyandsociety.org/vol10/iss2/art6.

Bell, E. E. (2006). Infusing race into the U.S. discourse on action research. In P. Reason & H. Bradbury (Eds.), *Handbook of action research: Participative inquiry and practice* (Concise ed., pp. 49–59). Thousand Oaks, CA: Sage.

Berkman, L. F., & Kawachi, I. (Eds.). (2003). *Neighborhoods and health.* New York: Oxford University Press.

Best, A., Hiatt, R. A., & Norman, C. (2005). *The language and logic of research transfer: Finding common ground* (Report of the National Cancer Institute of Canada Working Group on Translational Research and Knowledge Integration). Toronto: National Cancer Institute of Canada.

Brown, L. D., & Tandon, R. (1983). Ideology and political economy in inquiry: Action research and participatory research. *Journal of Applied Behavioral Science, 19*(3), 277–294.

Buchanan, D. R., Miller, F. G., & Wallerstein, N. (2007). Ethical issues in community-based participatory research: Balancing rigorous research with community participation in community intervention studies. *Progress in Community Health Partnerships: Research, Education, and Action, 1*(2), 153–160.

Cargo, M., and Mercer, S. L. (2008). The value and challenges of participatory research: Strengthening its practice. *Annual Review of Public Health, 29,* 325–350.

Coghlan, D. (2004). Action research in the academy: Why and whither? Reflections on the changing nature of research. *Irish Journal of Management, 25*(2), 1–10.

Collins, P. H. (2000). *Black feminist thought: Knowledge, consciousness, and the politics of empowerment* (2nd ed.). New York: Routledge.

Corburn, J. (2005). *Street science: Community knowledge and environmental health justice.* Cambridge, MA: MIT Press.

Cornwall, A., & Jewkes, R. (1995). What is participatory research? *Social Science & Medicine, 41,* 1667–1676.

Couto, R. A. (1987). Participatory research: Methodology and critique. *Clinical Sociology Review, 5,* 83–90.

De Koning, K., & Martin, M. (Eds.). (1996). *Participatory research in health: Issues and experiences* (2nd ed.). London: Zed Books.

Falk-Rafael, A. R. (2004). The effectiveness of feminist pedagogy in empowering a community of learners. *Journal of Nursing Education, 43*(3), 107–115.

Fals-Borda, O., & Rahman, M. A. (Eds.). (1991). *Action and knowledge: Breaking the monopoly with participatory action research.* New York: Apex Press.

Felix-Aaron, K., & O'Toole, T. P. (2003). Community-based participatory research [Special issue]. *Journal of General Internal Medicine, 18*(7).

Fixsen, D. L., Naoom, S. F., Blasé, K. A., Friedman, R. M., & Wallace, F. (2005). *Implementation research: A synthesis of the literature* (FMHI Publication no. 231). Tampa, FL., University of South Florida, Louis de la Parte Florida Mental Health Institute, National Implementation Research Network.

Flicker, S., & Savan, B. (2006). *A snapshot of CBR in Canada.* Toronto: Wellesley Institute.

Freire, P. (1970). *Pedagogy of the oppressed.* New York: Seabury Press.

Freire, P. (1973). *Education for critical consciousness.* New York: Seabury Press.

Freire, P. (1982). Creating alternative research methods: Learning to do it by doing it. In B. L. Hall, A. Gillette, & R. Tandon (Eds.), *Creating knowledge: A monopoly? Participatory research in development* (pp. 29–38). New Delhi: Society for Participatory Research in Asia.

Gaventa, J. (1981). Participatory action research in North America. *Convergence, 14,* 30–42.

Gaventa, J. (1993). The powerful, the powerless, and the experts: Knowledge struggles in an information age. In P. Park, M. Brydon-Miller, B. L. Hall, & T. Jackson (Eds.), *Voices of change: Participatory research in the United States and Canada* (pp. 21–40). Westport, CT: Bergin & Garvey.

Gebbie, K, Rosenstock, L., & Hernandez, L. M. (2003). *Who will keep the public healthy? Educating public health professionals for the 21st century.* Washington, DC: Institute of Medicine.

Gee, G. C., Spencer, M. S., Chen, J., & Takeuchi, D. (2007). A nationwide study of discrimination and chronic health conditions among Asian Americans. *American Journal of Public Health, 97*(7), 1275–1282.

Green, L. W. (2006). Public health asks of systems science: To advance our evidence-based practice, can you help us get more practice-based evidence? *American Journal of Public Health, 96*(3), 406–409.

Green, L. W. (2007). The Prevention Research Centers as models of practice-based evidence: Two decades on. *American Journal of Preventive Medicine, 33*(1), S6–S8.

Green, L. W., George, M. A., Daniel, M., Frankish, C. J., Herbert, C. P., Bowie, W. R., et al. (1995). *Study of participatory research in health promotion: Review and recommendations for the development of participatory research in health promotion in Canada.* Vancouver, BC: Royal Society of Canada.

Green, L. W., & Glasgow, R. E. (2006). Evaluating the relevance, generalization, and applicability of research: Issues in external validation and translation methodology. *Evaluation & the Health Professions, 29*(1), 126–153.

Green, L. W., & Mercer, S. L. (2001). Can public health researchers and agencies reconcile the push from funding bodies and the pull from communities? *American Journal of Public Health, 91,* 1926–1929.

Greenwood, D. J., & Levin, M. (1998). *Introduction to action research: Social research for social change.* Thousand Oaks, CA: Sage.

Hagey, R. S. (1997). Guest editorial: The use and abuse of participatory action research. *Chronic Diseases of Canada, 18*(1), 1–4.

Hall, B. L. (1981). Participatory research, popular knowledge, and power: A personal reflection. *Convergence, 14*(3), 6–19.

Hall, B. L. (1992). From margins to center: The development and purpose of participatory action research. *American Sociologist, 23*(4), 15–28.

Hall, B. L. (1999). Looking back, looking forward: Reflections on the International Participatory Research Network. *Forests, Trees and People Newsletter, 39,* 3–36.

Hall, B. L., Gillette, A., & Tandon, R. (Eds.). (1982). *Creating knowledge: A monopoly? Participatory research in development.* New Delhi: Society for Participatory Research in Asia.

Hall, G. (2001). Psychotherapy research with ethnic minorities: Empirical, ethical, and conceptual issues. *Journal of Consulting and Clinical Psychology, 69*(3), 502–510.

hooks, b. (1989). *Talking back: Thinking feminism, talking black.* Boston: South End Press.

Israel, B. A., Eng, E., Schulz, A. J., & Parker, E. A. (Eds.). (2005). *Methods in community-based participatory research for health.* San Francisco: Jossey-Bass.

Israel, B. A., Schulz, A. J., Parker, E. A., & Becker, A. B. (1998). Review of community-based research: Assessing partnership approaches to improve public health. *Annual Review of Public Health, 19,* 173–202.

James, S. A., Schulz, A. J., & van Olphen, J. (2001). Social capital, poverty, and community health: An exploration of linkages. In S. Saegert, J. P. Thompson, & M. R. Warren (Eds.), *Social capital and poor communities* (pp. 165–188). New York: Russell Sage Foundation.

Jones, L., & Wells, K. (2007). Strategies for academic and clinician engagement in community-partnered participatory research. *Journal of the American Medical Association, 297,* 407–410.

Kawachi, I., Kennedy, B. P., Lochner, K., & Prothrow-Stith, D. (1997). Social capital, income inequality, and mortality. *American Journal of Public Health, 87,* 1491–1498.

Krieger, J., Allen, C. A., Roberts, J. W., Ross, L. C., & Takaro, T. K. (2005). What's with the wheezing? Methods used by the Seattle-King County Healthy Homes Project to assess exposure to indoor asthma triggers. In B. A. Israel, E. Eng, A. J. Schulz, & E. A. Parker (Eds.), *Methods in community-based participatory research for health* (pp. 230–250). San Francisco: Jossey-Bass.

Krieger, N. (2000). Social epidemiology and health inequalities: A U.S. perspective on theories and actions. In I. Forbes (Ed.), *Health inequalities: Poverty and policy* (pp. 26–43). London: Academy of Learned Societies for the Social Sciences.

Krieger, N., Rowley, D. L., Herman, A. A., Avery, B., & Phillips, M. T. (1993). Racism, sexism, and social class: Implications for studies of health, disease, and well-being. *American Journal of Preventive Medicine, 9*(6), 82–122.

Lantz, P. M., Israel, B. A., Schulz, A. J., & Reyes, A. (2005). Community-based participatory research: Rationale and relevance for social epidemiology. In J. M. Oakes & J. S. Kaufman (Eds.), *Methods in social epidemiology* (pp. 239–266). San Francisco: Jossey-Bass.

LaVeist, T. A. (2005). *Race, ethnicity, and health: A public health reader.* San Francisco: Jossey-Bass.

Leung, M., Yen, I., & Minkler, M. (2004). Community-based participatory research: A promising approach for increasing epidemiology's relevance in the 21st century. *International Journal of Epidemiology, 33*(3), 499–506.

Lewin, K. (1946). Action research and minority problems. *Journal of Social Issues, 2,* 34–46.

Lewis, H. M. (2006). Participatory research and education for social change: Highlander Research and Education Center. In P. Reason & H. Bradbury (Eds.), *Handbook of action research: Participative inquiry and practice* (Concise ed., pp. 262–268). Thousand Oaks, CA: Sage.

Lykes, M. B. (1997). Activist participatory research among the Maya of Guatemala: Constructing meanings from situated knowledge. *Journal of Social Issues, 53,* 725–746.

Macaulay, A. C., & Nutting, P. A. (2006). Moving the frontiers forward: Incorporating community-based participatory research into practice-based research networks. *Annals of Family Medicine, 4,* 4–7.

Maguire, P. (2006). Uneven ground: Feminisms and action research. In P. Reason & H. Bradbury (Eds.), *Handbook of action research: Participative inquiry and practice* (Concise ed., pp. 60–70). Thousand Oaks, CA: Sage.

Marmot, M., & Wilkinson, R. G. (Eds.). (2006). *Social determinants of health* (2nd ed.). New York: Oxford University Press.

Merrifield, J. (1993). Putting scientists in their place: Participatory research in environmental and occupational health. In P. Park, M. Brydon-Miller, B. Hall, & T. Jackson (Eds.), *Voices of change: Participatory research in the United States and Canada* (pp. 65–84). Westport, CT: Bergin and Garvey.

Miller, R. L. & Shinn, M., (2005). Learning from communities: Overcoming difficulties in dissemination of prevention and promotion efforts. *American Journal of Community Psychology, 35*(3–4), 169–183.

Minkler, M. (2005). Community-based research partnerships: Challenges and opportunities. *Journal of Urban Health, 82*(2, Suppl. 2), 3–12.

Minkler, M., Blackwell, A. G., Thompson, M., & Tamir, H. (2003). Community-based participatory research: Implications for public health funding. *American Journal of Public Health, 93,* 1210–1213.

Minkler, M., Breckwich Vásquez, V., Chang, C. C., Blackwell, A. G., Thompson, M., & Rubin, V. (2008). *Promoting healthy public policy through community-based participatory research.* Oakland, CA: PolicyLink.

Minkler, M., Breckwich Vásquez, V., Tajik, M., & Petersen, D. (2008). Promoting environmental justice through community-based participatory research: The role of community and partnership capacity. *Health Education & Behavior, 35*(1), 119–137.

Morello-Frosch, R., Pastor, M., Sadd, J., Porras, C., & Prichard, M. (2005). Citizens, science, and data judo: Leveraging secondary data analysis to build a community-academic collaborative for environmental justice in southern California. In B. A. Israel, E. Eng, A. J. Schulz, & E. A. Parker (Eds.), *Methods in community-based participatory research for health* (pp. 371–392). San Francisco: Jossey-Bass.

Mosavel, M., Simon, C., van Stade, D., & Buchbinder, M. (2005). Community-based participatory research (CBPR) in South Africa: Engaging multiple constituents to shape the research question. *Social Science & Medicine, 61,* 2577–2587.

Neuhauser, L., Richardson, D., MacKenzie, S., & Minkler, M. (2007). Advancing transdisciplinary and translational research practice: Issues and models of doctoral education in public health. *Journal of Research Practice, 3*(2).

Northridge, M. E., Vallone, D., Merzel, C., Greene, D., Shepherd, P., Cohall, A. T., et al. (2000). The adolescent years: An academic-community partnership in Harlem comes of age. *Journal of Public Health Management and Practice, 6*(1), 53–60.

Omi, M. A. (2000). The changing meaning of race. In N. J. Smelser, W. J. Wilson, & F. Mitchell (Eds.), *America becoming: Racial trends and their consequences* (Vol. 1, pp. 243–263). Washington, DC: National Academies Press.

Park, P., Brydon-Miller, M., Hall, B. L., & Jackson, T. (Eds.). (1993). *Voices of change: Participatory research in the United States and Canada.* Westport, CT: Bergin & Garvey.

Petersen, D., Minkler, M., Breckwich Vásquez, V., & Baden, A. C. (2006). Community-based participatory research as a tool for policy change: A case study of the Southern California Environmental Justice Collaborative. *Review of Policy Research, 23*(2), 339–353.

Putnam, R. (2007). E pluribus unum: Diversity and community in the twenty-first century: The 2006 Johan Skytte Prize Lecture. *Scandinavian Political Studies, 30*(2), 137–174.

Reason, P., & Bradbury, H. (Eds.). (2006). *Handbook of action research: Participative inquiry and practice* (Concise ed.). Thousand Oaks, CA: Sage.

Reason, P., & Bradbury, H. (2008). *The SAGE handbook of action research: Participative inquiry and practice* (2nd ed.). Thousand Oaks, CA: Sage.

Rice, M. (2007). Lessons learned from the application of a participatory evaluation methodology to Healthy Municipalities, Cities and Communities initiatives in selected countries of the Americas. *Health Promotion & Education, 14*(2), 68–73.

Ritas, C. (2003). *Speaking truth, creating power: A guide to policy work for community-based participatory research practitioners.* Community-Campus Partnerships for Health. Retrieved Jan. 15, 2008, from http://depts.washington.edu/ccph/pdf_files/ritas.pdf.

Schwab, M., & Syme, S. L. (1997). On paradigms, community participation, and the future of public health. *American Journal of Public Health, 87,* 2049–2052.

Schulz, A. J., & Mullings, L. (Eds.). (2006). *Gender, race, class, and health: Intersectional approaches.* San Francisco: Jossey-Bass.

Smedley, B. D., Stith, A. Y., & Nelson, A. R. (Eds.), Institute of Medicine. (2003). *Unequal treatment: Confronting racial and ethnic disparities in health care.* Washington, DC: National Academies Press.

Stringer, E. T. (2007). *Action research* (3rd ed.). Thousand Oaks, CA: Sage.

Stringer, E. T., & Genat, W. (2004). *Action research in health practice.* Upper Saddle River, NJ: Merrill Prentice Hall.

Swantz, M.-L., Ndedya, E., & Masaiganah, M. S. (2006). Participatory action research in Tanzania, with special reference to women. In P. Reason & H. Bradbury (Eds.), *Handbook of action research: Participative inquiry and practice* (Concise ed., pp. 286–296). Thousand Oaks, CA: Sage.

Szreter, S., & Woolcock, M. (2004). Health by association? Social capital, social theory, and the political economy of public health. *International Journal of Epidemiology, 33,* 650–667.

Tervalon, M., & Murray-Garcia, J. (1998). Cultural humility versus cultural competence: A critical distinction in defining physician training outcomes in multicultural education. *Journal of Health Care for the Poor and Underserved, 9*(2), 117–125.

Thomas, S. B., & Quinn, S. C. (2001). Light on the shadow of the syphilis study at Tuskegee. *Health Promotion Practice, 1,* 234–237.

Viswanathan, M., Ammerman, A., Eng, E., Gartlehner, G., Lohr, K. N., Griffth, D., et al. (2004). *Community-based participatory research: Assessing the evidence* (Evidence Report/Technology Assessment No. 99; Prepared by RTI International-University of North Carolina). Rockville, MD: Agency for Healthcare Research and Quality.

Wallerstein, N. (1999). Power between evaluator and community: Research relationships within New Mexico's healthier communities. *Social Science & Medicine, 49,* 39–53.

Wallerstein, N., & Duran, B. (2006). Using community-based participatory research to address health disparities. *Health Promotion Practice, 7*(3), 312–323.

Wang, C. C., & Burris, M. A. (1994). Empowerment through photo novella: Portraits of participation. *Health Education Quarterly, 21,* 171–186.

Wells, K., & Norris, K. C. (Eds.). (2006). The Community Health Improvement Collaboration: Building community-academic partnerships to reduce disparities [entire issue]. *Ethnicity & Disease, 16*(1, Suppl. 1).

Westfall, J. M., VanVorst, R. F., Main, D. S., & Herbert, C. (2006). Community-based participatory research in practice-based research networks. *Annals of Family Medicine, 4*(1), 8–14.

Williams, D. R., Neighbors, H. W., & Jackson, J. S. (2003). Racial/ethnic discrimination and health: Findings from community studies. *American Journal of Public Health, 93*(2), 200–208.

Wing, S. (1998). Whose epidemiology, whose health? *International Journal of Health Services, 28,* 241–252.

W. K. Kellogg Foundation. (2008). *Kellogg Health Scholars Program.* Retrieved Apr. 7, 2008, from www.kellogghealthscholars.org.

W. K. Kellogg Foundation Community Health Scholars Program. (2001). *Stories of impact* [brochure]. Ann Arbor: University of Michigan, School of Public Health, Community Health Scholars Program, National Program Office.

CHAPTER

2

THE THEORETICAL, HISTORICAL, AND PRACTICE ROOTS OF CBPR

NINA WALLERSTEIN & BONNIE DURAN

If we do our [research] well, reality will appear even more unstable, complex, and disorderly than it does now.

J. Flax (1987, p. 643)

IN THE PAST few decades a new paradigm of *participatory research* has emerged, raising challenges to the positivist view of science. By the 1960s, simultaneous crises, within academia and sociopolitical movements, challenged relationships between universities and society and precipitated a global search for new social theories and practices of inquiry. Issues such as ownership of knowledge, the role of the researcher in engaging society, the role of community participation and agency, and the importance of power relations began to permeate the research process with the challenge to use knowledge to promote a more equitable society.

The long list of terms representing this new participatory research paradigm, which links applied social science and social activism, has been fairly daunting, and the nuanced differences between them are often difficult to decipher (see Chapter One). Some terms, such as *rapid assessment procedures, rapid rural appraisal,* and *participatory rural appraisal,* implemented primarily in developing nations, represent a methodological emphasis (De Koning & Martin, 1996a). Specific disciplines have produced their own terminology: *classroom action research, critical action research,* and *practitioner research* in the field of education (Kemmis & McTaggart, 2000); *action learning, action science, action inquiry,* and *industrial action research* in the fields of organizational psychology and organizational development (Argyris, Putnam, & Smith, 1985; Torbert & Taylor, 2008); *cooperative, mutual,* or *reflective practitioner inquiry* in psychology and human relations (Heron & Reason, 2006; Reason, 1994; Rowan, 2006); *constructivist* or *fourth-generation inquiry* in evaluation research (Lincoln, 2001); *emancipatory inquiry* in nursing (Henderson, 1995; Hills, 2001); and *popular epidemiology* and *street science* in public health (Brown, 1992; Corburn, 2005; Wing, 1998). Multiple concepts have come from the community development and social action literature, including *collaborative action research, participatory research, emancipatory* or *liberatory research,* and *dialectical inquiry* (Fals-Borda & Rahman, 1991; Hall, 1992; Hall, Gillette, & Tandon, 1982; Kemmis & McTaggart, 2000; Park, Brydon-Miller, Hall, & Jackson, 1993). A new term, *community-partnered participatory research,* places an even greater emphasis on partnering (Jones & Wells, 2007: see also Chapter Four), and *tribal participatory research* puts the focus on indigenous peoples (Fisher & Ball, 2003). In an exhaustive monograph on the different paradigms of collaborative social inquiry over the last twenty years, Trickett and Espino (2004) call for greater transparency of the assumptions, practice, and outcomes in the different traditions.

Despite their different emphases, however, as development studies theorist Robert Chambers (1992) notes, "these sources and traditions have, like flows in a braided stream, intermingled more and more" (p. 2). *Action research* and *participatory action research* (PAR), have often been used interchangeably in recent years to represent a convergence of principles (well articulated in Chapter Three); under these principles the community determines the research agenda and shares in the planning, data collection, analysis, and dissemination of the research (Israel, Eng, Schulz, & Parker, 2005; Israel, Schulz, Parker, & Becker, 1998; McTaggart, 1997; Reason & Bradbury, 2008; Stringer & Genat, 2004).

In the past ten years the use of the term *community-based participatory research* (CBPR) has gained respectability and attention in the health field. Like many of the terms previously mentioned, CBPR takes the perspective that participatory research involves three interconnected goals: research, action, and education (Hall, 1992). In a collaboration, shared principles result in a negotiation of information and capacities in mutual directions: researchers transferring tools for community members to use to analyze conditions and make informed decisions on actions to improve their lives, and community members transferring their expert content and meaning to researchers in the pursuit of mutual knowledge and application of that knowledge to their communities (Hatch, Moss, Saran, Presley-Cantrell, & Mallory, 1993). A majority of these terms can be traced to one of two historical traditions that represent two distinct approaches at opposite ends of a continuum: collaborative utilization-focused research with practical goals of system improvement, sometimes called the *Northern tradition,* and openly emancipatory research, which challenges the historical colonizing practices of research and political domination of knowledge by the elites, often called the *Southern tradition* (Brown & Tandon, 1983). This chapter will articulate the historical roots of these two traditions and discuss the contribution of theories of knowledge; postmodern, poststructural, postcolonial, and feminist theories; and theories of power in order to clarify points of convergence and difference within current theory and practice. This chapter ends with practical approaches for implementing Freirian dialogical education in community-based participatory research. Although the best of CBPR contains skills and dimensions from both traditions, this chapter argues that the paramount public health goal of eliminating disparities demands a research practice within the emancipatory perspective, a practice that fosters the democratic participation of community members to transform their lives.

HISTORICAL ROOTS

The initial user of the term *action research* within the Northern tradition was Kurt Lewin. In the 1940s, Lewin challenged the gap between theory and practice and sought to solve practical problems through a research cycle involving planning, action, and investigating the results of the action (Lewin, 1948/1997). He rejected the positivist belief that researchers study an objective world separate from the meanings understood by participants as they act in their world.

This tradition emanates most broadly from the sociological theory of Talcott Parsons and his predecessors, who viewed social progress as rational decision making based on applying ever-increasing scientific knowledge to real-world problems. With an emphasis on practitioners acting as coequals to the researchers in their research process, action science researchers in the fields of organizational development and social psychology have often worked in a consensus model, assuming that in organizations, for example, management and workers have equal power to influence quality improvement (Brown & Tandon, 1983; Argyris & Schön, 1996). The assumption has been that problems could be solved through institutional changes based on new knowledge, education, and transformational leadership that inspires a self-reflective community of inquiry (Peters & Robinson, 1984; Chisholm & Elden, 1993; Greenwood, Whyte, & Harkavy, 1993). In education, for example, teachers have been encouraged to become researchers in their classrooms to tackle questions previously left to academics (Stringer, 2007). In evaluation, constructivist-focused evaluators have focused on the use of knowledge for action, without having a political agenda (Lincoln, 2001).

Although a consensus model of action research can in practice be manipulated by those in power when they dominate the decision making, humanistic psychology researchers have created a cooperative inquiry strand within this model, a strand that adopts a firm belief in human agency and says that people can choose how they live through a process of reflexive inquiry. This strand insists on researcher and community member reciprocity, with no parties excluded or alienated from the research process as they exchange ideas and actions (Rowan, 2006).

Since the early 1970s, a second tradition of participatory research, arising within Latin America, Asia, and Africa and known collectively as the Southern tradition, has developed, receiving much of its impetus from the structural crises of underdevelopment, Marxist critiques by social scientists, liberation theology, and the search for new practice by adult educators and community developers among populations vulnerable to globalization. An outflow of education and social science academics from universities to work with land movements and community-based organizations transformed the concept that knowledge emanated from the academy and created an openness to knowledge learned from people's experience, or *vivencia,* as Latin American philosopher José Ortega y Gasset named it (Fals-Borda, 1991). Exiled Brazilian philosopher Paulo Freire, through the publication of *Pedagogy of the Oppressed* (1970) and other writings, which were banned during the Latin American military dictatorships in the 1970s, influenced the transformation of the research relationship from one in which communities were *objects of study* to one in which community members were *participating in the inquiry.* Freire's notion was that reality is not an objective truth or facts to be discovered but "includes the ways in which the people involved with facts perceive them. . . . The concrete reality is the connection between subjectivity and objectivity, never objectivity isolated from subjectivity" (1982, p. 29).

Rather than viewing research as neutral, participatory research intellectuals adopted the commitment to critical consciousness, emancipation, and social justice as they challenged their own roles in communities with the political ideology that "self-conscious people, those who are poor and oppressed, will progressively transform their environment by their own praxis" (Rahman, 1991, p. 13). Intellectuals were to be catalysts and supports of educational processes but not the vanguard of social change (Hall et al., 1982).

By 1976, progressive institutions outside academia began to take the lead, with the creation of the Participatory Research Group by the International Council for Adult Education in Toronto and its network of centers in India, Tanzania, the Netherlands, and Latin America (Hall, 2001). Other nodes of activity in the same tradition have included the Collaborative Action Research Group's work with Aborigines in Australia (Kemmis & McTaggart, 2000) and the Highlander Research and Education Center, in Tennessee, the oldest adult education and social change center in the United States (Horton & Freire, 1990; Horton, 1990; see also Appendix L). The first International Symposium on Action Research and Scientific Analysis dominated by professionals outside the United States was held in Cartagena, Colombia, in 1977, with the eighth held twenty years later and attracting two thousand delegates from sixty-one countries (Fals-Borda, 2006).

The Southern tradition has incorporated post-Marxist approaches that integrate cultural and social dimensions of oppression into theories of economic determinism (Laclau & Mouffe, 1985; Said, 1994). The interests of CBPR participants from U.S. communities of color often resonate with the Southern approach because these participants have recognized the colonizing role of research, education, and religion in their own communities. With indigenous peoples for example, public health and medical discourses have been used by economic and government bodies to "deauthorize" traditional ways of knowing, for the purposes of controlling Native populations and places. As recently as the 1950s and '60s, top public health journals were circulating "research" and medical discourse that characterized indigenous peoples as being primitive, lacking basic knowledge of child rearing and of hygiene, having exotic mental disorders, and being on the verge of dying out (Bahl, 1961; Breed, 1958; Gerken, 1940; Havighurst & Illkevitch, 1949; Hoffman, 1930). Reading these "research" papers based on misinformation and stereotypes may tell us more about the paternalistic and biased frame of mind of our profession than about the behaviors and beliefs of communities of color and other peoples disenfranchised by the system.

Placing each term used by the various disciplines at a specific point on the continuum between the problem-solving utilitarian approach and the emancipatory approach of CBPR is difficult because the actual research practice may vary with the local context, history, and ideology of the stakeholders. The same term may even be used with opposite meanings. *Participatory action research,* for example, has been used both to describe part of the emancipatory participatory research tradition (Rahman, 1985) and to describe part of the organizational development tradition (Whyte, 1991).

In general, however, action science, organizational action research, and the related traditions grounded in the Lewinian model are to be found at the end of the continuum focusing on pragmatic use of knowledge, with cooperative, psychological, and mutual inquiry being found closer to the middle of the continuum. The participatory research and PAR approaches associated with liberatory political Freirian goals and the Southern tradition are generally to be found clustered at the other end. Understanding the issues within the core concepts of participation, knowledge, and power and also Freire's thinking around praxis will enable each of us to reflect on our own practice within this continuum.

CORE CONCEPTS AND NEW THEORIES

Participation

Habermas (1974) observed that "in the process of enlightenment, there can only be participants" (p. 40). If we adopt Habermas's succinct statement in our CBPR work, the core question becomes, What do we mean by *participation*? Who is participating, for whom are we participating, in what spheres are we participating, to what ends are we participating, and perhaps most important of all, who or what is limiting participation in shaping our lives? In other words, where does the power lie (Bopp, 1994; Cornwall & Jewkes, 1995; Gaventa & Cornwall, 2008; Rifkin, 1996)?

For community-based participatory research, in particular, we need to ask, "If all research involves participation, what makes research participatory?" (Cornwall & Jewkes, 1995, p. 1668). In health, this question is critical, as international conferences since Alma Ata (in 1978) through Ottawa (in 1986) and Jakarta (in 1996) have declared the importance of community participation in improving health conditions. With health viewed as a resource originating from people within their social contexts rather than from the health care system, participation is seen as critical to reducing dependency on health professionals, ensuring cultural sensitivity of programs, facilitating sustainability of change efforts, and enhancing health in its own right (Jewkes & Murcott, 1998).

Despite the decades of using a value-based rhetoric of participation in development studies, public health, and participatory research, only relatively recently have researchers begun to question whether the reality of participation reflects the ideal. Some have questioned the authenticity of the participatory process (Tandon, 1988) or have viewed participation in a more limited fashion, as in the use of rapid rural appraisal to engage community members as informants (Cornwall & Jewkes, 1995). Others have suggested that participation is a developmental, emergent process that requires nurturing beyond the initial intentions (Goodman, 2001; Greenwood et al., 1993).

The most important issue for community-based participatory researchers is the relationship between outside researchers and community members (Brown & Vega, 1996; Jones & Wells, 2007). Habermas offers insights into these relationships through his theorizing about modernity (Habermas, 1987). To Habermas, modern societies have created two distinct worlds: the *systems* world of differentiated legal, economic, and political systems and the *life* world of families and cultural traditions in which individuals form and reproduce their identity and belief systems.

As the life world has increasingly become dominated by the systems world, people have begun to define themselves by their roles within systems. They become objects—clients and consumers—rather than subjects or democratic members of civil society. The results of being objectified can be seen in powerlessness, increases in mental disease, and the overall decline in people's belief that their participation makes a difference (as may, for example, be evidenced in decreased voting patterns). In applying CBPR, outside researchers may unwittingly become part of this dynamic, as universities often reinforce community member roles as clients and consumers.

Even within a CBPR practice that promotes authentic partnership, the actual practice between researchers and community members remains complex and involves making the power differences transparent, whether these differences are recognized or not. This means addressing such issues as who represents the community and university, who owns the data, and who represents the research project to the external world.

Although CBPR researchers expect that building collaborative relationships with community members will be sufficient to surmount any differences, power differentials can and often do remain substantial. Academic researchers almost always have greater access to resources, scientific knowledge, research assistants, and time than small community-based organizations do (Chataway, 1997). In a participatory evaluation study of healthy communities in New Mexico, lack of recognition of the power differences between communities and the evaluator inhibited collaboration and restricted use of research findings (Wallerstein, 1999).

One of the principles of CBPR involves recognizing that both outside researchers and community members have needs and agendas, which may sometimes be shared and at other times divergent or conflicting, especially if professional researchers pursue their career advancement at the expense of the community (Fine, 1994; Huberman, 1991; Lather, 1986). For example, community members might be more interested in jobs that research projects may bring to a community than in the knowledge production itself.

Increasingly, CBPR researchers interested in genuine partnership face communities, previously taken advantage of by researchers, that are now demanding their rights to determine what research is done and who will do it (De Bruyn, Chino, Serna, & Fullerton-Gleason, 2001). Historically, "helicopter research" in Indian Country (or "drive-by" research in urban settings), for example, was epitomized by the researcher flying in and taking information without leaving anything in return (Deloria, 1992). If CBPR practitioners fail to recognize the validity of these historical issues, they might be denied entry or have their research undermined through overt or hidden forms of resistance. In some tribal communities, institutional review boards directly control (and deny) access to researchers who are not fulfilling community needs, including the ability to publish findings. Good CBPR practice therefore demands a recognition of historical or current relationships and of potential natural skepticism resulting from historical patterns, and also an assurance that all parties will materially benefit from the knowledge produced (Duran & Duran, 1999; Duran, Duran, Brave Heart, & Davis, 1998; Fletcher, 2003; see also Appendix H).

At the same time, the contribution of CBPR researchers should not be undervalued. Academics often know of funding opportunities and have key expertise to offer about important health issues. They also face their own challenges for academic tenure and promotion, outcomes sometimes difficult to achieve in the context of building long-term relationships with communities (Goodman, 2001; see also Appendix E). Negotiation of a mutual code of collaborative working relationships and ethics (see Chapter Three) therefore becomes critical when adopting a participatory partnership (Fawcett, 1991; Gitlin & Russell, 1994; Perkins & Wandersman, 1990; see also Appendix G). Recently, researchers have developed instruments to evaluate the extent to which their research will serve the community and the extent of community participation in the research itself (Brown & Vega, 1996; Flicker, Travers, Guta, McDonald, & Meagher, 2007; George, Daniel, & Green, 1998–1999; see also Appendixes A, C, and G). These instruments, coupled with codes of ethics developed with and by local tribes and communities (Macaulay et al., 1998; Canadian Institutes of Health Research, 2008; see also Appendix H), provide a welcome opportunity to ensure that communities are a driving force in their own research. Codes of ethics may also need to be renegotiated periodically, as different research stages generate different levels of excitement, buy-in, or concerns about possible abuse of findings.

Who represents the community remains a key issue in participation. Often service providers are asked to serve on community advisory boards, yet they may or may not represent their constituents (Jewkes & Murcott, 1998). As Aiwa Ong (1991) has stated, there is a First World in every Third World community. If stakeholders reflect people who make up the power base of the First World, are they appropriate to fully represent local community residents (Green & Mercer, 2001)? As expressed throughout this book, CBPR represents the view that community members themselves need to be brought into the research process as decision-making participants. Least inclusive are participatory methods that seek input from community members solely as focus group or interview participants, with greater inclusion when advisory council members become facilitators, interviewers, or research coordinators within their own communities. Although a challenge, inclusion is greatest when advisory council members engage in decision making in all stages of the research, from beginning stages through data analysis, interpretation, and dissemination. The relationships that favor the community most are those that place funding and decision making within the community's lead agencies, which then subcontract to researchers (Duran & Duran, 1999).

A provocative book, *Participation: The New Tyranny?* (Cooke & Kothari, 2001), challenges the orthodoxy of participation, arguing that communities are too often viewed naively, concealing power relations and masking biases. Three tyrannies are proposed: the tyranny of decision making, in which community decision-making processes are overridden by development experts; the tyranny of the group, where group dynamics may reinforce the individuals in the community already in power; and the tyranny of methods. A method like participatory rural appraisal, for example, may use dialogue and visualization processes to honor local knowledge for local problem solving (De Koning & Martin, 1996b, p. 2) yet at the same time may obscure the need to challenge state or global institutional policies that override local determinants of well-being (Francis, 2001). These are important challenges and remind those of us working in the field that CBPR is not "reified out there, but constructed by a cadre of . . . professionals, be they academics, practitioners or policymakers, whose ability to create and sustain this discourse is indicative of the power they possess" (Cooke & Kothari, 2001, p. 15).

Unlike these authors, however, the authors of this chapter take a more optimistic stand, that reflexivity within ourselves and with our community collaborators can inspire a continual cycle of learning about our successes and about our failures. As Rifkin (1996) states, participation should not be seen as a magic bullet but as a complex and iterative process, which can change, grow, or diminish, based on the unfolding of power relations and the historical and social context of the research project.

Theories and Use of Knowledge

The creation and the use of knowledge are inherently the motivating forces behind all research; yet like participation, CBPR raises questions of by whom, about whom, and for what purpose this knowledge is defined (Cornwall & Jewkes, 1995; Gaventa & Cornwall, 2008; Hall, 1992; Tandon, 1988). Although positivist research paradigms consider knowledge creation to be a neutral and value-free activity, CBPR researchers have often drawn from more reflexive and interpretative modes of inquiry that explore the dialectic between researcher and what is being researched (Denzin & Lincoln, 2000; Poland, 1996; Reason, 1994).

CBPR critiques of positivists' search for objective truths have been pointed, stating that traditional inquiry discounts experiential knowledge, reinforces subjects' passivity, and obscures other voices (Gaventa & Cornwall, 2008; Wallerstein, 2007; see also Chapter Fourteen). In relation to public health theory, the critique of positivism finds that not only is it "not the only method for gaining valid knowledge, but it is a powerful ideology that thwarts the field's interests in alleviating suffering and promoting social justice" (Buchanan, 1998, p. 440). Indigenous researchers, taking the view that "one of the canons of good research is that it should never hurt the people studied" (Peacock, quoted in Crazy Bull, 1997), have posed this difference as knowledge for the sake of knowing (that is, for describing and categorizing objective reality) versus knowledge for the sake of decolonizing, healing, transforming, and mobilizing (Crazy Bull, 2004; Smith, 1999).

The emancipatory traditions of CBPR have drawn on critical social theory, which views knowledge as historically and socially constructed. Ideas about knowledge espoused by critical theorist Habermas are particularly relevant for CBPR and can be seen as three distinct aims of research (Habermas, 1971; Kemmis, 2008). *Empiricoanalytic reason* supports the aim of technical or instrumental control over problems, which is a rationale for the Northern tradition of utilitarian problem solving to make systems work better. *Practical reason* is normative in that actors orient themselves to living within common cultural and social values, a view that can inform both the Northern and Southern traditions. Dialogue around norms can, for example, support community and cultural renewal, and at the same time open the door for changes desired by community members. *Critical reason,* or *emancipatory reason,* reflects the research aim to better understand existing power struggles, that is, to understand how conflicts or power imbalances have come about based on human actions and what the future could be. These considerations in turn reflect central organizing principles of the Southern tradition (Habermas, 1971; Kemmis, 2008; Kemmis & McTaggart, 2000).

Freire provides a psychosocial understanding of how emancipatory knowledge can lead to having the power to make change. As people engage in dialogue with each other about their communities and the larger social context, their own internal thought patterns and beliefs about their social world change; their relationships to each other become strengthened; and ultimately, they enhance their capacities to reflect on their own values and to make new choices. These three dimensions have been called the "power of competence, connection, and confidence" (Park, 2006, p. 89).

Power Relations

Although knowledge is a major source of power and control, other material and institutional power relations are also central for understanding the dynamic relationships between researchers and communities. CBPR takes place not only in the context of the personal and historical relationships among researchers, their universities, and the communities where research is conducted but also in the much broader context of power relations involving the societal context in which the research takes place, the origins of the research, and the purpose of the research itself. CBPR researchers who hope to act on the most important problems in society, such as disparities based on race, class, gender, sexual orientation, or other identities, need to produce knowledge that clarifies and seeks to change unequal distributions of power and resources.

In addressing imbalances of power in society, participatory researchers may be aided by theories of political economy, which make up a broad, multidisciplinary framework that emphasizes how the structure of the economy and society affects the lives (and the health) of individuals (Alford & Friedland, 1985). A political economy view assumes that resources are allocated not according to merit or relative efficiency but on the basis of power. In the area of health and health care, it suggests that the behaviors and dynamics of both visible and behind-the-scenes players can be understood only in relation to these players' power and class position in society (Minkler, Wallace, & McDonald, 1994–1995; Navarro, 1984).

Gaventa (1980) and Gaventa and Cornwall (2008) identify four dimensions of power in CBPR, analyzing how power is exercised and who is excluded. The pluralist liberal democratic view assumes that power is a product of an open system of equal competing agendas, with lack of participation seen as a function of apathy or choice (Polsby, 1963). The second view argues that there is a hidden face to power in which some actors and issues are kept from open discussion through a mobilization of bias by powerful social norms or organizations against community interests (Bachrach & Baratz, 1962). CBPR researchers may unwittingly play into this bias in calling, for example, for evidence-based interventions. Although evidence-based practice is useful and can justify increased resources for community-based work, use of "evidence" language alone as an academic norm may inadvertently discredit the healing practices or beliefs in local cultures or the evidence that comes from practice (Green, 2006).

Stephen Lukes (1974) raises a third, and more insidious, dimension of power, one that excludes grievances by preventing conflicts or community ideas from even surfacing. Certain interests are favored without the need for conscious decisions or manipulation of language or policy (Minkler et al., 1994–1995; Wallace, Williamson, Lung, & Powell, 1991). Internalized oppression (see Chapter Five for more detail), for example, may contribute to a culture of silence in which people doubt they even have healing practices to offer.

All three of these dimensions—power as a function of equal competing agendas in an open system, as hidden power, and as the unspoken, hegemonic dominance of certain powerful groups—represent, in Foucault's framework (1977), repressive forms of power. Such power may be exercised through direct control or indirect language that shapes people's opportunities to fulfill their rights to have better education, employment, and living conditions. Emancipatory CBPR uncovers these mechanisms of control, biases, and internalized representations of reality, as a key strategy for change.

Foucault (1977, 1979) has best articulated the fourth perspective of power; in this view power is productive and based on relationships. Rather than seeing repressive power as monolithic, he conceptualizes power as a web of discourses and practices found in institutions, communities, and families and exercised through actions in multiple relationships. These power relationships are inherently unstable and therefore open to challenge.

For Foucault, knowledge symbolizes power. Repressive power, as expressed, for example, through the use of research language that is overly technical, can inhibit how communities may respond to researchers. As productive power, however, research knowledge can open the possibility of communities challenging existing limits and conceptualizing new practices (Foucault, 1980; Gaventa & Cornwall, 2008). As Deveaux (1999) has noted, "Where there is power, there is resistance" (p. 242). As community members learn about research, they can gain decision-making power in the research relationship and also enhance their capabilities to bring those decision-making skills to other community issues (Le Compte, 1995).

In CBPR, as noted earlier, the relationship between researchers and communities requires trust and mutual commitment over time. These relationships do not take place in a vacuum. When researchers walk into a community, they bring the history of the research institution and of other researchers with them. Relationships unfold within the particular historical and institutional context of trust or mistrust as well as through the personal connections between the partners (Minkler, 2004). In an analysis of community dialogue, Scott (1990) has outlined public and hidden discourse (see Chapter Five). In relation to research, *public transcripts* contain information in official language about what outside researchers bring to the table and what community members offer in return. Yet *hidden transcripts,* what community members fully think, may remain outside the purview of what is observed by the outside research team. Some of these hidden transcripts may also become public over time, as relationships evolve.

CBPR practice therefore must be about all partners asking questions within historical and current contexts and examining their own positions of power, whether by virtue of race or ethnicity, education, or community status, and being willing to negotiate these dynamics over time. As seen in Foucault's framework, positions of power can reverse, and the initial power of the researcher may give way to the knowledge and gatekeeper functions of community members. The researcher then becomes only one player in the telling and interpretation of stories (Buroway et al., 1991). If the goal is to create reciprocity, then both outside researchers and community members become, in the words of singer Chris Williamson, "the changer and the changed" (Lather, 1986, p. 263).

In CBPR, there is never a perfect equilibrium of power. All research efforts undergo cycles of participation and questioning by community members, bringing greater or lesser participation and greater or lesser ownership. In times of frustration, community members may retreat to hidden discourse, expressing concerns in private (especially if they speak a language different from that of the outside researchers) or simply pretending greater willingness to participate. In more open times, public discourse may represent more sharing and access to hidden discourse. This dialectic of collaboration and skepticism between research partners and community participants presents a continual challenge. As one community member has stated, however, a committed research relationship based on an underlying context of trust makes a difference; even if there is an incident where trust is challenged, the underlying relationship enables both parties to keep working together and to renegotiate shared power and trust.

FEMINISM, POSTSTRUCTURALISM, AND POSTCOLONIALISM

Feminist participatory researchers add critical dimensions to our understanding of the theory and practice of CBPR. In early critiques they challenged both the exclusion of women through the use of universal language of "the oppressed" and the lack of attention to gender differences in participation in data collection and analysis (Maguire, 1987).

Over the past forty years, feminism has shifted from studying women as a universal construct to understanding gender culturally and historically, with shifting identities of class, race and ethnicity, sexual orientation, and other areas of differences (Collins, 2000; Hesse-Biber, Gilmartin, & Lydenberg, 1999; Maguire, 2006; Olesen, 2000; Reid & Frisby, 2008). Gender is seen as central in power relations, with various mechanisms in use that can silence women, such as censorship, intimidation, marginalization, or trivialization (Devault, with Ingraham, 1999; Maguire, 2006).

Poststructuralism focuses on the ways that language and narratives construct reality and our view of social institutions, such as academia, public health, or medicine, and how these constructions are resisted by communities. Postcolonialism takes this further by using race or ethnicity as a primary lens through which to understand European colonization of other peoples and lands. To counter the dominant portrayals of the *other,* CBPR research within a postcolonial tradition seeks to uncover and honor community explanations and narratives of the condition of people's lives (Duran & Duran, 1995; Walters & Simoni, 2002). The role of the outside researcher in this context may therefore be largely to weaken the power of dominant culture explanations and create spaces for competing community ideas and practices to emerge. Empirically based youth interventions that research the effectiveness of resistance to peer pressure, for example, may be too individualistic for the cultural norms of some minority groups.

In CBPR, poststructuralist, postcolonialist, and feminist theory share certain methods and goals: analyzing personal lives in relation to the structures (both overt and hidden) that might control people's lives; celebrating strengths and agency, not just emphasizing victimization; working for goals of social justice (Maguire, 2006); and undermining the notion of the objectivity of science.

Issues within feminism and within racism (discussed in detail in Chapter Five), such as how women in general (or in some cases women of color) state their identities in different contexts, elucidate the complexities CBPR faces in understanding the richness of community life and change processes (Bell, 2006). African American women, for example, as detailed in Patricia Hill Collins's work (2000), can appear in public spaces to conform to societal roles yet in other contexts, such as church or family, be adopting more powerful roles. In complex ways, then, they are not accepting stories of themselves as the other but are creating new stories based on strong identities as sisters, mothers, or advocates— providing an illustration of Foucault's idea of productive power (Collins, 1999, 2000; Fine, Weis, Weseen, & Wong, 2000).

Postcolonial, postmodern, and poststructural theories have challenged the right of researchers to overstate their interpretations and thereby silence the community (Fine et al., 2000; Mohanty, 1988; Spivak, 1988). In CBPR processes, interpretation of data often falls to the outside researcher; participatory data analysis is very difficult to achieve. In the case of quantitative data, the knowledge and software needed for statistical analyses often are situated in universities or other research institutions. In the case of qualitative data, the mountain of transcripts to be examined may be daunting, and the iterative processes, even with specialized software, are time consuming. Yet when undertaken and done well, participatory analysis of both qualitative and quantitative data not only can improve external validity of the data but can force a different approach to publication as well (see Chapter Sixteen).

Michelle Fine (1994) articulates three researcher stances in relation to community voices and their publication: (1) *ventriloquy,* when researchers describe the other as objective truth, never using the word "I" in their interpretation and never connecting themselves to their analysis of the data; (2) *voices,* when researchers speak for the other, recording people's words and stories and presenting quotes from interview or focus group transcripts without a critical analysis of the context or history of people's experience; and (3) *activist feminist research,* when researchers develop a negotiated stance, being explicit about their own identity, and creating through dialogue with community members a context-based interpretation and portrayal of knowledge. This third stance cautions against simply presenting multiple community voices, because some voices may be more powerful than others or may reflect internalized oppression rather than fostering an emancipatory perspective (Fine, 1994; Le Compte, 1995). Fine et al. (2000) call on us as outside researchers to be wary of research intended to "help" communities and encourages us to engage in the difficult task of negotiating data interpretation and presentation with community members throughout the research process.

PAULO FREIRE AND PRAXIS

Although community-based participatory research rests solidly on our understanding of the complexities of participation, knowledge, and power relations, this orientation to research also cannot exist without its practical applications in the community. CBPR research, whether focused on disease causation or direct community improvement, always takes an intervention activist approach. To explore the actualities of CBPR practice and methods, therefore, it is helpful to return to Brazilian educator Paulo Freire, a major source of inspiration within the Southern emancipatory tradition.

Freire's starting point of concern for the powerless is reflected in his initial literacy teaching in the slums with the marginalized poor, who had what he termed a naive or magical consciousness that they could not be actors in their own fate. Using emotionally and socially charged words and pictures, Freire (1970, 1982) generated dialogue to facilitate people's transformation to *conscientization* (or critical consciousness) and *praxis* (action based on conscientization) in order to improve their lives. Exiled from Brazil at the time of the military coup in 1964, Freire fled to Chile, from which he was later also exiled. He worked for the World Council of Churches until he was able to return to Brazil in the early 1990s.

To Freire (1970) the purpose of education is human liberation, which means that people are the subjects of their own learning, not "empty vessels" filled by the knowledge of experts. To promote the learner as subject, Freire proposes a listening-dialogue-action approach (Wallerstein & Auerbach, 2004). The first step is listening to the generative themes or issues of community members in order to create a structured dialogue in which everyone participates as a co-learner to jointly construct a shared social reality. Individuals must be not only involved in efforts to identify their problems but also engaged in conscientization to analyze the societal context for these problems. The Portuguese word *conscientização* connotes both critical consciousness and personal engagement with the knowledge (Freire, 1970; Park, 2006). The goal of dialogue and conscientization is praxis, the ongoing interaction between reflection and the actions people take to promote individual and social change. It is only through actions and encountering barriers to change that people truly shape their knowledge of how the world works, linking their cognitive understanding with the visceral and emotional.

Much of the creativity of the Freirian approach, also called *popular* or *empowerment* education, lies in the development of *codes,* or physical forms of the themes generated by participants. These codes (sometimes called triggers or discussion catalysts) might be pictures, videos, role plays, and so on—any form that helps participants to "see" their reality with new eyes and develop alternative ways of thinking and acting. Multiple dialogue and communication methods—such as identifying issues through photodocumentary research and photovoice (see Chapter Nine), employing the techniques of Augusto Boal's *theater of the oppressed* (Boal, 1979) for characterizing conditions, and substituting video portrayals of research results for written reports—are expressions of this approach (Horton & Freire, 1990; Sohng, 1996). A Freirian, structured-questioning approach facilitates dialogue based on the triggers and thus can benefit the participatory process, especially during the research interpretation phase (Arnold, Burke, James, Martin, & Thomas, 1995; Hope & Timmel, 1999; Nadeau, 1996; Vella, 1995; Wallerstein & Auerbach, 2004). In the United States, the Highlander Research and Education Center has been an inspiration in this area with its comparable dialogue-based approach developed during its sixty-year history of participatory education and research on labor issues, civil rights, voting rights, youth, and environmental organizing (Horton, 1990; Lewis, 2006).

Freire's writings reinforce a deep belief in humanity and people's role in making change and as such have critical importance to CBPR:

> To be a good [participatory researcher] means above all to have faith in people; to believe in the possibility that they can create and change things. You need to love . . . to be convinced that the fundamental effort of community . . . education is the liberation of people, never their "domestication." This liberation begins to the extent that men [and women] reflect on themselves and their condition in the world—the world in which and with which they find themselves. To the extent that they are more conscientized, they insert themselves as subjects into their own history [adapted from Freire, 1971, p. 61].

In *Teaching to Transgress,* bell hooks (1994) builds on Freire and Thich Nhat Hanh (1987) to challenge us to examine the mutual process of "engaged pedagogy," or in our case engaged CBPR. Rather than expecting only that community members become immersed in the creation of their history, CBPR research is a process in which outside researchers also become transformed. When we bring our own understandings and interpretations, "it eliminates the possibility that we can function as all-knowing silent interrogators" (hooks, 1994, p. 21).

Freire returns to this theme of researcher engagement in a dialogue book with Ira Shor, where he discusses the risks and fears of transformation, acknowledging that resistance may be real, "but if you don't risk, you don't create anything. Without risking, for me, there is no possibility to exist" (Shor & Freire, 1987, p. 61). Concerns about becoming liberatory researchers may be based on our own previous socialization as researchers; our fears (often unspoken) that we will not be seen as experts, that we will be ignored, or in some cases, our fears or expectations that we will be devalued or dismissed.

In a grand tour of participatory action research, Kemmis and McTaggart (2000) call for transcending "either-or dichotomies" for a critical social science engaged in a "reflexive-dialectical view of subjective-objective relations and connections" (p. 576). They call for an eclectic and complex research practice that draws from Marxist critical theory, applied utilitarian problem solving, and poststructuralist and feminist approaches, all of which promote our understandings of personal and collective agency under specific local and global historical conditions. Ultimately, they situate the emancipatory tradition in CBPR in its aim to work with communities to "release themselves from the constraints of irrational, unproductive, unjust, and unsatisfying social structures that limit their self-development and self-determination" (p. 597). Freirian methodologies can be helpful in pointing researchers and communities to the dialogical processes that facilitate these complex understandings.

SUMMARY

Issues of participation, knowledge creation, power, and praxis are not abstract phenomena but rather authentic tensions that are enacted both in academia and in community settings. If, for example, we are not honest about our own power bases as researchers with education, resources, skills, and privilege (possibly due to race or ethnicity, gender, or other identities), there is little hope that we will be able to transform power dynamics. We need to understand how our personal biographies inform our ability to interpret the world, both in understanding the problems and in visioning community strengths. This is also true for our community partners. We further need to remember that we likely will not have full access to the phenomena being studied, though we can be open to mutual learning and to the notion that community knowledge can greatly enrich our understanding of the world.

A major challenge for those of us in the CBPR field lies in the potential limits of CBPR, given the realities of globalization, the imposition of Western cultural and economic structures on the rest of the world, and the difficulties for local communities in making meaningful change. *Scaling up* has become a buzzword in world institutions seeking to bring lessons from small communities to nation-states (Gaventa & Cornwall, 2008). Can CBPR be scaled up when so much depends on relationship building and commitment to collaborative work over time? Can realities be transformed at the local level in order to enhance health and contribute to a more equitable society? Although these questions are important, we must ensure that critiques and challenges of CBPR do not play into conservative strategies that dismiss the role of communities participating in change (or that, conversely, leave the work of change to local communities without adequate public government support). Another major challenge is in recognizing the potential consequences of our research. As we produce negotiated versions of community "truths" from our investigations, these meanings may in turn supercede the very perspectives we worked to uncover. In a dynamic world this is cause for both grave concern and celebration. In many ways CBPR relies on the process that N. Scott Momaday captured so beautifully: "We are what we imagine. Our very existence consists in our imagination of ourselves" (cited in Vizenor, 1978, p. vi).

Ultimately, CBPR is about knowledge creation and the value of practical and critical emancipatory reason for understanding power dynamics, for recognizing the interconnections between the personal and the social and between life worlds and system worlds, and for identifying the barriers to and facilitators of human actions that move toward the goal of social change. This can be a daunting and contradictory task but one full of promise and hope as we engage with community to promote more just societies.

QUESTIONS FOR DISCUSSION

1. What are the contributions of the various participatory research traditions (for example, Freirian theory and practice, feminist participatory research, Lewinian action research, and so forth) to community-based participatory research for health?

2. How does CBPR challenge and contribute to the fundamental role(s) of research?

3. As an opportunity for self-reflection, what is your particular theoretical approach to CBPR, or what are the components from which you draw?

4. How are the tensions embedded in the concepts of knowledge creation, purpose of research, participation, power, and praxis expressed in your own work? Or how might they be expressed in future work you hope to do?

KEY TERMS

Southern and northern traditions

Participatory research, action research, participatory action research

Theories of participation, knowledge, power, and praxis

Popular education empowerment

Poststructuralism, postcolonialism, and feminism

REFERENCES

Alford, R., & Friedland, R. (1985). *Powers of theory.* New York: Oxford University Press.

Argyris, C., Putnam, R., & Smith, D. M. (1985). *Action science: Concepts, methods, and skills for research and intervention.* San Francisco: Jossey-Bass.

Argyris, C., & Schön, D. A. (1996). *Organizational learning II.* Reading, MA: Addison-Wesley.

Arnold, R., Burke, B., James, C., Martin, D., & Thomas, B. (1995). *Educating for a change.* Toronto: Between the Lines.

Bachrach, P., & Baratz, M. S. (1962). The two faces of power. *American Political Science Review, 56,* 947–952.

Bahl, I. (1961). I couldn't have gotten along without Sam. *Nursing Outlook, 9*(6), 352–356.

Bell, E. E. (2006). Infusing race into the U.S. discourse on action research. In P. Reason & H. Bradbury (Eds.), *Handbook of action research: Participative inquiry and practice* (concise ed., pp. 49–59). Thousand Oaks, CA: Sage.

Boal, A. (1979). *Theatre of the oppressed.* London: Pluto Press.

Bopp, M. (1994). The illusive essential: Evaluating participation in non-formal education and community development processes. *Convergence, 27,* 23–45.

Breed, J. (1958). Better days for the Navajos. *National Geographic, 114,* 809–810.

Brown, L., & Vega, W. (1996). A protocol for community-based research. *American Journal of Preventive Medicine, 12*(4), 4–5.

Brown, L. D., & Tandon, R. (1983). Ideology and political economy in inquiry: Action research and participatory research. *Journal of Applied Behavioral Science, 19*(3), 277–294.

Brown, P. (1992). Popular epidemiology and toxic waste contamination: Lay and professional ways of knowing. *Journal of Health and Social Behavior, 33,* 267–281.

Buchanan, D. (1998). Beyond positivism: Humanistic perspectives on theory and research in health education. *Health Education Research, 13,* 439–450.

Buroway, M., Burton, A., Ferguson, A., Fox, K. J., Gamson, J., Gartrell, N., et al. (1991). *Ethnography unbound: Power and resistance in the modern metropolis.* Berkeley: University of California Press.

Canadian Institutes of Health Research. (2008). *CIHR guidelines for health research involving aboriginal people.* Retrieved Apr. 10, 2008, from http://www.cihr-irsc.gc.ca/e/29134.html.

Chambers, R. (1992). *Rural appraisal: Rapid, relaxed and participatory* (Discussion Paper No. 311). Brighton, U.K.: Institute for Development Studies.

Chataway, C. (1997). An examination of the constraints on mutual inquiry in a participatory action research project. *Journal of Social Issues, 4,* 747–766.

Chisholm, R., & Elden, M. (1993). Features of emerging action research. *Human Relations, 46,* 275–297.

Collins, P. H. (1999). Learning from the outsider within. In S. Hesse-Biber, C. Gilmartin, & R. Lydenberg (Eds.), *Feminist approaches to theory and methodology* (pp. 155–178). New York: Oxford University Press.

Collins, P. H. (2000). *Black feminist thought: Knowledge, consciousness, and the politics of empowerment* (2nd ed.). New York: Routledge.

Cooke, B., & Kothari, U. (Eds.). (2001). *Participation: The new tyranny?* London: Zed Books.

Corburn, J. (2005). *Street science: Community knowledge and environmental health justice.* Cambridge, MA: MIT Press.

Cornwall, A., & Jewkes, R. (1995). What is participatory research? *Social Science & Medicine, 41,* 1667–1676.

Crazy Bull, C. (1997). A Native conversation about research and scholarship. *Tribal College, 9*(1), 17.

Crazy Bull, C. (2004). Decolonizing research: Indigenous scholars can take over the research process. *Tribal College, 16*(2), 14.

De Bruyn, L., Chino, M., Serna, P., & Fullerton-Gleason, L. (2001). Child maltreatment in American Indian and Alaska Native communities: Integrating culture, history, and public health for intervention and prevention. *Child Maltreatment, 6*(2), 89–102.

De Koning, K., & Martin, M. (Eds.). (1996a). *Participatory research in health: Issues and experiences* (2nd ed.). London: Zed Books.

De Koning, K., & Martin, M. (1996b). Participatory research in health: Setting the context. In K. De Koning & M. Martin (Eds.), *Participatory research in health: Issues and experiences* (2nd ed., pp. 1–18). London: Zed Books.

Deloria, V. (1992). *God is red: A native view of religion.* Golden, CO: North American Press.

Denzin, N. K., & Lincoln, Y. S. (Eds.). (2000). *Handbook of qualitative research* (2nd ed.). Thousand Oaks, CA: Sage.

Devault, M., with Ingraham, C. (1999). Metaphors of silence and voice in feminist thought. In M. Devault, *Liberating method* (pp. 175–186). Philadelphia: Temple University Press.

Deveaux, M. (1999). Feminism and empowerment. In S. Hesse-Biber, C. Gilmartin, & R. Lydenberg (Eds.), *Feminist approaches to theory and methodology* (pp. 236–256). New York: Oxford University Press.

Duran, B., & Duran, E. (1999). Assessment, program planning, and evaluation in Indian country: Toward a postcolonial practice. In R. M. Huff & M. V. Kline (Eds.), *Promoting health in multicultural populations: A handbook for practitioners* (pp. 291–311). Thousand Oaks, CA: Sage.

Duran, E., & Duran, B. (1995). *Native American postcolonial psychology.* Albany: State University of New York Press.

Duran, E., Duran, B., Brave Heart, M.Y.H., & Davis, S. (1998). Healing the American Indian soul wound. In Y. Danieli (Ed.), *International handbook of multigenerational legacies of trauma* (pp. 341–353). New York: Plenum Press.

Fals-Borda, O. (1991). Some basic ingredients. In O. Fals-Borda & M. A. Rahman (Eds.), *Action and knowledge: Breaking the monopoly with participatory action research* (pp. 3–13). New York: Apex Press.

Fals-Borda, O. (2006). Participatory (action) research in social theory: Origins and challenges. In P. Reason & H. Bradbury (Eds.), *Handbook of action research: Participative inquiry and practice* (Concise ed., pp. 27–37). Thousand Oaks, CA: Sage.

Fals-Borda, O., & Rahman, M. A. (Eds.). (1991). *Action and knowledge: Breaking the monopoly with participatory action research.* New York: Apex Press.

Fawcett, S. (1991). Some values guiding community research and action. *Journal of Applied Behavior Analysis, 24,* 621–636.

Fine, M. (1994). Working the hyphens. In N. K. Denzin & Y. S. Lincoln (Eds.), *Handbook of qualitative research* (pp. 70–82). Thousand Oaks, CA: Sage.

Fine, M., Weis, L., Weseen, S., & Wong, L. (2000). For who? Qualitative research, representation, and social responsibilities. In N. K. Denzin & Y. S. Lincoln (Eds.), *Handbook of qualitative research* (2nd ed., pp. 107–132). Thousand Oaks, CA: Sage.

Fisher, P. A., & Ball, T. J. (2003). Tribal participatory research: Mechanisms of a collaborative model. *American Journal of Community Psychology, 32*(3–4), 207–216.

Flax, J. (1987). Postmodernism and gender relations in feminist theory. *Signs: Journal of Women and Culture in Society, 12,* 621–643.

Fletcher, C. (2003). Community-based participatory research relationships with aboriginal communities in Canada: An overview of context and process. *Pimatisiwin, 1*(1), 1–36.

Flicker, S., Travers, R., Guta, A., McDonald, S., & Meagher, A. (2007). Ethical dilemmas in community-based participatory research: Recommendations for institutional review boards. *Journal of Urban Health, 84*(4), 478–493.

Foucault, M. (1977). *Discipline and punish: The birth of the prison.* London: Allen Lane.

Foucault, M. (1979). *The history of sexuality* (Pt. 1). London: Allen Lane.

Foucault, M. (1980). *Power/knowledge: Selected interviews and other writings, 1972–1977* (C. Gordon, Ed.). New York: Pantheon Books.

Francis, P. (2001). Participatory development at the World Bank: The primacy of process. In B. Cooke & U. Kothari (Eds.), *Participation: The new tyranny?* (pp. 72–87). London: Zed Books.

Freire, P. (1970). *Pedagogy of the oppressed.* New York: Seabury Press.

Freire, P. (1971). To the coordinator of the culture circle. *Convergence, 4*(1), 61–62.

Freire, P. (1982). Creating alternative research methods: Learning to do it by doing it. In B. L. Hall, A. Gillette, & R. Tandon (Eds.), *Creating knowledge: A monopoly? Participatory research in development* (pp. 29–37). Toronto: Participatory Research Network.

Gaventa, J. (1980). *Power and powerlessness: Quiescence and rebellion in an Appalachian valley.* Urbana: University of Illinois Press.

Gaventa, J., & Cornwall, A. (2008). Power and knowledge. In P. Reason & H. Bradbury (Eds.), *The SAGE handbook of action research: Participative inquiry and practice.* (2nd ed., pp. 172–190). Thousand Oaks, CA: Sage.

George, M. A., Daniel, M., & Green, L. W. (1998–1999). Appraising and funding participatory research in health promotion. *International Quarterly of Community Health Education, 18,* 181–197.

Gerken, E. (1940). Development of a health education program. *American Journal of Public Health, 30,* 915–920.

Gitlin, T., & Russell, R. (1994). Alternative methodologies and the research context. In A. Gitlin (Ed.), *Power and method: Political activism and educational research* (pp. 181–202). New York: Routledge.

Goodman, R. (2001). Community-based participatory research: Questions and challenges to an essential approach. *Journal of Public Health Management and Practice, 7*(5), v–vi.

Green, L. W. (2006). Public health asks of systems science: To advance our evidence-based practice, can you help us get more practice-based evidence? *American Journal of Public Health, 96*(3), 406–409.

Green, L. W., & Mercer, S. L. (2001). Can public health researchers and agencies reconcile the push from funding bodies and the pull from communities? *American Journal of Public Health, 91,* 1926–1929.

Greenwood, D., Whyte, W. F., & Harkavy, I. (1993). Participatory action research. *Human Relations, 46,* 175–191.

Habermas, J. (1971). *Knowledge and human interests* (J. Shapiro, Trans.). Boston: Beacon Press.

Habermas, J. (1974). *Theory and practice* (J. Viertel, Trans.). London: Heinemann.

Habermas, J. (1987). *The theory of communicative action: Vol. 2. Lifeworld and system: A critique of functionalist reason* (T. McCarthy, Trans.). Boston: Beacon Press.

Hall, B. L. (1992). From margins to center: The development and purpose of participatory research. *American Sociologist, 23*(4), 15–28.

Hall, B. L. (2001). I wish this were a poem of practices of participatory research. In P. Reason & H. Bradbury (Eds.), *Handbook of action research: Participative inquiry and practice* (pp. 171–178). Thousand Oaks, CA: Sage.

Hall, B. L., Gillette, A., & Tandon, R. (1982). *Creating knowledge: A monopoly? Participatory research in development.* New Delhi: Society for Participatory Research in Asia.

Hatch, J., Moss, N., Saran, A., Presley-Cantrell, L., & Mallory, C. (1993). Community research: Partnership in black communities. *American Journal of Preventive Medicine, 9*(6), 27–31.

Havighurst, R., & Illkevitch, R. (1949). The intelligence of Indian children as measured by a performance scale. *Journal of Abnormal Social Psychology, 39,* 19–33.

Henderson, D. (1995). Consciousness raising in participatory research: Method and methodology for emancipatory nursing inquiry. *Advances in Nursing Science, 17*(3), 58–69.

Heron, J., & Reason, P. (2006). The practice of cooperative inquiry: Research "with" rather than "on" people. In P. Reason & H. Bradbury (Eds.), *Handbook of action research: Participative inquiry and practice* (concise ed., pp. 144–153). Thousand Oaks, CA: Sage.

Hesse-Biber, S., Gilmartin, C., & Lydenberg, R. (Eds.). (1999). *Feminist approaches to theory and methodology.* New York: Oxford University Press.

Hills, M. (2001). Using cooperative inquiry to transform evaluation of nursing students' clinical practice. In P. Reason & H. Bradbury (Eds.), *Handbook of action research: Participative inquiry and practice* (pp. 340–347). Thousand Oaks, CA: Sage.

Hoffman, F. L. (1930). Are the Indians dying out? *American Journal of Public Health, 20,* 609–614.

hooks, b. (1994). *Teaching to transgress.* New York: Routledge.

Hope, A., & Timmel, S. (1999). *Training for transformation* (Vols. 1–4). London, Intermediate Technologies Development Group.

Horton, M. (1990). *The long haul: An autobiography.* Garden City, NY: Doubleday.

Horton, M., & Freire, P. (1990). *We make the road by walking: Conversations on education and social change* (B. Bell, J. Gaventa, & J. Peters, Eds.). Philadelphia: Temple University Press.

Huberman, M. (1991). Linkage between researchers and practitioners: A qualitative study. *American Educational Research Journal, 27,* 363–391.

Israel, B. A., Eng, E., Schulz, A. J., & Parker, E. A. (Eds.). (2005). *Methods in community-based participatory research for health.* San Francisco: Jossey-Bass.

Israel, B. A., Schulz, A. J., Parker, E. A., & Becker, A. B. (1998). Review of community-based research: Assessing partnership approaches to improve public health. *Annual Review of Public Health, 19,* 173–202.

Jewkes, R., & Murcott, A. (1998). Community representatives: Representing the "community"? *Social Science & Medicine, 46,* 843–858.

Jones, L., & Wells, K. (2007). Strategies for academic and clinician engagement in community-partnered participatory research. *Journal of the American Medical Association, 297,* 407–410.

Kemmis, S. (2008). Critical theory and participatory action research. In P. Reason & H. Bradbury (Eds.), *The SAGE handbook of action research: Participative inquiry and practice* (2nd ed., pp. 121–138). Thousand Oaks, CA: Sage.

Kemmis, S., & McTaggart, R. (2000). Participatory action research. In N. K. Denzin & Y. S. Lincoln (Eds.), *Handbook of qualitative research* (2nd ed., pp. 567–605). Thousand Oaks, CA: Sage.

Laclau, E., & Mouffe, C. (2001). *Hegemony and socialist strategy: Towards a radical democratic politics.* New York: Verso.

Lather, P. (1986). Research as praxis. *Harvard Educational Review, 56,* 257–277.

Le Compte, M. (1995). Some notes on power, agenda, and voice: A researcher's personal evolution toward critical collaborative research. In P. McLaren & J. Giarelli (Eds.), *Critical theory and educational research* (pp. 91–112). Albany: State University of New York Press.

Lewin, K. (1997). *Resolving social conflicts and field theory in social science.* Washington, DC: American Psychological Association. (Original work published 1948)

Lewis, H. M. (2006). Participatory research and education for social change: Highlander Research and Education Center. In P. Reason & H. Bradbury (Eds.), *Handbook of action research: Participative inquiry and practice* (Concise ed., pp. 262–268). Thousand Oaks, CA: Sage.

Lincoln, Y. S. (2001). Engaging sympathies: Relationships between action research and social constructivism. In P. Reason & H. Bradbury (Eds.), *Handbook of action research: Participative inquiry and practice* (pp. 124–132). Thousand Oaks, CA: Sage.

Lukes, S. (1974). *Power: A radical view.* New York: Macmillan.

Macaulay, A., Delormier, T., McComber, A., Cross, E., Potvin, L., Paradis, G., et al. (1998). Participatory research with native community of Kahnawake creates innovative code of research ethics. *Canadian Journal of Public Health, 89,* 105–108.

Maguire, P. (1987). *Doing participatory research: A feminist approach.* Amherst: University of Massachusetts, Center for International Education.

Maguire, P. (2006). Uneven ground: Feminisms and action research. In P. Reason & H. Bradbury (Eds.), *Handbook of action research: Participative inquiry and practice* (Concise ed., pp. 60–70). Thousand Oaks, CA: Sage.

McTaggart, R. (1997). *Participatory action research: International contexts and consequences.* Albany: State University of New York Press.

Minkler, M. (2004). Ethical challenges for the "outside" researcher in community-based participatory research. *Health Education & Behavior, 31*(6), 684–697.

Minkler, M., Wallace, S., & McDonald, M. (1994–1995). The political economy of health: A useful theoretical tool for health education practice. *International Quarterly of Community Health Education, 15,* 111–125.

Mohanty, C. (1988). Under Western eyes: Feminist scholarship and colonial discourses. *Feminist Review, 30,* 60–88.

Nadeau, D. (1996). *Counting our victories: Popular education and organizing.* New Westminster, BC: Repeal the Deal Productions.

Navarro, V. (1984). Medical history as justification rather than explanation: A critique of Starr's "Social transformation of American medicine." *International Journal of Health Services, 14,* 511–528.

Nhat Hanh, T. (1987). *Being peace.* Berkeley, CA: Parallax Press.

Olesen, V. (2000). Feminisms and models of qualitative research. In N. K. Denzin & Y. S. Lincoln (Eds.), *Handbook of qualitative research* (2nd ed., pp. 158–174). Thousand Oaks, CA: Sage.

Ong, A. (1991). *The ethnography of resistance.* Berkeley: University of California Press.

Park, P. (2006). Knowledge and participatory research. In P. Reason & H. Bradbury (Eds.), *Handbook of action research: Participative inquiry and practice* (Concise ed., pp. 83–93). Thousand Oaks, CA: Sage.

Park, P., Brydon-Miller, M., Hall, B. L., & Jackson, T. (Eds.). (1993). *Voices of change: Participatory research in the United States and Canada*. Westport, CT: Bergin & Garvey.

Perkins, D. D., & Wandersman, A. (1990). "You'll have to work to overcome our suspicions": The benefits and pitfalls of research with community organizations. *Social Policy, 21*, 32–41.

Peters, M., & Robinson, V. (1984). The origins and status of action research. *Journal of Applied Behavioral Sciences, 20*, 113–124.

Poland, B. (1996). Knowledge development and evaluation in, of, and for healthy community initiatives: Part 1. Guiding principles. *Health Promotion International, 11*, 237–247.

Polsby, N. (1963). *Community power and political theory*. New Haven, CT: Yale University Press.

Rahman, M. A. (1985). The theory and practice of participatory action research. In O. Fals-Borda (Ed.), *The challenge of social change* (pp. 107–132). Thousand Oaks, CA: Sage.

Rahman, M. A. (1991). The theoretical standpoint of PAR. In O. Fals-Borda & M. A. Rahman (Eds.), *Action and knowledge: Breaking the monopoly with participatory action research* (pp. 13–24). New York: Apex Press.

Reason, P. (1994). Three approaches to participative inquiry. In N. K. Denzin & Y. S. Lincoln (Eds.), *Handbook of qualitative research* (pp. 324–339). Thousand Oaks, CA: Sage.

Reason, P., & Bradbury, H. (Eds.). (2008). *The SAGE handbook of action research: Participative inquiry and practice* 2nd. ed. Thousand Oaks, CA: Sage.

Reid, C., & Frisby, W. (2008). Continuing the journey: Articulating dimensions of feminist participatory research (FPAR). In P. Reason & H. Bradbury (Eds.), *The SAGE handbook of action research: Participative inquiry and practice* (2nd ed., pp. 93–105). Thousand Oaks, CA: Sage.

Rifkin, S. (1996). Paradigms lost: Toward a new understanding of community participation in health programmes. *Acta Tropica, 61*, 79–92.

Rowan, J. (2006). The humanistic approach to action research. In P. Reason & H. Bradbury (Eds.), *Handbook of action research: Participative inquiry and practice* (concise ed., pp. 106–116). Thousand Oaks, CA: Sage.

Said, E. (1994). *Culture and imperialism*. New York: Vintage Books.

Scott, J. (1990). *Domination and the arts of resistance: Hidden transcripts*. New Haven, CT: Yale University Press.

Shor, I., & Freire, P. (1987). *A pedagogy for liberation: Dialogues on transforming education*. Westport, CT: Bergin & Garvey.

Smith, L. T. (1999). *Decolonizing methodologies: Research and indigenous people*. London: Zed Books.

Sohng, S.S.L. (1996). Participatory research and community organizing. *Journal of Sociology and Social Welfare, 23*(4), 77–97.

Spivak, G. (1988). Can the subaltern speak? In L. Nelson (Ed.), *Marxism and the interpretation of culture* (pp. 271–313). Urbana: University of Illinois Press.

Stringer, E. T. (2007). *Action research* (3rd ed.). Thousand Oaks, CA.: Sage.

Stringer, E. T., & Genat, W. (2004). *Action research in health*. Upper Saddle River, NJ: Merrill Prentice Hall.

Tandon, R. (1988). Social transformation and participatory research. *Convergence, 21*(2), 5–18.

Torbert, W. R., & Taylor, S. S. (2008). Action inquiry: Interweaving multiple qualities. In P. Reason & H. Bradbury (Eds.), *The SAGE handbook of action research: Participative inquiry and practice* (2nd ed., pp. 239–251). Thousand Oaks, CA: Sage.

Trickett, E. J., & Espino, S.L.R. (2004). Collaboration and social inquiry: Multiple meanings of a construct and its role in creating useful and valid knowledge. *American Journal of Community Psychology, 34*(1–2), 1–69.

Vella, J. (1995). *Training through dialogue: Promoting effective learning and change in adults*. San Francisco: Jossey-Bass.

Vizenor, G. (1978). *Word arrows: Indians and whites in the new fur trade*. Minneapolis: University of Minnesota Press.

Wallace, S., Williamson, J., Lung, R., & Powell, L. (1991). A lamb in wolf's clothing? The reality of senior power and social policy. In M. Minkler & C. Estes (Eds.), *Critical perspectives on aging: The political and moral economy of growing old* (pp. 95–114). Amityville, NY: Baywood.

Wallerstein, N. (1999). Power between evaluator and community: Research relationships within New Mexico's healthier communities. *Social Science & Medicine, 49,* 39–53.

Wallerstein, N. (2007). Making traces: Evidence for practice and evaluation. In J. Green & R. Labonté (Eds.), *Critical perspectives in public health* (pp. 80–92). New York: Routledge.

Wallerstein, N., & Auerbach, E. (2004). *Problem-posing at work: A popular educator's guide.* Edmonton, AB: Grassroots Press.

Walters, K., & Simoni, J. (2002). Reconceptualizing Native women's health: An "indigenist" stress-coping model. *American Journal of Public Health, 92,* 520–524.

Whyte, W. (Ed.) (1991). *Participatory action research.* Thousand Oaks, CA: Sage.

Wing, S. (1998). Whose epidemiology, whose health? *International Journal of Health Services, 28,* 241–252.

CHAPTER

3

CRITICAL ISSUES IN DEVELOPING AND FOLLOWING CBPR PRINCIPLES

BARBARA A. ISRAEL, AMY J. SCHULZ, EDITH A. PARKER,
ADAM B. BECKER, ALEX J. ALLEN III, & J. RICARDO GUZMAN

Note: Portions of this chapter have been adapted from "Review of Community-Based Research: Assessing Partnership Approaches to Improve Public Health," by B. A. Israel, A. J. Schulz, E. A. Parker, & A. B. Becker, 1998, *Annual Review of Public Health, 19,* pp. 173–202. Adapted with permission of the publisher. The authors thank Sue Andersen for her valuable assistance in the preparation of this manuscript.

A DISPROPORTIONATE burden of morbidity and mortality has been shown to exist in communities with few economic and social resources and in communities of color (Smedley, Stith, & Nelson, 2003; LaVeist, 2005; House & Williams, 2000; Krieger, 2005; Marmot & Wilkinson, 2006). Addressing these disparities in health status is a major challenge for researchers, practitioners, community leaders, and the affected communities. Historically, research in such communities has rarely benefited and has sometimes actually harmed the people involved (Hatch, Moss, Saran, Presley-Cantrell, & Mallory, 1993; Thomas & Quinn, 1991), and interventions have often not been successful in improving health and well-being (Gebbie, Rosenstock, & Hernandez, 2003; Steuart, 1993; Susser, 1995). In addition, for the most part research has been conducted in ways that systematically exclude some people from having influence and power over the research process (Fals-Borda & Rahman, 1991; Hall, 1992; Hatch et al., 1993; Israel, Schulz, Parker, & Becker, 1998; Maguire, 2001; Wallerstein, 2006). To reduce these health disparities, researchers need to address such fundamental questions as these: What is the purpose of research? Who benefits from research? How are the results of research used? How can research contribute to reducing health disparities? And what role does research play in intervention and policy change and in knowledge generation?

There have been increasing calls and growing funding support for a greater use of participatory approaches to research as one strategy for considering these questions (Jones & Wells, 2007; Green et al., 1995; Hatch et al., 1993; Israel et al., 1998; Wallerstein, 2006). However, participatory approaches vary in the extent to which they address basic inequalities in the research content and process and in applying the knowledge gained to change efforts. The key principles of participatory research processes, referred to collectively here as *community-based participatory research* (CBPR), can serve as guidelines for those interested in this approach. However, it is also crucial to recognize that numerous issues arise in every local context and research partnership and that these issues need to be considered when developing and adhering to CBPR principles. The purpose of this chapter is to present a set of community-based participatory research principles derived from an integration of the literature and the collective experiences of the chapter authors, who have worked together on several CBPR efforts. In addition, this chapter presents case examples from our work with a CBPR partnership, the Detroit Community-Academic Urban Research Center (URC),[1] to illustrate and discuss critical issues in adopting and following these principles. Throughout the chapter, we emphasize the importance of flexibility, constant reflection, and critical analysis in applying and adapting these principles in different contexts.

CBPR DEFINITION AND KEY PRINCIPLES

Community-based participatory research in public health is a partnership approach to research that equitably involves, for example, community members, organizational representatives, and researchers in all aspects of the research process. The partners contribute "unique strengths and shared responsibilities" (Green et al., 1995, p. 12) to enhance understanding of a given phenomenon and the social and cultural dynamics of the community and to integrate the knowledge gained with action to improve the health and well-being of community members (Hatch et al., 1993; Schulz, Israel, Selig, & Bayer, 1998).

The following nine principles or characteristics seek to capture key elements of this approach.[2] These principles reflect the present state of knowledge in the field, and therefore they will continue to evolve as further community-based participatory research is conducted and evaluated. They are presented with the recognition that the extent to which any research endeavor can achieve any one or any combination of these principles will vary depending on the context, purpose, and participants involved in the process. Also, each principle may be located on a continuum, with the principle as described here representing an ideal goal toward which to strive (Cornwall, 1996; Green et al., 1995). Finally, although each principle is presented here as a distinct item, community-based participatory research is an integration of these principles.

1. CBPR recognizes community as a unit of identity The concept of community as an aspect of collective and individual identity is central to community-based participatory research (Israel et al., 1998). Units of identity—for example, membership in a family, friendship network, or geographical neighborhood—are all socially constructed dimensions of identity, created and re-created through social interactions (Hatch et al., 1993; Steuart, 1993). Community is characterized by identification with and emotional connection to other members, common symbol systems, shared values and norms, mutual (although not necessarily equal) influence, common interests, and joint commitment to meeting shared needs (Israel, Checkoway, Schulz, & Zimmerman, 1994; Sarason, 1984; Steuart, 1993). Communities of identity may be centered on a defined geographical neighborhood or be made up of members of a geographically dispersed group with a sense of common identity and shared fate (such as persons who share race or ethnicity or persons who identify as lesbian, gay, bisexual, or transgender). Furthermore, a city or other geographical area may not be a community in this sense of the term but rather an aggregate of individuals who do not share a common identity, or it may contain several different overlapping communities of identity within its boundaries. Community-based participatory approaches to research attempt to identify and to work with existing communities of identity and to strengthen a sense of community through collective engagement (Israel et al., 1994). Communities of identity contain many individual and organizational resources but may also benefit from skills and resources available from outside the immediate community of identity. Thus community-based participatory research efforts may involve individuals and groups who are not members of the community of identity. Such partnerships may include representatives from health and human service organizations, academia, community-based organizations, and members at large from another community.

2. CBPR builds on strengths and resources within the community Community-based participatory research seeks to identify and build on strengths, resources, and relationships that exist within communities of identity to address members' communal health concerns (Israel et al., 1998; McKnight, 1994; Steuart, 1993). These resources may include skills and assets of individuals (McKnight, 1994); networks of relationships characterized by trust, cooperation, and mutual commitment (Heaney & Israel, 2002); and mediating structures such as churches and other organizations where community members come together (Berger & Neuhaus, 1977). Community-based participatory research explicitly recognizes and seeks to support or expand social structures and social processes that contribute to the ability of community members to work together to improve health.

3. CBPR facilitates collaborative, equitable partnership in all research phases and involves an empowering and power-sharing process that attends to social inequalities In CBPR, to the extent desired, all parties participate in and share control over all phases of the research process, including problem definition, data collection, interpretation of results, and application of the results to address community concerns (De Koning & Martin, 1996; Green et al., 1995; Hatch et al., 1993; Israel, Schurman, Hugentobler, & House, 1992; Israel et al., 1998; Park, Brydon-Miller, Hall, & Jackson, 1993; Stringer, 2007). CBPR partnerships focus on issues and concerns identified by community members (De Koning & Martin, 1996; Green et al., 1995; Hatch et al., 1993; Israel, Eng, Schulz, & Parker, 2005a) and create processes that enable all parties to participate and share influence in the research. Recognizing that socially and economically marginalized communities often have not had the power to name or define their own experience, researchers involved with CBPR acknowledge the inequalities between themselves and community participants and the ways that inequalities among community members may shape their participation and influence in collective research and action (Blankenship & Schulz, 1996; Wallerstein, 2006). Attempts to address these inequalities involve explicit attention to the knowledge and expertise of community members and an emphasis on creating an empowering process that includes sharing information, decision-making power, resources, and support among members of the partnership (Israel et al., 1994; Israel et al., 1998; Jones & Wells, 2007).

4. CBPR promotes co-learning and capacity building among all partners Community-based participatory research is a co-learning process that facilitates the reciprocal transfer of knowledge, skills, and capacity (De Koning & Martin, 1996; Freire, 1973; Israel et al., 1998; Stringer, 2007). For example, researchers can learn from community members' administrative and management skills and from their *local theories*—understandings and commonly held beliefs about the community and broader social context (Elden & Levin, 1991), and community members acquire further skills in how to conduct research. The emphasis here is on enhancing the capacity of all partners involved, which will both improve the effectiveness of the CBPR effort and be applicable to other endeavors that partner organizations are involved in as well.

5. CBPR integrates and achieves a balance between research and action for the mutual benefit of all partners Community-based participatory research seeks to build a broad body of knowledge about health and well-being while also integrating and balancing that knowledge generation with community and social change efforts that address the concerns of the community involved (Green et al., 1995; Israel et al., 1998;

Maguire, 2001; Park et al., 1993). Information is gathered to inform action, and new understandings emerge as participants reflect on actions taken. CBPR may or may not incorporate a direct action component, depending on the decision made by the partners involved, but it does incorporate a commitment to the translation and integration of research results with community change efforts, with the intention that all partners involved will benefit (De Koning & Martin, 1996; Green et al., 1995; Schulz, Israel, et al., 1998).

6. CBPR emphasizes public health problems of local relevance and also ecological perspectives that recognize and attend to the multiple determinants of health and disease Community-based participatory research addresses public health problems that are of local relevance to the community involved, and it considers the concept of health from a positive model (Antonovsky, 1979; Hancock, 1993) that emphasizes physical, mental, and social well-being (World Health Organization, 1946). It also emphasizes an ecological model of health (Gottlieb & McLeroy, 1994; Israel et al., 1998; Stokols, 1996) that, as defined by Bronfenbrenner (1990), considers and encompasses the individual, the immediate contexts (such as family or social network) within which he or she lives, and the larger contexts (such as community or society) in which these immediate contexts are embedded. Accordingly, such approaches recognize and attend to, for example, biomedical, social, economic, cultural, and physical environmental factors as determinants of health and disease. Given this attention to multiple units of practice and the complex set of determinants of health and disease, CBPR efforts strive to achieve broad-scale social changes aimed at eliminating health disparities.

7. CBPR involves systems development through a cyclical and iterative process Community-based participatory research involves systems development, so that a system (for example, a partnership) develops the competencies to engage in a cyclical, iterative process that includes partnership development and maintenance, community assessment, problem definition, development of research methodology, data collection and analysis, interpretation of data, determination of action and policy implications, dissemination of results, action taking (as appropriate), specification of learnings, and establishment of mechanisms for sustainability (Altman, 1995; Israel et al., 1994, 1998; Stringer, 2007; Tandon, 1981).

8. CBPR disseminates findings and knowledge gained to all partners and involves all partners in the dissemination process Community-based participatory research seeks to disseminate findings and knowledge gained to all partners involved, in language that is understandable and respectful, and "where ownership of knowledge is acknowledged" (Bishop, 1994, p. 186; see also Gaventa, 1993; Hall, 1992; Israel et al., 1998; Parker et al., 2005; Schulz, Israel, et al., 1998). The ongoing feedback of data and use of results to inform action are integral to this approach (Israel, Schurman, & Hugentobler, 1992; Schulz et al., 2002). This dissemination principle also calls for the involvement of all partners as coauthors and reviewers of publications and copresenters at meetings and conferences.

9. CBPR requires a long-term process and commitment to sustainability Given the negative experiences of many communities with research projects and the time and effort needed to genuinely follow the principles described here, community-based participatory research requires a long-term process and commitment to sustainability on the part of all partners (Hatch et al., 1993; Israel, Eng, et al., 2005a; Jones & Wells, 2007). To establish and maintain the trust required to successfully conduct CBPR efforts and to accomplish the aims of reducing health disparities, this long-term commitment has to extend beyond a single research project or funding period. It needs to be a commitment to continue to work together even if funding is not available. Although there is no set time frame for the "long term," the emphasis in CBPR remains on the development of relationships and commitments that extend beyond any one funding period. Some goals, such as modifying local policies that affect, for example, the presence of environmental risks in a local community, may take a decade or more to realize. Although a specific partnership may reach a point at which it decides not to continue as a partnership, there should be a commitment to the relationships that exist between the individuals and organizations involved and agreement that the parties will continue to collaborate with and support each other as needed and as desired (Israel et al., 2006).

ISSUES IN DEVELOPING AND FOLLOWING CBPR PRINCIPLES

A substantial literature has examined the challenges and facilitating factors in conducting community-based participatory research (see, for example, Green et al., 1995; Israel et al., 1998, 2001; Lantz, Viruell-Fuentes, Israel, Softley, & Guzman, 2001; Israel et al., 2005b; Trickett & Espino, 2004) and the key components of equitable community-researcher partnerships (Baker, Homan, Schonhoff, & Kreuter, 1999; Israel, Schurman, & Hugentobler, 1992; Jones & Wells, 2007; Koné et al., 2000; Lasker, Weiss, & Miller, 2001). The purpose of this section is to discuss critical issues that can arise when CBPR participants are trying to adopt and follow the nine CBPR principles presented earlier. Drawing from the literature and our experiences, we put forth some issues in terms of recommended strategies, while other issues raise questions for which there is no single suggested strategy or resolution. In all instances, we suggest that these are important topics for CBPR partnerships to reflect on and address.

No One Set of CBPR Principles Is Applicable to All Partnerships Although we strongly support and work to apply the nine CBPR principles presented here, we recommend equally strongly that this set of principles not be adopted as is and imposed on other partnerships. Although we suggest that some core values underlying these principles may be applicable in most situations, all of these principles are not going to be applicable in all settings or in all cultures and communities. Furthermore, in keeping with the CBPR approach, any principles applied must be *owned* by the specific group and therefore will need to be adapted in order to take into account the local context of each partnership. It is important not to assume that everyone will understand and agree to a set of principles developed by others. Furthermore, the very process of partners jointly developing their partnership's principles provides an opportunity for much needed dialogue and sharing of perspectives that helps build trust and establish relationships.

Several of us were involved in developing an initial set of CBPR principles as part of a community-based public health (CBPH) initiative funded by the W. K. Kellogg Foundation that involved representatives from academia, health agencies, and community-based organizations in Detroit and Flint, Michigan (Schulz, Israel, et al., 1998). This process of developing the principles took over a year and a half, involving multiple constituencies in numerous meetings, negotiations, and revisions before the final principles were adopted by all the partners. Several years later, when the Detroit Community-Academic Urban Research Center partnership was established, these original principles were distributed and discussed over several URC board meetings. The final principles adopted by the URC were an adaptation of those initially developed by the CBPH partnership. One addition, for example, was language that placed greater emphasis on both knowledge generation and action that benefits the community.

Although the time spent to discuss the initial set of CBPR principles and then to adapt them for the URC was much shorter than the time it had taken to formulate the principles originally, it still took the URC partnership a long time to internalize and own the principles. The URC's internalization of the principles began to happen only as the partnership engaged in particular CBPR projects in which the partners faced implementing the principles on a day-to-day basis. Further, some of the language in the principles that sounded good to CBPR partners initially did not really have meaning until they faced particular decision points. To state this more generally, as participants gain additional insights, the understanding of the principles changes over time, and they need to be revisited and revised accordingly. Developing a set of CBPR principles therefore needs to occur within the context of a specific partnership and to be viewed as a fluid and evolving process.

Each CBPR Partnership Must Define Its "Community" The CBPR principles developed and implemented will vary in any given partnership, depending on how the "community" is defined and who is around the table representing the defined community (Israel et al., 1998; Koné et al., 2000). Recognizing that no single definition is applicable in all situations, the initial group involved in establishing a CBPR partnership needs to discuss a number of critical questions, such as the following: Who is the community? Who represents the community? Who has influence in the community, and how, if at all, are they involved? Who decides who the community partners will be in a CBPR effort? Are the community partners involved as individuals or as representatives of community-based organizations (CBOs)? If as individuals, do community members have a constituency that they represent and report to? If community members are representatives of CBOs, what is the connection or link between each CBO and the community in which it works? How *grassroots* are the community members and CBOs involved? Who are the representatives and participants involved in the partnership, and how do they compare to members of the community in terms of class (income and education level), gender, and race or ethnicity? Who has the time, resources, skills, and flexibility to sit on boards and committees and attend meetings and review documents as necessary? Who is defined as being "outside" the community and not invited to participate?

The Detroit URC and affiliated projects have been primarily involved with two communities that qualify as both geographical communities and communities of identity

(Israel et al., 1998; Koné et al., 2000). East Side Detroit is predominantly African American, and Southwest Detroit has Detroit's largest percentage of Latinos. It was initially decided by the academic and health department partners who established the URC that the community partners would be community-based organizations that are highly respected by the community in which they operate and that individual staff would serve on the URC board as representatives of their organizations (Israel et al., 2001). To the extent possible, individuals who held positions of leadership within the organization or were appointed by the organizational leadership were selected to serve on the board. Thus board members work in the communities involved but some do not actually live in these communities. In addition, if an individual leaves the represented organization, he or she no longer serves on the board and is replaced by another individual appointed by that organization.

Members of the board, even those who are from and still reside within the community, are sometimes somewhat different from community members at large, primarily in education level and income. In the latter instance, it is important to recognize that such differences do not mean that the persons are no longer community members. Those of us in academia and health agencies need to be careful not to impose a definition of what it means to be "from the community." Even in marginalized communities, not all members are going to be poor or have little formal education, and it is often those with more formal education and income who are best situated to participate in CBPR efforts, while at the same time having the inside view of what it is like to live in the community (Steuart, 1993).

In the URC-affiliated project, Community Action Against Asthma (Parker et al., 2005), the community partners were primarily representatives from community-based organizations, but the steering committee decided early on that one partner should be a community member who was a parent of a child with asthma, the focus of the project. Although we consider this a viable strategy, just as no one organization can represent a community, no one individual can represent a specific subpopulation. In situations like this it is also important to consider how to ensure that every individual is treated with respect and listened to, especially if representing what might be referred to as a stigmatized group (such as substance users or gang members) that is the focus of a CBPR effort. Furthermore, it is important to reflect on whether some groups are being excluded from sitting around the partnership table and to address this issue accordingly.

All Partners Must Decide What It Means to Have a "Collaborative, Equitable Partnership" and How to Make That Happen Perhaps one of the most critical principles of community-based participatory research is that it emphasizes creating and sustaining partnerships in which all members share control of the decision-making process. As an ideal to strive for, this is a core value of CBPR, but how does a CBPR effort ensure equity and shared influence and control? Every partnership needs to ask itself whether members are true *partners* or just *part* of the *partnership*—in other words, are all partners ready and able to share power? This requires considerable time and attention from all involved. Yet such attention to the partnership process may be frustrating for some, particularly if it is perceived to draw time and energy away from accomplishing the specific objectives of the CBPR effort (Israel et al., 2001; Lantz et al., 2001).

The Detroit Community-Academic Urban Research Center has engaged in a number of strategies to define and try to achieve a collaborative, equitable partnership (Israel et al., 2001). One of the procedures identified by community partners as contributing to shared influence and control is the URC's use of a consensus rather than a majority vote approach to decision making. Consensus decision making takes considerable time and has been known to hamper decision making in other situations (Johnson & Johnson, 2005). However, the URC board employs a slight variation, referred to as the 70 percent rule, that requires that all partners (100 percent) have to buy into a decision with at least 70 percent of their support. This approach has enabled board members to thoroughly examine issues and consider multiple perspectives prior to making a decision, giving everyone the opportunity to express opinions, influence the decisions made, and develop support for decisions reached without the expectation that everyone will be in complete agreement on all decisions (Israel et al., 2001).

Another approach that the URC takes is to work toward shared distribution of resources for the partners involved, including direct and indirect costs associated with grants (Israel et al., 2001; Lantz et al., 2001). Although the core funding and some of the URC-affiliated project funds go primarily to the university involved, in several projects a community-based organization is the fiduciary and lead organization, and in all instances the community partner organizations receive modest financial compensation. The board also reviews the budget for the core funding and influences decisions on budget-related matters. This is an area that has the potential to create conflicts in a partnership and requires ongoing consideration (Israel et al., 1998; Jones & Wells, 2007). Of course not all partner organizations have the interest in managing or capability to manage large-scale projects, and this may be an area in which to focus capacity-building efforts. In addition, there are other ways to distribute the benefits and rewards of participating in CBPR projects that need to be explored by a partnership (for example, the provision of technical assistance and educational opportunities as desired or attendance and presentation at professional meetings).

It is also important to acknowledge that although shared influence and control is a goal and equity is a basic premise of CBPR, some real inequities among partners are difficult to erase (especially those involving race, gender, and class). These inequities can and most likely do get played out to some extent even in a process that strives for equity among partners. If partners acknowledge and discuss these inequities, they may be better able to see how such differences affect the work of the partnership. Such an understanding can then lead to more effective processes for reducing the impact that power imbalances may have on the relationships among group members and the work of the partnership. For example, the steering committee members and village health workers of the East Side Village Health Worker Partnership had numerous discussions, at meetings and retreats and in more informal settings, about how race, class, gender, and other inequities influence their work and the communities with whom they work. At times such inequities were used for the mutual benefit of the partners involved. For example, there have been situations where community partners have requested that a university colleague attend a meeting to enhance the community partner's "credibility," and university partners have made similar requests of community partners.

Not Everyone Will Be Involved in the Same Way in All Activities   Another core value of CBPR is that all partners participate in all phases of the research process. Here again, it is important for CBPR partnerships to determine what that means for them, realizing that it may not mean that everyone is involved in the same way in all issues and activities. For example, in the East Side Village Health Worker Partnership, the steering committee played a major role in developing a conceptual framework of a stress process, designing a survey instrument and the administration method, interpreting the survey data, and applying the results to establish and implement intervention strategies (Schulz et al., 2002; Schulz, Israel, Parker, et al., 2003). The steering committee was not, however, involved in the actual process of data entry and data analysis for the survey questionnaire. Given the time demands and technical aspects of these two processes, different levels of involvement may be appropriate for different partners, while also recognizing that this may be an area where community partners are interested in enhancing their skills. However, it is crucial that the results of data analyses be fed back in ways that are understandable and useful and that all partners engage in the process of interpreting the data, which might include requesting that additional analyses be conducted. Given the multiple skills and expertise levels of the partners involved and the multiple demands on their time, choices need to be made on how best to draw on the diverse capabilities and interests that exist. This often means that the researchers are making some choices (have some power) in terms of what data are analyzed and what results are fed back, and this increases the need for self-critique and self-reflection among those partners who are taking the lead in these project components.

Establish Procedures for Dissemination   A number of questions related to the dissemination of CBPR findings need to be addressed. Who will be the coauthors of publications and copresenters at professional meetings? How is it decided who they are? What are their roles and responsibilities? What happens when only one partner is invited to present or submit an article? What are the priority publication outlets (journal articles or popular press, for example), and who makes those decisions? How is a balance reached between time spent developing reports to feed back results within the community and writing peer-reviewed publications? Here again, there is no one answer to these questions that will work for all partnerships. Rather, a partnership needs to engage in a process of developing procedures to ensure that the dissemination principle is followed.

The Community Action Against Asthma (CAAA) steering committee established a dissemination subcommittee, made up of an equal number of university and community partners, which met over several months to draft dissemination procedures. These procedures, which subsequently were brought to and modified by the full steering committee, spell out, for example, how participants will be selected as coauthors and co-presenters and what the expectations are for these roles (Parker et al., 2005). The development and application of such procedures across the projects has greatly expanded our discussion of these issues and has enhanced how we have dealt with them.

Although we recommend that written dissemination procedures be established, it is important that they not be perceived as formal or rigid. Flexibility is necessary and a willingness to respond quickly as requests arise that may not fit within the specified parameters. We also consider these to be evolving procedures that need to be revisited and revised as determined by each particular partnership. Although it may be ideal to address these questions during the early phases of a project, many of the issues may not seem relevant or compelling until a partnership has had to face them directly. What is most important here is to view this as an ongoing topic of conversation and deliberation, making changes as needed along the way.

Recognize and Value Priorities Identified by the Community Although community-based participatory research emphasizes the importance of examining and addressing the social determinants of health, at multiple levels of practice (individual, family, community), researchers need to be careful not to impose that approach on the partnership. Understandably, community partners may initially be most interested in addressing specific, tangible issues that seem more amenable to change than trying to address the broad-scale policies associated with social determinants of health. Indeed, an extensive literature in the community-organizing field indicates that an essential component of effective organizing efforts is winning tangible, small-scale changes in a relatively short period of time (Minkler & Wallerstein, 2005). As noted by Meredith Minkler and Cheri Pies (2005), one of the key ethical precepts of community organizing and community building is self-determination, that is, "starting where the people are" (Nyswander, 1956). This is also a major principle of community-based participatory research, with its emphasis on the local relevance of public health problems and community involvement in all aspects of the research process. It is important to understand that the choice here does not have to be either-or. Rather, although a CBPR effort begins by addressing specific priority issues identified by the community, over time, as part of the research and intervention process, the partnership members can engage in dialogue aimed at gaining a better understanding of the role of the social determinants of the specific issue selected and what can be done to affect those determinants.

The East Side Village Health Worker Partnership used a stress process model as a conceptual framework for addressing the social determinants of health on Detroit's East Side (Parker, Schulz, Israel, & Hollis, 1998; Schulz et al., 2002). Although the model was included in the initial grant proposal, in which there was not much community involvement, it was never presented to the community per se. Instead, a locally defined stress process model was developed by the steering committee over a series of meetings (Schulz, Parker, et al., 1998). Based on this stress process model and subsequent in-depth interviews and survey questionnaires conducted with community members, the village health workers prioritized the issues they wanted to address. These included strengthening socially supportive relationships, enhancing relationships with the police, increasing safety for children, improving accessibility and appropriateness of health services, and fostering environments conducive to diabetes management and prevention. Although each of these issues has underlying social determinants, the initial strategies in which the partnership engaged emphasized short-term activities aimed at addressing these concerns (Halloween parties for children, "pamper me" events for women, participating in Police Week). These successful events have led to an increased sense of community competence, and through ongoing conversations with the village health workers and steering committee members, some participants also seemed ready to engage in broader-scale policy and social changes (Schulz et al., 2002).

Work with the Cultural Diversity of the Partners Involved Community-based participatory research partnerships are likely to involve partners who differ in ethnicity and race, gender, social class, sexual orientation, community or academic role, and academic discipline. The multiple perspectives represented require the development of a common language, trust, and mutual respect; an understanding of the various cultures; and the recognition that different participants may have different goals and agendas and also different experiences with and degrees of commitment to CBPR. Participants will also be contending with conflicting loyalties and multiple demands on their time, and they will vary in what they can contribute to the CBPR effort (Israel et al., 1998; Israel, Parker, et al., 2005; Koné et al., 2000; Northridge et al., 2000). As noted earlier, each CBPR partnership also has to consider how structural inequities contribute to the cultural differences that exist within it. Although the development of cultural competency is particularly germane for researchers working in community settings, as the following examples indicate there are also important differences within and across communities of identity that need to be considered.

The Community Action Against Asthma project was the first URC-affiliated project to simultaneously involve participants from both East Side and Southwest Detroit and also to involve researchers from the discipline of environmental health science as well as the field of health behavior and health education. Initially, some of the researchers who had less experience with CBPR were perceived by the community partners as being somewhat aloof and interested only in their research findings and not in the community members themselves. In addition, some of the Latino community partners from Southwest Detroit interpreted some of the comments from partners from the East Side, a predominantly African American community, as stereotypical and discriminatory toward Latinos. Cultural competency workshops, small-group meetings, and other strategies may be effective means of ensuring that the cultural diversity that exists is respected and celebrated (Parker et al., 2003; see also Chapter Five).

Differences also occur across research disciplines. On several occasions, for example, environmental scientists and social scientists involved in CAAA have used the same words with very different meanings. In one instance the term *qualitative data* was used by the environmental scientists to mean any data not calibrated by a machine; thus the results of a closed-ended survey were considered qualitative data. In the social sciences, however, *qualitative data* describes the results of a research paradigm involving open-ended data collection approaches. Similarly, the use of the term *scale* by a social scientist at a meeting discussing the results of a factor analysis and the formation of indices from a survey questionnaire caused some confusion among the environmental health scientists, who use the term *scale* to refer to an instrument that measures substances in the environment. The recognition of these language differences has contributed some levity and humor to our conversations but also a commitment to ongoing work to develop a mutually understandable language.

Develop Procedures to Ensure CBPR Principles Are Followed As a CBPR partnership establishes trust and a track record of successfully conducting research and interventions, there are likely to be other researchers and community organizations that want the partnership to work with them in response to, say, a funding agency's call for particular proposals or a community's specifically identified problem. However, the would-be partners' rationale for reaching out to the partnership may not be in the partnership's or community's best interest. For example, some researchers may see working with the partnership as a way to get access to subjects, and some community-based organizations may see the partnership as a mechanism to obtain access to resources. It is important that partnerships develop a process and procedures for disseminating their CBPR principles to potential collaborators and ensuring that new projects adhere to these principles. Such procedures may be perceived by others as gatekeeping mechanisms that "keep others out." Communicating that the principles are a means to "open the gate" appropriately remains an ongoing challenge.

In the URC a subcommittee (or sometimes the entire board) reviews each request for a new project; the review may include a presentation by the interested parties to the full board. An expedited review process, making use of e-mail and conference calls, has also been adopted. Although these procedures have worked well—and have also resulted in a number of in-depth conversations about the principles and what they mean—at times the process has upset colleagues wanting to work with the URC. In one instance, a faculty member not affiliated with the URC requested a letter of support for a grant proposal from a faculty member who is affiliated, and did not understand the need to wait and get approval from the URC board. In another case a community-based organization interested in joining one of the CBPR projects did not understand why a community partner could not make that happen.

Partnership Size Must Be Decided by and Appropriate for the Community A question that we are frequently asked is, "What is the most appropriate or effective number of partners to include in a community-based participatory research effort?" No firm answer can be found in the literature; rather, the specific context and goals have to be considered, and the initial partners involved have to decide what is most appropriate in their particular situation. Our own experience leads us to recommend that a CBPR partnership start small, beginning with partner organizations from only one or two communities of identity (Israel et al., 2001). Such an approach has the advantage of building on existing relationships and trust and the likelihood of identifying mutually agreed upon goals while also recognizing the considerable research evidence that the most effective size for problem-solving groups is eight to twelve members (Johnson & Johnson, 2005). If there are preestablished, long-standing relationships in the community of identity, a partnership might be effective with a somewhat larger initial number of partners. Furthermore, it is also important to realize that there are limits to the skills, resources, and time available from members in smaller groups, and thus a slightly larger core group may be needed (ideally not more than twelve to sixteen partner organizations) and that identifying other mechanisms to involve additional persons may be necessary as well.

In our own work we often use what could be considered a Venn diagram approach to participation. At the center of a series of overlapping circles is a core group of project partners who are members of and make up the decision-making group for the CBPR partnership. In addition, we often need specific work groups or action teams in which other individuals or organizations are invited to participate (as members of an outer, nonoverlapping circle) along with members of the core group. Another approach that we use could more closely be represented using a concentric circle diagram, in which the core partners in the CBPR effort are represented in the center circle, and other organizations are invited to participate in a more limited way (outer circle). For example, in the Community Action Against Asthma project, the steering committee is composed of representatives from thirteen partner organizations, and as part of a community-organizing component of the project, a more loosely affiliated interorganizational network of organizations with similar interests in environmental triggers of asthma was established. The organizations in this network were kept informed of the work of the project and some organizations were involved in specific community-organizing efforts as appropriate.

In general we recommend that the core group of CBPR partners remain fairly small, recognizing that there are multiple approaches to expanding to include others as needed. It is important for all involved to recognize that partnership size is fluid and evolving and is a critical topic for the partnership's consideration. In an existing partnership that is considering adding new members, it is helpful to develop a set of criteria for membership and for the existing partners to discuss and agree on the needs of the partnership that new members would help to meet; the expectations, roles, and responsibilities of new members; and the procedures for adding new members. It is useful to spell out such criteria and procedures in writing, but at the same time we caution against being too formal and rigid, as that could undermine the very strength of a community-driven participatory process.

Recognize That CBPR Principles Alone Do Not Dictate Research Design and Methodology We see some confusion in the field that is manifested in the suggestion that community-based participatory research approaches by definition dictate the types of research design and methods that are appropriate. Community-based participatory research is not a method per se, and there is no one design or method appropriate for all CBPR efforts. Instead, each partnership has to decide what works best for its research question and intervention goal in its particular community context. For example, although qualitative methods provide in-depth understanding of a given phenomenon and give voice to those who are often not listened to, CBPR partnerships and communities may also be interested in knowing how widespread opinions are on a given issue. In our East Side Village Health Worker Partnership, in addition to conducting group dialogues and in-depth interviews on the stress process, we also conducted a random sample survey with community residents (Schulz, Parker, et al., 1998).

Furthermore, from a research design perspective, even though the use of a control group that receives no direct benefit from the research is neither appropriate nor, we would suggest, ethical in the context of CBPR, there are other viable designs. For example, the Community Action Against Asthma project was designed as a staggered intervention in which half of the children (and their households) enrolled in the project were randomly selected to receive the intensive phase of the intervention during the first year and the second half were selected to receive the intervention during the second year. This allowed us to evaluate the intervention effects by comparing wave 1 and wave 2 participants, a fairly standard research design. Although this was agreed on by the partners involved, we also need to mention that many participants assigned to wave 2 were troubled by the delay in receiving the intervention and by the multiple requests to provide data during the first year, in which they did not receive any direct benefits.

Continually Evaluate How Well CBPR Principles Are Followed To develop and maintain an effective CBPR partnership and to enhance participants' understanding of the factors that contribute to this effectiveness, it is necessary to conduct an ongoing evaluation of the extent to which and in what ways the CBPR principles are being followed (Israel et al., 2001; Israel, Lantz, McGranaghan, Kerr, & Guzman, 2005; Parker et al., 2002; Schulz, Israel, & Lantz, 2003). Such an evaluation needs to be an integral part of the partnership, with members involved in all aspects of the evaluation and with the results fed back on a regular basis and used to make changes in how the partnership operates, as appropriate.

Since its founding, the Detroit Community-Academic Urban Research Center has conducted an evaluation to assess URC board members' perceptions and experiences of the board's activities, processes, and progress, including accomplishments, adherence to CBPR principles, challenges, and facilitating factors (Israel et al., 2001; Israel, Lantz, et al., 2005; Lantz et al., 2001). An evaluation subcommittee of the board initially guided this assessment, which has included multiple data collection methods (for example, in-depth interviews with board members, mailed closed-ended survey questionnaires, and field notes). Each year the results of this evaluation have been fed back and discussed at URC board meetings and have enhanced members' understanding of the CBPR principles adopted and how to effectively follow them (Israel et al., 2001; Israel, Lantz, et al., 2005; Lantz et al., 2001). In addition to this evaluation of the overall URC board, a number of the affiliated projects engage in a similar ongoing assessment of their partnerships (Parker et al., 2002; Schulz, Israel, Parker, et al., 2003; Schulz et al., 2002).

SUMMARY

As discussed throughout this chapter, if researchers, practitioners, and community members are to address the growing disparities in health status between marginalized communities and those with greater social and economic resources, they need more equitable approaches to research, approaches that involve both action and knowledge generation that are beneficial to and reflective of the communities involved. Community-based participatory research is one approach that engages diverse partners in strategies aimed at obtaining multiple perspectives in order to address community-identified concerns. Our set of community-based participatory research principles can be used as guidelines by all those interested in this approach; however, we reiterate that no one set of existing principles is appropriate for all communities and all situations. Similarly, we want to emphasize that there is not just one approach to CBPR. As partnerships consider the issues raised here, each partnership will develop its own approach to inquiry and change, along with principles that are appropriate for its own partners working together in their specific context. What is crucial is the long-term commitment to reducing fundamental inequalities that exist throughout the systems in which we all live and work.

QUESTIONS FOR DISCUSSION

1. In what ways do the principles discussed in this chapter add to our understanding of CBPR's theoretical base? How do they reflect this theory?

2. The chapter authors state that "no one set of CBPR principles is applicable to all partnerships." Think of a partnership you are familiar with or that you have read about. Is there a principle on the list that might need to be modified in some way to better meet the needs of this partnership? Is there a principle you think would be worth proposing that is not in the authors' list?

3. The Detroit Community-Academic Urban Research Center (URC) that is described in this chapter made a conscious decision to include as partners community-based organizations rather than less formal, grassroots groups. What might the URC have added by making this decision? Might there be downsides to this decision?

KEY TERMS

CBPR principles   Health disparities   Partnerships

NOTES

1. The Detroit Community-Academic Urban Research Center (URC) partnership was established in 1995 as part of the Urban Research Centers Initiative of the Centers for Disease Control and Prevention (Grant No. U48/CCU515775), and has subsequently received funding from the W. K. Kellogg Foundation, The Skillman Foundation, and the University of Michigan. The Detroit URC develops, implements, and evaluates interdisciplinary, collaborative, community-based participatory research and intervention projects that aim to eliminate health disparities and improve the health of residents in Southwest, East Side, and Northwest Detroit. Since the Detroit URC was established its partners have included eleven community-based organizations (Butzel Family Center, Community Health and Social Services Center, Communities in Schools, Detroit Hispanic Development Corporation, Detroiters Working for Environmental Justice, Friends of Parkside, Kettering/Butzel Health Initiative, Latino Family Services, Neighborhood Service Organization, Rebuilding Communities, Inc./Warren-Conner Development Coalition, and Southwest Counseling and Development Services), the Detroit Department of Health and Wellness Promotion, the Henry Ford Health System, and the University of Michigan Schools of Public Health, Nursing, and Social Work. The experiences of the Detroit URC board and of those involved in affiliated projects have greatly contributed to the ideas presented here.

2. This discussion includes excerpts and revised portions from a set of CBPR principles originally presented by Israel et al. (1998), pp. 177–180.

REFERENCES

Altman, D. G. (1995). Sustaining interventions in community systems: On the relationships between researchers and communities. *Health Psychology, 14,* 526–536.

Antonovsky, A. (1979). *Health, stress, and coping: New perspectives on mental and physical well-being.* San Francisco: Jossey Bass.

Baker, E. A., Homan, S., Schonhoff, R., & Kreuter, M. W. (1999). Principles of practice for academic/practice/community research partnerships. *American Journal of Preventive Medicine, 16*(3), 86–93.

Berger, P. L., & Neuhaus, R. J. (1977). *To empower people: The role of mediating structures in public policy.* Washington, DC: American Enterprise Institute for Public Policy Research.

Bishop, R. (1994). Initiating empowering research? *New Zealand Journal of Educational Studies, 29,* 175–188.

Blankenship, K. M., & Schulz, A. J. (1996, August). Approaches and dilemmas in community-based research and action. Paper presented at the annual meeting of the Society for the Study of Social Problems, New York.

Bronfenbrenner, U. (1990). *The ecology of human development: Experiments by nature and design.* Cambridge, MA: Harvard University Press.

Cornwall, A. (1996). Towards participatory practice: Participatory rural appraisal (PRA) and the participatory process. In K. De Koning & M. Martin (Eds.), *Participatory research in health: Issues and experiences* (2nd ed., pp. 94–107). London: Zed Books.

De Koning, K., & Martin, M. (1996). *Participatory research in health: Issues and experiences* (2nd ed.). London: Zed Books.

Elden, M., & Levin, M. (1991). Cogenerative learning: Bringing participation into action research. In W. F. Whyte (Ed.), *Participatory action research* (pp. 127–142). Thousand Oaks, CA: Sage.

Fals-Borda, O., & Rahman, M. A. (Eds.). (1991). *Action and knowledge: Breaking the monopoly with participatory action research.* New York: Apex Press.

Freire, P. (1973). *Education for critical consciousness.* New York: Continuum.

Gaventa, J. (1993). The powerful, the powerless, and the experts: Knowledge struggles in an information age. In P. Park, M. Brydon-Miller, B. Hall, & T. Jackson (Eds.), *Voices of Change: Participatory Research in the United States and Canada* (pp. 21–40). Westport, CT: Bergin & Garvey.

Gebbie, K., Rosenstock, L., & Hernandez, L. M. (2003). *Who will keep the public healthy? Educating public health professionals for the 21st century.* Washington, DC: Institute of Medicine.

Gottlieb, N. H., & McLeroy, K. R. (1994). Social health. In M. P. O'Donnell & J. S. Harris (Eds.), *Health promotion in the workplace* (pp. 458–493). Albany, NY: Delmar.

Green, L. W., George, M. A., Daniel, M., Frankish, C. J., Herbert, C. P., Bowie, W. R., et al. (1995). *Study of participatory research in health promotion: Review and recommendations for the development of participatory research in health promotion in Canada.* Vancouver, BC: Royal Society of Canada.

Hall, B. L. (1992). From margins to center: The development and purpose of participatory research. *American Sociologist, 23*(4), 15–28.

Hancock, T. (1993). The healthy city from concept to application: Implications for research. In J. K. Davies & M. P. Kelly (Eds.), *Healthy cities: Research and practice* (pp. 14–24). New York: Routledge.

Hatch, J., Moss, N., Saran, A., Presley-Cantrell, L., & Mallory, C. (1993). Community research: Partnership in black communities. *American Journal of Preventive Medicine, 9*(6), 27–31.

Heaney, C. A., & Israel, B. A. (2002). Social networks and social support. In K. Glanz, B. K. Rimer, & F. M. Lewis (Eds.), *Health behavior and health education: Theory, research and practice* (3rd ed., pp. 185–209). San Francisco: Jossey-Bass.

House, J. S., & Williams, D. R. (2000). Understanding and reducing socioeconomic and racial/ethnic disparities in health. In B. D. Smedley & S. L. Syme (Eds.), *Promoting health: Intervention strategies from social and behavioral research* (pp. 81–124). Washington, DC: National Academies Press.

Israel, B. A., Checkoway, B., Schulz, A. J., & Zimmerman, M. A. (1994). Health education and community empowerment: Conceptualizing and measuring perceptions of individual, organizational, and community control. *Health Education Quarterly, 21,* 149–170.

Israel, B. A., Eng, E., Schulz, A. J., & Parker, E. A. (2005a). Introduction. In B. A. Israel, E. Eng, A. J. Schulz, & E. Parker (Eds.), *Methods in Community-Based Participatory Research for Health* (pp. 3–26). San Francisco: Jossey-Bass.

Israel, B. A., Eng, E., Schulz, A. J., & Parker, E. A., (Eds.). (2005b). *Methods in community-based participatory research for health.* San Francisco: Jossey-Bass.

Israel, B. A., Krieger, J. W., Vlahov, D., Ciske, S., Foley, M., Fortin, P., et al. (2006). Challenges and facilitating factors in sustaining community-based participatory research partnerships: Lessons learned from the Detroit, New York City, and Seattle urban research centers. *Journal of Urban Health, 83,* 1022–1040.

Israel, B. A., Lantz, P. M., McGranaghan, R., Kerr, D., & Guzman, J. R. (2005). Documentation and evaluation of community-based participatory research partnerships: The use of in-depth interviews and closed-ended questionnaires. In B. A. Israel, E. Eng, A. J. Schulz, & E. A. Parker (Eds.), *Methods in community-based participatory research for health* (pp. 255–277). San Francisco: Jossey-Bass.

Israel, B. A., Lichtenstein, R., Lantz, P. M., McGranaghan, R. J., Allen, A., Guzman, J. R., et al. (2001). The Detroit Community-Academic Urban Research Center: Lessons learned in the development, implementation, and evaluation of a community-based participatory research partnership. *Journal of Public Health Management and Practice, 7*(5), 1–19.

Israel, B.A., Parker, E. A., Rowe, Z., Salvatore, A., Minkler, M., Lopez, J., et al. (2005). Community-based participatory research: Lessons learned from the Centers for Children's Environmental Health and Disease Prevention Research. *Environmental Health Perspectives, 113,* 1463–1471.

Israel, B. A., Schulz, A. J., Parker, E. A., & Becker, A. B. (1998). Review of community-based research: Assessing partnership approaches to improve public health. *Annual Review of Public Health, 19,* 173–202.

Israel, B. A., Schurman, S. J., & Hugentobler, M. K. (1992). Conducting action research: Relationships between organization members and researchers. *Journal of Applied Behavioral Science, 28,* 74–101.

Israel, B. A., Schurman, S. J., Hugentobler, M. K., & House, J. S. (1992). A participatory action research approach to reducing occupational stress in the United States. In V. Di Martino (Ed.), *Preventing Sress at Work: Conditions of Work Digest* (Vol. 2, pp. 152–163). Geneva: International Labor Office.

Johnson, D. W., & Johnson, F. P. (2005). *Joining together: Group theory and group skills* (9th ed.). Boston: Allyn & Bacon.

Jones, L., & Wells, K. (2007) Strategies for academic and clinician engagement in community-partnered participatory research. *Journal of the American Medical Association, 297,* 407–410.

Koné, A., Sullivan, M., Senturia, K. D., Chrisman, N. J., Ciske, S. J., & Krieger, J. W. (2000). Improving collaboration between researchers and communities. *Public Health Reports, 115,* 243–248.

Krieger, N. (2005). *Embodying inequality: Epidemiological perspectives.* Amityville, NY: Baywood.

Lantz, P. M., Viruell-Fuentes, E., Israel, B. A., Softley, D., & Guzman, J. R. (2001). Can communities and academia work together on public health research? Evaluation results from a community-based participatory research partnership in Detroit. *Journal of Urban Health, 78,* 495–507.

Lasker, R. D., Weiss, E. S., & Miller, R. (2001). Partnership synergy: A practical framework for studying and strengthening the collaborative advantage. *Milbank Quarterly, 79,* 179–205.

LaVeist, T. A. (2005). *Minority populations and health: An introduction to health disparities in the United States.* San Francisco: Jossey Bass.

Maguire, P. (2001). Uneven ground: Feminisms and action research. In P. Reason & H. Bradbury (Eds.), *Handbook of action research: Participative inquiry and practice* (pp. 59–69). Thousand Oaks, CA: Sage.

Marmot, M., & Wilkinson, R. G. (Eds.). (2006). *Social determinants of health* (2nd ed.). New York: Oxford University Press.

McKnight, J. L. (1994). Politicizing health care. In P. Conrad & R. Kern (Eds.), *The Sociology of health and illness: Critical perspectives* (4th ed., pp. 437–441). New York: St. Martin's Press.

Minkler, M., & Pies, C. (2005). Ethical issues in community organization and community participation. In M. Minkler (Ed.), *Community organizing and community building for health* (pp. 116–134). New Brunswick, NJ: Rutgers University Press.

Minkler, M., & Wallerstein, N. (2005). Improving health through community organization and community building. In M. Minkler (Ed.), *Community organizing and community building for health* (pp. 26–50). New Brunswick, NJ: Rutgers University Press.

Northridge, M. E., Vallone, D., Merzel, C., Greene, D., Shepard, P., Cohall, A. T., et al. (2000). The adolescent years: An academic-community partnership in Harlem comes of age. *Journal of Public Health Management and Practice, 6*(1), 53–60.

Nyswander, D. (1956). Education for health: Some principles and their application. *California Health, 14,* 65–70.

Park, P., Brydon-Miller, M., Hall, B. L., & Jackson, T. (Eds.). (1993). *Voices of change: Participatory research in the United States and Canada.* Westport, CT: Bergin & Garvey.

Parker, E. A., Israel, B. A., Williams, M., Brakefield-Caldwell, W., Lewis, T. C., Robins, T., et al. (2003). Community action against asthma: Examining the partnership process of a community-based participatory research project. *Journal of General Internal Medicine, 18*(7), 558–567.

Parker, E. A., Robins, T. G., Israel, B. A., Brakefield-Caldwell, W., Edgren, K. K., & Wilkins, D. J. (2005). Developing and implementing guidelines for dissemination: The experience of the Community Action Against Asthma project. In B. A. Israel, E. Eng, A. J. Schulz, & E. A. Parker (Eds.), *Methods in community-based participatory research for health* (pp. 285–306). San Francisco: Jossey-Bass.

Parker, E. A., Schulz, A. J., Israel, B. A., & Hollis, R. (1998). Detroit's East Side Village Health Worker Partnership: Community-based lay health advisor intervention in an urban area. *Health Education & Behavior, 25*(1), 24–45.

Sarason, S. B. (1984). *The psychological sense of community: Prospects for a community psychology.* San Francisco: Jossey-Bass.

Schulz, A. J., Israel, B. A., & Lantz, P. M. (2003). Instrument for evaluating dimensions of group dynamics within community-based participatory research partnerships. *Evaluation and Program Planning, 26,* 249–262.

Schulz, A. J., Israel, B. A., Parker, E. A., Lockett, M., Hill, Y., & Wills, R. (2003). Engaging women in community-based participatory research for health: The East Side Village Health Worker Partnership. In M. Minkler & N. Wallerstein (Eds.), *Community-based participatory research for health* (pp. 293–315). San Francisco: Jossey-Bass.

Schulz, A. J., Israel, B. A., Selig, S. M., & Bayer, I. S. (1998). Development and implementation of principles for community-based research in public health. In R. H. MacNair (Ed.), *Research strategies for community practice* (pp. 83–110). New York: Haworth Press.

Schulz, A. J., Parker, E. A., Israel, B. A., Allen, A., DeCarlo, M., & Lockett, M. (2002). Addressing social determinants of health through community-based participatory research: The East Side Village Health Worker Partnership. *Health Education & Behavior, 29*(3), 326–341.

Schulz, A. J., Parker, E. A., Israel, B. A., Becker, A. B., Maciak, B. J., & Hollis, R. (1998). Conducting a participatory community-based survey for a community health intervention on Detroit's East Side. *Journal of Public Health Management and Practice, 4*(2), 10–24.

Smedley, B. D., Stith, A. Y., & Nelson, A. R. (Eds.), Institute of Medicine. (2003). *Unequal treatment: Confronting racial and ethnic disparities in health care.* Washington, DC: National Academies Press.

Steuart, G. W. (1993). Social and cultural perspectives: Community intervention and mental health. *Health Education Quarterly, 1*(Suppl.), S99–S111.

Stokols, D. (1996). Translating social ecological theory into guidelines for community health promotion. *American Journal of Health Promotion, 10,* 282–298.

Stringer, E. T. (2007). *Action research* (3rd ed.). Thousand Oaks, CA: Sage.

Susser, M. (1995). The tribulations of trials: Intervention in communities. *American Journal of Public Health, 85,* 156–158.

Tandon, R. (1981). Participatory evaluation and research: Main concepts and issues. In W. Fernandes & R. Tandon (Eds.), *Participatory research and evaluation* (pp. 15–34). New Delhi: Indian Social Institute.

Thomas, S. B., & Quinn, S. C. (1991). The Tuskegee Syphilis Study, 1932 to 1972: Implications for HIV education and AIDS risk education programs in the black community. *American Journal of Public Health, 11,* 1498–1505.

Trickett, E. J., & Espino, S.L.R. (2004). Collaboration and social inquiry: Multiple meanings of a construct and its role in creating useful and valid knowledge. *American Journal of Community Psychology, 34*(1–2), 1–69.

Wallerstein, N. (2006). Challenges for the field in overcoming disparities through a CBPR approach. *Ethnicity & Disease, 16,* S1146–S1148.

World Health Organization. (1946). *Constitution.* New York: Author.

CHAPTER

4

BRINGING EXPERIMENTAL DESIGN TO COMMUNITY-PARTNERED PARTICIPATORY RESEARCH

LORETTA JONES, PAUL KOEGEL, & KENNETH B. WELLS

Note: The authors thank the members of Building Wellness, the Community Partners in Care steering council members, and Keith Norris for their contributions to this work. Support for this work was provided by the UCLA/RAND NIMH Center for Research on Quality in Managed Care (P30 MH068639), Community Partners in Care (R01 MH078853), the UCLA in LA Initiative (Witness for Wellness Project, funded by UCLA Center for Community Partnerships), RAND Health, EXPORT (5P20MD000240), and the Centers for Disease Control and Prevention (99IPA06350).

COMMUNITY-PARTNERED participatory research (CPPR) is a form of community-based participatory research (CBPR) that builds the capacity of a partnership comprising community and academic stakeholders in order to address a signature issue of shared concern, such as a public health problem (Jones & Wells, 2007). CPPR emphasizes an equal partnership with true power sharing and collaboration in all phases of the work, including partner capacity building and research elements. Over the last twelve years a partnership consisting of community members; leaders of community-based organizations; and researchers from the Centers for Disease Control and Prevention (CDC), RAND, the University of California, Los Angeles (UCLA), Charles R. Drew Medical University, and the University of Southern California (USC) have been developing the capacity to plan and implement experimental designs as an evaluation strategy within CPPR projects. Our focus within that partnership has been on clinical depression, a topic that has drawn a high level of interest among grassroots community members, some of whom have personal concerns in relation to depression. Their perspectives, voiced as their leadership has emerged, have added a distinctly personal urgency to the identification of social justice concerns that underlies CPPR projects. Our participant mix has offered a remarkable opportunity to learn how to level the playing field when planning rigorous experimental designs with a CPPR partnership that includes personally vulnerable individuals as co-planners. This context has forced us to be clear about how to make design choices with an eye toward both achieving methodological rigor and fulfilling equitable partnership principles. Further, these contextual issues have made us more aware of the tension between taking the time needed to prepare for next steps and responding to real, unmet needs of vulnerable populations.

In this chapter we discuss our partnership's experience with planning randomized trials studies within a CPPR framework. We first define CPPR in more detail. We then discuss the value and importance of applying randomized designs in community-partnered participatory research. Next we describe how a planning phase for a pilot study led to the formulation of a four-phase framework for randomized CPPR trials. Finally, we describe how we are following that framework in the planning phase of a new National Institutes of Health–funded, randomized comparison trial that is being conducted within a CPPR framework.

USING CPPR AS A FRAMEWORK

The goals of community-partnered participatory research overlap with and derive from the classical features of CBPR (Israel, Eng, Schulz, & Parker, 2005; Leung, Yen, & Minkler, 2004; see also Chapters One through Three). These goals include community program development, collaborative research conducted by a partnership of academic and community participants, and capacity building for partnered planning and implementation of research-informed programs.

The CPPR approach stresses equal sharing of resources and decision-making authority in all project phases and activities across community and academic partners and perspectives. Additionally, it emphasizes the gains of collaboration in building capacity and achieving goals of both community and academic partners.

The method of CPPR features the following project structure and processes:

1. Development of a leadership council that gathers community and academic leaders to frame an issue and establish, support, and coordinate the efforts of the project

2. Formation of work groups in the relevant areas to develop, implement, and evaluate the impact of action plans, which are also reviewed at key points with a coordinating council and broad selection of community representatives

3. Integration of the work groups' action plans into a set of products created with input from all partnership, or coalition, stakeholders

4. Joint analyses of project data

5. Dissemination of products and findings by the coalition to local and, as appropriate, national academic, community, and policy stakeholders

These CPPR project processes and activities are conceptualized as occurring in three stages: *vision* (developing a mission and framework), *valley* (developing, implementing, and evaluating action plans), and *victory* (product development, dissemination, and celebration). Complex projects may have different subcomponents in different stages at the same time, which must then be integrated into a whole through the leadership council.

CPPR initiatives are implemented through a set of guiding principles that help the members establish and maintain mutual respect and trust and also equality of power sharing and productivity. These principles are formalized in a written agreement signed by the community and academic coalition stakeholders and by the individual members in leadership roles, and they are reinforced through trainings and documents (Jones & Wells, 2007).

This structure for project development and implementation adhering to documented principles gives CPPR a place within the broad range of CBPR and community-based research approaches. Some experts suggest that equal power sharing is rare even in such initiatives (Israel et al., 2005; Wallerstein, 1999; see also Chapters Five, Fourteen, and Twenty-One). For example, other approaches may involve getting technical assistance from researchers to help a community approach a problem or inviting community advisers into a funded project that academics have initiated. The CPPR model involves a high degree of joint leadership at every step, including the choice of study topic and approach, which must balance community and academic partners' priorities and expertise.

A key feature of CPPR initiatives is the emphasis on joint community and academic leadership and ownership. The coalition and work groups are headed by one or more community leaders and one or more academic leaders, who work together to guide all initiative phases. This structure requires equal respect for academic and community expertise and perspectives, and much of the work-group time in a CPPR initiative is spent sharing and understanding diverse perspectives within and across community and academic stakeholders. Through this sharing, academic members are encouraged to consider themselves part of the community, with a vested interest in the project and evaluation outcomes. Similarly, community members are encouraged to consider themselves part of the academic and evaluation team, with a vested interest in the scientific outcomes. This sharing means that a central goal of CPPR—to build capacity among partnership members—works in both directions. Community partners build the capacity to conduct rigorous research on problems of interest to the community and translate results into action. Academic partners often build their understanding of community life and the real-world context in which interventions have to be situated. Both community and academic partners develop critical leadership skills. Achieving these goals requires a consistent focus in all phases of work on relationship building, which can be fraught with conflict that must be guided through partnered leadership to resolution, for example, by promoting sharing, insight, and forgiveness.

THE FIT BETWEEN DESIGNS AND PROJECTS

This partnered leadership makes CPPR a particularly suitable framework for blending CBPR principles and methods with rigorous health services research approaches, including randomized, controlled designs. The negotiation of issues and approaches in a CPPR effort facilitates the partnership's consideration of rigorous designs, including randomized trials—provided that the community members are supported in a fair consideration of the pros and cons and the implications of the alternative designs, including what they offer the community as a product.

There are several reasons why we consider it important to explore the application of randomized designs:

1. To address community issues with strong evaluation data that support causal inference

2. To expand the scope of designs that the community and the partnership are comfortable using routinely within a CPPR framework—that is, to develop a legacy or history of community partnership in a full range of research designs

3. To find the best way of answering high-priority questions for the community

4. To develop an improved body of research on the impact of CPPR as an approach to building community-planning capacity in health

Yet community-based participatory research initiatives have seldom used experimental or other rigorous research designs (Buchanan, Miller, & Wallerstein, 2007). A recent review of CBPR studies in health identified only sixty studies, about one-third of which were intervention studies; only a few of these used rigorous designs such as experiments (Viswanathan et al., 2004). Some recent examples of experimental pilot studies and main studies that use a CBPR framework for intervention development as well as study design development, implementation, and analyses are the PRAISE! Project, which focused on improving dietary practices through African American churches; a pilot study of using a workbook-journal to improve psychosocial outcomes for women with breast cancer; a comparison of a faith-based weight loss program to a traditional weight-loss program; and a comparison of different complementary medicine interventions to improve end-of-life care for persons infected with HIV (Ammerman et al., 2003; Angell et al., 2003; Corbie-Smith et al., 2003; Fitzgibbon et al., 2005; Williams et al., 2005). Several of these projects were conducted within a CBPR framework and generated interventions either making use of community input or based largely on community ideas. Some studies compared study challenges and strategies and modifications made with community input to the key principles of CBPR defined in Israel et al. (2005; see also Chapter Three). Most studies were not designed specifically to evaluate the added value of using a CBPR framework for intervention versus using a more standard top-down or expert-driven intervention to improve health outcomes. Such an evaluation is a goal of the NIH-funded trial discussed later in this chapter.

There are many plausible reasons for the paucity of CBPR studies using experimental designs. Even in the absence of experimental designs, research that engages the community is time consuming, so use of rigorous designs may reduce research feasibility. Evaluations of CBPR initiatives often rely heavily on qualitative and mixed-method approaches that are not typical primary methods for a randomized trial. Further, in many underserved, predominantly minority communities, there is distrust of research in general and especially of experiments. As a result of historical abuses such as the infamous Tuskegee study of untreated syphilis in black men, which continued for decades after an effective treatment became available (Thomas & Quinn, 2001), the term *experiment* has acquired highly negative connotations, suggesting people being treated like "guinea pigs" or devalued and considered something less than human. The applied randomized designs typical of the larger health services research studies, such as the group-level randomized design, are complex to design, implement, and analyze. Within a CPPR framework, virtually all of the decisions necessary to design such a trial would need to be made with input from all interested partners, enabled by adequate training to appreciate both the options and the implications for the community. In the absence of this investment in capacity building, the community may not judge the resulting findings to be fair or valid. Randomized trials can require elaborate participant consent forms, which may similarly require resources to enable fair participation at the individual level. As we learned from experience in the Witness for Wellness project, these are significant challenges that are likely to require painstaking, resource-intensive negotiation and collaboration among the partners (Chapter Five and Appendixes A, C, and H).

EXPERIMENTAL DESIGN LESSONS FROM THE BUILDING WELLNESS PILOT

The Witness for Wellness project developed from initial efforts to apply the CPPR framework to reducing the impact of clinical depression on underserved communities of color (Bluthenthal et al., 2006). The goals, principles, and work-group structure of Witness for Wellness are illustrated in Figure 4.1.

The central partnership structure is represented by the bus, which invites people to enter or leave the project as they need to, to accommodate their changing life needs and priorities. The work of the initiative is represented by the road, and the goal (wellness, or freedom from depression) is the distant but visible destination. The route is marked by three signposts representing work groups: Talking Wellness, a group that addresses the

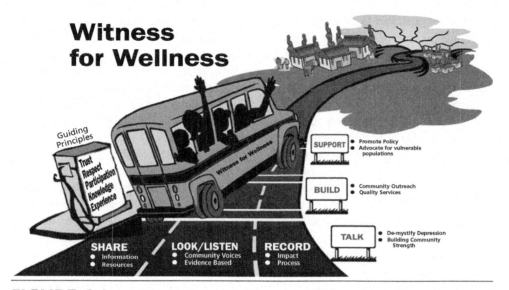

FIGURE 4.1   *Witness for Wellness Logo*

Source: Witness for Wellness project (Bluthenthal et al., 2006). Used with permission of the Witness for Wellness Executive Committee.

stigma of mental illness and recognizes and builds on community strengths (Chung et al., 2006), Building Wellness, a group that seeks to improve outreach and services quality (Jones et al., 2006), and Supporting Wellness, a group that develops or supports policy that enables improved services and advocacy that protects vulnerable populations (Stockdale et al., 2006). Each work group was asked to identify priority action items and to implement and evaluate the impact of its plans. The top priority of the Building Wellness (BW) group was developing a practical tool to support screening, education, and referral for depression through case workers serving minority communities. This practical action plan received broad community support (Jones et al., 2006).

In reviewing options for an evaluation design, the BW work group selected a randomized, controlled trial because community members wanted evidence that would convince local service providers to adopt the program if successful. The academic investigators thought that a pilot randomized trial could lead to a successful NIH grant that would represent a next step for the partnership. The pilot received limited funding from a UCLA in LA community partnership grant and collateral support from a National Institute of Mental Health (NIMH) UCLA/RAND center, programs at Charles R. Drew Medical University, and RAND Health. What resulted, given the effort to develop the trial with equal participation in all components and limited resources for such an ambitious effort, was a more than two-year planning and capacity-building process that has so far yielded an intervention toolkit and evaluation measures but not yet produced the completed evaluation. Yet this planning process stimulated new community services partnerships and resulted in a funded NIMH grant that builds on the idea for the pilot and on the toolkit and lessons learned from developing the pilot. The recognition that the planning process itself had both policy and scientific outcomes that are equivalent to those expected from a full, completed CPPR project stimulated the central thesis of this chapter, that a randomized trial can be seen as having four project phases, each of which is its own full CPPR study. Below we first summarize the overall Building Wellness pilot planning experience through three lessons learned, and then we present the four-phase model for rigorous CPPR evaluation that resulted from these lessons.

Lesson 1: Establish a Framework and Expectations

A clear and comprehensive framework and set of expectations to guide the work of developing a randomized trial using a CPPR perspective is needed at the outset. Because our partnership had little experience in designing this type of project, Building Wellness lacked such a framework and had unrealistic expectations about the time frame for trust development and the technical capacity building necessary to achieve a completed randomized trial with equal participation in all phases. Metaphorically speaking, we were constructing the boat as we were setting sail. Consequently, the leadership was not fully prepared at the outset to set work-group expectations or to suggest strategies to achieve efficiencies to remain on schedule, especially given limited resources and high expectations. Given experience and a framework, we believe we could have helped academic and community partners avoid some of the frustrations of prolonged planning and achieve more regular, short-term victories along the course of planning. Alternately, the intervention development and design and the planning and capacity building could have profitably been viewed as sufficient cause for celebration.

An example is helpful in illustrating how the lack of a framework sometimes became a problem. In the first phase of pilot development, the BW work group developed three action plans, including identifying a depression screening measure, developing a toolkit for education, and developing referral sources for mental health care. The depression screening committee reviewed existing, brief, self-report screeners and identified four for group evaluation of cultural appropriateness/readability, effectiveness as a screening tool, and cost/feasibility, using a modified Delphi consensus process to integrate community input into ratings (Patel, Koegel, Booker, Jones, & Wells, 2006; see also Chapter Nine). Although all the selected screeners were deemed acceptable, one was preferred by the work group because its language was simpler. Subsequently, the academic co-leaders discovered that there were costs associated with using the preferred screener because it was proprietary. This problem was referred to the Witness for Wellness Council leadership for a policy decision, and the council decided that the project could not afford to pay for a screener.

This decision disappointed community members who had worked hard to understand the features of the screeners and provide their input. The resulting tensions in the group led to clearer expectations that all scientific and financial issues relevant to selecting a study measure would be fully identified in advance. There were some differences of opinion as to whether this was a responsibility of academic members or whether this step should also be conducted in partnership even if that meant further delays to develop the partnered technical capacity for that step. Most important, the discussion and disagreements led to a greater appreciation by all participants of the complexity of the scientific and practical issues, more transparent expectations, and greater insight into the importance of deliberation to reach good joint decisions. Although such difficult interactions may be unavoidable and even desirable in developing an effective community-academic research collaboration, a more comprehensive framework might have helped participants to anticipate the need for time and leadership support to resolve issues in the planning phase. The project did take the time to resolve the issues with extensive, partnered leadership support—a "victory" from a CPPR perspective—but the project fell further behind schedule. This is only one example of bumps in the road that our bus hit. Indeed, we were somewhat naive about how many times this cycle would be needed to plan a randomized, controlled pilot study.

Another example of such a challenge occurred at a later stage, when Building Wellness members began to design a Web site to disseminate the complete intervention toolkit during the pilot. Many community members were interested in learning something about Web site design and enjoyed this application of their creative skills. Over a period of about six months, work-group members studied Web sites, reviewed with technical experts how Web sites were set up and how functions were programmed, and had brainstorming sessions on Web site design. They also collaborated with experienced Web-design artists in considering video clips of images (such as a helping hand reaching out) and page layouts, and they drafted introductory language for the various Web pages for the functions and components of the toolkits. During this phase there was relatively little academic input because the community members wanted more independence after the intensity of selecting the screener and considering design options, activities that relied heavily on academic expertise.

This phase of Web design led to many creative ideas and images and a sense of community accomplishment for those involved. However, it did not result in a completed Web site because of changes in availability of academic technical staff, perhaps too great an effort on the part of the designer to accommodate community input on technical matters, and a need to incorporate the clinical content of the intervention into the Web-site design. Therefore a separate, second-phase Web design was required, with some new and some continuing community leaders and stronger partnered academic input to ensure a balance of community voice and necessary technical and clinical expertise. In other words, because of the extended time it took to learn how to collaboratively develop a Web-based intervention tool and to allow community and academic members to express their expertise and preferences, some members got off and others got on the bus. This shift in people and direction resulted in delays that were sometimes discouraging to participants and consumed extra resources. However, we had learned our lesson from the screener discussions, so we capped this phase of work by supporting work-group members from both the first and second phases of development in making presentations to the full committee, to the Witness for Wellness Council, and to participants at a project retreat, as well as to two sets of community providers, all of whom were enthusiastic about the tool. This constituted a project *victory lap,* and led to the next lesson.

Lesson 2: Time and Resources Are Investments

The time and resources required to negotiate the experimental design among the partners should be viewed as investments in the partnership. In a CPPR project a major part of building capacity is building trust in the partnership to solve complex problems. This takes time for relationship building and for negotiating a division of labor, and it takes sensitivity to community and academic participants' priorities for their work tasks. In an experimental study these negotiations can take even more time than they might ordinarily because the decisions are complex, the stakes for community and academic participants may be high, and sensitivities to the implications of decisions may also be intense. However, negotiation and shared decision making on every issue of experimental design helps partners to build a foundation of trust as well as the technical competence that enables partnerships to move ahead. Our subsequent experience showed us that initial investments of time and resources can expedite planning the next experimental design within the partnership. We caution, however, that not all delays or complexities may be due to community members' adjusting to the technical demands of rigorous research. The greatest source of delay in the BW project was—and remains—the need to adjust study implementation to community realities, particularly taking into account the ethical implications of intervention design decisions, as discussed in the next section.

Even apart from these particular problems, disagreements, and negotiations, however, many aspects of the joint development of the Building Wellness pilot, enjoyable though they were, made heavy use of resources and time. For example, the measures and survey operations work group required considerable time to develop pre- and postsurveys with community input for three levels of stakeholders (administrators, providers, and clients). With assistance from community reviewers and their own extensive experience with prior studies, the academic co-leads for the Building Wellness work group drafted measures for outcomes, services use, and knowledge of depression and treatment. Community members reviewed the measures and gave extensive input, ranging from rewording measures or adding items to suggesting shifts in emphasis for the survey as a whole, such as including a focus on homelessness as a comorbidity and an outcome. Work-group members practiced administering the client survey to each other, producing extensive notes on the experience and timing each administration—information that led the academic team to make some changes in the instrument. Community members and experienced survey researchers jointly considered the feasibility of training grassroots community members to conduct the outcome surveys for the project. As a result of those discussions, job descriptions were drafted, collaboratively, and posted. An academic staff member was recruited to develop Web- or laptop-based versions of the surveys and to carry out translation and back-translation for Spanish versions. A desire for further training on such matters helped stimulate the formation of a methods "book club" for academic and community partnership members, who initially read methods sections from CBPR textbooks (Israel et al., 2005; Minkler & Wallerstein, 2003).

As a result of these activities the planning phase for our group's first experimental trial conducted under a CPPR framework took over two years but resulted in a greatly expanded partnership capacity for research overall. One community member, for example, became a research specialist in a community-based organization, and community and academic partners gave presentations on interim steps at national conferences. Some stages were exasperating for all; others were viewed as going by too quickly or possibly allowing insufficient time for full input or understanding. In the end the trump card was the decision to delay implementation until an agency agreement was in place to ensure that those who screened positive for depression would receive a clinical assessment. In the face of this delay, viewed as inevitable once encountered, the investment in partnership development was viewed as both worthwhile and as holding its own community and scientific value, even though that value was not one overtly intended for this project. This realization led to the next lesson.

Lesson 3: A Planning Phase Can Be a Productive Project

The planning phase for a randomized design under a CPPR perspective should be considered its own first-phase CPPR project, one that creates valuable products and outcomes in its own right. This planning can be viewed as a civic learning enterprise, and its own desirable outcomes can include building the partnership's capacity for research and for completing community and academic products. During the planning, as reviewed earlier, community members and academic leaders come on and get off the bus, participating in the learning experience for community benefit, whether or not they participate in the actual trial implementation. Outcomes can include improved understanding of academic and community priorities and strengths, shared knowledge gain, increased capacity for rigorous research, development of products such as interventions or measures, and even expanded service capacities. The realization that the planning phase can have its own intended and unintended, or "surprise," outcomes helps all involved to see some balance between the time and resource demands of this phase of the work and the potential gains for all stakeholders. As they develop the vision, valley, and victory for the planning phase, leaders of projects can help academic and community members to anticipate this balance and to realize positive outcomes.

An example from the Building Wellness pilot illustrates how we came to learn this lesson. The evaluation work group reviewed options for a design, including the pros and cons of using a randomized, controlled trial with various potential control groups versus using an observational study of experiences under the intervention without a control group. Community meetings and discussions indicated high enthusiasm for a design that would ensure future use of the intervention if it were found to be successful. The next decision concerned the control group. The intervention would involve use of the toolkit by a community case worker plus a voucher for referral for clinical assessment. The question was whether the control condition should consist just of the usual caseworker services or if it should offer the usual caseworker services plus a voucher for referral. At first community members preferred the comparison of the intervention to usual care, because they thought it was more likely that the toolkit would emerge as superior. However, when it was pointed out by academics that this would lead to uncertainty about whether the toolkit or the voucher improved access, the community members, to achieve a purer test of the toolkit, preferred the version of the control condition that included the voucher. At the same time, however, there was widespread concern among community and academic members about low service availability for the target population in South Los Angeles and known difficulties in accessing services in a timely manner even with a referral. Academics were concerned that this could pose ethical problems while community participants emphasized that these problems existed in reality and that data were needed to support advocacy for expanding services. At some point in this discussion, academic and community members realized that they were in a kind of role reversal in terms of typical expectations of academic and community perspectives.

The group then presented the draft design and toolkit to administrators and providers from South Los Angeles service agencies identified by the referral work group as willing to have their names listed on the BW pilot Web site. Agency leaders thought it was unacceptable to screen for need without ensuring access to at least a clinical assessment, and because the screening would be done by the research team for intervention and control, ensuring access would require a voucher for a clinical assessment and willing agencies to provide the assessments of the participants screening positive for depression. This requirement for ensured access fit with the preferred scientific design (using a voucher for both conditions) identified in the prior community-academic dialogue. The lead mental health agency for the target area agreed to provide free assessments to a limited number of clients but requested a partner agency to share the load. After much exploration we found one community free clinic that would accept such a charge if the local mental health agency would support assessment and provision of treatment at its local site, as an off-site extension of the mental health services. A series of meetings and telephone calls over several months led to a memorandum of understanding to support this relationship. However, the agencies also expressed concern that the arrangement would not be sustainable without a policy change and suggested waiting for such an opportunity. After several additional months, an opportunity was identified to meet new agency goals of expanding mental health services for Medicare patients under the conditions of the memorandum, offering a sustainable partnership after the pilot. Although achieving those policy conditions required an additional nine-month delay of the pilot, the memorandum of understanding and ensuing sustainable partnership were significant outcomes of the planning for the Building Wellness pilot in their own right, impressing work-group members and representing an important services delivery outcome of the planning.

Thus community planning for a rigorous pilot became a community action initiative for new services delivery capacity locally. As a result, the delays in implementing the pilot were of less material consequence for the community than we might have expected from the delay in implementation, because planning alone achieved key community goals of the pilot.

Moreover, the outcomes of the planning phase also included important scientific accomplishments over and above the capacity building of the partnership for research. The extensive planning process, which we documented and shared in presentations and publications (Jones & Wells, 2007), provided the necessary preliminary experience in community engagement and represented the equivalent of an intervention development grant. This supported an R01 proposal to NIMH to compare community engagement and technical assistance as implementation approaches for evidence-based, depression care toolkits, including using traditional clinicians and social service agencies as providers. Lessons from the Building Wellness pilot planning phase were incorporated into the proposal. The R01 was funded at about the same time as policy changes, promoted through the partnership's earlier efforts, enabled an expanded services partnership capacity. Thus the planning phase led to achieving community and scientific goals as well as development of the partnership's research capacity. After much discussion and negotiation within our partnership, we are now planning to scale down the Building Wellness pilot to a feasibility pilot of the toolkit, to inform this new R01. The fact that this particular pilot planning process was prolonged allowed us to develop the insight that such planning is in fact its own CPPR initiative with opportunities for community, scientific, and partnership outcomes.

Building on this insight, we suggest that a randomized trial conducted within a CPPR framework has four phases, each representing a distinct CPPR initiative with its own vision (mission), valley (work groups and action plans), and victory (products and celebration). These four phases are planning, trial implementation, evaluation (analysis), and dissemination.

In light of this framework, a randomized trial can be viewed as a civic learning enterprise, with community and academic members and leaders coming on and getting off the bus but also participating in the learning experience for community benefit during each of the four phases from planning through dissemination. From this perspective, products and capacity building can result from each phase—just as new community services solutions were implemented during the planning phase of the Building Wellness pilot. Further, this framework makes it likely that any interested persons or agencies in the community can find a place somewhere in the phases that suits them. Conversely, when these phases are not recognized as CPPR projects in their own right, then their outcomes will not be captured as either community victories or accomplishments of a type of partnered research, and this can lead to frustrated expectations, possibly negative views of rigorous research, and perceptions that community-based research cannot be rigorous.

We anticipate that each subsequent phase will be at least as complex as the planning phase. For example, during trial implementation, we will need to engage the broader community in a sense of ownership of the work and trust in the safe conduct of the trial. Similarly, we will need to collaboratively implement the interventions and collect outcomes data with respect for and adherence to community and scientific standards and norms. In the classic tradition of science, the trial is the primary scientific work and the findings the products of interest. From the perspective of CPPR, there are many other potential products, such as how the community uses the findings and intervention resources later on, whether new service capacities are developed or the burden of illness is reduced in the community, or whether capacities are developed among community and academic stakeholders. To this end, the third phase (collaborative analysis) may lead particularly to development of the partners' capacities for research and data presentations, whereas the fourth phase (dissemination) may lead to translation into policy implications or changes in community structures, such as sustainable services partnerships.

Viewing randomized trials conducted under a CPPR perspective as a multiphase process, where each phase has its own goals and outcomes, has implications for the way such trials are designed and funded and the way researchers and community members are engaged and trained to conduct them. Further, this perspective has implications for the relevant products of such trials and for anticipating the level of support required to implement and complete trials.

Each phase requires support in applying the CPPR principles. For example, the overall project leadership council needs to guide the initiative within and across phases. The work groups need to be appropriately defined and constructed to accomplish each phase. Civic and academic leaders need to be recruited and aligned with work-group tasks to ensure successful implementation and uses of the initiative at each phase. Further, the CPPR perspective can define the relevant community capacity outcomes. As randomized trials will likely be used to test an intervention, specialized work groups (such as those used for the Building Wellness pilot) may be needed to develop and later implement the intervention during the trial. Intervention development may require special skills (such as clinical supervision) and then a different team may be required to successfully develop that one phase. Distinct teams with distinct responsibilities may also be desirable scientifically, to reduce any bias that might accumulate if one team both developed or implemented an intervention and then also collected evaluation data on its outcomes. We are now applying the specific lessons learned from the BW pilot and following the four-phase model for a randomized pilot under CPPR in the Community Partners in Care (CPIC) study, which itself resulted from the BW pilot. Early experience with the planning phase of that trial is described in the following section.

APPLYING THE LESSONS: CPIC

Community Partners in Care (CPIC) is a new, randomized, controlled trial of CPPR as an implementation intervention for evidence-based depression care in communities of color in Los Angeles. Currently in the planning phase, the entire study, in addition to being a trial of CPPR, is being conceptualized and implemented using a CPPR framework. To our knowledge, this is one of the first randomized, controlled outcome trials of the effectiveness of a CBPR-based dissemination approach compared to the effectiveness of an alternative, expert-driven dissemination approach (see also Buchanan et al., 2007).

The trial draws on the lessons from Building Wellness—in particular that as in civil rights, it takes everybody to plan a change. In this case having community agencies and members working jointly with academic partners is necessary to develop a sustainable plan for implementing evidence-based, quality improvement programs for care for depression in the community.

The subject of the implementation interventions (community engagement versus technical assistance) is two evidence-based depression quality improvement programs, Partners in Care and We Care. When implemented in primary care and other community settings, these programs have been shown to achieve substantial gains in health and employment outcomes over periods ranging from one to nine years for minorities, and to reduce health outcome disparities relative to whites (Miranda, Azocar, Organista, Dwyer, & Areane, 2003; Miranda, Chung, Green, et al., 2003; Miranda, Duan, Sherbourne, et al., 2003; Wells, Sherbourne, Miranda, et al., 2007; Wells, Sherbourne, Schoenbaum, et al., 2004, Sherbourne, Edelen, Zhou, et al., 2008).

The study is being jointly conducted by lead community partners (Healthy African American Families, QueensCare Faith and Health Partnerships, the Los Angeles Urban League, COPE Health Solutions, and the Los Angeles County Department of Mental Health Services) and by academic partner institutions (RAND Health, UCLA Semel Institute Health Services Research Center, Charles R. Drew Medical University, and University of Southern California Mental Health Disparities Research Center).

The conceptual framework for the study is displayed in Figure 4.2. Approaches generated by community organizations and their planning and academic resources are integrated through a CPPR-based planning process and set of principles to arrive at intervention solutions that are evaluated through comparisons to the alternative, expert-based approach. Unlike prior studies that focus on a given system of care such as primary care or employer-based services, this study considers the range of relevant institutions in a community providing services to depressed clients, which may include social service agencies; primary care, mental health, and substance abuse agencies; and other community organizations such as faith-based organizations—encompassing the potential sources of support identified by community participants in the Witness for Wellness project (Bluthenthal et al., 2006). This affords a challenge to intervention design and implementation as it stretches the available toolkits for supporting implementation of a quality improvement intervention.

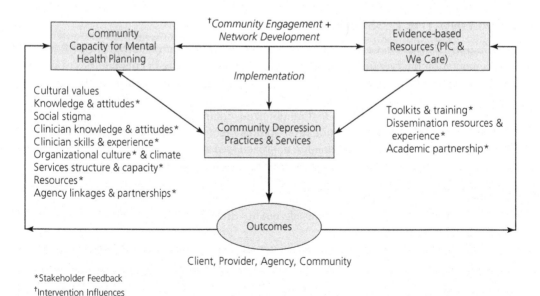

FIGURE 4.2   *Conceptual Framework for Community Partners in Care*
Source: Bluthenthal et al., 2006.

Community Partners in Care will be implemented in three underserved communities in Los Angeles—South Los Angeles, Hollywood, and East Los Angeles. The partnership will recruit a set of diverse community agency partners and then randomly assign individual sites drawn from these organizations, stratified by neighborhood and agency type, to either (1) a community engagement and network development intervention that uses CPPR methods to develop a *community plan* for the training, implementation, and oversight of the PIC/We Care interventions; or (2) a comparison group that receives a brief, expert consultation through a training conference and has access to the materials through a Web site. After collaborative analyses of impact, the community organizations will receive either training or reinforcement of training in using the "winning" model, the one that leads to greater outcome improvement and more sustainable adoption of the toolkits by administrators and providers. This *wait-list* training will also constitute the first step of the dissemination phase.

We also added an initial, or prestudy, phase for proposal development for the Community Partners in Care study, a phase that was fully developed using a CPPR framework. We developed the proposal in response to a new NIMH announcement seeking research on dissemination and implementation of evidence-based interventions. We submitted an initial proposal, which received a good but not fundable score, and we were funded on the resubmission. In submitting the proposal, it became clear that the three-year history of partnership work in Building Wellness (and a similar partnership with QueensCare around implementing nurse-led depression interventions in nonclinical settings in Hollywood) enabled us to move forward expeditiously. We were able to agree quickly on a division of labor because we had spent three years understanding the skills and capabilities of each participant organization and its place within the broader study vision. An overall division of funds was discussed, with a desirable goal of one-third to data (for all partners), one-third to community, and one-third to academic partners—but no hard-and-fast rule was established and the partners had sufficient trust to agree to let the budget follow the work. The final budget was very close to this proposed split.

The main proposal challenge was how to design a study that would be assessed on its technical rigor but would represent the community perspective as fully as possible. For example, considering our BW pilot experience, we identified one key area—site recruitment and survey training—where we had not previously had much experience in partnered development and implementation. We prioritized this area for extensive partnership development, training, and relationship development across community and academic partners. Further, we relied heavily on academic staff with extensive experience in working with the community members in the BW pilot for matters such as developing budgets and coordinating resumes, because of the trust they had developed. When the BW community members reacted to a first draft with concerns that the community perspective was underrepresented, there was sufficient trust for all to believe that this would be rectified in revision. The final rewrite emphasized the strength of partners and the selected communities and included examples of collaborative work and insights such as references to stories included in this chapter. Underpinning a successful partnership is the assumption that participants will work in good faith to resolve problems and will honor processes for negotiating a resolution (Israel et al., 2005; see also Chapter Twenty-One and Appendix C). Our partnership members had sufficient trust to develop the proposal together, through a combination of delegation, prioritization for joint development, and cross-review. In addition, all were glad to use what they had learned in the BW pilot to take a next step.

THE ROAD AHEAD FOR CPIC

At the time of this writing, we are about four months into the planning phase of CPIC, with site recruitment to begin in four to six weeks. Relative to the beginning of the Building Wellness pilot, all phases of CPIC planning have had more extensive community leadership. The lead statistician is routinely identifying early opportunities for community members to have final say on design decisions (such as how communities are defined in each geographical region). We have a more successful set of delegation procedures to systematically identify and then integrate both community and scientific perspectives on intervention design, anticipating the need for iterative negotiation and revision. We have set up monthly targets not only for products and decisions, as is typical of randomized design planning, but for broad community input. For example, our first input session in the intervention sites involved one hundred community members, thirty of whom were monolingual Spanish speakers. A second session is planned to gain community policy support, and a third will focus on integrating the community engagement intervention. We are identifying each community event as a project victory that is building the community's awareness of depression and the community and academic partners' capacities to address it, while also solving project design issues. We are counting on our Building Wellness pilot experience in collaborative instrument development to guide a nearly nine-month process of developing the client surveys, expanded to allow the iterations that indicate we are serious about community input. These strategies are permitting the community engagement to be more consistent across phases so the partnership can conduct the planning and point toward implementation with greater assurance. Of course the greater resources of an R01 help enormously in this regard, although we still had not specifically requested funds for all of these development activities in the proposal and are receiving in-kind contributions from community and academic institutional partners. This latter fact underscores once again the importance of an active institutional and policy advisory board for such a project.

This partnered planning process will also generate the necessary ambassadors who will give communities voice and leadership to help ensure the trial's implementation and future impact from the findings. We have observed that the planning phase alone can result in bringing rigorous science deeply into underserved communities of color. The challenge is to construct this bridge without becoming locked into concerns about historical research abuses and institutional racism, and to overcome such expectations through ensuring community co-leadership, taking the time to achieve transparency in decisions, and bringing the benefits of evidence-based programs into communities with high levels of unmet need. To accomplish this balance, such efforts must attend carefully to core principles of ethical clinical research as applied to community trials (Chen, Jones, &

Gelberg, 2006). That is, trials must achieve a good balance of social and scientific value; attend to scientific validity through rigorous methods; develop fair subject selection strategies; ensure a favorable risk-benefit ratio; foster independent review; ensure meaningful and complete informed consent; and communicate and instill mutual respect for potential and enrolled participants in the trial to the many community and research partners involved in all four phases. We think there is much potential for realizing these principles for randomized trials conducted within a CPPR framework, because of the greater potential for scientific validity coupled with community input, each supported by respectful deliberation.

This form of science translation within a community-academic partnership context embodies a central goal of the Clinical and Translational Science Awards (CTSAs) of the National Institutes of Health reflecting the new direction of program announcements for grants promoting use of community-based participatory research in medically underserved groups (U.S. Department of Health and Human Services, 2008; see also Chapters One and Twenty-One and Appendix B).

SUMMARY

Our planning efforts for Community Partners in Care are currently addressing a series of questions that go beyond the lessons of Building Wellness: How can we best implement the CPPR perspective within each phase of the study from planning through dissemination? What is the appropriate expectation for the vision, valley, and victory for each phase? For example:

- How can we frame the operations of CPPR within the community engagement and network development intervention condition to enable an effective trial?
- How can we best blend CPPR principles with more traditional, theory-based network development or quality improvement approaches?
- How can we ensure support for community members to participate in design, data collection, and analyses?
- How will we obtain the community and policy support to achieve successful recruitment and, later, impact of findings and to solve critical implementation problems along the way?

In addressing these questions we are formulating plans to monitor the process of conducting the trial and adhering to CPPR principles in all four phases, for both community and academic participants. For example, we are conducting an implementation evaluation to examine adherence to CPPR principles in intervention implementation. In this way, we hope to provide information on how CPPR can inform the design of randomized trials while we also examine how these same principles can affect implementation of evidence-based interventions to improve depression care. Over time, it is our intent to provide fuller information and technical assistance on how a CPPR perspective can inform each phase of a randomized trial and can also support uses of the trial findings and products in building capacity to achieve and maintain healthy communities.

QUESTIONS FOR DISCUSSION

1. The authors write that the primary challenge in writing their NIH grant proposal was "how to design a study that would be assessed on its technical rigor but would represent the community perspective as fully as possible." What strategies and activities used in this study appeared to address this concern?

2. The logo in Figure 4.1 captures the notion discussed in this chapter of a fluid approach to participation, one in which community and academic partners get "on and off the bus" as needed yet still provide real input and derive real benefit from their involvement. What might be some of the advantages and some of the challenges of this "bus" approach?

3. This chapter focuses on the development phase of a health services research, randomized controlled trial (RCT) using CPPR principles. What additional challenges might emerge during the implementation phase? Discuss examples of some interventions in health services research or beyond (for example, in the areas of policy change or community development) that would be either easier or more difficult to conduct as randomized, controlled trials.

KEY TERMS

Community-partnered participatory research

Planning for randomized trials

Stages of community-based research

Capacity building

REFERENCES

Ammerman, A., Corbie-Smith, G., St. George, D.M.M., Washington, C., Weathers, B., & Jackson-Christian, B. (2003). Research expectations among African American church leaders in the PRAISE! Project: A randomized trial guided by community-based participatory research. *American Journal of Public Health, 93,* 1720–1727.

Angell, K. L., Kreshka, M. A., McCoy, R., Donnelly, P., Turner-Cobb, J. M., Graddy, K., et al. (2003). Psychosocial intervention for rural women with breast cancer. *Journal of General Internal Medicine, 18*(7), 499–507.

Bluthenthal, R., Jones, L., Fackler-Lowrie, N., Ellison, M., Booker, T., Jones, F., et al. (2006). Witness for wellness: Preliminary findings from a community-academic participatory research mental health initiative. *Ethnicity & Disease, 16*(1, Suppl. 1), S18–S34.

Buchanan, D. R., Miller, F. G., & Wallerstein, N. (2007). Ethical issues in community-based participatory research: Balancing rigorous research with community participation in community intervention studies. *Progress in Community Health Partnerships: Research, Education, and Action, 1*(2), 153–160.

Chen, D. T., Jones, L., & Gelberg, L. (2006). Ethics of clinical research within a community-academic partnered participatory framework. *Ethnicity & Disease, 16*(1, Suppl. 1), S118–S135.

Chung, B., Corbett, C. E., Boulet, B., Cummings, J. R., Paxton, K., McDaniel, S., et al. (2006). Talking wellness: A description of a community-academic partnered project to engage an African American community around depression through the use of poetry, film, and photography. *Ethnicity & Disease, 16*(1, Suppl. 1), S67–S78.

Corbie-Smith, G., Ammerman, A. S., Katz, M. L., St. George, D.M.M., Blumenthal, C., Washington, C., et al. (2003). Trust, benefit, satisfaction, and burden: A randomized controlled trial to reduce cancer risk through African-American churches. *Journal of General Internal Medicine, 18*(7), 531–541.

Eng, E. (2004, November). *What defines community-based participatory research: A review and synthesis.* Paper presented at the 132nd annual meeting of the American Public Health Association, Washington, DC.

Fitzgibbon, M. L., Stolley, M. R., Ganschow, P., Schiffer, L., Wells, A., Simon, N., et al. (2005). Results of a faith-based weight loss intervention for black women. *Journal of the National Medical Association, 97*(10), 1393–1402.

Israel, B. A., Eng, E., Schulz, A. J., & Parker, E. A. (Eds.). (2005). *Methods in community-partnered participatory research for health.* San Francisco: Jossey-Bass.

Jones, A., Charla, F., Butler, B. T., Williams, P., Wells, K. B., & Rodriguez, M. (2006). The Building Wellness project: A case history of partnership, power sharing, and compromise. *Ethnicity & Disease, 16*(1, Suppl. 1), S54–S66.

Jones, L., & Wells, K. (2007). Strategies for academic and clinician engagement in community-participatory partnered research. *Journal of the American Medical Association, 297,* 407–410.

Leung, M., Yen, I., & Minkler, M. (2004). Community-based participatory research: A promising approach for increasing epidemiology's relevance in the 21st century. *International Journal of Epidemiology, 33*(3), 499–506.

Minkler, M., & Wallerstein, N. (Eds.). (2003). *Community-based participatory research for health.* San Francisco: Jossey-Bass.

Miranda, J., Azocar, F., Organista, K. C., Dwyer, E., & Areane, P. (2003). Treatment of depression among impoverished primary care patients from ethnic minority groups. *Psychiatric Services, 54*(2), 219–225.

Miranda, J., Chung, J. Y., Green, B. L., Krupnick, J., Siddique, J., Revicki, D. A., et al. (2003). Treating depression in predominantly low-income young minority women: A randomized controlled trial. *Journal of the American Medical Association, 290*(1), 57–65.

Miranda, J., Duan, N., Sherbourne, C., Schoenbaum, M., Lagomasino, I., Jackson-Triche, M., et al. (2003). Improving care for minorities: Can quality improvement interventions improve care and outcomes for depressed minorities? Results of a controlled randomized trial. *Health Services Research, 38*(2), 613–630.

Patel, K. K., Koegel, P., Booker, T., Jones, L., & Wells, K. B. (2006). Innovative approaches to obtaining community feedback in the Witness for Wellness experience. *Ethnicity & Disease, 16*(1, Suppl. 1), S35–S42.

Sherbourne, C. D., Edelen, M. O., Zhou, A., Bird, C., Duan, N., & Wells, K. B. (2008). How a therapy-based quality improvement intervention for depression affected life events and psychological well-being over time: A 9-year longitudinal analysis. *Medical Care, 46*(1), 78–84.

Stockdale, S., Patel, K., Gray, R., Hill, D. A., Franklin, C., & Madyun, N. (2006). Supporting wellness through policy and advocacy: A case history of a working group in a community partnership initiative to address depression. *Ethnicity & Disease, 16*(1, Suppl. 1), S43–S53.

Thomas, S. B., & Quinn, S. C. (2001). Light on the shadow of the syphilis study at Tuskegee. *Health Promotion Practice, 1,* 234–237.

U.S. Department of Health and Human Services. (2008). *Request for applications.* Retrieved April 15, 2008, from http://grants.nih.gov/grants/guide/rfa-files/RFA-RM-07–007.

Viswanathan, M., Ammerman, A., Eng, E., Gartlehner, G., Lohr, K. N., Griffth, D., et al. (2004). *Community-based participatory research: Assessing the evidence* (Evidence Report/Technology Assessment No. 99; Prepared by RTI International, University of North Carolina). Rockville, MD: Agency for Healthcare Research and Quality.

Wallerstein, N. (1999). Power between evaluator and community: Research relationships within New Mexico's healthier communities. *Social Science & Medicine, 49,* 39–53.

Wells, K., Sherbourne, C., Duan, N., Unutzer, J., Miranda, J., Schoenbaum, M., et al. (2005). Quality improvement for depression in primary care: Do patients with subthreshold depression benefit in the long run? *American Journal of Psychiatry, 162*(6), 1149–1157.

Wells, K. B., Sherbourne, C. D., Miranda, J., Tang, L., Benjamin, B., & Duan, N. (2007). The cumulative effects of quality improvement for depression on outcome disparities over 9 years: Results from a randomized, controlled group-level trial. *Medical Care, 45*(11), 1052–1059.

Wells, K., Sherbourne, C., Schoenbaum, M., et al. (2004). Five-year impact of quality improvement for depression: Results of a group-level randomized controlled trial. *Archives of General Psychiatry, 61*(4), 378–386.

Williams, A., Selwyn, P. A., McCorkle, R., Molde, S., Liberti, L., & Katz, D. L. (2005). Application of community-based participatory research methods to a study of complementary medicine interventions at end of life. *Complementary Health Practice Review, 10*(2), 91–104.

PART

2

POWER, TRUST, AND DIALOGUE

WORKING WITH DIVERSE COMMUNITIES IN CBPR

As Angela Cornwall and Rachel Jewkes (1995) suggest, participatory research is funda-
mentally about "the who question"—who defines the problem? And who generates,
analyzes, represents, owns, and acts as a result of the information? The central issues in

how we answer these questions are ultimately issues of power and control. In Part Two, this volume continue to surface these issues, with a related set of questions that serve as threads that run throughout the book:

- *Who is the "community"?*
- *What roles can (or should) outsider researchers play in CBPR?*
- *How do we create processes that build community leadership without making people "strangers in their own communities"?*
- *How can we openly confront and attempt to address power differentials based on race, class, gender, and professional hierarchy?*
- *How can race and racism in particular be addressed more centrally in CBPR?*

The continued centrality of race and ethnicity and of racism in the social fabric of contemporary United States and of interlocking oppressions based on race and ethnicity, class, and gender (Mullings & Shulz, 2006) makes a special focus on these topics critical to any in-depth look at community-based participatory research (CBPR) for health. Chapter Five examines the difficult issues of race and ethnicity, racism, and white privilege that must be confronted when CBPR involves communities of color. Camara Jones's (2000) three-tiered model of racism (institutionalized, personally mediated, and internalized) is presented, providing an important context for understanding the dynamic interactions possible among these tiers within CBPR practice. The intimate interdependence between racism and power is then examined, with special attention to Michael Foucault's (1980) differentiation between repressive power—power that limits the opportunity structures for people of color—and productive power, power that creates norms, truths, and knowledge and through them both enables dominant control and provides the opportunity for subordinate communities to challenge power structures and bring about change. Concepts such as historical trauma and hidden and public transcripts, the critical role of language in cultural translation, and the important yet often unspoken role of white privilege in the CBPR relationship are each explored and illustrated in this chapter. The chapter authors then examine how understanding racism in all of its forms can help CBPR partners, regardless of their own race or ethnicity, build "alliances across differences." Such alliances will by definition be uncomfortable at times. Yet as Vivian Chávez and her colleagues conclude, in this very discomfort and in embracing "the conflict that characterizes cross-cultural work" (Gutierrez & Lewis, 2005, p. 244), CBPR partners will be better positioned to dance—and continually learn to dance—in the multicultural context that characterizes so much of our work.

As Richard Couto (1987) has argued, although a core function of participatory research is to surface and validate the community's knowledge, "in practice, this is very difficult to do without some person, outside the community, with professional credentials, lending assistance or credence to local knowledge and claims about its validity" (p. 85). Issues of power, potential conflict, and development of partnerships once again are deeply embedded in this reality.

In Chapter Six, sociologist Randy Stoecker describes three contrasting roles that outside academics may play in community-based participatory research—the roles of initiator, consultant, and collaborator. Determining which of these roles may be most appropriate in a given CBPR effort requires addressing key questions from the onset: What is the project attempting to do? What skills does the outside academic bring to the project and the partnership? And how much participation does the community actually need and want? Guideposts for the effective and ethical engagement of outside academics in CBPR are offered in this chapter, as is a perspective on the ways outsider roles may change over the life of the project as community needs, capacities, and desires grow and change. Finally, the author reminds us that doing participatory research is in fact not an end in itself but a means to an end—community-driven social change.

Part Two concludes with two case studies that illustrate many of the themes and challenges discussed in the preceding chapters. In Chapter Seven, Ann Cheatham-Rojas and Eveline Shen describe and analyze a case study of participatory research with Cambodian girls in a southern California community around the youth-identified issue of sexual harassment in the public schools. Issues of power, trust, and dialogue are examined both in the context of the partnership itself and in the broader community as the girls learned to understand and engage with the school and school district power structure to bring about change through an action-oriented CBPR process. Lessons and insights for others engaged in CBPR partnerships with youths are offered, as is an updated look at longer term outcomes of the work.

In Chapter Eight, the final chapter in this part, Kristen Clements-Nolle and Ari Bachrach present a case study of the myriad benefits and challenges of involving one of the nation's most hidden—and heavily stigmatized—populations in a CBPR partnership, and the centrality of trust and dialogue in this context. The San Francisco–based Transgender Community Health Project adhered to the principles of participatory research in a strong epidemiological study of and with the transgender population. Both the dramatic findings of this study and the substantial changes in research, policy, and practice it continues to catalyze a decade after its completion, underscore the power of methodologically rigorous and ethically sound CBPR with hidden populations.

REFERENCES

Cornwall, A., & Jewkes, R. (1995). What is participatory research? *Social Science & Medicine, 41,* 1667–1676.

Couto, R. A. (1987). Participatory research: Methodology and critique. *Clinical Sociology Review, 5,* 83–90.

Foucault, M. (1980). *Power/knowledge: Selected interviews and other writings, 1972–1977* (C. Gordon, Ed.). New York: Pantheon Books.

Gutierrez, L. M., & Lewis, E. A. (2005). Education, participation, and capacity building in community organizing with women of color. In M. Minkler (Ed.), *Community organizing and community building for health* (2nd ed., pp. 240–253). New Brunswick, NJ: Rutgers University Press.

Jones, C. P. (2000). Levels of racism: A theoretic framework and a gardener's tale. *American Journal of Public Health, 8,* 1212–1215.

Mullings, L., & Schulz, A. J. (2006). Intersectionality and health: An introduction. In A. J. Schulz & L. Mullings (Eds.), *Gender, race, class, and health: Intersectional approaches* (pp. 3–17). San Francisco: Jossey-Bass.

CHAPTER

5

THE DANCE OF RACE AND PRIVILEGE IN CBPR

VIVIAN CHÁVEZ, BONNIE DURAN, QUINTON E. BAKER,
MAGDALENA M. AVILA, & NINA WALLERSTEIN

DANCING PROVIDES a provocative analogy for exploring the interplay of race and ethnicity, racism, and privilege that often goes unacknowledged in community-based participatory research (CBPR). Like dancing, CBPR has the potential for making research partners feel exhilarated, awkward, controlled, and free. The dance involves being aware of differences and respecting that although some people appear to be "natural" dancers, others need more time and instruction as they experiment with movement. Dancers complement each other's steps, sometimes leading, sometimes following; they are aware of each other, navigating the dance floor while trying not to step on each other's toes. And when toes do get stepped on, dancers must be self-reflective enough to learn from the experience and not be defensive, to decide whether to continue dancing or to take a seat, and to know that these dynamic processes are normal and inevitable, however rewarding or hurtful they may be.

Dancing, like CBPR, comes in a myriad of forms and styles, depending on the dance partners' styles and interests and the music being played. Moreover, when dance takes place in the United States, which is, perhaps more than any other industrialized country in the world, distinguished by the size and diversity of its racial and ethnic populations (Smelser, Wilson, & Mitchell, 2000), it takes on a racialized character. Dancers from different cultures must learn each other's movements, rhythms, and meanings. To dance is to express our social and cultural context without imposing an absolute "correct way" to dance.

Admittedly, dancing may not be the best analogy for CBPR, as it does not begin to capture the issues of pain and structural oppression that are a part of racism and privilege and therefore often at play in research relationships. Nevertheless, dancing goes back as far in history as research and curiosity. In the words of Zora Neale Hurston, "Research is formalized curiosity. It is poking and prying with purpose. It is a seeking that s/he who wishes may know the cosmic secrets of the world and they that dwell therein" (Walker, 1979, p. 49).

The construct of race and ethnicity, though problematic, is used throughout this chapter because of its historical importance in the American psyche. Furthermore, the trilogy of race and ethnicity, racism, and white privilege is underscored throughout this chapter not because it is more important than other dimensions, such as social class or gender, but because it has often been neglected in CBPR and other areas of research. Race is not a biological construct that reflects innate differences but rather a social construct that captures the impact of racism. As such, the variable of *race* measures a combination of social class, culture, and biogenic factors (LaVeist, 2005; Lin & Kelsey, 2000). As a rough though imperfect proxy for socioeconomic status, race captures the social classification that governs the distribution of risks and opportunities in a race-conscious society such as the United States (Jones, 2000, 2001). The meaning of race in the United States cannot be seen simply as an objective fact or treated as an independent variable (Omi, 2000). Contemporary immigration to the United States is a factor in the changing meaning of race. Between 2000 and 2005, 7.9 million documented and undocumented immigrants came to the United States—more than during any previous five-year period in the nation's history—and the immigrant population topped thirty-five million (Camarota, 2005). As Michael Omi (2000) comments, "The massive influx of new immigrant groups has destabilized specific concepts of race, led to a proliferation of identity positions, and challenged prevailing modes of political and cultural organization" (p. 245).

This chapter will build on the principles of CBPR (see Chapter Three) to examine the hard issues of race and ethnicity, racism, and white privilege that every community-based participatory researcher, whether white or a person of color, should consider when doing CBPR with communities of color. We begin with an overview of a useful framework for understanding racism that addresses institutional and personally mediated racism and also internalized oppression. We then discuss the powerful role of language and the potential errors that arise in translating cultural constructs in research and practice. Third, we explore the concept of white privilege (Cooper, 1989; Hurtado, 1996; Krieger, Williams, & Zierler, 1999; McIntosh, 1998) and how this power imbalance often obstructs trust and community building during participatory research. We conclude with suggestions for building alliances across difference and offer a set of recommendations CBPR researchers can draw on in attempting to better address the issues of race, racism, and privilege that often float at the periphery of participatory research (Blair, Cahill, Chopyak, & Cordes, 2000).

FRAMEWORK OF OPPRESSION AND RACISM

Although most often talked about in relation to the oppressed (such as women, the poor, and people of color), race, class, and gender are part of the whole fabric of experience for all groups. These variables exist within interlocking hierarchies that create systems of privilege as well as of disadvantage (Andersen & Collins, 1995; Mullings & Schulz, 2006). The complexity of social relations, social issues, and social justice is infused with race, class, and gender (Andersen & Collins, 1995; Mullings & Schulz, 2006). These processes are dynamic and change by time and place, with individual vulnerability to oppression increasing to the degree that the interlocking systems of oppression increase. That is, the less power a person has in society, the more *at risk* that person is for health and social problems (Garrett, 2000; Hogue, Hargraves, & Collins, 2000). A focus on the intersection of these multiple systems of inequality explains how people can simultaneously experience oppression along one dimension (such as class) and privilege along another (such as gender)—consider, for example, a wealthy white woman or a poor Latino male. The primary roots of oppression worldwide are economic, social, cultural, and gender inequalities reproduced by an institutionalized system of power imbalance between and among groups of people (Marmot & Wilkinson, 2006). Although oppression may look similar across cultures and generations, its mechanisms are historically and locally determined and change over time and place, depending on domination and resistance.

Some scholars and activists have defined racism as "prejudice plus power" (Omi, 2000); others posit racism as a life-threatening illness (James, 1994; Krieger, Rowley, Herman, Avery, & Phillips, 1993; Williams, 1997). Recognizing the multiple mechanisms of oppression and drawing on the work of Jones (2001), Omi (2000), Sherover-Marcuse (1986), Tilley (1990), Foucault (1980), and others, we offer three interrelated theories of how racism and privilege may manifest in community-based participatory research projects. These theories involve a three-tiered framework for racism, an analysis of power as repressive versus productive, and an understanding of discourse in communities, which may be public or may be hidden to the researcher.

Three-Tiered Racism Framework

Camara Jones (2000) has developed a framework for understanding racism as institutionalized, personally mediated, and internalized. Institutionalized racism manifests itself in both material conditions and access to power. Examples of material conditions include differential access to quality education, adequate housing, gainful employment, appropriate medical facilities, and a clean environment. With regard to power, institutionalized racism includes differential access to information, including one's own history, resources, and voice, and differential representation in government and the media.

Personally mediated racism refers to prejudice, discrimination, stereotypes, and judgments based on assumptions about the abilities, motives, and intentions of others according to their race. As Jones (2001) notes, this "is what most people think of when they hear the word racism. . . . It manifests as lack of respect, suspicion, devaluation, scapegoating, and dehumanization" (p. 300).

Internalized racism does not need an outside judge of character. It is characterized by people's own belief in the negative messages they receive about their race or ethnicity. The core of this perspective is that "an oppressive society re-creates itself in its victims' hearts" (Sherover-Marcuse, 1986, p. 4). Internalized oppression addresses subjectivity, questions of power, and the part each person plays in the evolution of his or her own life story. It acknowledges that oppression does not come only from an external intersection of multiple systems of inequality; the enemy is also within.

The interaction of institutionalized racism, personally mediated racism, and internalized racism produces a racial climate that can manifest itself in community-based participatory research in the following manner. In many major U.S. cities, whites have fled to suburbia, abandoning the inner city to turf battles among different racial minorities for housing, public services, and economic development (Omi, 2000). Racial segregation of neighborhoods, created through institutionalized policies or norms, has limited educational or employment opportunities for communities of color. With more than 80 percent of whites living in virtually all-white neighborhoods and nearly nine in ten white suburbanites living in communities that are less than 1 percent African American (Omi, 2000), a degree of isolation exists that can lead to a skewed perception of what other people experience and a reinforcement of personally mediated stereotypes. This skewed perception is bolstered by images, descriptions, and depictions fostered by cultural institutions such as the mass media. After all, if one does not know many African Americans or does not personally experience discrimination and one's only knowledge comes from second- or third-hand sources, it is likely that one will find the notion of widespread mistreatment unbelievable. Finally, the isolation of people of color can lead to internalized racism; that is, people internalize their lack of opportunities as self-blame.

These three levels of racism may also be played out in the relationship between researchers and communities. First, on the institutional level, structural factors inform the class and ethnic makeup of the CBPR collaborators. Given differential access by race to goods, services, and opportunities in society, CBPR often involves university researchers who are white working in communities of color where social and health problems are identified. People and communities of color are those being studied, not those doing the studying. Clarence Spigner (2000) extends this point further, noting contradictions within CBPR itself: "The research establishment is overwhelmed by well-meaning non-minorities who recognize racism and its consequences on health, but only greater representation of people-of-color in the health establishment can ameliorate the inherent contradictions of 'participatory democracy' fundamental to the process of community-based participatory research" (p. 259). As Marianne Sullivan and her colleagues (2001) suggest, diversifying academic research faculty and bringing about other forms of institutional change must be seen as important goals of CBPR if we are to successfully overcome this problem. However, even though it is crucial to take steps in this direction, it is also important to note that institutionalized racism works to establish the dominant culture and its way of doing things, including traditional forms of research, as the yardstick that measures and establishes credibility.

On the second level, personally mediated racism may manifest in stereotypical projections between public health professionals as outsiders and community members as insiders. When the outsider does not share the lived experiences of community members, assumptions are often made by both parties and preconceived ideas may go unchallenged (Hatch, Moss, Saran, Presley-Cantrell, & Mallory, 1993; Perkins & Wandersman, 1990; Minkler, 2004). In the case of the outside researchers, these assumptions tend to focus on finding deficits rather than community resources because the framework in health and human service systems charges system workers to assess problems rather than recognize solutions (McKnight, 1995). This deficit model promotes the idea that solutions must come from outside the community, a view supported as well by those looking for someone to come in and "save" the community from itself.

Third, on the level of internalized oppression and racism, researchers of color face their own experiences with racism and privilege as *outsider-insiders*. People of color involved in CBPR may not be able to identify their community's assets due to feelings of internalized oppression that make them undervalue community resources. Before community members can name the gifts, talents, and resources in their community, they themselves have to believe these assets exist. Finally, internalized oppression may also lead community residents to value white researchers and dismiss both educated members of their own community of color and the learning and teaching available in that community from the residents themselves.

Repressive and Productive Power

To understand racism more clearly, it is important to understand the multiple ways that power is manifested in both the dominant society and subordinate communities. Foucault differentiates between power that represses others and power that produces *others*. Repressive power structures, like institutional forms of racism, operate through direct control over people's opportunities in relation to education, employment, living conditions, and other factors that contribute to health or disease. Productive power, exercised by mainstream institutions including those of public health, creates and reproduces the symbols and hierarchies of structural power that normalize and mask repressive relationships—for example, believing that "research" must be carried out in the conventional manner taught by professional experts at major universities. Repressive and productive power is not monolithic, however; it is built into webs of relationships and practices found in institutions, communities, and families that are inherently unstable and therefore susceptible to challenge (Foucault, 1980).

Productive power as expressed by subordinate communities offers the possibility of challenging oppressive structures, through the capacity of communities to bring about outcomes and effects in the world (Tilley, 1990, p. 287). This community productive power, emanating from lived experience, is the origin of race- and ethnicity-centered interventions and indigenous theories of health and illness, which represent a counterhegemonic challenge to outside definitions of community problems and solutions. In other words, if hegemony is the assumption that the dominant culture controls the ideological sectors of society—culture, religion, education, and the media—in a manner that disseminates values to reinforce its position (Scott, 1985), then counterhegemony is the interruption of this practice from the grassroots perspective.

One example of counterhegemonic theory is the concept of historical trauma, which has gained popularity among Native American community-based health practitioners and consumers (Brave Heart & De Bruyn, 1998; Duran, Duran, & Brave Heart, 1998). The theory of historical trauma posits that traumatic assaults on past generations, most notably the colonization of the Americas, created a psychological and physical health effect among the descendents of those affected. The historical events of the colonization are among the important root causes of both high rates of physical and psychological health disparities and of weak mainstream political will to ameliorate them.

Community-based participatory researchers working in communities of color, and particularly in native communities, would be well advised to be conversant with historical trauma and related theories. The advantage of engaging with such approaches is that they speak directly to the lived experience of individuals and groups and may therefore be more widely accepted as the basis for research and intervention emanating from the community.

Hidden and Public Transcripts

The relationship between community members and outside researchers in CBPR is based on dialogue, mutual respect, and sharing of lived realities (Ansley & Gaventa, 1997; Cornwall & Jewkes, 1995; Israel, Eng, Schulz, & Parker, 2005). However, though researchers may believe they have access to community norms and ideas, they may have access only to what is considered public. James Scott (1985) theorizes that there are four levels of community dialogue: public discourse, hidden transcripts, coded defiance, and open defiance. Public discourse is the official, institutionalized language; public discourse about health takes as its basis the authority of public health systems. Hidden transcripts, in contrast, are produced by subordinates gathering outside the gaze of power and constructing a sharply critical political and cultural discourse. As Makani Themba suggests (1999), much rap music is a form of hidden transcript, providing members of an oppressed group with a critical venue for "expressing rage at the status quo as well as holding a candid discussion of social issues" (p. 22). There may be many hidden transcripts in any given community, and outsiders rarely have access to all of them. Coded counterhegemonic discourse involves disguise and anonymity; it is the veiled expression, typically by subordinate groups, of hidden transcripts during public discourse. In the case of CBPR, where researchers and community members have entered into collaborative understanding, open expression of conflict may be rare. Yet among themselves, as noted in Chapter Two, community researchers of color may express defiance, make jokes, and express tensions not safe to bring up in the presence of their white counterparts from university or professional environments.

With internalized oppression, community partners in research may often self-censor and conform to what is presented. They may nod their heads and say yes in resignation—when the heart feels no—as a result of having been led to believe that they are "deficient" and dare not challenge. When community research participants feel that they are not truly equal partners, the range of allowable forms of self-expression is limited. Community-based ethnographic research on substance abuse and substance abusers (Bourgois, Lettiere, & Quezada, 1997) describes how community members who are paid to participate in studies anticipate what the researcher wants and may speak those words in order to maintain the relationship and not disturb the peace: "Street addicts usually do not want to appear stupid or offensive to a friendly interviewer. In fact they usually have at least a partially internalized society's normalizing judgments and are depressed, ashamed, or ambivalent about their marginality. . . . [One respondent said he] liked the researcher administering the interview protocol, so he tried to respond in what he thought was a socially appropriate manner" (p. 166).

This interaction involves a dialectic of resistance between outside research partners and community participants with very real ethical dilemmas involved in speaking truth to power. There may be fear of speaking out about personal and community oppression because of the risk of creating stereotypes and misinformation in outside researchers' minds, which then might be generalized to all communities of color. Furthermore, people from communities of color learn very early not to reveal true information to white people because they do not believe that whites want to hear the truth or because they fear that the truth will not be heard. As Scott (1985) has aptly pointed out, "power-laden situations are nearly always inauthentic. . . .The greater the disparity in power between the two parties, the greater the proportion of the full transcript that is likely to be concealed" (p. 286).

Community-based participatory research must go beyond the surface issues of making research questions culturally and linguistically appropriate and relevant. Research participants have obvious and compelling reasons to seek refuge behind public transcripts when in the presence of power. Similarly, outside researchers in the presence of "subordinates" often adopt a public transcript that consists of expected gestures and words. As subordination requires a credible performance of humility and deference, so domination requires a credible performance of mastery and power.

CBPR must be about asking questions about and examining the power dynamics that exist when some people speak and others are silent. Drawing on Freire's (1970) work, CBPR can transform the culture of silence among oppressed groups. Community members take risks in sharing their personal stories and speaking with outside researchers. Even in CBPR, time constraints sometimes lead outside or university researchers who do not know the importance of a community story to stop the telling of that story and to opt for more closed-ended matters. This way of conducting research silences community members and impedes their full participation in the research process. In addition, it limits the information gathered to whatever the outside researcher thinks is relevant. This in turn leads to research results and interventions that lack an authentic community "voice." Solutions are consequently developed with incomplete and inadequate information from a limited, outside researcher's perspective. Cynthia Chataway (1997), a white female university researcher, also notes that doing all the talking and presenting of opinions and facts may get in the way of participatory research. She suggests that withholding information can allow space for the "other" to speak and act, bringing a balance of power to the relationship that forces the other to speak outside of the public transcript. Chataway's description of silencing herself to avoid dominating the research relationship is an important one for CBPR researchers who are outside or university members of the team to consider. However, a word of caution: withholding information can in some cases be manipulative. The important issue is that outside researchers must learn to value what community participants have to say, listen to everyone in a meaningful way, and not speak as the "expert." Once again, a dance is involved; balancing silence and speaking creates the space for community members to express themselves.

TRANSLATING CULTURE

How do you say *empowerment* in Spanish? What does empowerment mean for African Americans? The answers to these questions are crucial in CBPR because the concept of empowerment is an important goal. Practitioners have been grappling with questions about translating *empowerment* and communicating cultural constructs since the first time this word appeared in the literature (Erzinger, 1994). The question of how to say *empowerment* in Spanish matters to CBPR researchers concerned about the development of culturally and linguistically relevant data collection. Data collection instruments rely not only on literal translations but also on a deeper translation of meaning, concepts, and cultural constructs. Empowerment operationalized from a multicultural perspective is played out in a range of ways that challenge researchers to make evident the need to remember the sixth principle of CBPR for health (see Chapter Three), that it focuses on problems of local relevance and attends to the social, economic, and cultural conditions that influence health status. The issue of empowerment raises the question of whether many public health concepts are relevant, meaningful, and translatable across cultures. For example, since collectivism, or family or group centeredness, is a sociobehavioral orientation in many communities of color (Aguirre-Molina, Molina, & Zambrana, 2001; Halgunseth, 2004; Spigner, 2000), are the constructs of health education theories that focus on the individual applicable to people who identify with collective, cooperative models? The answer to this question matters, as it may affect every step of the research process, from problem definition to instrument development, data collection, analysis, and dissemination of research findings.

It is a key principle of CBPR that research must be produced, interpreted, and disseminated to community members in clear, useful, and respectful language. Nonetheless, academia has its own language and assumptions that often clash with those of a majority of the people in the communities where research is conducted. As professionally trained outside researchers, we often take for granted knowledge of words, acronyms, and concepts that are familiar to us, assuming that others who do not understand will ask for an explanation. The commitment to disseminate research and communicate back with the community where the data were gathered requires that CBPR researchers go outside the usual boundaries of academic convention. Often the frame of reference for disseminating research findings is guided by "acceptable" standards of academia, such as publication in peer-reviewed journals or presentation at professional meetings (see Chapter Six). However, even with community members involved, specialized professional language often prescribes how health issues and community needs should be introduced and studied, findings posed and disseminated, and strategies recommended. To be true to the principles of CBPR, projects must be designed in which research is only a piece of the work to be undertaken. Successful CBPR projects acknowledge the role of history; specifically, that the relationship between researchers and community members begins not with the project itself but centuries ago, with the advent of slavery and other forms of exploitation.

Another important point at the nexus of language and culture is that researchers of color are often expected to serve as translators, ventriloquists, and spokespersons (Trinh, 1989). Often researchers of color are not in the role of primary investigator but act in a secondary capacity to bridge the gap between communities of color and institutions of research, bringing knowledge across in both directions. Researchers who speak the language of the community become privy to the hidden transcripts in communities of color and might come across information that on both ethical and practical grounds may best be kept confidential. It is important to respect that relationships are primary and integral to the goals of CBPR. A researcher who learns and publishes information that should have remained confidential can cause considerable conflict and pain within the community if and when this breach of confidence comes to light. It will also make it far more difficult to establish the previous level of trust again in that community and thus will limit access to crucial information and data. The abuse of trust in communities has been a recurring reality that must be taken seriously if outside researchers are committed to a long-term relationship (Flicker, Travers, Guta, McDonald, & Meagher, 2007; Hatch et al., 1993; Perkins & Wandersman, 1990). The violation of trust historically affects questions of accountability. And this brings to bear a significant question: To whom is the outside researcher accountable?

WHITE PRIVILEGE

Although there are multiple sources of overlapping privilege, it is especially important in the United States to confront the experience of privilege that goes with being of the dominant race (Cooper, 1989; Hurtado, 1996; Krieger et al., 1999; McIntosh, 1998; Omi, 2000). The experience of the dominant group often serves as the point of reference, the *norm,* and is compared with that of people who are disadvantaged along a continuum of oppression and powerlessness (McIntosh, 1998).

Experiences of bias and discrimination mask the ways in which systems of privilege work. The racialization process for whites is evident on college campuses, as white students encounter a heightened awareness of race that calls their own identity into question (Omi, 2000). Research on white Americans suggests that they do not experience their ethnicity as a definitive aspect of their social identity unless they work or live in diverse communities. Omi (2000) remarks: "Whites tend to locate racism in color consciousness and find its absence in color-blindness. In so doing, they see the affirmation of difference and racial identity among racially defined minority students as racist. Black students, by contrast, see racism as a system of power, and correspondingly argue that they cannot be racist because they lack power" (p. 257).

In essence there seem to be "two languages of race" (Blauner, 1994), one in which members of communities of color see the centrality of race in history and everyday experience and another in which whites see race as a peripheral reality and do not perceive themselves as racist.

Unconscious racism—being able to ignore issues surrounding race—is a key aspect of white privilege (McIntosh, 1998). Being white, male, and of the middle or upper class provides unearned advantages. White privilege, however, is independent of feelings of racism. Whereas in the past, white privilege was asserted through blatantly racist acts and political policies, today the mechanisms of white privilege are more complex and firmly entrenched. Even when they may perceive a lack of "racist feelings," whites may reproduce the system of white privilege in several ways: (1) by feeling that they are getting only what is due to them, what they deserve (meritocracy) (Mills, 1998); (2) by mistakenly seeing the prevalent white culture as culturally neutral; (3) by not recognizing that their privilege is not automatically shared by or conferred on others; and (4) by not having to contend with internalized oppression (Cooper, 1989; Hurtado, 1996; Krieger et al., 1999; McIntosh, 1998; see also Appendix I).

The advantage of not having to deal with race is denied to people of color who are constantly reminded of their "disadvantaged status." Jerry Tello tours the country giving seminars on cultural competency and systems change for health and human services personnel. He notes that it is vital that people of color not forget where they came from. "The minute you forget and get comfortable, someone will remind you," whether it is with the innocent question, "Where are you from?" or more poignantly, "Who are you here with?" or, "Why are you here?" (personal communication with J. Tello, 1995). Similarly, Paulo Freire (1973) expressed early on his concern that leadership training and by extension professional or academic training in research makes people of color "strangers in their own community."

For professionally trained researchers who are white or otherwise advantaged, privilege is one of the most important and difficult arenas in CBPR to address, as it in part defines who they understand themselves to be. The outcomes and mechanisms of institutionalized racism are easier to uncover because these are not personal. To look internally at privilege conferred due to education, race, sexual orientation, gender, or institutional affiliation means a long-term commitment to engage in deep inner work researchers may not be prepared to do. To this end Melanie Tervalon and Jane Murray-Garcia (1998) suggest the application of *cultural humility,* which they define as involving a lifelong commitment to self-evaluation and self-critique in order to redress power imbalances and to develop and maintain mutually respectful dynamic partnerships based on mutual trust. Cultural humility proves to be an essential tool for building community partnerships and organizing for change (Cohen, Chávez, & Chehimi, 2007). The concept and practice of cultural humility connotes tremendous self-reflection, the ability to recognize our own cultural beliefs and assumptions to break through commonly held assumptions and stereotypes getting in the way of truly being able to be "competent" or "sensitive" in another's culture. In this way, the suggestion to apply cultural humility is akin to the admonition, "physician heal thyself."

BUILDING ALLIANCES ACROSS DIFFERENCES

Hugh Vasquez, Nell Myhand, and Allan Creighton, authors of *Celebrating Diversity, Building Alliances* (2002), emphasize the hope in the momentum that has created an increased demand for justice. People are willing to find ways of working together with partners who may be different from themselves in order to see justice happen. These authors underscore that it is our human nature to want to be close to other people and to break down all the divisions that exist among us. The first step is the desire to examine what the systemic and personal barriers are. Makani Themba (1999) adds to the hopefulness with a reality test. "Racism," she says, "is like the gorilla in the living room. It's running through the place making noises and everyone is trying to sit politely and ignore it" (p. 157). Themba also notes that the privileges and pain associated with racism make it vital to remember that racism is a system that is much larger than the sum of the individuals whom it affects. In order to address racism, she notes, we have to understand its systemic nature and learn how to build new, less comfortable alliances. Similarly, as Lorraine Gutierrez and Edith Lewis (2005) suggest, we must "recognize and embrace the conflict that characterizes cross-cultural work" (p. 244).

The larger context in which the dance of racism and privilege takes place makes it necessary that we continue to work against structural or institutionalized racism, because as long as it is present any CBPR is severely limited in what it can hope to achieve. As Camara Jones (2000) points out, "Institutionalized racism is the most fundamental of the three levels [of racism] and must be addressed for important change to occur" (p. 1214). The dance analogy suggests that CBPR is not only about dancing; it is also about continuously learning to dance while accepting the invariability of continued mistakes along the way. Failing to dance—that is, failing to address racism and privilege—will inevitably lead to power imbalances and lack of coordination between white researchers and community researchers. "Power imbalances often stand in the way of developing effective working relationships grounded in trust" (Sullivan et al., 2001, p. 136).

RECOMMENDATIONS FOR RESEARCH AND PRACTICE

In addition to the suggestions implicit in the basic principles of CBPR, such as having community partners involved in all phases of the research process, the following set of recommendations, drawn from a variety of sources (Chávez et al., 2004; Duran & Duran, 1999; Jones, 2001; Omi, 2000; Mullings & Schulz, 2006; Spigner, 2000; Themba, 1999; Wallerstein, 1999), puts special emphasis on reducing racism and privilege in CBPR.

- Practice cultural humility. Learn more about your own cultural lens. What are your operating values and belief systems? Where do they come from? And how do they interact when you are working with culturally diverse communities?
- Acknowledge the diversity within racial and ethnic groups. Expand data collection to include questions on ancestry, migration history, and language. Researchers need to be attentive to the increasing heterogeneity of racial and ethnic groups and may need to rethink the types of research questions asked.

- Acknowledge that race is a social construct, not a biological determinant, and model race as a contextual variable in multilevel analyses.
- Address the present-day existence and impacts of racism (institutionalized, personally mediated, and internalized), not only as variables to measure but also as lived experiences within the research process. The complex nature of race relations in the United States following the civil rights era requires that we move beyond discussing race and racism as a black-white phenomenon to encompassing multiple racial and ethnic groupings in our discourse.
- Examine the role of racism in diminishing the health of the entire population, not just the health of members of low-income communities of color. Emphasize the intersectionality of race, gender, age, and class to examine how different categories engage with racism and with each other.
- Encourage people from communities of color to pursue higher education. They will bring new perspectives to CBPR and will raise new questions. Bringing about institutional change, such as diversifying academic research faculty, is an important goal of CBPR.
- Use the research process and outcomes to mobilize and advocate for change to reduce disparities and enhance race relations.
- Listen, listen, and listen. Pay close attention to both hidden and public transcripts, and speak about white privilege and racism.
- Accept that outsiders cannot fully understand community and interpersonal dynamics. Do not, however, let this stop you from taking part in the dance.
- Recognize that privilege, especially white privilege, is continually operating to some degree and creating situations of power imbalance. Such an understanding is crucial in honest, ongoing communication that builds trust and respect.
- Build true multicultural working relationships, and in a partnership mode, develop guidelines for research data collection, analysis, publication, and dissemination of research findings.

SUMMARY

CBPR attempts to change the paradigm in which research is conceived and operationalized. Racism and privilege are major challenges to this paradigm shift. Understanding the roots of oppression and its relationship to trust and community building are part of the dance that is indispensable to doing this work. So is addressing the challenge of creating true equal partnerships in CBPR in a world of injustice. Having as collaborators working-class people of color who consider themselves equal partners and are considered equal partners in the research process requires ongoing effort.

The effort to understand racism and all its consequences is work done in the context of relationships. To empower a community, we must become a community, supporting and challenging each other as we implement culturally competent, power- and race-sensitive inquiry. Dancing forward, following the flow of the dance of race and privilege in community-based participatory research, outside researchers must become comfortable with not always taking the lead but often dancing side by side with the community and sometimes following the community's lead.

QUESTIONS FOR DISCUSSION

1. Race, racism, and white privilege are some of the hardest issues in our society to acknowledge and address. How does Camara Jones's three-tiered definition of racism help you understand these issues? What has been your experience as a person of color or as a white person at these different levels?

2. How do racism and other intersecting oppressions, that is, class, gender, or sexual orientation, connect with issues of power in community research settings? Explore how repressive and productive power and how hidden and public transcripts affect the CBPR research process.

3. Take any of the recommendations listed earlier, such as practicing cultural humility. How can you practice this recommendation within a CBPR framework to build authentic partnerships, acknowledging and working with the differences that are present?

KEY TERMS

Racism	White privilege	Internalized oppression
Power	Culture	Cultural humility

REFERENCES

Aguirre-Molina, M., Molina, C., & Zambrana, R. (Eds.). (2001). *Health issues in the Latino community.* San Francisco: Jossey-Bass.

Andersen, M. L., & Collins, P. H. (1995). *Race, class, and gender: An anthology* (2nd ed.). Belmont, CA.: Wadsworth.

Ansley, F., & Gaventa, J. (1997, January-February). Researching for democracy and democratizing research. *Change,* pp. 46–53.

Blair, R., Cahill, K., Chopyak, J., & Cordes, C. (2000). *Common problems, uncommon resources: Exploring the social and economic challenges of community-based research.* Atlanta: Community Research Network.

Blauner, B. (1994). Talking past each other: Black and white languages of race. In F. Pincus & H. Ehrlich (Eds.), *Race and ethnic conflict: Contending views on prejudice, discrimination, and ethnoviolence* (pp. 18–28). Boulder, CO: Westview Press.

Bourgois, P., Lettiere, M., & Quezada, J. (1997). Social misery and the sanctions of substance abuse: Confronting HIV risk among homeless heroin addicts in San Francisco. *Social Problems, 44,* 155–173.

Brave Heart, M.Y.H., & De Bruyn, L. M. (1998). The American Indian holocaust: Healing historical unresolved grief. *American Indian and Alaska Native Mental Health Research, 2,* 60–82.

Camarota, S. (2005). *Immigrants at mid-decade: A snapshot of America's foreign-born population in 2005.* Washington, DC: Center for Immigration Studies.

Chataway, C. (1997). An examination of the constraints on mutual inquiry in a participatory action research project. *Journal of Social Issues, 4,* 747–766.

Chávez, V., Israel, B. A., Allen, A. J., III, Lichenstein, R., DeCarlo, M., Schulz, A. J., et al. (2004). A bridge between communities: Video-making using principles of community-based participatory research. *Health Promotion Practice, 5*(4), 395–403.

Cohen, L., Chávez, V., & Chehimi, S. (Eds.). (2007). *Prevention is primary: Strategies for community well-being.* San Francisco: Jossey-Bass.

Cooper, T. (1989). The rewards of racial prejudice. *Journal of Housing, 46*(3), 105–107.

Cornwall, A., & Jewkes, R. (1995). What is participatory research? *Social Science & Medicine, 41,* 1667–1676.

Duran, B., & Duran, E. (1999). Assessment, program planning, and evaluation in Indian country: Toward a postcolonial practice. In R. M. Huff & M. V. Kline (Eds.), *Promoting health in multicultural populations: A handbook for practitioners* (pp. 291–311). Thousand Oaks, CA: Sage.

Duran, B., Duran, E., & Brave Heart, M.Y.H. (1998). Native Americans and the trauma of history. In R. Thornton (Ed.), *Studying Native America: Problems and prospects in Native American studies* (pp. 60–78). Madison: University of Wisconsin Press.

Erzinger, S. (1994). Empowerment in Spanish: Words can get in the way. *Health Education Quarterly, 21,* 417–419.

Flicker, S., Travers, R., Guta, A., McDonald, S., & Meagher, A. (2007). Ethical dilemmas in community-based participatory research: Recommendations for institutional review boards. *Journal of Urban Health, 84*(4), 478–493.

Foucault, M. (1980). *Power/knowledge: Selected interviews and other writings, 1972–1977* (C. Gordon, Ed.). New York: Pantheon Books.

Freire, P. (1970). *Pedagogy of the oppressed.* New York: Seabury Press.

Freire, P. (1973). *Education for critical consciousness.* New York: Continuum.

Garrett, L. (2000). *Betrayal of trust: The collapse of global public health.* New York: Hyperion.

Gutierrez, L. M., & Lewis, E. A. (2005). Education, participation, and capacity building in community organizing with women of color. In M. Minkler (Ed.), *Community organizing and community building for health* (2nd ed., pp. 240–253). New Brunswick, NJ: Rutgers University Press.

Halgunseth, L. C. (2004). Continuing research on Latino families: El pasado y el futuro. In M. Coleman & L. H. Ganong (Eds.), *Handbook of contemporary families: Considering the past, contemplating the future* (pp. 333–351). Thousand Oaks, CA: Sage.

Hatch, J., Moss, N., Saran, A., Presley-Cantrell, L., & Mallory, C. (1993). Community research: Partnership in black communities. *American Journal of Preventive Medicine, 9*(6), 27–31.

Hogue, C.J.R., Hargraves, M. A., & Collins, K. S. (2000). *Minority health in America: Findings and policy implications from the Commonwealth Fund Minority Health Survey.* Baltimore: Johns Hopkins University Press.

Hurtado, A. (1996). *The color of privilege: Three blasphemies on race and feminism.* Ann Arbor: University of Michigan Press.

Israel, B. A., Eng, E., Schulz, A. J., & Parker, E. A. (Eds.). (2005). *Methods in community-based participatory research for health.* San Francisco: Jossey-Bass.

Israel, B. A., Schulz, A. J., Parker, E. A., & Becker, A. B. (1998). Review of community-based research: Assessing partnership approaches to improve public health. *Annual Review of Public Health, 19,* 173–202.

James, S. A. (1994). John Henryism and the health of African-Americans. *Cultural Medical Psychiatry, 18,* 163–182.

Jones, C. P. (2000). Levels of racism: A theoretic framework and a gardener's tale. *American Journal of Public Health, 8,* 1212–1215.

Jones, C. P. (2001). Invited commentary: "Race," racism and the practice of epidemiology. *American Journal of Epidemiology, 4,* 299–304.

Krieger, N., Rowley, D. L., Herman, A. A., Avery, B., & Phillips, M. T. (1993). Racism, sexism, and social class: Implications for studies of health, disease, and well-being. *American Journal of Preventive Medicine, 9*(6), 82–122.

Krieger, N., Williams, D. R., & Zierler, S. (1999). "Whiting out" white privilege will not advance the study of how racism harms health. *American Journal of Public Health, 5,* 782–783; Discussion, 784–785.

LaVeist, T. A. (2005). *Minority populations and health: An introduction to health disparities in the United States.* San Francisco: Jossey-Bass.

Lin, S. S., & Kelsey, J. L. (2000). Use of race and ethnicity in epidemiologic research: Concepts, methodologic issues, and suggestions for research. *Epidemiology Review, 22,* 187–202.

Marmot, M., & Wilkinson, R. G. (Eds.). (2006). *Social determinants of health* (2nd ed.). New York: Oxford University Press.

McIntosh, P. (1998). White privilege: Unpacking the invisible knapsack. In M. McGoldrick (Ed.), *Re-visioning family therapy: Race, culture, and gender in clinical practice* (pp. 147–152). New York: Guilford Press.

McKnight, J. (1995). *The careless society: Community and its counterfeits.* New York: Basic Books.

Mills, C. W. (1998). *Blackness visible: Essays on philosophy and race.* Ithaca, NY: Cornell University Press.

Minkler, M. (2004). Ethical challenges for the "outside" researcher in community-based participatory research. *Health Education & Behavior, 31*(6), 684–697.

Mullings, L., & Schulz, A. J. (2006). Intersectionality and health: An introduction. In A. J. Schulz & L. Mullings (Eds.), *Gender, race, class and health: Intersectional approaches* (pp. 3–17). San Francisco: Jossey-Bass.

Omi, M. A. (2000). The changing meaning of race. In N. J. Smelser, W. J. Wilson, & F. Mitchell (Eds.), *America becoming: Racial trends and their consequences* (Vol. 1, pp. 243–263). Washington, DC: National Academies Press.

Perkins, D. D., & Wandersman, A. (1990). "You'll have to work to overcome our suspicions": The benefits and pitfalls of research with community organizations. *Social Policy, 21*(1), 32–41.

Scott, J. (1985). *Weapons of the weak.* New Haven, CT: Yale University Press.

Sherover-Marcuse, R. (1986). *Emancipation and consciousness: Dogmatic and dialectical perspectives in the early Marx.* Malden, MA: Blackwell.

Smelser, N. J., Wilson, W. J., & Mitchell, F. (Eds.). (2000). *America becoming: Racial trends and their consequences* (Vol. 1). Washington, DC: National Academies Press.

Spigner, C. (2000). African Americans, democracy, and biomedical and behavioral research: Contradictions or consensus in community-based participatory research? *International Quarterly of Community Health Education, 3,* 259–284.

Sullivan, M., Koné, A., Senturia, K., Chrisman, N., Ciske, S., & Krieger, J. W. (2001). Researcher and researched-community perspectives: Toward bridging the gap. *Health Education & Behavior, 2,* 130–149.

Tervalon, M., & Murray-Garcia, J. (1998). Cultural humility versus cultural competence: A critical distinction in defining physician training outcomes in multicultural education. *Journal of Health Care for the Poor and Underserved, 9*(2), 117–125.

Themba, M. N. (1999). *Making policy, making change: How communities are taking law into their own hands.* Berkeley, CA: Chardon Press.

Tilley, C. (1990). Michel Foucault: Towards an archaeology of archaeology. In C. Tilley (Ed.), *Reading material culture: Structuralism, hermeneutics, and post-structuralism* (pp. 281–347). Malden, MA: Blackwell.

Trinh, T. M. (1989). *Woman, native, other.* Indianapolis: Indiana University Press.

Vasquez, H., Myhand, N., & Creighton, A. (2002). *Celebrating diversity, building alliances: A curriculum for making the peace in middle school.* Alameda, CA: Hunter House.

Walker, A. (Ed.). (1979). *I love myself: A Zora Neale Hurston reader.* New York: Feminist Press.

Wallerstein, N. (1999). Power between evaluator and community: Research relationships within New Mexico's healthier communities. *Social Science & Medicine, 49,* 39–53.

Williams, D. R. (1997). Race and health: Basic questions, emerging directions. *Annals of Epidemiology, 5,* 322–333.

CHAPTER

6

ARE ACADEMICS IRRELEVANT?

APPROACHES AND ROLES FOR SCHOLARS IN CBPR

RANDY STOECKER

The word "academic" is a synonym for irrelevant.

SAUL ALINSKY (1946/1969, P. IX)

I REMEMBER the moment my academic career changed. I was a graduate student, sitting in the Cedar-Riverside Project Area Committee (PAC) office to interview Tim Mungavan about this amazing Minneapolis neighborhood that had instituted a radical,

Note: This chapter is adapted from "Are Academics Irrelevant?" by R. Stoecker, 1999, *American Behavioral Scientist, 42*(5), 840–854. Copyright 1999 by Sage Publications, Inc. Reprinted by permission of Sage Publications, Inc.

grassroots, community-controlled redevelopment program. Tim, the group's architect and organizer, leaned back in his chair, put his feet up on his desk, and looked me sternly in the eye. He said, "We have students and reporters coming through all the time, asking neighborhood people to give their time and answer their questions. And we don't get so much as a copy of a paper from them. If I agree to talk with you, then I want you to agree that you'll give us a copy of the paper you write" (Stoecker, 1994, p. 25). Tim tells the story of how I then tried to make myself relevant, and he set me to work cleaning the PAC's storeroom, thinking that if I stuck with it after that, I might really be serious. I stuck, at least partly because the storeroom was a treasure trove of neighborhood information. My relationship with the neighborhood continues to this day.

When I got my first academic job at the University of Toledo, I met Dave Beckwith, a community organizer with the Center for Community Change and the University of Toledo Urban Affairs Center. Dave handed me a list of community-generated research needs almost the day I arrived. I negotiated with him and other activists to do a resource and needs assessment of Toledo's community-based organizations. This project, involving neighborhood activists throughout, built a coalition that brought in over $2 million to support those groups. As time went on, however, I found myself working with bankers, foundation officials, and large nonprofits that did not share my desire to transform all power structures to participatory democracies and community-controlled economies. I consequently became involved in a factional power struggle that destroyed the coalition built by that first project (Stoecker, 1997). Then I was in two very different participatory research projects in 1996. The first project I initiated. It began with academics, never made the transition to community control, and died. The second began with community members, and I became involved as one of many. This project is thriving (Stoecker & Stuber, 1999). Since then, when the original version of this chapter was written, I have worked increasingly closely with a number of community organizers helping me to clarify my role in community-based participatory research (CBPR), most recently at the University of Wisconsin in Madison. I have also been working with the Bonner Foundation's Community Research Project, which is building CBPR programs in more than a dozen universities, and have begun to see the diversity of CBPR-related approaches out there (Stoecker, 2001). All of this has confirmed what I wrote in the original version of this chapter and reinforces in me the haunting question of how I, as an academic, can become relevant.

OPTIONS FOR THE ACADEMIC

I have now made a career of CBPR, and I do finally feel relevant when I am working with community groups. But I still worry. The original goal of participatory research was for the members of the community to do things themselves and become self-sufficient knowledge providers and social change producers (Gaventa, 1991, 1993). Now, with people like me doing CBPR, are we furthering or hindering the long-term goals of community-controlled knowledge production and progressive social change? As Heaney (1993) has argued:

> However well-intentioned and zealous the efforts of individual faculty who have brought participatory research into the academic arena, one can only question by what

compromises such researchers are likely to survive. . . . Having made our work acceptable in academic terms, we see that work now being incorporated into academic cur-
ricula. Our papers have become required readings for professional researchers who are
expected to master the theory and methods of participatory research. It is not difficult to
imagine the day when Third World governments and community organizations will hire
only professional participatory researchers trained and certified by graduate institutions
[pp. 43–44].

Participatory researchers seem to do increasingly well in the university (Cancian,
1993; Gedicks, 1996). But there are often compromises. Graduate students trying to do
CBPR are still forced to take control of the research in order to get credit to graduate
(Heaney, 1993). The reward system of universities discourages collaboration, and community members have to make time and even money sacrifices to collaborate in research,
while academics get rewards (Hall, 1993; see also Appendix D). And in many institutions, community research is still seen as a kind of "community housework" that is not
socially valued and hence does not receive much attention (Hubbard, 1996).

So how, as academics, do we keep our eyes on the twin prizes of community-
controlled knowledge and progressive social change while still doing relevant work?
Today academics seem to adopt three roles when approaching CBPR: the initiator, the
consultant, and the collaborator.

The Initiator

One thing that most distinguishes CBPR from more conservative approaches is the belief
that the research question should be generated by the community, not the researcher
(Brown & Tandon, 1983; Deshler & Ewert, 1995). However, Peter Reason (1994) notes
that "paradoxically, many PAR [participatory action research] projects would not occur
without the initiative of someone with time, skill, and commitment, someone who will
almost inevitably be a member of a privileged and educated group" (p. 334). Researchers
usually initiate the contact with community organizations, even if they do consequently
respond to requests coming from the community (Maguire, 1987).

Some also see the researcher as an educator or leader who helps the community overcome its false consciousness. This is tricky, however, because "for the alternative ideology
to result from a collective effort throughout the research process, all forms of indoctrination
and ideological imposition had to be ruled out" (de Roux, 1991, p. 50). Mohammad Anisur
Rahman (1991) accuses some PAR practitioners of placing themselves in a vanguard role.
And Stringer (1996) cautions, "When we try to 'get' people to do anything, insist that they
'must' or 'should' do something, or try to 'stop' them from engaging in some activity, we
are working from an authoritative position that is likely to generate resistance" (p. 43).

Can an academic adopt an initiator approach that is truly empowering? Mary Brydon-
Miller (1993) describes how her initial research led to a *community accessibility committee* that began taking action on its own. In this case the research process strengthened
people's awareness of their own skills and resources, requiring the researcher to take on
more of a process-facilitating role and less of a product-producing role. Conversely, in a
CBPR project I initiated, we were never able to switch control over to the community, as

too many of our academic members lacked skills in community organizing and process facilitating (Stoecker & Stuber, 1999).

The Consultant

In the strictest sense the original participatory research model says that community members should do the research themselves (Gaventa, 1991, 1993). However, in many cases academics find themselves consulting with community groups (Stoecker, 2001). The community commissions the research, and the academic carries it out while being held accountable to the community. In some cases the accountability process can be intense, with the researcher getting community input at each stage of the research project. I have used the consultant approach regularly, at the community's request. To ask already overburdened community members to do the research when they could be doing other more important things contradicts the social change goal of CBPR. A community group armed with a PhD-authored study may also be more influential than a group with research authored by someone not regarded as following scientific standards (Beckwith, 1996).

John Gaventa (1993), however, critiques both the initiator and the consultant approaches. Because not just material wealth but also intellectual knowledge is power, we need to change both material relations and knowledge relations. Consequently, "to the extent that the research still remains in the hands of the researcher, a real transfer of ownership of knowledge may not have occurred. The dichotomy between those who produce knowledge and those who are most affected by it still exists. Eventually, the researcher may decide to leave, taking the skills, experience, and newly acquired knowledge along with him or her" (pp. 33–34).

The Collaborator

The Policy Research Action Group (PRAG) in Chicago (see, for example, PRAG, 2008, and Appendix L) pioneered the practice of *collaborative research* (Nyden, Figert, Shibley, & Burrows, 1997). In this approach, "it is recognized that the researcher may have certain technical expertise and the community leader may have knowledge of community needs and perspectives. Rather than either side using these resources to gain control in a research relationship, they need to be combined to provide a more unitary approach to research" (Nyden & Wiewel, 1992, p. 45). In contrast to those who fear that CBPR practitioners might further disempower the community, the PRAG model wonders if CBPR sometimes makes the researcher subservient to the community, and thus less useful than he or she might otherwise be.

But collaboration is hard. Rahman (1991) worries that it is not easy to establish a truly equal relationship at the outset with people who are traditionally victims of a dominating structure. Community members are not used to the "talk" world of academics, and they are often skeptical of it. And real collaboration takes a lot of time—for meetings, for accountability processes, for working through the inevitable conflicts—a commodity that may be in especially short supply for community group members. The collaborative approach may be less efficient than the consultant approach in that it asks community members to participate in ways they are not interested in or do not have time for. Patricia

Maguire (1987) reminds us, "While researchers may be able to invest their total work time in a [CBPR] project, participants continue their regular life activities" (p. 46). But does collaborative participation go far enough in changing existing knowledge relations? If the collaboration generates new knowledge and understanding for both community members and academics, then perhaps so, but if the collaboration is just each group doing what it does best, then maybe not.

RECOMMENDATIONS FOR THE ACADEMIC

The three CBPR approaches available to academics—initiator, consultant, and collaborator—seem unsatisfactory and fraught with tensions. The problem, however, is not with the approaches but with a conception that CBPR is a research project. It's not. It is a social change project of which the research is only one piece. As such, it has three goals:

- Learning knowledge and skills relevant to the task at hand
- Developing relationships of solidarity
- Engaging in action that wins victories and builds self-sufficiency

"Doing research" is not, in itself, a goal. Research is only a method to achieve these broader goals. And that is where the crux of the issue lies. One way to get unstuck from thinking about CBPR as primarily research is to work from a project-based model. The project-based model (Stoecker, 2005) starts with diagnosing a social issue or problem—what is the cause of the problem or issue, whom does it affect and how, and what is its history? The next step is to develop a prescription—a new policy or practice or program. Then the group implements the prescription and, finally, starts the process of evaluating its effectiveness. At each stage of this four-step process there are information issues. The diagnosis stage may require a needs assessment or asset mapping. The prescription stage may require policy analysis or a best practices study. The implementation stage may or may not have research, but sometimes, as in a community theater project, the actual program also requires some research to make it happen. And the evaluation, of course, is research intensive, though in a project-based context the evaluation is done to improve the program, not to report to outsiders. Note, however, that no research is done outside of the context of the social change focus itself, and no research is even designed until the group has some basic understanding of what changes it wants to create.

In this project-based model, then, the researcher role is only one of many, and we need to consider the other roles that make for successful CBPR.

Roles in Social Change

Achieving the social change goals of CBPR requires that four roles be fulfilled: leader or *animator,* community organizer, popular educator, and participatory researcher.

Part translator, part facilitator, part self-esteem builder, the leader's role may be the most general and combines parts of the other roles, but in essence the leader is an indigenous or adopted community member who helps people develop a sense that they and their issues are important. For Rahman (1991), this *animator* has "a sense of commitment and a desire to live and work in the villages; innovativeness in work and a willingness to experiment with new approaches; communication skills, in particular the ability to dialogue, discuss and listen to the people; flexibility and a readiness to learn from one's own and others' experiences; and intellectual ability and emotional maturity" (p. 96).

The community organizer, a role many associate with Saul Alinsky (1946/1969, 1971; see also Beckwith & Lopez, 1997), is often confused with the researcher in CBPR—devaluing organizer skills and misleading academics as to what the real tasks are. Two important CBPR authors describe researchers in ways that better fit the community organizer. Ernie Stringer (2007) portrays the "researcher" as a catalyst who stimulates people rather than imposes on them, emphasizes process over product, enables people to do things themselves, starts where people are, helps people plan and act and evaluate (rather than advocates for them), and focuses on human development as well as solutions to problems. Peter Park (1993) says that a community's "sense of the problem may not always be externalized as a consensually derived and objectified target of attack in the community, although there may be suffering, a sense of malaise and frustration, and anger. For this reason, the situation characteristically requires outside intervention in the guise of a researcher . . . to help formulate an identifiable problem to be tackled" (p. 8). The tragedy of conflating the organizer and researcher roles, which I have painfully learned, is that only a few academics are good organizers. Those trained in the 1960s social movements have real organizing skills. Those of us not trained in active mobilizations know *how* to do research. But we only know *about* organizing. I am among the latter group—too young to have gotten on-the-job training and too geographically isolated from the good organizing efforts out there today. My most successful CBPR experiences, then, have been working with those who are good organizers (Stoecker, 1999; Stoecker & Beckwith, 1992).

The popular educator, discussed earlier, facilitates the learning process. This is not a teacher who is assumed to have knowledge that he or she gives to people who are assumed to be ignorant. Rather, it is a facilitator who helps people discover for themselves what they already know and create new knowledge (Freire, 1970; Horton & Freire, 1990; Williams, 1996). As a consequence, people develop greater self-confidence along with greater knowledge. Ideally, in such a setting the expert knowledge of the educator combines with the experiential knowledge of community members, creating entirely new ways of thinking about issues (Fear & Edwards, 1995).

Finally, the participatory researcher knows how to find the references quickly, can construct a survey blindfolded, and can create a research process either with strong guidance from community members or in collaboration with them. The role of participatory researcher in this context is stripped of the other tasks of the initiator approach and is limited to conducting the research. But this role is also about more than being technically skilled. It is also about being committed to transformation of the social relations of knowledge production and to democratic participation in the research process.

One person might occupy multiple roles. For example, a researcher who is a good organizer can be an initiator. Also several people might occupy the same role, especially in the research process, where a variety of people might collectively make research decisions.

Guideposts for the Academic

It is important to understand the relationship between the academic approaches to CBPR (initiator, consultant, collaborator) and the roles in social change (community leader, community organizer, popular educator, participatory researcher). The academic engages with the community as an initiator, a consultant, or a collaborator. In doing so, he or she may fill one or more social change roles. For example, an academic who engages with the community as an initiator may be filling not just the participatory researcher role but perhaps the others as well. An academic who engages as a consultant may need to fill only the participatory researcher role.

We should ask three questions whenever we enter a CBPR situation, to help us determine which of the approaches (initiator, consultant, or collaborator) fits the community best. The answers will depend on whether one is working with an organized community or an unorganized community (Maguire, 1993).

What Is This CBPR Project Trying to Do? Some CBPR projects begin in a less well-organized community and are actually community-organizing projects—using the research to bring people together and build skills and relationships. The Appalachian Alliance conducted a massive eighty-county, six-state study that continues to inform communizing efforts (Horton, 1993). Yellow Creek Concerned Citizens, fighting toxic industrial waste polluting their water, found that doing their own health survey "gave them a reason and an incentive to call at every household along the fourteen-mile length of the creek, and sit down and discuss with them the problems they were experiencing. [It also] broadened and strengthened the leadership within the group. The prime activists in the health survey were women who became better informed and more vocal and confident through their work with the survey. . . . Now, you have to remember that none of us were trained health scientists, and some of the people who were doing this research had not graduated from high school" (Merrifield, 1993, pp. 78, 80).

If you are entering a less organized, low-resource community, members may not have filled the leader, organizer, educator, and researcher roles. If that is the case, see the discussion of the second question, What are your skills? Because depending on which social change roles are already filled and which ones can be filled by others, you may find yourself occupying the rest. Less organized communities, when they lack members who can fill the roles of leader, educator, organizer, and researcher, need an initiator researcher. These situations are the most difficult for the academic to enter, because they require so many skills beyond simply doing research.

Some projects create special difficulties. A coalition, in its early stages, is no different from any other relatively unorganized community, even if its individual member organizations are stable. Complications also arise with service organizations. If the research project is to "study" the service population but the only people making decisions are service providers, it violates the most fundamental characteristic of CBPR—that the people affected help to control the research.

Other CBPR projects may come from already well-organized communities that realize they need research to achieve their goals. For instance, I received a call from a neighborhood group concerned about outside landlords' and real estate agents' attempts to transform their neighborhood so that fewer residents would be homeowners and more would be student renters. The group wanted to document how many rental houses the neighborhood had. They had done the research themselves and sought technical advice only on their research process. In this situation the consultant researcher approach fit well, as the group did not need ongoing assistance.

What Are Your Skills? Researchers with good organizing skills can potentially walk into any community so long as they are aware of the basic issues confronting any organizer, such as whether the organizer has insider or outsider status, is sponsored or invited, and understands the preexisting community members' skills and leaders. Researchers with organizer skills can practice an initiator approach in less organized communities, helping people define their needs and organizing action research projects to fill those needs.

If those are not your skills, however, be critically reflective of yourself and the community and ask:

- How organized is this community?
- To what extent are the functional roles of leader, organizer, educator, and researcher filled?
- To what extent can the unfilled social change roles be filled by others?
- Which of the unfilled social change roles can I play?

If you are only comfortable researching, then you are probably limited to a consultant approach and are thus limited to working only with well-organized communities. Be wary of communities with lots of internal conflict or weak organizational structures unless there are others who are effective at filling the other roles (Simonson & Bushaw, 1993). If you are not good at facilitating discussion in the classroom, you will not be good at it on the streets either. Communicating abstract academic ideas so that people think about their practical implications, discussing research in a way that helps people organize action, and helping people build confidence in their own knowledge are special skills indeed.

If you are comfortable with the leader and popular educator roles, then you may use the collaboration approach. Here also, be wary of less well-organized groups, because any group needs some degree of organization to collaborate. Interpreting and communicating with a diverse membership is also central to the collaborator approach and can occur only after the academic has been "adopted" into the community. In contrast to the researcher's stance in traditional research, "going native" is the most desirable condition in CBPR. True collaboration may even mean dramatically altering the character of the research, as tastes for research differ, and you may find yourself doing theater, storytelling, and other forms of creative education (Comstock & Fox, 1993).

There are other skill issues to be aware of. First, are there some kinds of research you are good at and others that you are not? CBPR has a habit of changing midstream, sometimes requiring dramatic shifts in the research process. When I began researching Toledo philanthropic foundations for a neighborhood coalition, I expected to do interviews but found myself copying numbers from poorly microfiched foundation tax returns. Second, how are your writing skills? Academics are often asked to write, both because a PhD author is still seen as having credibility in some quarters and because academics are seen as having time and writing skills. But if your writing looks like a journal article, no one will read it, and no one will use it. In a participatory evaluation project I recently facilitated, I wrote the group's final report using framed sidebars, varied fonts, graphics, and other magazine-like qualities. Group members told me it helped them actually read the report.

Third, what are your time constraints? Deadlines in the real world are not like those in academia. Missing a deadline means missing a grant opportunity, missing a government hearing, missing a legislative vote. You cannot make up those kinds of misses, and you cannot get extensions. And consistent with Saul Alinsky's (1971) rules of community organizing, a CBPR project that drags on is a drag. Find out ahead of time what the group's deadlines are, and either commit to them or stay out of the project. And remember, there's no spring break in the real world.

How Much Research Participation Does the Community Need and Want? This may be the most contentious issue in CBPR today. Rahman's (1991) and Gaventa's (1993) concern that we change the social relations of both material production and knowledge production must be heeded. At the same time, we must worry that overemphasizing participation can undermine the need to act quickly and forcefully.

For well-organized communities with a sense of empowerment that are moving on an issue, participation in every aspect of the research may not make sense. Often these groups could do their own research but have more important things to do. Having an outside academic facilitate and even do the research does not hinder community members from learning new skills and does not maintain knowledge inequality. In these cases, a consultant approach may be perfectly acceptable. In cases where the research will be ongoing, a collaborator approach may be more desirable. An initiator approach will likely not work because an outsider academic pushing an agenda will be seen as an attempt to undermine the community.

With less organized communities, the research process is also a community-organizing process. In these cases, participation must be organized and maximized. If there are no organizers available and the researcher has organizer skills, the initiator researcher approach may be appropriate. It is extremely important, however, that the initiator researcher strictly follow good organizer practice that builds community control as the project progresses and makes the research serve the community organizing.

There are mixed cases, however, where it is less clear what to do. Those difficult middle cases, where there is some degree of organization and a looming deadline, often require a trade-off between efficiency and democracy, which is no different from the tension between democracy and efficiency that affects any community-organizing or development project (Stoecker, 1994). My former colleagues and I found this in a CBPR project building a community network in Toledo, Ohio (Stoecker & Stuber, 1999). As the grant deadline approached, we had to decide whether to fill in some blanks with less participation than we wanted or miss the deadline. We chose to fill in the blanks, building in opportunities for later participation in the event the grant arrived. Another even more difficult case arises when the researcher does most of the project when the target population cannot participate. This is especially the case with undocumented populations who have no rights of assembly to meet or attend demonstrations and who cannot be safely identified in the research process (Hondagneu-Sotelo, 1993).

The most important thing is for communities to consciously choose which decision points to control and which to let a researcher control. These decision points are

- Defining the research question
- Designing the research
- Implementing the research design
- Analyzing the research data
- Reporting the research results
- Acting on the research results

The community must always define the research question. The academic can use an initiator approach to help develop the question, perhaps by surveying the community's information needs, but should not choose the question itself.

The academic can design the research, but community involvement in this step can prevent many a foolish decision. When my colleagues and I developed an eight-page survey for community groups as part of an Internet access study, our community participants pointed out that anything over two pages would be ignored.

Community involvement in implementing the design will serve only two specific objectives—to help individuals build specific skills and to help them build relationships with one another. If the research process will not also be a community-organizing process, it may be more effective for the researcher to do the research. Also, as other contributors to this volume make clear, community involvement in implementing the design can significantly lengthen the time it takes to collect data, since the individuals carrying out the research may need extensive training. The only unsuccessful CBPR project I have been involved in was one in which community members conducted interviews without any training or preparation for that role. We were working with a neighborhood whose members spoke predominantly Spanish, and neither of us researchers was a strong Spanish speaker, so we used our small grant to pay community members to interview each other. We were unprepared for the social stresses that prevented them from completing the interviews quickly and for the problems created by lack of training. In retrospect, providing training for community team members in interviewing techniques and in coping with the social stresses they experienced, though adding to the project's timetable, would have increased the quality of data collected while also addressing CBPR's commitment to individual and community capacity building (see Chapter Three).

Analyzing the data, if it cannot be done collaboratively, should at least be done with strict accountability to the community. One method is to present or show rough drafts of the analysis to community members, who can then modify the findings and interject new data. Even in my graduate school research of the Cedar-Riverside neighborhood, I quickly learned that I got more information from people's reactions to my written reports than I did from the original interviews.

Who should take responsibility for reporting the results is another tricky issue. There may be a strategic purpose, as I have noted, for having "PhD" on the cover of the report. But many communities are also very concerned that academics not use community research to enhance their own careers. Some communities demand ownership of the data and the results, whereas others have little concern about this. But you should at least talk with the community about issues of authorship in the event that they have not thought about it. Never attempt to publish an article from the research without the community's permission.

Organizing action can be the weakest part of a CBPR project, often because the researcher sees the project as research rather than as community organizing and the roles of leader, educator, and organizer have been neglected. But this phase is also the most important part of the project, and another one where community control is paramount. A researcher who is a good organizer can help the community think about what strategies and tactics might be possible, but the community has to make strategic and tactical choices based on what its members can and are willing to do.

There are cases where the academic is irrelevant and where we can do little or nothing to contribute to a community project. But neither should we sell ourselves short. Even where the academic is not needed, you may be able to help by documenting the struggle so that others may learn from it. As a graduate student academic in Cedar-Riverside, I was of little use to the community members who first got me thinking about CBPR. I had no expert knowledge in anything that they did not have more of. I ended up being relevant, however, in documenting the neighborhood's struggle and spreading the word of what happened so that the neighborhood could remember itself and others could adapt its model.

Finally, this chapter is written by an academic speaking mostly to other academics. In Exhibit 6.1, Dave Beckwith offers recommendations for academics who want to help.

The last may be the most important. We academics, so concerned with doing the right thing and so trained to evaluate everything from every angle before we act, often end up paralyzed. If we have real respect for the communities we work with, we will

---

EXHIBIT 6.1 **An Organizer's Recommendations for Academics**

- Be quick.
- Listen.
- Don't just listen, participate.
- Know the sources.
- Use your priestly power for good.
- Be creative.
- Use people.
- Help us get ahead of the curve.
- Look to all your work for opportunities to help.
- *Pecca fortiter* ("sin bravely")!

Source: Beckwith, 1996.

understand that they will tell us when we make mistakes, and they will not let us lead them astray. We must learn from our own mistakes and successes, but if we are doing CBPR in the right way, our mistakes and successes will both be shared. And that is the comfort, ultimately, of being relevant.

SUMMARY

Academically trained researchers wanting to increase their relevance in the "real world" of community may find in CBPR a promising avenue for doing so. But the road is bumpy and fraught with obstacles, and time, commitment, and a willingness to acknowledge one's mistakes and missteps must prevail. Above all, though, academics must be comfortable admitting how much they don't know—and how much they have to learn by collaborating with the community.

That collaboration can take one of several forms, with the outside researcher as initiator, consultant, or true collaborator. But regardless of the role taken, the academic must realize that CBPR is first and foremost about social change; research is just one part of a much larger whole. With that in mind, and with an attitude of humility and real respect for how much the community has to teach us, CBPR can indeed be an exhilarating path.

QUESTIONS FOR DISCUSSION

1. The author discusses three roles for academics in CBPR: the initiator, the consultant, and the collaborator. Some have argued, though, that the consultant role may not qualify as appropriate in "true" CBPR.

   a. Where do you stand in this argument, and how would you defend your position?

   b. Have you played any of these roles in the context of community-based research?

   c. If not, which role(s) might you be comfortable playing and under what circumstances?

2. The author writes that CBPR is not simply a research project, but rather "a social change project of which the research is only one piece." Others, for example Shawna L. Mercer, Lawrence Green, and their colleagues (see Appendix C), suggest that the goals of CBPR may be "education and taking action *or* effecting change" (emphasis added) indicating that social change need *not* necessarily be part of every CBPR endeavor. What might some convincing arguments be on either side of this debate?

3. This chapter ends with community organizer Dave Beckwith's (1996) list of recommendations for academics who want to help. Please review the list, shown in Exhibit 6.1.

   a. Is there anything you would add? Anything you would subtract or change?

   b. The chapter author offers his view that the last item on the list, "*pecca fortiter* ('sin bravely')!" may be the most important because "[w]e academics, so concerned with doing the right thing and so trained to evaluate everything from every angle before we act, often end up paralyzed." Do you agree? And how would you defend your position?

KEY TERMS

Community research
Initiator
Collaborator

Social change
Community organizing

REFERENCES

Alinsky, S. D. (1969). *Reveille for radicals.* New York: Vintage Books. (Original work published 1946)

Alinsky, S. D. (1971). *Rules for radicals.* New York: Vintage Books.

Beckwith, D. (1996). Ten ways to work together: An organizer's view. *Sociological Imagination, 33,* 164–172.

Beckwith, D., & Lopez, C. (1997). *Community organizing: People power from the grassroots.* COMM-ORG: The On-Line Conference on Community Organizing and Development. Retrieved Mar. 17, 2006, from http://comm-org.utoledo.edu/papers97/beckwith.htm.

Brown, L. D., & Tandon, R. (1983). Ideology and political economy in inquiry: Action research and participatory research. *Journal of Applied Behavioral Science, 19*(3), 277–294.

Brydon-Miller, M. (1993). Accessibility self-advocacy at an independent living center: A participatory research approach. In P. Park, M. Brydon-Miller, B. L. Hall, & T. Jackson (Eds.), *Voices of change: Participatory research in the United States and Canada* (pp. 125–143). Westport, CT: Bergin & Garvey.

Cancian, F. M. (1993). Conflicts between activist research and academic success: Participatory research and alternative strategies. *American Sociologist, 24,* 92–106.

Comstock, D. E., & Fox, R. (1993). Participatory research as critical theory: The North Bonneville, USA, experience. In P. Park, M. Brydon-Miller, B. L. Hall, & T. Jackson (Eds.), *Voices of change: Participatory research in the United States and Canada* (pp. 103–124). Westport, CT: Bergin & Garvey.

de Roux, G. I. (1991). Together against the computer: PAR and the struggle of Afro-Colombians for public services. In O. Fals-Borda & M. A. Rahman (Eds.), *Action and knowledge: Breaking the monopoly with participatory action research* (pp. 37–53). New York: Apex Press.

Deshler, D., & Ewert, M. (1995). *Participatory action research: Traditions and major assumptions.* Ithaca, NY: Cornell Participatory Action Research Network.

Fear, K., & Edwards, P. (1995). Building a democratic learning community within a PDS. *Teaching Education, 7*(2), 12–24.

Freire, P. (1970). *Pedagogy of the oppressed.* New York: Seabury Press.

Gaventa, J. (1991). Toward a knowledge democracy: Viewpoints on participatory research in North America. In O. Fals-Borda & M. A. Rahman (Eds.), *Action and knowledge: Breaking the monopoly with participatory action research* (pp. 121–133). New York: Apex Press.

Gaventa, J. (1993). The powerful, the powerless, and the experts: Knowledge struggles in an information age. In P. Park, M. Brydon-Miller, B. L. Hall, & T. Jackson (Eds.), *Voices of change: Participatory research in the United States and Canada* (pp. 21–40). Westport, CT: Bergin & Garvey.

Gedicks, A. (1996). Activist sociology: Personal reflections. *Sociological Imagination, 33,* 55–72.

Hall, B. L. (1993). Introduction. In P. Park, M. Brydon-Miller, B. L. Hall, & T. Jackson (Eds.), *Voices of change: Participatory research in the United States and Canada* (pp. xiii–xxii). Westport, CT: Bergin & Garvey.

Heaney, T. W. (1993). "If you can't beat 'em, join 'em": The professionalization of participatory research. In P. Park, M. Brydon-Miller, B. L. Hall, & T. Jackson (Eds.), *Voices of change: Participatory research in the United States and Canada* (pp. 41–46). Westport, CT: Bergin & Garvey.

Hondagneu-Sotelo, P. (1993). Why advocacy research? Research and activism with immigrant women. *American Sociologist, 24,* 56–68.

Horton, B. D. (1993). The Appalachian Land Ownership Study: Research and citizen action in Appalachia. In P. Park, M. Brydon-Miller, B. L. Hall, & T. Jackson (Eds.), *Voices of change: Participatory research in the United States and Canada* (pp. 85–102). Westport, CT: Bergin & Garvey.

Horton, M., & Freire, P. (1990). *We make the road by walking: Conversations on education and social change* (B. Bell, J. Gaventa, & J. Peters, Eds.). Philadelphia: Temple University Press.

Hubbard, A. (1996). The activist academic and the stigma of "community housework." *Sociological Imagination, 33,* 73–87.

Maguire, P. (1987). *Doing participatory research: A feminist approach.* Amherst: University of Massachusetts, Center for International Education.

Maguire, P. (1993). Challenges, contradictions, and celebrations: Attempting participatory research as a doctoral student. In P. Park, M. Brydon-Miller, B. L. Hall, & T. Jackson (Eds.), *Voices of change: Participatory research in the United States and Canada* (pp. 157–176). Westport, CT: Bergin & Garvey.

Merrifield, J. (1993). Putting scientists in their place: Participatory research in environmental and occupational health. In P. Park, M. Brydon-Miller, B. L. Hall, & T. Jackson (Eds.), *Voices of change: Participatory research in the United States and Canada* (pp. 65–84). Westport, CT: Bergin & Garvey.

Nyden, P., Figert, A., Shibley, M., & Burrows, D. (Eds.). (1997). *Building community: Social science in action.* Thousand Oaks, CA: Pine Forge Press.

Nyden, P., & Wiewel, W. (1992). Collaborative research: Harnessing the tensions between researcher and practitioner. *American Sociologist, 23*(4), 43–55.

Park, P. (1993). What is participatory research? A theoretical and methodological perspective. In P. Park, M. Brydon-Miller, B. L. Hall, & T. Jackson (Eds.), *Voices of change: Participatory research in the United States and Canada* (pp. 1–20). Westport, CT: Bergin & Garvey.

Policy Research Action Group. (2008). *Policy Research Action Group: Welcome.* Retrieved Apr. 18, 2008, from http://www.luc.edu/curl/prag.

Rahman, M. A. (1991). The theoretical standpoint of PAR. In O. Fals-Borda & M. A. Rahman (Eds.), *Action and knowledge: Breaking the monopoly with participatory action research* (pp. 13–23). New York: Apex Press.

Reason, P. (1994). Three approaches to participative inquiry. In N. K. Denzin & Y. S. Lincoln (Eds.), *Handbook of qualitative research* (pp. 324–339). Thousand Oaks, CA: Sage.

Simonson, L. J., & Bushaw, V. A. (1993). Participatory action research: Easier said than done. *American Sociologist, 24,* 27–38.

Stoecker, R. (1994). *Defending community: The struggle for alternative redevelopment in Cedar-Riverside.* Philadelphia: Temple University Press.

Stoecker, R. (1997). The imperfect practice of collaborative research: The "Working Group on Neighborhoods" in Toledo, OH. In P. Nyden, A. Figert, M. Shibley, & D. Burrows (Eds.), *Building community: Social science in action* (pp. 219–225). Thousand Oaks, CA: Pine Forge Press.

Stoecker, R. (1999). Making connections: Community organizing, empowerment planning, and participatory research in participatory evaluation. *Sociological Practice, 1,* 209–232.

Stoecker, R. (2001). *Community-based research: The next new thing.* Retrieved May 28, 2007, from http://comm-org.utoledo.edu/drafts/cbrreportb.htm.

Stoecker, R. (2005). *Research methods for community change: A project-based approach.* Thousand Oaks, CA: Sage.

Stoecker, R., & Beckwith, D. (1992). Advancing Toledo's neighborhood movement through participatory action research: Integrating activist and academic approaches. *Clinical Sociology Review, 10,* 198–213.

Stoecker, R., & Stuber, A.C.S. (1999). Building an information superhighway of one's own: A comparison of two approaches. *Research in Politics and Society, 7,* 291–309.

Stringer, E. T. (2007). *Action research* (3rd ed.). Thousand Oaks, CA: Sage.

Williams, L. (1996). First enliven, then enlighten: Popular education and the pursuit of social justice. *Sociological Imagination, 33,* 94–116.

CHAPTER

7

CBPR WITH CAMBODIAN GIRLS IN LONG BEACH, CALIFORNIA

A CASE STUDY

ANN CHEATHAM-ROJAS & EVELINE SHEN

Note: We would like to acknowledge and thank HOPE members Theary Chhay, Rotha Dom, Sothavy Meas, Ra Rok, Cheath Monica Ching, Mary Im, Molica Pov-Meas, Socheata Sun, Sophea Lun, Sothearith Chhay, and the many other HOPE members who contributed to this work. Thanks also go to Gina Acebo, Que Dang, Judy Han, Diep Tran, Betty Hung, Sopharn Lun, Rina Mehta, and Karen Chan. Many other individuals, groups, and organizations offered support that was essential to the success of this project, including the Cambodian Association of America, United Cambodian Community, Mount Carmel Cambodian Center, Cambodian Association of America, Student Leaders Against Sexual Harassment, Californians for Justice, California State University, Long Beach, Long Beach Sexual Assault and Crisis Agency, National Institute of Environmental Health Sciences, Khemara Buddhikaram Cambodian Buddhist Temple, Joanne O'Bryne, Doris Kagin, Francis Calpotura, Meredith Minkler, Leonard Syme, Dawn Phillips, Bobbie Smith, Jenny Oropeza, Alan Lowenthal, and Betty Karnette.

THE PAST DECADE has seen growing appreciation of the potential of youths for active involvement in critically analyzing and helping to address complex health and social issues, including violence, deteriorating schools, HIV/AIDS, substance abuse, and reproductive health (Checkoway, Dobbie, & Richards-Schuster, 2003; Wallerstein, Sanchez, & Velarde, 2005; Wilson et al., 2007). Increasingly, moreover, these partnership efforts with youths employ strengths-based approaches in which youths are helped to recognize and further develop their own assets as critical thinkers and problem solvers (Amsden & VanWynsberghe, 2005; Cargo, Grams, Ottoson, Ward, & Green, 2003; Ozer et al., 2008; Wilson et al., 2007). The Long Beach community-based participatory research project on sexual harassment, mounted by Asian Communities for Reproductive Justice (ACRJ), formerly known as Asians and Pacific Islanders for Reproductive Health, was one such project, with a goal of having project research and organizing driven by young people themselves, by youths with the power to make important decisions and take action into their own hands. These youths were not helping the project but developing it themselves, within a defined structure and theoretical framework.

This chapter will first describe ACRJ and its Health, Opportunities, Problem-Solving, and Empowerment (HOPE) projects and then discuss the community-based participatory research (CBPR) process that took place in Long Beach, California, as HOPE members worked to study and address the problem of sexual harassment. Following a look at the theory and principles that guided the project and the context in which it took place, the youths' identification of sexual harassment as an issue they wished to explore and address is described. The research and action components of the project are then discussed, including the policy changes that occurred as a result of this work and the subsequent development by the ACRJ's Long Beach Project of a new, autonomous organization, Khmer Girls in Action. The chapter concludes with a discussion of some of the special challenges of working with youths, especially low-income youths of color, in CBPR; the approaches and strategies that worked best; and lessons for other such projects conducted with and by youths.

ACRJ AND THE HOPE PROJECTS

Asian Communities for Reproductive Justice is a social, political, and economic justice organization fighting for the liberation of Asian and Pacific Islander women and girls in the arena of reproductive justice. ACRJ asserts that a woman experiences reproductive justice when she has the power and resources to make healthy choices for herself and her family at home, at work, in school, and in all other areas of life. This means living in a home free from sexual and physical violence, living and working without fear of sexual harassment, and living without hatred due to sexual identity.

ACRJ's expanded definition of reproductive justice extends to having all forms of work and labor valued and having the right to earn an equitable and livable wage, to eat safe and affordable food, and to determine and gain access to comprehensive health care for oneself and one's family. Finally, it includes the right to have the support and commitment of the government and private institutions for having or not having a child and the right to live in an environment that supports these choices (Asians and Pacific Islanders for Reproductive

Health, 2001). To work toward a world in which women have reproductive justice, ACRJ strives to challenge the different ways in which racism, sexism, patriarchy, and poverty structurally and institutionally affect women's reproductive health and freedom.

Central to ACRJ's early work were two HOPE projects for Southeast Asian girls (aged fourteen to eighteen) in Long Beach and Oakland, California. These projects attempted to address the underlying causes of health, economic, social, and political disparities by building more collective power to hold institutions accountable for practices that affect community health and the quality of life of residents. The four core strategies in the HOPE approach were leadership development, popular education, community-based participatory research, and community building.

The CBPR project described in this chapter was part of the Long Beach HOPE project, which worked exclusively with Cambodian girls. ACRJ decided to work with this population because Asian immigrant refugee communities have some of the nation's highest poverty and welfare rates. Cambodians in the United States are overwhelmingly concentrated in the lowest-paying jobs, and close to 30 percent live in poverty (Reeves & Bennett, 2004). Although figures vary due to underreporting, more than 30,000 Cambodians are believed to live in Long Beach, making up the largest Cambodian community outside Cambodia (Quintiliani & Needlam, 2007). Because many Southeast Asians living in the United States have not yet gained U.S. citizenship and cannot vote, there is a general lack of involvement with mainstream political activity among them. Yet younger members of this population proved ripe for involvement in community organizing and CPBR around an issue of deep personal and collective concern. The CBPR project described in this chapter involved more than forty HOPE members in different capacities for over two years, with five involved through the entire process and fourteen participating for a year or more.

SETTING THE STAGE FOR PARTICIPATORY RESEARCH

The CPBR process in this study was somewhat unusual in that the "outside" researchers, the ACRJ staff, included experienced community organizers and popular educators as well as an academically trained researcher, all of whom were working very closely with the Cambodian community in Long Beach. The staff's roles were to provide theory, political analysis, experience, and technical assistance with research, organizing skills, and perspectives on social movements. Staff provided guidance by asking challenging questions, facilitating training sessions, and employing popular education techniques (described later in this chapter) to help the girls in issue selection and analysis. At the same time, the ACRJ staff members were up front about the fact that the girls had the responsibility and power to make decisions and take actions that would ultimately uphold the values and mission of ACRJ and HOPE. As Margaret Le Compte (1995, p. 91) has argued, "Issues of power, agenda and voice are givens" in collaborative research but must be openly addressed and acknowledged. Dealing explicitly with issues of power in CBPR does not mean that power is always equally shared but rather that power dynamics are not hidden and that efforts at democratizing power take place to the extent possible.

Before beginning the project in Long Beach, ACRJ staff developed a list of values and ideals capturing their vision of CBPR, which would help in providing direction for the process. These values and ideals included using population education and the action-reflection cycle; continually revisiting the problem and tracking its changes; developing checkpoints for success; valuing and encompassing different ways of learning and using accessible language; having staff provide structure, process, and guidance, while knowing that their specific CBPR roles (initiator, consultant, collaborator, and so on; see Chapter Six) would continually change; and teaching the girls to navigate the outside community, academic, and professional realms.

As Barbara Israel and her colleagues note in Chapter Three, the core values and principles associated with CBPR should, ideally, be tailored to the particular group or project. Several core values and guiding principles were established specifically for this project, stating that there would be

- Mutual learning
- An emphasis on the process, not just the outcome
- New definitions of success (making success not solely dependent on the outcome)
- Youth ownership
- Integrity
- Faith that girls can make changes
- Shared authority, accountability, and ownership between HOPE members and ACRJ
- A valuing of every experience (including disappointment)
- Explicit information about the skills and experiences that staff and HOPE members bring
- Opportunities for HOPE members to be trainers

Consistent with these principles, HOPE members were given the support needed to develop a critical understanding of the issues they faced, based on an analysis of their own knowledge and experience. They then used this understanding to develop informal theory and a reproductive justice analysis, to do research, and to take action to change structures that impinged on their reproductive freedom.

Providing Support for the Process

For all HOPE members to undertake the CBPR process effectively, it was essential to have not only their understanding and full commitment but also the support of their parents, extended families, and communities. Several HOPE members found that their families were either apathetic about their participation or hesitant to allow it at all, making full participation impossible. In contrast, members who had the support of their families were much more likely to remain with the project throughout.

HOPE members often needed considerable personal support, beyond that provided by their families, in order to engage effectively in this work. ACRJ staff offered such support, providing tutors, help in talking with teachers about schoolwork and grades, referrals to therapists, and help in getting to doctor's appointments to deal with possible pregnancies and other medical problems that the girls were uncomfortable about dealing with through their families. In one instance ACRJ helped secure a loan for a member's mother so that she could pay the rent and her daughter could continue participating in the program.

The provision of a small stipend for each member helped demonstrate respect and appreciation of her time and work and allowed many to continue with the project at age sixteen, when they might otherwise have been obligated by financial necessity to stop to find employment.

One of the four key strategies of HOPE was community building, which is also a necessary precursor to effective CBPR. ACRJ recognized that expecting the girls to come to numerous meetings and training sessions and to work on research, analysis, and organizing was realistic only if opportunities were also provided for having fun and building trust and relationships within their group. Providing time and space for team-building activities, including cultural events, informal discussions, and other social interaction opportunities (Walter, 2005), helped to energize the HOPE members and to build the motivation and interpersonal trust and support needed to engage effectively in CBPR.

Many different community-building activities occurred prior to and in conjunction with the CBPR project, including writing workshops, potlucks with Cambodian food, team-building games, sleepovers, and "rap sessions." These last proved particularly popular, and a safe environment, with structure and ground rules, was developed within which the girls could share openly about their personal lives.

Training for Participation in CBPR

To facilitate its CBPR work with HOPE, ACRJ created training sessions designed to empower and develop grassroots organizing skills and political analysis and to foster leadership. As described later in this chapter, and consistent with the philosophy of Paulo Freire (1970), popular education lies at the heart of ACRJ's training, and this approach continued throughout the entire participatory research process. Using a Freirian dialogical method, *teacher learners,* in this case ACRJ staff, posed questions to the HOPE members, challenging them to draw on their own knowledge and experience to generate common themes, look at underlying causes and consequences, and come up with action plans for addressing shared concerns.

Emphasizing the feminist principle that "the personal is political" and using reproductive freedom as the core component of the training, ACRJ staff helped HOPE members see the structural and environmental causes of problems rather than internalizing these problems.

To help the members become accustomed to the language and concepts of CBPR before they began their project, for example, staff led discussions of the various ways research is used by society and helped the girls differentiate between being exploited for research purposes and participating to make a contribution to their communities. Members learned about marketing research and about academic and medical research that has hurt people, such as the Tuskegee study in which African American men were denied access to syphilis cures so that scientists could study the long-term consequences of the disease (Thomas & Quinn, 1991). The girls were engaged in dialogue about research in which they had already participated or with which they were familiar and about the ways CBPR differed from more traditional approaches to research. Such dialogue helped the HOPE members develop a clear understanding of why a CBPR process was being employed and what they might gain by using CBPR to study and help bring about change in an area of concern to them.

Training sessions were also held to help HOPE members understand the differences between reproductive health and reproductive justice. The impact of war and violence in Cambodia on their mothers and grandmothers; unsafe conditions in the garment industry, in which many of their mothers worked; racial profiling in the welfare-to-work system; and stereotypes of Asian women as exotic, passive, obedient, and quiet were discussed as social factors affecting Cambodian girls and women, and their reproductive freedom, in Long Beach.

Finally, the training sessions also helped place the CBPR work the members were going to begin in the context of community organizing and social movements and offered skill building in community organizing and in understanding power and power relationships. One session used the particularly effective tool of the *power flower* (see Figure 7.1). During this training session, each girl looked at a copy of the flower power and colored in both the outer petals that represented categories in which she was in the dominant group and the inner petals that represented categories in which she was not in the dominant group. Through a series of follow-up questions, the girls were helped to understand the areas in which they did and did not have power, both individually and as a group. They

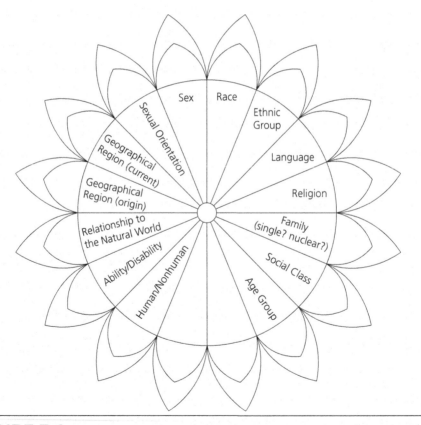

FIGURE 7.1 *The Power Flower*
Source: Arnold, Burke, James, Martin, & Thomas, 1991, p.13. Reprinted with permission.

were asked to imagine how the world would be different if everyone had a chance to hold power and to discuss what happens when people who hold a lot of power abuse it (through racist or homophobic acts, for example).

The power flower proved particularly valuable once the girls had selected and begun working on their issue (sexual harassment) and helped them avoid self-blame for situations that they now realized reflected broader power dynamics. This training also encouraged them to view various types of oppression as interlocking and introduced the important contributions of feminist and antiracist scholars (Collins, 2000; hooks, 1989) in furthering understanding in this area.

IDENTIFYING SEXUAL HARASSMENT AS AN ISSUE

As noted earlier, the issue identification process employed by ACRJ involves the use of popular education strategies to help members talk about their individual lives and then collectivize those experiences as they begin to see that many of their individual difficulties share the same societal roots. In addition, and in accord with the ideas of Charlotte Bunch (1983) and Lee Staples (2004), who point out that a good issue is one that fits within a broader social agenda, ACRJ staff facilitated the issue selection process with attention to ACRJ's explicit agenda for reproductive justice. Staff provided a structure of analysis, theory, coaching, facilitation, and resources so that members could consider the various issues they were concerned about in terms of, among other things, whether and how they fit within this broad structure.

Numerous other criteria were used in issue selection. These included a potential issue's ability to challenge traditional gender (or racial or class or other) divisions of labor and social roles, to stimulate leadership development among low-income Asian and Pacific Islander girls, to assert a new perspective on who gets defined as an expert and whose voices get heard, and to influence the understanding and approach to social change of Asian and Pacific Islanders and of progressive social movements and organizations.

The issue of sexual harassment, which became the central focus of the CBPR process, was an ideal one from ACRJ's perspective: it came from the community, was clearly connected to the organization's broader reproductive justice agenda, and lent itself to a careful analysis of the sociostructural roots of the problem.

Sexual harassment was first discussed when two of the HOPE members told the group of an incident that had occurred in their social studies class as these HOPE members were sharing photos of their recent participation in a demonstration in the state capital. The teacher confiscated the pictures and went on to extensively criticize, to the class, the HOPE program and its activities in Sacramento. The teacher remarked to the two HOPE members, "If those gang-whores and sluts would only keep their jeans on, we would not need abortion programs like yours." Other members of the class who were friends of the girls were then told by the teacher to "write an essay about why bilingual education should not exist."

Critical learning comes from the scrutiny of everyday life (Sohng, 1996). Although the HOPE members did not initially identify this incident as sexual harassment, staff-led dialogue and training helped the girls to identify the racism, sexism, classism, and sexual harassment embedded in this incident. The members were asked to go back to the power flower and think about which petals of the flower the teacher was drawing on when he made the statement about "sluts" and "gang-whores." Using Freirian problem posing, the staff also asked whether there were any equivalent terms to *sluts* and *whores* for men. They also led a decoding of the word *gang* and how it is typically used in reference to young people of color who are poor, reflecting ageism, racism, and classism. Through this process, HOPE members developed a sophisticated analysis of the power dynamics involved in the incident experienced and further understood that the teacher's actions were indeed a potent example of sexual harassment.

As dialogue continued, HOPE members realized that they were being sexually harassed on a daily basis and often blaming themselves for the incidents that occurred. Staff again played a key role in initiating a process that Vio Grossi (1981) has termed *disindoctrination* and that helps people to detach themselves from myths imposed on them by the power structure that keep them from seeing their own oppression.

After additional popular education training sessions that helped the HOPE members understand internalized oppression, the social factors contributing to sexual harassment, and the consequences of such abuse, the girls were eager to move into action. They came up with recommendations for the prevention of further incidents of sexual harassment in the schools and arranged to meet with the school principals and separately with a district superintendent.

Although these meetings failed to get the desired results, subsequent debriefings provided excellent opportunities for the girls to use their critical reflection and analysis skills. For example, one of the principals had commented in the meeting, "I am just like you. I put on my pants the same way, but I am a man and you are a woman." This statement was considered in relation to the power flower, and it became clear that this individual was not just like the HOPE members. He held far more power than the girls on multiple dimensions (including gender, race, and class), in addition to holding a position that granted him final decision-making power for the school he headed.

RESEARCHING THE PROBLEM

For the HOPE members, both the critical reflection process and the failure of the initial meetings to achieve the desired outcomes reinforced the need to move into the next phase of the CBPR process—studying the problem of sexual harassment in greater detail.

Staff posed questions to assist the members in brainstorming what they wanted to learn about sexual harassment, and forty questions emerged. In addition to wishing to learn about the prevalence of such harassment and whether the perpetrators were teachers, staff, or students, HOPE members wanted answers to such questions as these: "How does sexual harassment affect students' ability to learn and participate in school?" "What do students and teachers already know about sexual harassment?" and, "Is sexual harassment related to other health issues, such as sexually transmitted diseases (STDs), depression, pregnancy, drug and alcohol use, and smoking?" The members' earlier training through ACRJ had made them familiar with a variety of research methods, including written surveys, interviews, photojournals, document review, and observation.

As Peter Reason (1994) notes, participatory research may use methods that look more "orthodox," making sense of them from the community perspective. In this instance, the HOPE members decided that written questions would be the most efficient means of getting the most questions answered about their sensitive and important topic.

The members then worked on writing the survey, with technical assistance from staff. An initial brainstorming session, in which members identified many potential ways in which sexual harassment at school could affect students, was particularly helpful in suggesting possible areas for questioning. These areas (for example, possible impacts on mental and physical health, self-esteem, grades, work habits, participation in class, and suicidal thoughts) were among the items explored by the survey.

The HOPE members' insider knowledge of sexual harassment and related issues in their community also enabled them to come up with critical questions that outside researchers would not know to ask. For example, although having someone urinate in front of you is not a form of sexual harassment that is either common knowledge or cited in the literature, it was a critical issue for students in this community. The criteria used by the HOPE members in deciding whether or not to include a survey question were that the question would elicit information helpful to the development of their organizing campaign, would not be repetitive, and would produce new knowledge for future use.

To reduce the possibility of error, the questions about physical and mental health were taken from the Behavioral Risk Factor Surveillance System, which has been in use since 1984. These questions have undergone several reliability and validity studies and been modified accordingly (Centers for Disease Control and Prevention, 2002). In addition to learning about the use of standardized questions like these, the HOPE members learned about pretesting and did their own pretesting of the survey. As a result of what they learned, they shortened the final instrument considerably and eliminated male students from the target population.

The target population for the survey was determined to be female students at the Long Beach high school the HOPE members attended. A nonprobability sample design was used and a quota sample taken. To obtain as large and diverse a group of participants as possible, the HOPE members placed themselves in strategic locations throughout the high school to distribute the survey. Completed surveys were returned by more than four hundred girls, or more than 25 percent of the target population.

Although ACRJ staff had anticipated that the HOPE members themselves would be heavily involved in the subsequent data analysis stage of the project, the data collection had been so labor intensive that the girls wanted a break. Indeed, an important staff role at this point and other points involved reminding the HOPE members how much they had accomplished through their work to date, having them think about what would be lost if they gave up, and engaging them in the kind of community-building activities that could help balance their task-oriented work with attention to their more social needs (Walter, 2005). By agreeing to analyze the data themselves, ACRJ staff were both respecting the wishes of the HOPE members and providing the break they had desired.

The HOPE members did let staff know, however, the forms of data they wanted from the survey for use in the subsequent organizing phase of the project. The survey results provided strong evidence of the nature and widespread scope of the sexual harassment that HOPE members had so often personally experienced. Some highlights of the survey findings were that over 87 percent of those surveyed had experienced sexual harassment. Sixteen percent had been harassed by a teacher or staff person, 54 percent did not know that a grievance procedure existed or how to file a complaint about sexual harassment, and 35 percent talked less in class because of sexual harassment. Although there was a possibility of bias due to the nonprobability design of the survey, the analysis of findings suggested a possible association between sexual harassment and health and also between sexual harassment and the ability to learn and succeed in school.

MOVING INTO ACTION

With the survey work complete, the focus of the CBPR work turned to action for social change, within the conceptual framework of ACRJ's unique organizing theory. In addition to emphasizing the centrality of culture and identity and seeing political education as crucial to the support of strategic organizing and development, this theory stresses that framing and reframing ideas is a main goal of the organizing and CBPR process. Sexual harassment was thus framed as an issue of school safety for girls, healthy sexuality, equitable education, environmental justice, and reproductive justice.

The most effective direct action organized by HOPE to reduce sexual harassment was the Community Forum on School Safety. In preparation for this event, at which HOPE members would release their study results and their recommendations for action, visits to allies were made by HOPE members and staff to ask these allies to cosponsor the forum, sign on to the platform of recommendations, speak at the event, and contribute money. Actively building a large base of partners in this way enabled the forum to become a venue for reframing the moral and practical dimensions of sexual harassment.

Families and friends of HOPE members, community members, and more than twenty representatives of community organizations attended the forum. In addition the attendees included two Long Beach school board members, the principals of the girls' high school, the Long Beach School District superintendent, a representative of the state legislature, a representative of the city council, and reporters from the mass media.

As planned, HOPE members used the forum to release the dramatic results of their survey and, with support of ACRJ staff, to present their tenets, or recommendations, for ensuring a safe learning environment for girls in Long Beach. These tenets were that all students have the right to a safe learning environment not compromised by gender discrimination, that eliminating sexual harassment should be a priority in order to ensure girls' right to learn in a safe school environment, that a more student-friendly grievance procedure should be adopted and publicized, and that training on sexual harassment should be instituted for teachers and students.

The forum was successful in shining a spotlight on and reframing the issue of student safety with a gender focus. In their media advocacy, HOPE members and their ACRJ staff supporters were also able to link their issues with the heightened concern over school safety as a result of the Columbine, Colorado, school shootings in April 1999. Releases to the press therefore included such statements as this: "Students, parents, and community members want to see an effective response to sexual harassment, a threat just as real to girls' safety as guns, drugs, and gangs. This is a real danger to female students, and we want to see some accountability."

School officials adopted every one of the recommendations advocated by the HOPE members and their allies. The following fall, all 4,500 students at the high school were required to watch a video on sexual harassment during preregistration, and all were given educational materials about students' rights with respect to sexual harassment. Antiharassment posters designed and produced by HOPE members were displayed in almost every classroom and in many public spaces throughout the school, and a student-friendly version of the sexual harassment grievance procedure was provided to all students.

On a broader level a community advisory board, including representatives of the school district and of local community groups, was formed to work on issues of sexual harassment in the Long Beach schools. As a result of the board's work, training on sexual harassment is provided to all tenth-grade health classes, teachers now receive in-service training on sexual harassment, peer counselors are getting training on how to counsel students who are sexually harassed, and a mechanism has been developed to monitor and address incidents of sexual harassment. Successful efforts to make these changes effective districtwide were indeed a major outcome of the project.

ACRJ also has increased its work on the national level through EMERJ (Expanding the Movement for Empowerment and Reproductive Justice), a national initiative to build and strengthen the reproductive justice movement. Launched in January 2007, EMERJ is increasing coordination and collaboration among reproductive justice groups across the country and improving their strategic planning efforts. EMERJ is designed to build a strong and vibrant reproductive justice movement that in the long term is capable of (1) organizing people, money and information; (2) shifting people's worldview and ideology; (3) shifting policy; and (4) shifting public perception and public will. Through these various developments, ACRJ has contributed to the fight for reproductive justice on the local, state, and national levels.

KHMER GIRLS IN ACTION: A YOUTH-LED ORGANIZATION IS BORN

In 2001, the Long Beach Project of ACRJ spun off from ACRJ and became a separate organization, Khmer Girls in Action (KGA). KGA's mission is to contribute to the movement for social, economic, and political justice by building a strong, progressive, and sustainable community institution led by Southeast Asian women and girls. KGA believes that the most effective way to create sustainable, ongoing change in a community is to support and foster the self-determination of its members. An important part of its mission is, in fact, to "challenge the ideology that Asian women cannot be leaders in this struggle" (KGA, 2008). KGA actively pursues its mission through three "core strategies: leadership development, community organizing, and cultural production. All of KGA's programming components foster and encourage analysis of gender, class, race, sexuality, and culture." Further, and again in its own words, KGA "engages members to develop organizing strategies that are sensitive to the cultural and political conditions of Southeast

Asian communities" (KGA, 2008). While continuing to address reproductive health and justice, KGA also puts a heavy accent on immigrant and refugee rights and "cultural production," through which members document their community history and experiences and then draw on this background to help bring about change. As suggested previously, although much of KGA's work is with and by Cambodian girls and women, the organization also emphasizes the importance of broader community partnerships (KGA, 2008). KGA worked with numerous other organizations, for example, to defeat a November 2006 state ballot initiative that would have required parental consent for abortions.

LESSONS LEARNED

Although the CBPR case study described in this chapter was clearly a success, a number of important lessons were learned along the way that in retrospect could have further increased project effectiveness. For example, the dearth of social justice groups in Long Beach and the fact that the youth culture in that community did not include activism or social change work suggests that it might have been helpful early in the process to bring in other groups that do organizing with youths. Such groups from the Los Angeles area could have provided a much needed sense of support for the members. Forging such connections might also have given the members other people to turn to during hard times or when they just wanted more local advice, particularly from other youths engaged in this kind of work.

It would also have been more effective to have a senior organizer who was local, understood the community, and had experience running organizing campaigns, rather than having a consultant from ACRJ's Northern California office fill the organizer role. Although ACRJ's position as an Asian and Pacific Islander–focused feminist organization was clearly important, this experience underscored ACRJ's need for a larger pool of trained and culturally competent organizers, familiar with CBPR, who could undertake such work in their own locales.

Lessons were also learned about the need to plan for attrition, particularly in work with youths. This entire CBPR process took two years. Although five members were involved from beginning to end, many others played important roles for shorter time periods. It would have been helpful to plan for attrition from the beginning and to recruit more people initially to prevent loss of momentum when key individuals had to leave the project.

ACRJ also learned from this process that youths need to feel that their work is connected to that of other youths and to see it moving forward. The importance of being shown and reminded of the results of one's work in order to foster continued engagement has been stressed in community organizing and CBPR in many venues (see, for example, Staples, 2004; El-Askari & Walton, 2005). But as this case study suggests, it may be particularly important in work with youths. In addition, as noted earlier, young people, more than other community members in CBPR efforts, may need a great deal of one-on-one work and support that ensures their personal needs are met so they can continue to participate in the project. Learning to maintain balance in the provision of such resources is a critical and ongoing challenge for adults engaged with youths in CBPR and related activities (Checkoway, Dobbie, & Richards-Schuster, 2003; Wallerstein, Sanchez, & Velarde, 2005; Wilson et al., 2007).

In a conservative community like Long Beach, in which organizing is not a part of the culture, the heightened importance of building allies and being well prepared in advance of meetings and events was also underscored. In this project the conservative school administration was not prepared for an organizing effort involving important elements of the community and the mass media. Administrators were caught off guard, and this appeared to contribute to the HOPE members' and allies' successes in getting their recommendations for change accepted. Thinking ahead about the kind of culture that exists where CBPR is being attempted is critical, because this culture will affect the types of support needed for community-based participatory research.

With some important exceptions, such as work done in the context of the National Black Women's Health Project (2008), the reproductive rights movement has been heavily white and middle class (Rosen, 2000). An important lesson learned from this case study is that in order to involve women of color, low-income women, or youths, it is necessary to discover people's self-interests and their community's interests. Done correctly, CBPR can be an ideal avenue for surfacing and acting on these interests. Within the reproductive rights movement, CBPR that truly "starts where the people are" will require working on a variety of issues beyond access to abortion.

SUMMARY

A traditional approach to improving the reproductive health of Cambodian youths in Long Beach might have been to provide sex education, abstinence promotion, or free condoms. The CBPR process described in this case study involved going considerably deeper to enable youths in the community to identify, study, and address the root causes of reproductive health problems. At the same time, the CBPR process produced powerful new data on the prevalence of the problem of sexual harassment and its possible association with reproductive and mental health problems.

During the CBPR process, the research and its results moved HOPE members and helped them see that far from being simply an individual problem, sexual harassment was affecting many people. They saw as well that by studying and addressing this issue, they could give something back to the community and make improvements for other students and female family members as well as for themselves. Because "the methods used to validate knowledge claims must also be acceptable to the group controlling the knowledge validation process" (Collins, 2000, p. 204), having the research results from their survey gave the HOPE members considerable leverage. The survey captured the attention of the school authorities and the media in ways that individual accounts had not. The research also provided credibility and legitimacy to the organizing work.

The girls' major role in designing the research and making all of the major decisions, within the overarching framework provided by ACRJ, was a critical aspect of this CBPR process, The research gave the HOPE members facts and figures that they could in turn use to interest other organizations in serving as powerful allies in their campaign. When HOPE members could say that 87 percent of the more than four hundred students surveyed had been harassed, the issue was raised to the community level, and more people got involved. When the community truly controls the CBPR process, community members may be better positioned to understand problems and make a difference. When community members then form their own autonomous organization, as Khmer Girls in Action did in Long Beach, the prospects for sustainable change are further enhanced.

QUESTIONS FOR DISCUSSION

1. The chapter authors describe popular education as lying "at the heart" of their organization's trainings and continuing on through the entire participatory research process. What are some central tenets of popular education and how are they illustrated in this case study?

2. The authors used the power flower exercise (see Figure 7.1 and the accompanying discussion) to help CBPR participants reflect on areas in which they feel that they are members of a dominant or subordinate group or category. Try doing this exercise yourself, and then answer these questions: How did you feel doing the exercise? Were there any surprises? Would you consider using this exercise with a school or community group with which you were working in a CBPR partnership? Why or why not?

REFERENCES

Amsden, J., & VanWynsberghe, R. (2005). Community mapping as a research tool with youth. *Action Research, 3*(4), 257–281.

Arnold, R., Burke, B., James, C., Martin, D., & Thomas, R. *Educating for a change.* Toronto: Between the Lines Press, 1991.

Asians and Pacific Islanders for Reproductive Health. (2001). *HOPE project for girls: A reproductive freedom tour of Oakland.* Oakland, CA: Author.

Bunch, C. (1983). The reform tool kit. In J. Friedman (Ed.), *First harvest: The Institute for Policy Studies, 1963–1983* (pp. 204–208). New York: Grove Press.

Cargo, M., Grams, G., Ottoson, J., Ward, P., & Green, L. (2003). Empowerment as fostering positive youth development and citizenship. *American Journal of Health Behavior, 27*(Suppl. 1), S66–S79.

Centers for Disease Control and Prevention. (2002). *Health-related quality-of-life measures.* Atlanta: National Center for Chronic Disease Prevention and Health Promotion.

Checkoway, B., Dobbie, D., & Richards-Schuster, K. (2003). Involving young people in community evaluation research. *Community Youth Development, 4*(1). Retrieved May 23, 2007, from http://www.cydjournal.org/2003Spring/checkoway.html.

Collins, P. H. (2000). *Black feminist thought: Knowledge, consciousness, and the politics of empowerment* (2nd ed.). New York: Routledge.

El-Askari, G., & Walton, S. (2005). Local government and resident collaboration to improve health: A case study in capacity building and cultural humility. In M. Minkler (Ed.), *Community organizing and community building for health* (2nd ed., pp. 254–271). New Brunswick, NJ: Rutgers University Press.

Freire, P. (1970). *Pedagogy of the oppressed.* New York: Seabury Press.

hooks, b. (1989). *Talking back: Thinking feminism, talking black.* Boston: South End Press.

Khmer Girls in Action. (2008). *History.* Retrieved Apr. 20, 2008, from http://kgalb.org/history/history.html.

Le Compte, M. (1995). Some notes on power, agenda, and voice: A researcher's personal evolution toward critical collaborative research. In P. McLaren & J. Giarelli (Eds.), *Critical theory and educational research* (pp. 91–112). Albany: State University of New York Press.

National Black Women's Health Project. (2008). Home page. Retrieved Apr. 20, 2008, from http://www. blackwomenshealth.org.

Ozer, E. J., Cantor, J., Cruz, G. W., Fox, B., Hubbard, E., & Moret, L. (2008). The diffusion of youth-led participatory research in urban schools: The role of the prevention support system in implementation and sustainability. *American Journal of Community Psychology, 41*(3–4), 278–289.

Quintiliani, K., & Needlam, S. (2007). Cambodians in Long Beach, California: The making of a community. *Journal of Immigrant and Refugee Health Status, 5*(1), 29–53.

Reason, P. (1994). Three approaches to participative inquiry. In N. K. Denzin & Y. S. Lincoln (Eds.), *Handbook of qualitative research* (pp. 324–339). Thousand Oaks, CA: Sage.

Reeves, T. J., & Bennett, C. E. (2004). We the people: Asians in the United States. Census 2000 Special Reports. U.S. Department of Commerce, Economics and Statistics Administration, U.S. Census Bureau. Retrieved May 22, 2008, from www.census.gov/prod/2004pubs/censr-17.pdf.

Rosen, R. (2000). *The world split open: How the modern women's movement changed America.* New York: Viking Penguin.

Sohng, S.S.L. (1996). Participatory research and community organizing. *Journal of Sociology and Social Welfare, 23*(4), 77–97.

Staples, L. (2004). *Roots to power: A manual for grassroots organizing* (2nd ed.). New York: Praeger.

Thomas, S. B., & Quinn, S. C. (1991). The Tuskegee syphilis study, 1932 to 1972: Implications for HIV education and AIDS risk education programs in the black community. *American Journal of Public Health, 11,* 1498–1505.

Vio Grossi, F. (1981). The socio-political implications of participatory research: Yugoslavia: International Forum on Participatory Research. *Convergence, 14*(3), 34–51.

Wallerstein, N., Sanchez, V., & Velarde, L. (2005). Freirian praxis in health education and community organizing: A case study of an adolescent prevention program. In M. Minkler (Ed.), *Community organizing and community building for health* (2nd ed., pp. 218–236). New Brunswick, NJ: Rutgers University Press.

Walter, C. (2005). Community building practice: A conceptual framework. In M. Minkler (Ed.), *Community organizing and community building for health* (2nd ed., pp. 66–78). New Brunswick, NJ: Rutgers University Press.

Wilson, N., Dasho, S., Martin, A. C., Wallerstein, N., Wang, C., & Minkler, M. (2007). Engaging young adolescents in social action through photovoice. *Journal of Early Adolescence, 27*(2), 241–261.

CHAPTER

CBPR WITH A HIDDEN POPULATION

THE TRANSGENDER COMMUNITY HEALTH PROJECT A DECADE LATER

KRISTEN CLEMENTS-NOLLE & ARI MAX BACHRACH

Slowly and often painfully conventional researchers are coming to realize that working with the poor and voiceless is infinitely more rewarding than working on them.

CORNWALL & JEWKES, 1995

Note: We would like to thank the research associates (Nikki Calma, Carla Clynes, Matt Rice, Nashanta Stanley, and Doan Thai), field coordinators (Vince Guilin, Robert Guzman, and Scott Ikeda), and Transgender Community Advisory Board members (Connie Amarthitada, Nadia Cabezas, Crystal Catamco, Tamara Ching, Patrick Forte, Sage Foster, Liz Highleyman, Russell Hilkene, Carry Kissel, Jade Kwan, Yosenio Lewis, Lauren Michaels, Margaret Morvay, Major, Chenit Ong-Flaherty, Elise Shiver-Russell, Zak Sinclair, Claire Skiffington, Tammy Jean Spirithawk, Viny Tango, Gina Tucker, Adela Vasquez, Kiki Whitlock, and Willy Wilkinson) for all their dedication and hard work.

COMMUNITY-BASED participatory research (CBPR) is increasingly being recognized as a useful approach in epidemiology. For many years, environmental epidemiologists have embraced the principles of CBPR (Brown, 1992; Brugge & Hynes, 2005; Lantz, Israel, Schulz, & Reyes, 2005; Wing, 1998) and more recently, CBPR has been used in epidemiological studies of cancer screening (Nguyen et al., 2006), HIV/AIDS (Rhodes, Yee, & Hergenrather, 2006), and physical activity (Pazoki, Nabipour, Seyednezami, & Imami, 2007). However, as Schwab and Syme (1997) noted over a decade ago, community participation in the research process represents a major paradigm shift for epidemiology

> It implies working across disciplines, and with the population itself, in defining variables, designing instruments, and collecting data (qualitative and quantitative) that reflect the ecological reality of life in that population, as people experience it. This collaboration is not easy. It calls for cross-disciplinary patience, as well as cultural sensitivity and competence, to overcome the differences of race, class, and age that generally exist between public health specialists and populations we are here to serve. Epidemiologists would not be required to surrender rigor, but they would be required to share power! [p. 2050]

This new paradigm is well suited for research with oppressed and marginalized populations who have historically been left out of the research process and may not trust outside investigators (Hall, 1981; Corburn, 2005). Collaborating with local people in all aspects of the research process can build community confidence and trust, improve internal study validity, and facilitate the use of study results to improve community health. This chapter describes how CBPR was successfully used in an epidemiological study with perhaps the most socially marginalized population in the United States: the transgender community. After a brief introduction to this hidden population and a summary of the study results, we will illustrate how CBPR guided the development and implementation of our research efforts.

We frame our case study within the CBPR principles originally outlined by Barbara Israel and her colleagues (Israel, Schurman, & Hugentobler, 1992) and further described in Chapter Three: community-based participatory research is participatory, is cooperative, is a co-learning process, involves systems development, is an empowering process through which participants can increase control over their lives, and achieves a balance between research and action. We conclude with recommendations for other researchers who wish to use CBPR to conduct research with other marginalized and hidden populations.

THE TRANSGENDER COMMUNITY AND THE CBPR STUDY

Transgender is an inclusive term used to describe persons who do not conform to social gender norms associated with their physical sex (Gender Education and Advocacy, 2001). The transgender community is made up of a diverse group of individuals who may also self-identify as transsexual, transvestite, intersex, bigender, male (born female), or female (born male). Transgendered persons live their lives to varying degrees as their chosen gender, but in so doing, they endure severe social stigmatization as well as discrimination in housing, health care, and employment (Feinberg, 2001; Green, 1994; Lombardi, 2001).

A transgendered person may change his or her name and gender on all personal and legal identification, such as a birth certificate, Social Security card, and driver's license. To enhance the secondary sex characteristics of their chosen gender, male-to-female (MTF) transgendered individuals often take estrogen, antiandrogens, and progesterone, and female-to-male (FTM) persons take testosterone. Some transgendered individuals also choose to have sex reassignment or gender confirmation surgeries. However, many lack the considerable financial resources to pay for such surgeries, which are rarely covered by health insurance.

The size of the transgender population in the United States is unknown because national and local data collection forms include only male and female gender categories. Similarly, we have little epidemiological data to document the health of transgendered persons. Of particular concern in San Francisco, California, was the lack of information available on HIV infection in this hidden population. In the mid-1990s, anecdotal reports from members of the transgender community and health care providers suggested that HIV/AIDS might be a significant problem for transgendered persons. However, no large epidemiological studies with the transgender community had been conducted in San Francisco or elsewhere to determine the prevalence of HIV and associated risk behaviors.

To address this limitation, researchers from the San Francisco Department of Public Health and members of the transgender community worked together to conduct the first large epidemiological study with transgendered persons: the Transgender Community Health Project. Although the primary objective of the study was to obtain an estimate of HIV prevalence and risk behaviors among transgendered persons in San Francisco, the study also addressed access to health and prevention services and a range of psychosocial health issues.

From July 1 through December 31, 1997, a total of 392 MTF and 123 FTM transgendered persons were recruited, interviewed, and tested for HIV. Over one-third (35 percent) of MTF participants were found to be infected with HIV. African Americans and individuals with a history of injection drug use, multiple sex partners, and less education were significantly more likely than other participants to be HIV positive. Among FTM participants, HIV prevalence (2 percent) and risk behaviors were much lower. However, FTMs who have sex with gay and bisexual men may be at risk due to low condom use. About two-thirds of MTF and over half of FTM participants were classified as depressed, and 32 percent of each population had attempted suicide (Clements-Nolle, Marx, Guzman, & Katz, 2001). As will be further described in the following case study, these alarming results greatly influenced policy, prevention, and health care for transgendered persons in San Francisco.

CBPR Is Participatory and Cooperative
The Transgender Community Health Project was initiated and driven by community concerns and priorities. Frustrated with data collection forms that offered only binary (male or female) gender classifications and keenly aware of the number of transgendered persons becoming infected with HIV, a group of transgendered individuals became vocal about the lack of epidemiological HIV data for their community. Members of this group attended several San Francisco Health Commission and Department of Public Health

meetings and wrote letters stating the need to conduct a transgender HIV prevalence and risk behavior study. Eventually, as a result of this persistent community organizing, the San Francisco HIV Prevention Planning Council made such a study a priority.

In 1995, researchers from the health department asked these same community members to collaborate in the development of a transgender research grant application. This grant proposal was funded by the state of California's Office of AIDS and the Centers for Disease Control and Prevention in 1996. At this time, ten more MTF and FTM transgendered volunteers were recruited to help plan and implement formative research for the proposed epidemiological study.

The formative research consisted of thirty key informant interviews, eleven focus groups (with one hundred transgendered persons altogether), and four months of ethnographic community mapping. The transgender community collaborators played a particularly important role in developing the focus group questions, cofacilitating each focus group, and assisting in the analysis and publication of the focus group data (Clements-Nolle, Wilkinson, Kitano, & Marx, 2001). In addition, several community members worked very closely with health department researchers to conduct ethnographic mapping in neighborhoods thought to have high concentrations of transgendered persons. This helped to determine the time of day and locations when recruitment should take place to ensure a diverse sample of MTF and FTM individuals for the epidemiological study.

In 1997, a full community advisory board (CAB) was established to assist in the design and implementation of the quantitative study protocols. To ensure diversity and a range of experience among CAB members, some members were recruited through street outreach and others were recruited by writing letters to agencies that served the target population. This resulted in a twenty-four-member CAB that consisted almost entirely of MTFs and FTMs who were homeless, current sex workers, health care providers, or social service providers. The CAB members worked together to develop a mission statement and a set of agreements that were then used to facilitate each meeting. The agreements outlined the need to respect one another's differences and helped the CAB create a safe space where people from various backgrounds could feel comfortable contributing to the research process.

The CAB initially met twice a month and then monthly to develop protocols, sampling plans, data collection instruments, and human subject applications; pilot-test the instruments; interview and hire the research team; develop transgender-specific education and referral materials; and oversee participant recruitment and data collection activities. The expertise that the CAB members provided in developing the survey instrument was invaluable. Several CAB members met with health department researchers in between meetings to develop culturally appropriate ways to ask sexual behavior questions of MTFs and FTMs who might or might not have undergone sexual reassignment surgery. The resulting survey has served as a model for other jurisdictions conducting transgender studies.

The CAB also decided that interviewing and HIV testing should be conducted at seven community-based organizations located in the key neighborhoods identified by the ethnographic mapping. The CAB felt that rotating recruitment across neighborhoods would help ensure a diverse sample of participants and facilitate referrals to the very agencies where the interviewing and HIV testing were being conducted.

In May 1997, three MTFs (African American, Filipina, and Latina) and three FTMs (one Vietnamese and two whites) were hired as research associates. All of these research associates had strong ties with their respective communities, which helped the study gain access to the various racial and ethnic, socioeconomic, and gender subpopulations within the transgender community. The research associates helped to finalize the study instruments and were responsible for recruiting, interviewing, HIV-testing, providing referrals, and presenting the study results. They quickly became aware that many of the agencies and clinics to which they referred study participants were not sensitive to the needs of transgendered people. To address this limitation, the research associates planned and conducted numerous transgender, in-service training sessions at local agencies and clinics.

The research associates also believed that existing HIV prevention and referral materials did not reflect the reality of transgender identity and served to further alienate the community. Therefore the research associates worked closely with CAB members to develop transgender-specific HIV education and referral materials. Created by and for members of the transgender community, these materials addressed issues specific to transgendered persons (for example, how to inject hormones safely) and used transgender-specific images (for example, a MTF transgendered person who had not undergone surgery was shown putting a condom on her penis). Such images validated transgender identity and expressed the importance of self-protection.

In December 1997, the research associates presented preliminary study results to participants, collaborating agencies, the HIV Prevention Planning Council, and the HIV Health Services Council. During the first six months of 1998, the CAB met every other month to develop the full analysis plan; review and interpret the results; and decide the content of reports, publications, and press releases. Community involvement began to drop off during this quantitative analysis phase. Some CAB members felt alienated by discussions of analysis, and others were simply not as interested in this phase of the research. The group members decided that they trusted the health department researchers to clean, code, and analyze the data, and the CAB met only quarterly for the rest of the year, to interpret results and guide data dissemination.

In 1999, the CAB resumed monthly meetings to plan a large community forum where the research associates presented the study results. The community forum was held at Glide Memorial Church in the Tenderloin (a low-income neighborhood from which a large number of study participants had been recruited) and was attended by about two hundred people. The CAB asked that reporters not be invited to the forum because of the tendency of the media to sensationalize stories regarding the transgender community. An exception was made for a public radio station that presented a very objective summary of the study results.

After the community forum the CAB membership changed. Several original CAB members had moved out of the area, and others felt that their work was completed. A frontline staff member and a program director from each agency serving the transgender community were asked to join the CAB to begin the process of translating the study results into action. The new eighteen-member CAB met bimonthly in 2000 and quarterly in 2001 to ensure that the research findings were widely distributed and used to secure funding for new HIV services, develop new categories for gender classification, and develop a transgender behavioral risk assessment instrument to be used by agencies providing HIV prevention for transgendered clients.

CBPR Is a Co-Learning Process

The health department researchers and transgender community members came to the table with different, but equally important, knowledge and skills. Throughout each phase of the research project, the two groups challenged and learned from each other, and this reciprocal transfer of knowledge was an especially valuable component of the Transgender Community Health Project.

The transgendered CAB members and research associates spent many hours educating the health department researchers about issues specific to the transgender community, such as the importance of self-identity and the psychosocial reasons for risk taking that were crucial to appropriate study design, measurement, and data interpretation. Relying on local knowledge improved the quality of the research and, as will be seen later, facilitated the use of the results for program and policy development. The CAB members were trained in research methodology, and the research associates attended more than thirty-five training sessions on topics including HIV counseling, interviewing techniques, protection of human research subjects, research ethics, infection control, street outreach, suicide prevention, and referrals. In addition several research associates and CAB members acquired new skills by presenting the study results at local and national conferences and by coauthoring study publications.

Cross-training between MTF and FTM community members also occurred. Although both groups were part of the larger transgender community, it immediately became clear that their issues were different. For example, MTFs were very concerned about employment discrimination and the high prevalence of sex work in their community, whereas for FTMs the tendency to have unprotected sex as a way to feel sexually validated as male was a more pressing issue. MTF and FTM community members learned a great deal from each other, and the emerging differences profoundly informed the development of the sampling frame, questionnaire, and data analysis plan.

CBPR Involves System Development

According to Israel and her colleagues (1992), CBPR develops the competencies to diagnose and analyze problems and to plan, implement, and evaluate interventions aimed at meeting identified needs. Members of the CAB who worked at community-based organizations were able to use the results from the Transgender Community Health Project to develop new or improve existing interventions at their agencies. For example, the finding that more unprotected sex occurred with main rather than casual or paying partners prompted several agencies to include the main partners of transgendered clients in their risk reduction interventions.

CAB members also decided to develop a simplified data collection instrument that could be used to evaluate interventions at the agency level. Health department researchers helped the CAB members develop a transgender-specific, behavioral risk assessment and conducted several trainings on human subjects and survey administration. In this way individuals at community-based organizations were empowered to generate their own client-level data, rather than always relying on information gathered from outside researchers.

CBPR Is an Empowering Process

The CAB members often refer to the Transgender Community Health Project as "the study we conducted." As one CAB member remarked, "This time we weren't the clowns, we were the researchers. We weren't asked to do a show or be in a float" (Vasquez, 2001). The CAB members were intimately involved in all phases of the research study, and their feelings of study co-ownership were evident from the outset. As CAB member Willy Wilkinson (2000) later wrote: "I remember the feeling of excitement and commitment that permeated the room. For the first time ever, the responsibility to define and document our community's needs was in our hands, and we were going to do whatever it took to do it right, even if it meant frustration, struggle, and disagreement along the way. This process of community empowerment and self-determination cannot be forced or faked; it came because we were given the opportunity to meet as a community and grapple to define our lives and realities." Feelings of community ownership were also apparent when the research associates presented the study findings to local agencies, boards, and planning councils. In addition, the research associates were guest lecturers for university courses and made presentations at local and national conferences. Through this process the research associates emerged as positive role models in the transgender community and acquired valuable skills that they later used to pursue higher-level employment.

The Transgender Community Health Project also empowered the research associates to be themselves in a work environment. For some, this was the first opportunity they had been given to present themselves professionally as they expressed themselves personally. In addition, although many of the research associates had long histories of educating social service providers and the world around them about transgender issues, the study provided monetary and professional validation for this work. The research associates were considered experts in topics that are not typically valued in traditional work environments. Their collective knowledge of topics like sex work, hormones, and monolingual immigrant communities has been recognized by many as a key to the study's success.

CBPR Balances Research and Action

The primary objective of the Transgender Community Health Project was to obtain a sound estimate of HIV prevalence and risk behaviors among transgendered persons in San Francisco. However, the research was also conducted in relation to the kind of commitment to action that is a hallmark of participatory research (Cornwall & Jewkes, 1995; Hall, 1981; Israel, Eng, Schulz, & Parker, 2005).

As soon as the HIV prevalence data were confirmed, the results were returned to the community. First, a presentation was made to study participants, collaborating agencies, and local planning councils, and then a large forum was held where a community report was released. The research associates and CAB members participated in every presentation and offered program and policy recommendations based on their review of the study data.

The release of findings from the Transgender Community Health Project occurred long before the intricate analyses necessary for publication were complete. Using these initial data, both the health department and local agencies were able to secure additional funds for HIV prevention and health services for transgendered persons. This resulted in the development and implementation of new programs for transgendered individuals in San Francisco more than two years before the first publication from the study went to press.

The study results have also been used by human rights groups to argue for improved health care and greater discrimination protection for transgendered persons. Recently, the San Francisco Health Services System Board asked for specific data from the Transgender Community Health Project on health issues and gender confirmation surgery, and the board used these materials in making its landmark decision to offer transgender health care (including sex reassignment surgery) to San Francisco city employees.

Other examples of the balance between research and action are evident when reviewing the accomplishments of the research associates and the CAB members. The in-service agency training sessions that were conducted by research associates throughout the study had a substantial impact on improving services for transgendered individuals in San Francisco. Although the training was originally developed for agencies to which the Transgender Community Health Project made frequent referrals, the research associates quickly began to receive requests for training from agencies throughout the Bay Area. Several of the research associates still do transgender in-service trainings.

CAB members attended several San Francisco HIV Prevention Planning Council meetings and successfully convinced the council to adopt new categories for classifying transgendered persons for data collection and service provision. Today, not only are such categories used by all community-based organizations who contract with the San Francisco Department of Public Health to provide HIV prevention, but many large HIV/AIDS data reporting systems in San Francisco now report data separately for transgendered persons. As noted later, efforts also are under way to encourage federal agencies, such as the Centers for Disease Control and Prevention (CDC), to adopt similar data collection categories.

PROJECT IMPACT OVER TEN YEARS

Even though data collection for the Transgender Community Health Project ended a decade ago, the study continues to contribute to research, education, and action. The research associates have all remained involved in research and health services for transgendered persons. Some are pursuing advanced degrees in health-related fields, and several have moved into program management positions. The community collaborators also continue to work closely with the San Francisco Department of Public Health on HIV prevention, health service, and research initiatives. The original CAB that was established to design and implement the Transgender Community Health Project continues to meet monthly. This group advises the health department and the HIV Prevention Planning Council on issues related to transgender sensitivity, service gaps, and emerging research needs. Transgender sensitivity trainings have continued in San Francisco, including annual trainings for medical providers and recent trainings for teachers and staff at local high schools. In addition, the health department recently received funding from the federal Health Resources and Services Administration (HRSA) to develop "best practice" guidelines for HIV/AIDS health services for transgender individuals. These guidelines have further contributed to the department's efforts to affect changes in programs, practices, and policies that can improve transgender health and quality of life.

The Transgender Community Health Project has inspired continued transgender research at the health department, including HIV incidence (Kellogg, Clements-Nolle, Dilley, Katz, & McFarland, 2001), HIV testing (Schwarcz & Scheer, 2004), and qualitative research with the partners of transgender persons (Coan, Schrager, & Packer, 2005). The standardized transgender behavioral risk assessment that was originally developed by the CAB is still used by agencies funded to provide HIV prevention services to transgender clients. In addition, San Francisco continues to lead the nation by collecting and reporting HIV/AIDS data for transgender individuals (separate from other males and females). These data have been instrumental for epidemiological forecasting, community planning, and resource prioritization efforts.

Local efforts have also influenced initiatives at the national level. Transgender Community Health Project data and training materials were recently used by the American Psychological Association when it developed a transgender module for its national train-the-trainer program. This program focuses on improving local psychologists' ability to respond to people infected and affected by HIV. Community members from San Francisco also joined representatives from other states for consultation meetings with the CDC and HRSA focused on improving HIV prevention and health services for transgender populations. And although the transgender identity is still not required in national HIV/AIDS reporting, the CDC recently coordinated a meeting with transgender community members and researchers to guide the development of a transgender behavioral surveillance pilot project. Finally, local community activists used data from the Transgender Community Health Project when advocating for the inclusion of the transgender identity in the hate crimes bill and employment nondiscrimination act recently debated in Congress.

The Transgender Community Health Project and its ten-year legacy of continued research, education, and action is an example of the lasting impact of CBPR. As a transgendered research associate (Ari Bachrach) reflects on the study, it is clear that the study also had a profound effect on the community members who were involved:

> It's hard to separate the personal and professional impact the study has had on me, because being a transperson seeking employment does not allow for that kind of distinction. [The Transgender Community Health Project] was such a unique opportunity because I was valued for the skills I had and I was empowered to feel like an expert because of my lived experience. Whenever I have to make employment transitions it is a source of great stress to me, in large part because of the complexity of navigating new environments as a visibly non-gender-conforming person. It's easy to fall into internalized transphobia. I use my experience at TCHP to remind me that I deserve to be treated with respect.
>
> Working within my community in such a directly beneficial way was a really valuable experience because the study was so formative and groundbreaking in terms of improving services for trans-populations. Feeling personally valued in a work situation and knowing that my work directly impacted the ways the entire community was treated individually and systemically, in such lasting ways, is profound. The many benefits in my own life and the community continue to unfold. I feel so lucky to have had this amazing opportunity.

SUMMARY

The Transgender Community Health Project is a partnership between San Francisco Department of Public Health researchers and transgendered community members that was initiated in response to community concerns in 1996 and is still continuing today. This epidemiological study provided valuable data on a hidden population with a complex array of social, physical, and mental health needs. Community collaborators worked closely with health department researchers to ensure that the study results were released in a timely manner and were used to effect social change and improve health outcomes for transgendered persons.

The Transgender Community Health Project helped secure funding for new health and prevention services, improve gender discrimination protection, change the gender categories on existing data collection forms, build agency capacity for data collection, and increase the transgender sensitivity of community-based organizations. In addition, researchers from Los Angeles, New York, Boston, and Seattle have asked for assistance in conducting similar studies in their local jurisdictions. In time, the results of such studies may provide a broader understanding of HIV and other public health issues among transgendered individuals throughout the United States.

The overall success of the Transgender Community Health Project can likely be attributed to its effective engagement of CBPR. This research approach is very helpful for conducting epidemiological research with marginalized and hidden populations who have historically been excluded from the research process and have little trust of outside researchers (see Chapter Four). By encouraging community participation in all phases of the research process, CBPR can demystify research, facilitate co-learning and capacity building, build community trust, improve study validity, and help ensure that the data generated will be used to influence program and policy change. However, researchers interested in using CBPR should realize that this approach requires flexibility, patience, and a long-term commitment.

A central tenet of CBPR is the need to address community-identified concerns (Cornwall & Jewkes, 1995). Outside researchers may find that they must abandon predetermined research objectives that are not congruent with community priorities. This may be difficult for a researcher who wants to respond to a request for proposals from an agency with specific research goals and objectives that it is willing to fund. In addition, CBPR's emphasis on returning data to the community and involving community collaborators as copresenters and coauthors may conflict with rules specified by academic or funding institutions. If the flexibility to negotiate research objectives and data dissemination rules is lacking, CBPR may not be an appropriate or feasible approach.

Funding agencies and researchers also need to be aware that using an equitable and collaborative research approach can be very time consuming. If this process is rushed, important issues may be missed, and community members may become frustrated and disillusioned. As described in Chapter Three, CBPR involves a long-term commitment that typically extends beyond a given funding period. Many communities have had negative experiences with outside researchers, who typically seem to disappear as soon as they have obtained their data (Green & Mercer, 2001; see also Chapter Five and Appendix H). If they do not make a commitment to stay involved until the data are used to effect change, outside researchers may have a difficult time obtaining the community trust necessary for CBPR.

Fortunately, support and funding opportunities for participatory approaches in research that aims to decrease inequities in health status are increasing (Green & Mercer, 2001; Minkler, Blackwell, Thompson, & Tamir, 2003; see also Appendix B). Such support may give researchers the flexibility and time needed to employ CBPR approaches with populations who are disproportionately affected by health and social problems but have had little opportunity to share their experience and knowledge. By recognizing the profound contribution that local experts can make to the research process, CBPR has the potential to contribute to the improved community health and social well-being of marginalized and hidden populations.

QUESTIONS FOR DISCUSSION

1. A particularly impressive aspect of the Transgender Community Health Project was its effective use of a community advisory board (CAB). Yet as the authors of this chapter acknowledge, such involvement can be highly labor intensive, slowing down the timetable for the actual research. How might you use this case study to advocate for the use of an active CAB in an epidemiological study your colleagues hope to undertake with another marginalized community? (Note: They're very concerned about the time issue!)

2. The chapter authors describe how the outcomes of the Transgender Health Project have continued to be felt long after the study has ended. Thinking back to these outcomes, which one(s) may have been the most important in terms of changing programs, policies, or practices? What evidence of individual and community capacity building can you point to, and how would you rank that among the project outcomes?

3. If you were to design a CBPR effort with another marginalized community, what might be the single most important lesson from this project that you would hope to bring with you? What might you do differently?

KEY TERMS

Transgender   Epidemiology

REFERENCES

Brown, P. (1992). Popular epidemiology and toxic waste contamination: Lay and professional ways of knowing. *Journal of Health and Social Behavior, 33,* 267–281.

Brugge, D., & Hynes, H. P. (Eds.). (2005). *Community research in environmental health: Studies in science, advocacy and ethics.* Burlington, VT: Ashgate.

Clements-Nolle, K., Marx, R., Guzman, R., & Katz, M. (2001). HIV prevalence, risk behaviors, health care use, and mental health status of transgender persons: Implications for public health intervention. *American Journal of Public Health, 91,* 915–921.

Clements-Nolle, K., Wilkinson, W., Kitano, K., & Marx, R. (2001). HIV prevention and health service needs of the transgender community in San Francisco. In W. Bockting & S. Kirk (Eds.), *Transgender and HIV: Risks, prevention, and care* (pp. 69–88). Binghamton, NY: Haworth Press.

Coan, D. L., Schrager, W., & Packer, T. (2005). The role of male sexual partners in HIV infection among male-to-female transgendered individuals. In W. Bockting & E. Avery (Eds.), *Transgender health and HIV prevention: Needs assessment studies from transgender communities across the United States* (pp. 21–30). Binghamton, NY: Haworth Medical Press.

Corburn, J. (2005). *Street science: Community knowledge and environmental health justice.* Cambridge, MA: MIT Press.

Cornwall, A., & Jewkes, J. (1995). What is participatory action research? *Social Science & Medicine, 41,* 1667–1676.

Feinberg, L. (2001). Trans health crisis: For us it's life or death. *American Journal of Public Health, 91,* 897–900.

Gender Education and Advocacy. (2001). *Gender variance: A primer.* Retrieved May 13, 2008, from www.gender.org/resources/dge/gea01004.pdf.

Green, J. (1994). *Investigation into discrimination against transgendered people: A report by the Human Rights Commission.* San Francisco: City and County of San Francisco.

Green, L. W., & Mercer, S. L. (2001). Can public health researchers and agencies reconcile the push from funding bodies and the pull from communities? *American Journal of Public Health, 91,* 1926–1929.

Hall, B. L. (1981). Participatory research, popular knowledge, and power: A personal reflection. *Convergence, 14*(3), 6–19.

Israel, B. A., Eng, E., Schulz, A. J., & Parker, E. A. (Eds.). (2005). Introduction to methods in community-based participatory research for health. In Israel, Eng, Schulz and Parker (Eds.) *Methods in community-based participatory research for health.* (pp. 3–29). San Francisco, CA: Jossey-Bass.

Israel, B. A., Schurman, S. J., & Hugentobler, M. K. (1992). Conducting action research: Relationships between organization members and researchers. *Journal of Applied Behavioral Science, 28,* 74–101.

Kellogg, T. A., Clements-Nolle, K., Dilley, J., Katz, M. H., & McFarland, W. (2001). Incidence of human immunodeficiency virus among male-to-female transgendered persons in San Francisco. *Journal of Acquired Immune Deficiency Syndromes, 38,* 380–384.

Lantz, P. M., Israel, B. A., Schulz, A. J., & Reyes, A. (2005). Community-based participatory research: Rationale and relevance for social epidemiology. In J. M. Oakes & J. S. Kaufman (Eds.), *Methods in social epidemiology* (pp. 239–266). San Francisco: Jossey-Bass.

Lombardi, E. (2001). Enhancing transgender health care. *American Journal of Public Health, 91,* 869–872.

Minkler, M., Blackwell, A. G., Thompson, M., & Tamir, H. (2003). Community-based participatory research: Implications for public health funding. *American Journal of Public Health, 93,* 1210–1213.

Nguyen, T. T., McPhee, S. J., Gildengorin, G., Nguyen, T., Wong, C., Lai, K. Q., et al. (2006). Papanicolaou testing among Vietnamese Americans: Results of a multifaceted intervention. *American Journal of Preventive Medicine, 21,* 1–9.

Pazoki, R., Nabipour, I., Seyednezami, N., & Imami, S. R. (2007). Effects of a community-based healthy heart program on increasing healthy women's physical activity: A randomized controlled trial guided by community-based participatory research (CBPR). *BMC Public Health, 7,* 216.

Rhodes, S. D., Yee, L. J., & Hergenrather, K. C. (2006). A community-based rapid assessment of HIV behavioural risk disparities within a large sample of gay men in southeastern USA: A comparison of African American, Latino, and white men. *AIDS Care, 18,* 1018–1024.

Schwab, M., & Syme, S. L. (1997). On paradigms, community participation, and the future of public health. *American Journal of Public Health, 87,* 2049–2052.

Schwarcz, S., & Scheer, S. (2004). HIV testing behaviors and knowledge of HIV reporting regulations among male-to-female transgenders. *Journal of Acquired Immune Deficiency Syndromes, 37,* 1326–1327.

Vasquez, A. (2001, March 7). Panel presentation, Transgender Community Health Project, PAR class, School of Public Health, University of California, Berkeley.

Wilkinson, W. (2000). *The Transgender Community Health Project: Participatory action research with a hidden population.* Unpublished manuscript, School of Public Health, University of California, Berkeley.

Wing, S. (1998). Whose epidemiology, whose health? *International Journal of Health Services, 28,* 241–252.

3

SELECTING ISSUES AND EVALUATING OUTCOMES WITH COMMUNITIES

One of the greatest challenges in community work involves differentiating between problems and issues. A problem, as community organizer Mike Miller once argued, is what an outsider looking in would identify as something "wrong" with a community and in need of fixing. An issue, in contrast, is something the community identifies and feels strongly enough about that it is willing to work on it to bring about change.

One of the hallmarks of community-based participatory research is, of course, its commitment to starting with an issue that the community, rather than the outside expert, identifies. In the ideal case, community members will have identified such an issue on their own and will have approached the outsider about working collaboratively with them. Often, however, as suggested in Part Two, it is the outside researcher who has the time and resources to play the role of initiator in a potential CBPR project. In such cases, the outsider may use a variety of methods to help community members identify an issue about which they care deeply and around which a CBPR effort might take place.

In Chapter Nine, the first chapter in Part Three, Meredith Minkler and Trevor Hancock describe and illustrate a host of such techniques and methods, ranging from risk mapping and walking or windshield (driving) tours to Delphi techniques and the development of neighborhood health indicators. Yet such issue selection efforts must be accompanied by equal attention to helping communities identify their strengths and resources—assets that can help them in collaboratively studying shared issues and engaging in subsequent community problem solving. Many of the issue selection techniques and methods explored in this chapter are equally useful as means of helping communities identify their strengths.

In Chapter Ten, Marita Jones and her colleagues from the Shiprock Area Indian Health Service Unit, New Mexico, illustrate how Internet-based tools used in the context of CBPR played a key role in two health promotion initiatives for and with widely dispersed Native communities in the United States. The roles of a variety of Web-based technologies in promoting distributed learning and community capacity while also facilitating participatory evaluation and knowledge creation are illustrated. Despite some very real challenges that also are noted, the chapter concludes that Internet-based tools hold particular promise for engaging youths, residents of rural areas, and any dispersed populations who wish to create shared learning communities.

In Chapter Eleven, Caroline Wang and Cheri Pies describe and illustrate the use of photovoice as still another approach that has gained wide currency in CBPR with a wide range of communities and populations. Drawing on a variety of theoretical and practice approaches, photovoice involves providing inexpensive cameras and training to often marginalized groups, who capture their own images of what matters in their world and develop a collective new voice for sharing their issues and strengths (Wang & Burris, 1994). Chapter Eleven explores the use of photovoice by a county health department in California and the ways it can significantly broaden and deepen a health department's understanding of community-perceived needs and assets. Ethical and practical challenges in the use of photovoice methodology also are discussed.

One of the greatest challenges for those involved in community-based work is determining how to evaluate the results of such efforts without disempowering communities in the process. The development of the field and practice of participatory evaluation has been critical in this regard, combining a commitment to high-quality inquiry with an equally strong emphasis on the principles of empowerment and capacity building (Fetterman & Wandersman, 2005; Coombe, 2005). In Chapter Twelve, Jane Springett and Nina Wallerstein trace the conceptual and practice roots of participatory evaluation, its relationship to participatory research, and its increasingly central role in the evaluation of health promotion initiatives. The relationship between the evaluator and the evaluated, the selection of appropriate tools and methods, the emergent nature of the evaluative process itself, and the contradictions inherent when "different agendas are being overtly brought together" are among the thorny issues surfaced and explored. The chapter concludes with a brief case study of the participatory evaluation of New Mexico's Youth Link project, illustrating both the challenges and the value added when such an approach to evaluation is employed.

REFERENCES

Coombe, C. (2005). Participatory evaluation: Building community while assessing change. In M. Minkler (Ed.), *Community organizing and community building for health* (2nd ed., pp. 405–418). New Brunswick, NJ: Rutgers University Press.

Fetterman, D. M., & Wandersman, A. (2005). *Empowerment evaluation: Principles in practice.* New York: Guilford Press.

Wang, C. C., & Burris, M. A. (1994). Empowerment through photo novella: Portraits of participation. *Health Education Quarterly, 21,* 171–186.

CHAPTER

COMMUNITY-DRIVEN ASSET IDENTIFICATION AND ISSUE SELECTION

MEREDITH MINKLER & TREVOR HANCOCK

WHEN RESIDENTS of Tillery, North Carolina, began to suspect that the chronic sore throats, itchy eyes, and other health problems besetting their community were tied to the use of open lagoons and other practices of the hog production industry, they began their own "barefoot epidemiology" to document what was taking place. Impressed by their efforts, a journalist connected their organization, Concerned Citizens of Tillery (CCT), with researchers at the University of North Carolina's School of Public Health, and an exemplary, decade-long, community-based participatory research (CBPR) project got under way (Wing, Grant, Green, & Stewart, 1996; Tajik & Minkler, 2007).

The Tillery partnership, which is presented in Chapter Fifteen, is in many ways an ideal case. The issue around which CBPR took place came directly from the community, which subsequently began its own study and then partnered with both a university and the local health department to conduct the more detailed research needed and to advocate for change. Yet in many cases it is outside researchers or practitioners, rather than communities themselves, who wish to embark on a CBPR project. As Randy Stoecker suggests in Chapter Six, in such cases the outsider frequently plays the role of initiator, approaching community organizations about the possibility of a collaboration and setting the process in motion. In other instances, typified by the Healthy Communities approach, a neighborhood or community may decide that it wishes to create a better and healthier environment for its citizens and embark on a process of identifying its assets and studying and addressing the things it hopes to change.

This chapter examines the processes of community-driven issue selection, giving particular attention to the roles that outside researchers or practitioners may play in facilitating this process. In keeping with the emphasis in CBPR on recognizing and building on community capacity, however, it is equally concerned with the often similar processes through which communities may be helped to identify and build on their resources. The chapter begins with a brief review of the core principles guiding a participatory and strengths-based approach to community asset identification and issue selection. Next it presents a variety of methods and approaches for assisting communities in identifying their assets and resources as well as their concerns and issues. It then reviews some key criteria, adapted from the field of community organizing, that may usefully guide community issue selection in CBPR. Finally, it highlights the challenge that arises when categorical funding and other factors constrain issue selection in a participatory research effort. Using as an example the federal Healthy Start program to reduce infant mortality, this chapter illustrates how even within such constraints, a commitment to community participation and empowerment can lead to high-level community involvement in deciding on the issues on which collective research and action will take place.

CORE PRINCIPLES AND CONSIDERATIONS

The approaches to community identification of assets and issues described in this chapter are grounded in a conceptual framework that builds on three core principles. First, and central to the other two, is the principle that reminds us to "start where the people are." Articulated by health education leader Dorothy Nyswander (1956) over fifty years ago, starting where the people are is critical not only for demonstrating to communities our faith in them but also in ensuring that the issues we jointly address are the ones that really matter. As sociologist John McKinlay is fond of saying, we professionals frequently suffer from an unfortunate malady known as "terminal hardening of the categories." We get the kinds of answers we are comfortable dealing with because we ask the kinds of questions that will give us those answers. In community health research, for example, residents may be told that HIV/AIDS or heart disease is a major health problem in their community and asked their opinions about various preventive health approaches. Although this may yield some valuable information, it may miss the fact that different issues, such as drugs, violence, or unemployment, may be of far greater concern to the community. Starting where the people are would have us shelve more traditional approaches, in which the researcher enters the community with his or her research topic and methods predetermined. Instead, and consistent with the principles of CBPR, it would have us foster a dialogical process through which the community's felt concerns heavily shape and determine the topic chosen, how it is explored, and to what ends (Hall, 1992).

As suggested in Chapter Five, starting where the people are also means listening for and honoring what James Scott (1990) has called the *hidden transcripts,* or private discourse, of an oppressed community. Hidden transcripts may take the form of stories, jokes, dreams, and fantasies and the kind of "plain talk" that cannot be safely expressed within earshot of the dominant group. Although much of the content of hidden transcripts is, by definition, not for public consumption by researchers and others outside the group, methodical listening and a willingness to take seriously the messages conveyed can be an important avenue for improving one's understanding of an oppressed group. Makani Themba (1999) points to rap music as "one of very few venues for expressing rage at the status quo as well as holding a candid discussion of social issues" (p. 22). Despite the commodification of and contradictions within some rap music, its ability to "chronicle the lived experience" of a sizable group of African American and other youths in America make it a powerful medium for CBPR participants committed to better understanding an oppressed group. Methodical listening to rap music and keen attention to other cultural expressions can form the basis for the dialogue that lies at the heart of CBPR.

Another dimension of "starting where the people are" involves a second core principle—recognize and begin with community strengths and assets, rather than problems. In their classic indictment of traditional "needs-based" approaches to health and human welfare, Kretzmann and McKnight (1993) argue that well-meaning professionals and bureaucracies frequently hurt communities by characterizing them as "bundles of pathologies" or problems to be solved. Although such characterizations may be useful in attracting outside funding, they may also do substantial damage by reinforcing a deficit mentality in which both community members and outsiders view the community in terms of its problems—needs and deficiencies to be "fixed" by outside experts (McKnight & Kretzmann, 1992).

The past two decades have witnessed a growing appreciation of the importance of a more balanced perspective, which begins by helping communities identify and build on their strengths (Chávez, Minkler, Wallerstein, & Spencer, 2007). *Community asset identification* is used here as a broad concept to capture a variety of different processes through which communities themselves, often with the assistance of outside professionals, engage in the collection of such information. As Sharpe, Greany, Lee, and Royce (2000) have argued, "An assets orientation does not imply ignoring needs and problems or throwing out rational, strategic planning." But "by involving community members in visual, intuitive, and nonlinear processes of self-assessment and discovery, assets-oriented approaches invite more creativity in assessment and planning than collection and perusal of statistical data alone can engender" (p. 206).

The third and final principle embedded in community-driven approaches to asset identification and issue selection involves the heavy accent that CBPR places on authentic dialogue. As discussed in Chapter Two, the type of dialogue described by Paulo Freire (1970, 1973) helps people "look at the 'whys' of their lives, inviting them to critically examine the sources and implications of their own knowledge" (Sohng, 1996, p. 86). In so doing, it facilitates co-learning by community members and researchers and, as Sohng points out, avoids presupposing a frame of reference that is in fact the researcher's rather than the community's. Dialogical approaches thus lead to a far richer and deeper understanding of both community strengths and locally identified problems and issues than traditional researcher-as-interviewer-and-interrogator methods alone are likely to achieve.

The discussion in this chapter draws on each of these principles—starting where the people are, emphasizing and building on community strengths and assets, and using the power of dialogue—as they help inform community-driven, rather than researcher-driven, identification of community assets and selection of issues for community-based participatory research.

TOOLS FOR IDENTIFYING COMMUNITY RESOURCES AND ISSUES

A host of tools and approaches to help communities identify their strengths and assets and also the problems or issues they wish to address have been developed and refined over the past three decades. Although a full discussion of each approach is beyond the scope of this chapter, the following descriptions do provide an overview of several of the most promising approaches and suggest resources for acquiring more detailed information on each.

Walking and Windshield Tours

Crucial to identifying both community assets and potential issues or problems is seeing one's community "through fresh eyes." One effective way of beginning this process is by walking, wheeling, or driving slowly through the community on both weekends and weekdays, at different times of the day, observing and recording one's observations (Eng & Blanchard, 1990; Sharpe et al., 2000). In CBPR, both community residents and outside researchers may take part in this process, working individually or in teams and later sharing their impressions and observations. Although tape recorders, cameras, and even video recorders may be employed, windshield and walking tours typically result simply in handwritten notes or maps that highlight key observations. Such tours can provide valuable impressionistic data about things like the condition and types of local housing, the extent and nature of social interactions, the presence of vacant lots and commercial and recreational facilities, and the general maintenance of buildings, yards, and common grounds (Day, Boarnet, Alfonzo, & Forsyth, 2006; Eng, Briscoe, & Cunningham, 1990; Sharpe et al., 2000). Looking at the content of bulletins boards in community centers, libraries, houses of worship, and local stores or the public notices stapled to utility poles or fences can provide clues to local "hot" issues in the community, and community safety audits (discussed later) are another form of walking tour that can yield valuable information.

Interviews with Formal and Informal Leaders and "Regular Folks"

Community assessment frequently relies on interviews with key informants, but as Sung Sil Lee Sohng (1996) has cautioned, this approach necessarily limits each interaction's frame of reference to that of the interviewer and further misses the co-learning that can come with an approach that is more dialogical. Yet there is clearly a place for thoughtful interviewing in community assessment, particularly when questions are formulated to invite participants to share their pride in their community and their vision for it as well as their concerns and felt needs.

Interviews may be conducted with both formal leaders and informal ones—those *natural helpers* to whom people go for advice or help and who are often key behind-the-scenes players in helping neighborhoods function effectively. As Peggy Shepard (2007) suggests, such individuals should include not only the leaders of tenant associations, churches, and the like, but also the "go-to people" in the community. Valente and

Pumpuang (2007) review ten methods for the identification of formal and informal opinion leaders, several of which hold special relevance for CBPR. They include *positional methods,* to identify individuals who hold formal leadership positions, such as clergy or elected officials; *judge's ratings,* wherein knowledgeable persons identify and rate potential individuals on their leadership qualities; *snowball techniques,* through which already identified formal or informal leaders nominate others who in turn are asked for their suggestions until a core group of names has emerged; and various *sociometric methods,* through which community networks are mapped and all individuals are asked to whom they go for advice. For the purposes of CBPR and other community-building efforts, however, it is particularly important to identify those informal leaders, including long-time residents, who can answer a series of questions like this (see also Israel, 1985; Eng, Briscoe, & Cunningham, 1990; Sharpe et al., 2000; Valente & Pumpuang, 2007):

- Whom do people in this neighborhood go to for help or advice?
- Whom do children go to?
- When this community has had a problem in the past, who has been involved in working to solve it?
- Who gets things done in this community?

Interviews with "regular folks" also are critical to identifying a core group of informal leaders, who then should be interviewed and, ideally, involved as CBPR participants. Interviewers may also ask residents such varied questions as these (see also Duhl & Hancock, 1988; Eng & Blanchard, 1990; Hancock & Minkler, 2005; National Coalition for Healthier Cities & Communities/National Civic League (2003); Israel, 1985; Sharpe et al., 2000):

- What do you like best about living in this neighborhood?
- What would you most like to see changed?
- What are some of the things other people are proud of in the community?
- Is this a good neighborhood in which to raise kids? (Why or why not?)
- When challenges or problems arose in the past, did the community come together to meet them? If so, can you give an example? How well did this collaboration work?
- Where in the community do kids go for fun or just to hang out?
- If youths get into a fight in this community, are adult residents likely to intervene?
- Do people in the neighborhood socialize with one another often? Do you socialize with others here?
- How would you characterize the relationships between members of different racial or ethnic groups in the neighborhood?

The answers to such questions can provide a wealth of initial data and stories about a community and may be compiled in narrative form or in charts summarizing key findings (Sharpe et al., 2000).

Modified Delphi Process

The *Delphi survey* is a method for getting an opinion from a large group; group members do not need to meet but can still benefit from feedback and interaction. First, materials are reviewed and rankings elicited, after which differences in rankings are discussed, materials modified, and a second round of voting undertaken, often with a median or other statistical marker used to suggest consensus (Patel, Koegel, Booker, Jones, & Wells, 2006). One of the chapter authors (Trevor Hancock) used a modified version of this method in Toronto in the early 1980s. For each of two health areas, a panel of approximately one hundred community leaders from all walks of life identified key health issues in the community. More recently, a modified Delphi technique was employed in the Los Angeles–based Witness for Wellness project, a mental health–focused partnership between an African American, community-based organization and researchers at a local medical school and the RAND Corporation (Patel et al., 2006). Project work groups each presented their goals and action plans to over forty work group members, who then each rated the various plans on six criteria: *clarity, feasibility, impact, reach, appropriateness, and feeling* (a "respondent's gut reaction to the plan") (pp. S1–S37). As Patel and her colleagues note, despite some initial concerns about feeling judged, community partners expressed high satisfaction with the method, particularly in view of its transparency and the ease with which results could be shared and understood.

The advantages of a Delphi or modified Delphi technique are that it enables a wide variety of individuals to participate in a way that is not too time consuming and that it allows both the list of issues and the rank ordering of those issues to be determined by the participants themselves.

Community Capacity Inventories

As this chapter has suggested, an important alternative to the *community needs assessments* traditionally relied on in fields like public health and social welfare is capacity-focused efforts, which form a critical part of CBPR. The simplest such approaches often involve creating a *community capacity inventory,* typically by developing a written list of the skills and talents of individual community members and of the associations and other resources of the neighborhood as a whole. Although a simple survey can help gather the material for this list, the information gleaned from windshield and walking tours, interviews, and other assessment methods described in this chapter can be used as well. Similarly, community newspapers or directories may contain references to dozens of individual and neighborhood resources and can also constitute important community assets in themselves. For a detailed guide to undertaking a comprehensive community capacity inventory, see Kretzmann and McKnight's *Building Communities from the Inside Out* (1993).

As McKnight and Kretzmann (1992) have pointed out, conducting a capacity inventory can be an important way of drawing attention to the gifts of "labeled" or stigmatized people as well as members of such often forgotten groups as elders and children. In the Healthy Neighborhoods project in West Contra Costa County, California, facilitators taped to the wall of a community center large pieces of paper with headings such as "child care provision," "artistic abilities," "cooking for large groups," and "non-English-speaking ability." Residents who previously had seen themselves as lacking any talents and special skills soon were signing their names under several skill categories (El-Askari & Walton, 2005). Of particular importance in the aftermath of several state level anti-immigrant ballot initiatives was turning "speaking a language other than English" from a liability into a strength through this process (El Askari & Walton, 2005; Minkler, 2000).

Community Asset Maps

Closely related to community capacity inventories are *community asset maps,* created by community members themselves as they "map" local resources, abilities, and other building blocks for community growth and change (McKnight & Kretzmann, 1992). A community asset map is a visual representation of the physical assets of a community—library, playgrounds, schools, parks, houses of worship—that may constitute important physical and social support structures for achieving community goals. Asset maps are often drawn first by individuals or teams who walk or ride through their neighborhood and indicate the assets they observe on their own hand-drawn maps. Then they share their individual perceptions, and using push pins on a large street map, land use map, or collectively drawn asset map, they then develop a map that represents the collective views of the group about community strengths, or building blocks.

Although asset mapping is sometimes conducted by outsiders with minimal contact with residents, it becomes a potent tool in CBPR when community members play an active role in the process. Sharpe and her colleagues (2000) thus describe how the visual mapping of a South Carolina neighborhood by outsiders at first suggested that a local church was an important community meeting place. Through dialogue with residents, however, it became apparent that nearly all the church's members lived outside the neighborhood, leaving local residents with little sense of identification with the institution. Asset mapping efforts that are driven by local residents are better able to accurately map community-perceived strengths and resources and thus to be a strong resource in CBPR. Finally, community asset mapping has proven an excellent method for use with low literacy populations and with youths, where the "community" may be a school, a neighborhood, or other shared space (Amsden & VanWynsberghe, 2005; Wilson et al., 2007).

Risk Mapping

The technique known as *risk mapping* was first developed by workers in an auto plant in Italy in the 1960s. Using a blueprint of the factory's production line and drawing on it circles of varying sizes and colors to indicate the different workplace hazards, the workers then had their findings verified by a group of scientists. The risk-mapping method was adapted and used by Mexico City health and safety activists in the 1970s and by the 1980s had achieved popularity in the United States as well. Health departments, university-based occupational health centers, community-based organizations concerned with environmental health issues, and unions are among the entities that have effectively used this approach (Mujica, 1992; see also Appendix J), which is now widely employed in the field of occupational health.

Risk mapping need not involve a shared work setting to be an effective tool in CBPR. Residents of a housing complex (such as an apartment building or a single-room-occupancy hotel) or pupils in a school can focus on shared spaces such as multipurpose rooms, hallways, and elevators to collectively identify hazards to which they are exposed. Community members sharing such a space are asked to draw a floor plan of the site, indicating boundaries, doorways, windows, and other key features. Colored markers then are used to identify different types of hazards (physical, chemical, and so on), as described in Appendix J (see also Mujica, 1992). Community members then discuss the various risks identified on their map, decide on those they most wish to address, and develop plans for further studying and taking action to address the chief hazards of concern to the group.

A variant of the risk map is the community safety audit conducted by groups of women who examine potential threats to safety in their neighborhood by walking through it in a group at night, identifying poorly lit areas and other safety hazards (Wekerle & Whitzman, 1995). The problem areas thus identified can then be used as a basis for study and action to bring about change.

Community Dialogues or Guided Discussions

Engaging community members in dialogues or guided discussions about their communities has become an increasingly popular means of community assessment and issue selection. Within this broad category of approaches, focus groups are among the most popular, typically involving six to twelve diverse community members under the direction of a trained moderator. In a confidential and nonthreatening discussion about their community, members address a series of questions designed to elicit their beliefs about the strengths of their neighborhoods and the changes they would like to see. Whether tape-recorded and transcribed or summarized through detailed handwritten notes, the output of focus groups can provide a wealth of information for thematic analysis and use in subsequent community-driven asset assessment and issue selection (Krueger & Casey, 2000).

Nominal group process (Delbecq, Van de Ven, & Gustafson, 1975) is a second small-group method with considerable appeal for community assessment and issue selection. A structured process designed to foster creativity, encourage conflicting opinions, and prevent domination by a few vocal individuals, nominal group process is especially helpful in encouraging the participation of marginal group members (Hancock & Minkler, 2005; Siegel, Attkisson, & Cohn, 1977).

The *community dialogues* approach, developed by the National Coalition for Healthier Cities & Communities/National Civic League (2003), represents a method that can involve either small groups or literally hundreds of individuals in diverse settings in a process of discussing their hopes and dreams for their communities and the issues about which they are concerned. Sample dialogue questions include the following:

- What do you believe are the two or three most important characteristics of a healthy community?
- What makes you most proud of our community?
- What are some specific examples of people or groups working together to improve the health and quality of life of our community?
- What do you believe is keeping our community from doing what needs to be done to improve health and quality of life?
- What would excite you enough to become involved (or more involved) in improving our community?

Voting with Your Feet

An interesting and simple way to assist a group in identifying its priorities is to ask group members to list their priorities and then to move into smaller work groups representing the priorities that have been identified. Because people cannot be in more than one place at a time, the level of commitment to each of the listed priority issues becomes apparent very quickly. An issue that is deemed very important (such as poverty) may in fact fail to attract any people to a work group forming to deal with it, perhaps because the issue is too big and people feel helpless in the face of it. Conversely, if most of the people in the room were to move into one particular group, this would indicate that a lot of time and energy should be committed to that issue and that those people could form the core of a work group. (The fact that an issue receives no support from the participants on a particular day does not mean it is not an important issue but rather that the people in the room that day are not the right ones to deal with it.)

Developing Community Indicators

Growing attention has been focused on the development and use of *community health indicators* (CHIs), measures that characterize a neighborhood or community as a whole, rather than the individuals or subgroups of which it is comprised (Cheadle, Wagner, Koepsell, Kristal, & Patrick, 1992; Hancock, Labonté, & Edwards, 1999). Such indicators take several forms and may be thought of as "a community analogue to health-risk appraisal for individuals" (Patrick & Wickizer, 1995, p. 72). The number, type, and visibility of "No Smoking" signs in workplaces, the proportion of space in grocery stores devoted to fresh fruits and vegetables (see Chapter Twenty-One), and the proportion of a community's children under age two with up-to-date immunizations are all examples of potent community health indicators. Equally important, however, are such indicators as transportation, including transit access and bikeable streets, and *voting power*, the percentage of residents who voted in the last presidential election (Costa, Palaniappan, Wong, et al., 2002). Sustainable Seattle (1995) has pioneered the use of *provocative indicators,* such as the number of salmon in a creek—indicators that although perhaps not directly related to health say something interesting—and perhaps at times troubling—about the community.

Although indicators are often created and employed by outside professionals, the very process of developing CHIs can be an important part of CBPR. Constituting as they do a limited set of quantitative and qualitative measures that reflect the current health status of the complex system that a community represents, CHIs can also suggest how the community's health status, broadly defined, is changing over time (Bauer, 2003). Ideally, as Hancock and his colleagues (1999) have pointed out, good community indicators should reflect six key determinants of health: environmental quality, economic activity, social cohesion and "civicness," equity (including power), sustainability, and livability. They should further capture four process dimensions—education, participation, empowerment and civil rights, and government performance—as well as the outcome of health status. Finally, to be relevant to both policymakers and the general public, community indicators should have these key qualities:

- Face validity—they make sense to people
- Theoretical and empirical validity—they measure an important health determinant or dimension

▪ Social value—they measure things people care about

▪ Valency—they are powerful and carry social and political punch [Hancock, Labonté, & Edwards, 2000]

The West Oakland Environmental Indicators Project (Pacific Institute, 2002; Costa et al., 2002) in California offers a potent example of how a CBPR health indicators project can help a community to bring about change. Community-driven identification of indicators and gathering of relevant scientific data produced powerful findings (for example, that West Oakland residents face seven times the toxic pollution of the city as a whole, and children in this community have asthma hospitalization rates seven times higher than that of the state's children as a whole). Presented in the form of a colorful booklet with a "toxic tour" accompanying its release, the findings have now also been used to develop a partnership with the Environmental Protection Agency (EPA) to further study and address the neighborhood's environmental problems.

Visioning Processes

Community dialogues and the creation of healthy community indicators are often part of a larger *visioning process* through which a group of community members "collectively define a shared dream of what their community can become" (Sharpe et al., 2000, p. 209). Varying in length and format from a daylong retreat to a yearlong process with multiple phases, the process of visioning typically involves both small-group work and large-group convenings under the leadership of trained facilitators. The visioning workshop process has been extensively used in healthy community projects. Groups with as many as one hundred or more participants are taken through a process of guided imagery in which they see their community at some point in the future when it is as healthy as it could be. Then, working in small groups of six to eight, they are asked to draw a group picture of what they saw in their mind's eye. These pictures are then shared with the group as a whole, and themes evident in most of the pictures are identified. These common themes can then be the basis for issue development, because they reflect the factors that the participants recognize as being most important and fundamental to the health of their community (Hancock, 1993).

One of the benefits of this approach is that it is a great leveler; the university president probably does not draw any better than the truck driver—both probably draw like six-year-olds and not as well as the street youths! Moreover, individuals do not need to be literate to participate because the process is all verbal and visual—no writing is permitted on the drawings—at least not until the point where common categories are identified, and even then symbols can be used.

In the Clark County Community Voices 2010 project, in Vancouver, Washington, teen mothers, members of a Russian church group, and participants in a local senior organization were among a wide variety of community members who took part in a yearlong visioning process. Through focus groups, they addressed such questions as, "What do you most like about your community?" "What are your hopes for your community's children twenty years from now?" and, "Where would you put your energy to make the community a better place?" (Lasker, Abramson, & Freedman, 1998).

As in the other community dialogue approaches described in this chapter, the processes involved in this activity can constitute a critical phase of CBPR, while the identification of community-perceived strengths and issues in need of redress can form an important basis for subsequent research and praxis.

Creative Arts

Growing appreciation of the role that the arts can play in helping communities identify their strengths and assets as well as their shared problems and concerns (McDonald, Sarche, & Wang, 2005) is grounded in part in the philosophy and methods of Paulo Freire. As he asked, rhetorically, "How is it possible for us to work in a community without feeling the spirit of the culture that has been there for many years, without trying to understand the soul of the culture?" (Horton & Freire, 1990, p. 131).

A variety of techniques have been used to capture visual and oral expressions of the history, sources of pride, and shared concerns of a people. Key among these are community murals, vision workshop drawings, poetry and arts workshops, plays about the community's history and present issues, and videotapes capturing a wealth of perspectives on community life. As Marian McDonald and colleagues (2005) observed, "Cultural forms of expression rooted in community help not only to give voice to concerns but to establish the collective life, whether through celebrations, ritual or grief" (p. 352). Further, they can help a community break down walls of social isolation and share collective visions—shared experiences that can be particularly important in oppressed or marginalized communities.

Illustrating this message the photovoice process described in Chapter Eleven provides community members with a powerful means of documenting, through their own photographs, community assets and problems that in turn can form the basis of dialogue, collective analysis, and action for social change. This process has been successfully used by such diverse groups as rural women in China (Wang & Burris, 1994), youths in low-income multicultural neighborhoods (Wilson et al., 2007), and homeless people (Wang, Cash, & Powers, 2000), and has demonstrated considerable promise with these diverse populations (see Chapter Eleven).

ISSUE SELECTION IN CBPR

The approaches just described can produce a wealth of stories and data by and about a community and its resources, strengths, perceived problems or needs, and dreams for the future. The outside researcher or professional can often play a valuable role in helping community members learn about and use one or more of these methods and then critically reflect on what they have learned about their community as a basis for the next steps in the CBPR process.

Because the methods described in this chapter are likely to reveal a wide range of problems of concern to the community, however, a critical step in CBPR is to help community members *turn problems into issues,* to identify those concerns they feel deeply enough about to systematically study and take action on. In this process the outsider can play a valuable role in asking the kinds of questions that can help community members decide on a specific issue or concern that can in turn form the basis of collective study and action for social change.

Community organizers provide a variety of guidelines and criteria for issue selection that can be adapted to CBPR. Borrowing from organizer Lee Staples (2005, p. 175), for example, and using community rather than community organization as the frame of reference, residents engaged in CBPR may evaluate the pros and cons of an issue they are considering by dialoguing about the following questions:

- Is the issue consistent with the long-range goals or agenda of the community (as identified, for example, through a visioning process)?
- Will the issue unify or be divisive?
- Will the issue contribute to community capacity building?
- Will the process of CBPR on this issue provide a good educational experience for leaders and community members, developing their consciousness, independence, and skills?
- Will the community receive credit for a victory?
- Will working on this issue result in new partnerships or alliances?
- Will CBPR on this issue result in concrete action for change and produce new issues for subsequent CBPR efforts?
- Will CBPR on this issue lead to an improved health or social outcome for the community?
- Is the issue important enough to people that they are willing to work on it?

As suggested by this list, a good issue for a CBPR effort will be consistent with the community's overall vision of itself as a healthy community and will help it move toward that vision. Similarly, and while recognizing that communities are not homogeneous in their goals and values (Labonté, 2005), a good issue will be selected through a democratic process that helps the community avoid the kind of divisiveness that can weaken it rather than strengthen it (Staples, 2005). A good issue will not only appeal to a broad range of community members but also provide multiple opportunities for participation in the CBPR process. Similarly, a good issue will attract new leaders and provide both leaders and members of the community with opportunities for developing a variety of skills and abilities that contribute to capacity building on the individual, organizational, and community levels. Ideally, the issue chosen will also attract external funding and other outside supports that can further expand the community's resource base (Staples, 2005). An issue may attract other potential community or institutional partners too, whose participation may further enhance aspects of the CBPR process while contributing to local capacity building.

Like community organizing, CBPR for health is ultimately concerned with bringing about social change that will promote the health and well-being of the community. The issue selection process should therefore also involve dialogue about whether and how participatory research on the issue under consideration is likely to bring about conditions that will make the community a better and healthier place in which to live. An issue that excites people but has little or no prospect of leading to actions that ultimately improve community health will not be a good issue for CBPR.

In sum, many factors need to be considered by communities as they decide on the issue or issues that will drive a CBPR effort. By fostering a dialogue using the types of questions and guiding considerations discussed here, the outside researcher or professional can play an important role in helping community members with this critical stage in the CBPR process.

WHEN PREEXISTING GOALS CONSTRAIN ISSUE SELECTION

This chapter has been written from the perspective that communities can and should have a major role in determining the problem or issue to be studied and addressed through a CBPR process. Yet as earlier chapters have made clear, achieving true community-driven issue selection is often difficult in practice. Public health researchers thus frequently approach a community concerned about its high rates of HIV/AIDS or substance abuse and wishing to collaborate in studying the problem and developing a community-based intervention. Similarly, funding mandates may sharply circumscribe the areas within which issue selection may take place.

The federal government's landmark initiative to eliminate disparities in health represents a good case in point. When the Centers for Disease Control and Prevention (CDC) made substantial funds available for eliminating health disparities, it earmarked six *areas of focus* within which such efforts must take place: cancer screening and management, cardiovascular disease, child and adult immunizations, diabetes, HIV/AIDS, and infant mortality (U.S. Department of Health and Human Services, 1998). Serious disparities in both health access and health outcomes continue to exist by race and ethnicity in all six of these areas. Yet for communities upset over drugs in their children's playgrounds, violence, or high unemployment rates, none of these six may be an issue of central concern. Similarly, the Delphi process used in Toronto, as described earlier, led to the identification of unemployment, poverty, and stress as the major threats to the health of the communities. Clearly, these are community priorities, but they do not usually fall within the mandate of a health department, even one as progressive as Toronto's then was. This led to some interesting reflections and some innovative actions.

These examples illustrate a classic dilemma. On the one hand, making funds available to conduct CBPR can be a boon to communities, providing resources and stimulating partnerships that can help them tackle major health problems. On the other hand, limiting funding or other support to particular content areas within health, narrowly defined, may violate the basic principle of community-driven issue selection.

For communities and their professional allies engaged in CBPR within the constraints imposed by initiatives like the federal effort to eliminate health disparities, some useful lessons may be learned from such related efforts as the National Healthy Start Program (NHSP) to reduce infant mortality. When the NHSP commenced in 1991, the United States ranked twenty-second in the world in infant mortality, and the black infant death rate was more than twice the white rate. The program's goal was to reduce infant mortality by half over a five-year period in fifteen demonstration sites, plus an additional eighty sites added by the late 1990s. Although specifically targeting infant mortality, however, program guidelines also emphasized the need for "substantive and informed" community participation through consortia and other means designed to foster community-driven approaches at every stage of the process (Health Resources and Services Administration, 1991, p. 4). As a consequence, community consortia often engaged participants in studying and addressing the issues they identified. In Cleveland, for example, residents successfully took on a local hospital's use of an incinerator that was creating an environmental hazard, while in Chicago, consortium participants studied the new welfare reform time limits and work requirements and worked to get waivers in place for mothers with special needs children (Minkler, Thompson, Bell, & Rose, 2001).

Taking a cue from such examples, CBPR projects that begin in response to problem-specific, community-based health initiatives can, with creativity and attention to the interconnections between many health and social issues, often *broaden the net* so that issues of primary concern to the community become a driving force for the collaborative research and action undertaken.

SUMMARY

This chapter has provided a broad overview of the core principles underlying community-driven asset identification and issue selection and their relevance for CBPR. It has also described and illustrated by example a number of tools and approaches that communities may find useful for recognizing and building on their strengths and for collectively identifying issues about which they feel strongly enough to engage in systematic inquiry and action. However, this overview of tools and methods has also intentionally omitted an important and growing category of approaches, those that use computer technology in assessing community resources and potential issues for CBPR. It is to these increasingly potent tools for assessment and issue selection that this volume turns in the next chapter.

QUESTIONS FOR DISCUSSION

1. This chapter describes the first principle in community-driven issue selection as "starting where the people are." Thinking back on your own experiences or case studies with which you are familiar, can you give an example of a time when this principle was followed? What were the results?

2. The chapter authors suggest using questions like these to identify the natural leaders with whom researchers might partner: "Whom do people in this neighborhood go to for help or advice?" "Whom do children go to?" "When this community has had a problem in the past, who has been involved in working to solve it?" "Who gets things done in this community?" In groups of three, ask each other these questions, thinking of your own neighborhood, school cohort, or office community as a case in point. Then reverse roles. How did you feel asking (and being asked) these questions? What questions might usefully be added to the list?

3. Review the section of this chapter titled "Risk Mapping," then using that description of risk mapping and following the numbered steps in Appendix J, pair up with one to three partners to draw a risk map for a shared space (for example, a popular

coffee shop, the student or employee lounge, or a shared living or working place) or a hypothetical place of a type you have worked in previously (for example, a hospital waiting room or fast-food restaurant). Spend a total of fifteen minutes on the exercise. Then discuss your reactions and whether and how you might use this method as part of a CBPR effort.

KEY TERMS

Community capacity

Natural helpers

Asset mapping

Community health indicators

REFERENCES

Amsden, J., & VanWynsberghe, R. (2005). Community mapping as a research tool with youth. *Action Research, 3*(4), 257–281.

Bauer, G. F. (2003). Sample community health indicators on the neighborhood level. In M. Minkler & N. Wallerstein (Eds.), *Community-based participatory research for health* (pp. 438–445). San Francisco: Jossey-Bass.

Chávez, V., Minkler, M., Wallerstein, N., & Spencer, M. S. (2007). Community organizing for health and justice. In L. Cohen, V. Chávez, & S. Chehimi (Eds.), *Prevention is primary: Strategies for community well-being* (pp. 95–121). San Francisco: Jossey-Bass.

Cheadle, A., Wagner, E. A., Koepsell, T. D., Kristal, A., & Patrick, D. (1992). Environmental indicators: A tool for evaluating community-based health promotion programs. *American Journal of Preventive Medicine, 8,* 345–350.

Costa, S., Palaniappan, M., Wong, A. K., Hays, J., Landeiro, C., & Rongerude, J. (2002). *Neighborhood knowledge for change: West Oakland environmental indicators project.* Oakland, CA: Pacific Institute.

Day, K., Boarnet, M., Alfonzo, M., & Forsyth, A. (2006). The Irvine-Minnesota Inventory to measure built environments: Development. *American Journal of Preventive Medicine 30,* 144–152.

Delbecq, A., Van de Ven, A. H., & Gustafson, D. H. (1975). *Group techniques for program planning: A guide to nominal group and Delphi processes.* Glenview, IL: Scott, Foresman.

Duhl, L., & Hancock, T. (1988). *A guide to assessing healthy cities.* Copenhagen: FADL.

El-Askari, G., & Walton, S. (2005). The Healthy Neighborhoods Project: A local health department's role in catalyzing community development. *Health Education & Behavior, 25,* 146–159.

Eng, E., & Blanchard, L. (1990). Action-oriented community diagnosis: A health education tool. *International Journal of Community Health Education, 11*(2), 93–110.

Eng, E., Briscoe, J., & Cunningham, A. (1990). The effect of participation in water projects on immunization. *Social Science & Medicine, 30,* 1349–1358.

Freire, P. (1970). *Pedagogy of the oppressed.* New York: Seabury Press.

Freire, P. (1973). *Education for critical consciousness.* New York: Continuum.

Hall, B. L. (1992). From margins to center: The development and purpose of participatory action research. *American Sociologist, 23*(4), 15–28.

Hancock, T. (1993). Seeing the vision, defining your role. *Healthcare Forum Journal, 36*(3), 30–36.

Hancock, T., Labonté, R., & Edwards, R. (2000). Indicators that count: Population health indicators at the community level. Report # HP-10–0207. Toronto: University of Toronto/ParticipAction, Centre for Health Promotion.

Hancock, T., & Minkler, M. (2005). Community health assessment or healthy community assessment: Whose community? Whose health? Whose assessment? In M. Minkler (Ed.), *Community organizing and community building for health* (2nd ed., pp. 138–157). New Brunswick, NJ: Rutgers University Press.

Health Resources and Services Administration. (1991). *Guidance for the Healthy Start Program.* Washington, DC: Author.

Horton, M., & Freire, P. (1990). *We make the road by walking: Conversations on education and social change* (B. Bell, J. Gaventa, & J. Peters, Eds.). Philadelphia: Temple University Press.

Israel, B. A. (1985). Social networks and social support: Implications for natural helper and community level interventions. *Health Education Quarterly, 12,* 66–80.

Kretzmann, J. P., & McKnight, J. L. (1993). *Building communities from the inside out: A path toward finding and mobilizing a community's assets.* Chicago: ACTA.

Krueger, R. A., & Casey, M. A. (2000). *Focus groups: A practical guide for applied research* (3rd ed.). Thousand Oaks, CA: Sage.

Labonté, R. (2005). Community, community development, and forming of authentic partnerships: Some critical reflections. In M. Minkler (Ed.), *Community organizing and community building for health* (2nd ed., pp. 82–96). New Brunswick, NJ: Rutgers University Press.

Lasker, R. D., Abramson, D. M., & Freedman, G. R. (1998). *Pocket guide to cases of medicine and public health collaboration.* New York: Center for the Advancement of Collaborative Strategies in Health/New York Academy of Medicine.

McDonald, M., Sarche, J., & Wang, C. C. (2005). Using the arts in community organizing and community building. In M. Minkler (Ed.), *Community organizing and community building for health* (2nd ed., pp. 346–364). New Brunswick, NJ: Rutgers University Press.

McKnight, J. L., & Kretzmann, J. P. (1992). *Mapping community capacity.* Evanston, IL: Northwestern University, Center for Urban Affairs and Policy Research.

Minkler, M. (2000). Participatory action research and healthy communities. *Public Health Reports, 115,* 191–197.

Minkler, M., Thompson, M., Bell, J., & Rose, K. (2001). Contributions of community involvement to organizational-level empowerment: The federal Healthy Start experience. *Health Education & Behavior, 28,* 783–807.

Mujica, J. (1992). Coloring the hazards: Risk maps, research, and education to fight health hazards. *American Journal of Industrial Medicine, 22,* 767–770.

National Coalition for Healthier Cities & Communities/National Civic League (2003), Dialogue questions. In M. Minkler & N. Wallerstein (Eds.) *Community-Based Participatory Research for Health* (pp. 465–468). San Francisco, CA: Jossey-Bass.

Nyswander, D. (1956). Education for health: Some principles and their application. *Health Education Monographs, 14,* 65–70.

Pacific Institute. (2002). *Pacific Institute releases new report on West Oakland.* Retrieved Apr. 27, 2007, from www.pacinst.org/reports/environmental_indicators.

Patel, K. K., Koegel, P., Booker, T., Jones, L., & Wells, K. (2006). Innovative approaches to obtaining community feedback in the Witness for Wellness experience. *Ethnicity & Disease, 16*(1, Suppl. 1), S35–S42.

Patrick, D. L., & Wickizer, T. M. (1995). Community and health. In B. C. Amick, S. Levine, A. R. Tarlov, & D. C. Walsh (Eds.), *Society and health* (pp. 46–92). New York: Oxford University Press.

Scott, J. (1990). *Domination and the arts of resistance: Hidden transcripts.* New Haven, CT: Yale University Press.

Sharpe, P. A., Greany, M. L., Lee, P. R., & Royce, S. W. (2000). Assets-oriented community assessment. *Public Health Reports, 113,* 205–211.

Shepard, P. (2007, Nov. 5). *Environmental health leadership training.* Presentation to the 135th annual meeting of the American Public Health Association, Washington, DC.

Siegel, L. M., Attkisson, C. C., & Cohn, I. H. (1977). Mental health needs assessment: Strategies and techniques. In W. A. Hargreaves & C. C. Attkisson (Eds.), *Resource materials for community mental health program evaluation* (2nd ed., pp. 46–65). Washington, DC: U.S. Government Printing Office.

Sohng, S.S.L. (1996). Participatory research and community organizing. *Journal of Sociology and Social Welfare, 23*(4), 77–97.

Staples, L. (2005). Selecting and cutting the issue. In M. Minkler (Ed.), *Community organizing and community building for health* (2nd ed., pp. 173–192). New Brunswick, NJ: Rutgers University Press.

Sustainable Seattle. (1995). *Indicators of sustainable communities.* Retrieved Oct. 5, 2007, from http://www.sustainableseattle.org.

Tajik, M., & Minkler, M. (2007). Environmental justice research and action: A case study in political economy and community-academic collaboration. *International Quarterly of Community Health Education, 26*(3), 215–232.

Themba, M. N. (1999). *Making policy, making change: How communities are taking law into their own hands.* San Francisco: Jossey-Bass.

U.S. Department of Health and Human Services. (1998). *Call to action: Eliminating racial and ethnic disparities in health.* Washington, DC: Author/Grantmakers in Health.

Valente, T. W., & Pumpuang, P. (2007). Identifying opinion leaders to promote behavioral change. *Health Education & Behavior, 34*(6), 881–896.

Wang, C. C., & Burris, M. A. (1994). Empowerment through photo novella: Portraits of participation. *Health Education Quarterly, 21,* 171–186.

Wang, C. C., Cash, J. L., & Powers, L. S. (2000). Who knows the streets as well as the homeless? Promoting personal and community action through photovoice. *Health Promotion Practice, 1,* 81–89.

Wekerle, G., & Whitzman, C. (1995). *Safe cities: Guidelines for planning, design, and management.* New York: Van Nostrand Reinhold.

Wilson, N., Dasho, S., Martin, A. C., Wallerstein, N., Wang, C., & Minkler, M. (2007). Engaging young adolescents in social action through photovoice. *Journal of Early Adolescence, 27*(2), 241–261.

Wing, S., Grant, G., Green, M., & Stewart, C. (1996). Community-based collaboration for environmental justice: Southeast Halifax environmental awakening. *Environment and Urbanization, 8,* 129–140.

CHAPTER

10

USING WEB-BASED TOOLS TO BUILD CAPACITY FOR CBPR

TWO CASE STUDIES OF AMERICAN INDIAN LEADERSHIP DEVELOPMENT

**MARITA JONES, SHELLEY FRAZIER, CHRIS PERCY,
JEFFREY L. STOWELL, KRISTINE MALTRUD, & NINA WALLERSTEIN**

FOR MORE THAN a decade, Internet-based technology has been altering the community-based participatory research (CBPR) landscape, presenting new opportunities for research, learning, and community participation (Schultz, Fawcett, Francisco, & Berkowitz, 2003). Originally envisioned as a way to connect citizens and communities to a vast array of "how-to" information and supports for community-based action and research, the Internet has become a powerful tool in communities' efforts to actually *take* action and to collect and disseminate CBPR learning in ways previously perceived to be impractical or impossible (Fawcett, Schultz, Carson, Renault, & Francisco, 2003; see also Appendix D). The net effect has been an increase in the number of participating communities, the quality of that participation, the value to participating communities, and the quality of research and learning (Agre & Schuler, 1997). The Internet has allowed CBPR participants to enhance the values of participatory research that have become guiding principles for CBPR (Green et al., 1995; see also Chapter Three); and has strengthened the potential for community-based participatory and empowerment evaluation (Fetterman & Wandersman, 2004, 2007; see also Chapter Twelve; Fawcett et al., 2003; Wallerstein, 2000). Specifically, the Internet has enabled increasing participation of *both* community members and research and evaluation experts through enhanced tools for live and threaded discussion, storytelling, and other methodologies that previously required researchers and community members to be together in the same room or connected through less robust technologies. Methodologies, such as functional Internet supports that customize the collecting and sharing of information, cultural adaptations of existing tools (Fawcett et al., 2000), adaptation of information for youth and adult learning styles; and multilanguage translation have allowed the field of CBPR to increasingly realize its tradition of culturally based co-learning (Freire, 1973; Horton & Freire, 1990).

As Internet use has increased—today close to 75 percent of the U.S. population is on line (Pew Trusts, 2008)—Internet-based health education has also expanded. In the last decade this education has taken place through patient chat rooms, bulletin boards, small-group patient education interventions, Internet-based case management, and more recently, cultural adaptations. In a pilot Internet adaptation of the Stanford Diabetes Self-Management Program (Stanford University School of Medicine, 2008), Native peer leaders recruited participants over the Internet, provided education over the Internet, and conducted a follow-up focus group through an interactive list serve (Jernigan, 2007). Acceptance was high, with participants stating that the program complemented clinic-based providers and diabetes educators, particularly for most people who came from rural and reservation settings.

With this growth in interest, an increasingly rich array of CBPR resources is becoming available on the Internet (also see Appendix L). A community-based participatory research e-mail community (2008) was created through a partnership between Community-Campus Partnerships for Health (2008) and the Wellesley Institute. The Community Campus Partnerships for Health through the Institutional Partnerships for Prevention Research Group (2008) also offers an extensive CBPR curriculum. Several nonprofit organizations and CBPR collaboratives provide substantial online CBPR resources, including publications from the Community Research Network of the LOKA Institute (2008), the Institute for Community Research (2008), the Community-Based Collaboratives Research Consortium (2008), Living Knowledge (2008), the Southeast Community Resource Center (2008), and the Johns Hopkins Urban Health Institute (2008). Finally, the Work Group for Community Health and Development (2008a) at the University of Kansas has developed an online participatory evaluation system for local communities (see Appendix D) and has also produced a 7,000-page *community tool box* (CTB) (Work Group for Community Health and Development, 2008b), providing tools for CBPR partners in planning, leadership, group process, and other capacity development (Fawcett et al., 2000).

The public sector has been slower to buy into CBPR than the nonprofit world; however, there are exceptions. An extensive CBPR conference summary is available on line, convened in 2001 by the Agency for Healthcare Research and Quality (2001). Also, the Centers for Disease Control and Prevention (CDC) (2008) has online CBPR resources, as does the National Institutes of Health (NIH) (2008).

Although the Internet has increased the capacity of CBPR, barriers such as the *digital divide,* the gap between those who have access to quality computer and Internet technology and those who do not, continue to exist (Norris, 2001). Two recent surveys, however, found that this divide is narrowing, with 74 percent of whites, 61 percent of African Americans, 80 percent of English-speaking Hispanics (Pew Trusts, 2008); and 69 percent of Native Americans (Heuertz, Gordon, Moore, & Gordon, 2002) stating that they used the Internet. Despite this apparent level of access, many rural and poor communities and neighborhoods still lack quality Internet access (owing to bandwidth or computer hardware limitations) or any Internet access at all. Equally important is the computer skills gap across generations of *researchers* and *community participants,* which can often limit the possibilities for effective collaborative Internet tool use.

Finally, the security or perceived security of information shared in confidence among CPBR participants becomes of increasing concern in a digital age. Ensuring the security of information so that the processes or results of CPBR are not misused is paramount if the field is to continue to progress in using Internet-based tools and supports.

INTRODUCTION TO CASE STUDIES

Since 2003, the Health Promotion/Disease Prevention (HP/DP) Policy Advisory Committee, made up of tribal leaders and representatives of American Indian and Alaska Native health organizations, has worked together with the Indian Health Service to establish a comprehensive HP/DP plan to support the development of tools, resources, and training for local community wellness initiatives based on cultural and traditional teachings.

This plan aims to reach the diverse population of more than 4.1 million Native people, representing over 566 tribes and urban Indian groups across the nation. Compared to the U.S. population as a whole, Native people face a lower life expectancy, substantially higher obesity rates, and a 231 percent higher diabetes mortality rate. These outcomes are coupled with conditions of poverty and the lowest per capita health care expenditures for any U.S. population group. In seeking to improve their own health, Native people are turning to traditional teachings of balance and of integrated mind, body, and spirit, which have served them well for hundreds of years of survival, as well as to advocacy for greater resources for prevention, health promotion, and health care.

Internet-based tools have recently begun to play a central role in two key health promotion initiatives rooted in cultural and traditional teachings: the Healthy Native Communities Fellowship and Just Move It. A consideration of how these tools have been useful in these programs—providing a means for shared learning, support, motivation, networking, and participatory evaluation—can provide lessons for others involved in healthy communities work and community-based participatory research.

CASE 1: HEALTHY NATIVE COMMUNITIES FELLOWSHIP

Established in 2004, the Healthy Native Communities Fellowship (HNCF) is a corner-stone of the HP/DP initiative. Started as a yearlong program to work with community teams who wished to expand their ability to mobilize Native communities to promote health and wellness, the fellowship is grounded in Native cultural, social, spiritual, and intellectual perspectives and consists of

- Four weeklong, face-to-face retreats.
- Fellow Space: an action-learning process in which fellow teams practice their skills in their home communities between retreats in order to involve home teams and engage broader community support.
- Coaching by HNCF staff to assist fellows in implementing new skills.
- An online learning community called the HNCF Workstation, where fellows connect via the Internet for discussions, use of a resource library, and networking through posting success stories and other documentation of actions and change during their fellowship year and beyond. Support is then provided to the fellow alumni through Internet communication and coaching for three to five years after they graduate from the fellowship.

Fourteen to fifteen teams from across the nation, comprising forty to fifty individuals altogether, participate in the fellowship each year. Team members, drawn from tribal governments, police, spiritual leaders, and elders and from the fields of education, health, environment, and business and the like, represent a cross-section of their community. The four directions of the *medicine wheel* form the framework for the fellowship curriculum (see Figure 10.1). An action-learning model inspired by the work of Paulo Freire guides fellows as they start with personal and team listening and assessment, using tools such as team and individual learning plans and a personal medicine wheel to generate goals for personal transformation and healing that will support their own changing roles in communities. The curriculum continues with an emphasis on listening, dialogue, planning, action, and reflection skills for community development and change within each fellow's specific cultural, spiritual, political, and economic contexts.

The HNCF WorkStation is a customized, online, Internet-based learning community designed to provide fellows with information and tools for communicating, sharing, learning, and evaluating in relation to local community change efforts, with a goal of creating an intentional *family* among fellows and faculty. Not only is this workstation used at the retreats but fellows have access to it in between retreats and alumni maintain their membership after they graduate (Healthy Native Communities Partnership, 2008b). Continual access is an important feature. As one fellow has said, "The workstation is wonderful. I can access it any time when this session is over and other times when I wish. I can log on and leave word with staff and other fellows."

The first contact for the fellowship is through a teleconference for the teams and the HNCF coaches one month prior to the first retreat. Introductory hands-on training is conducted demonstrating workstation use, including how to access posted announcements

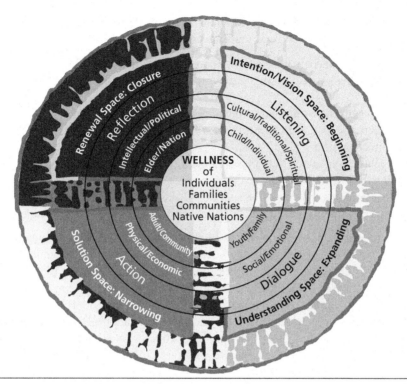

FIGURE 10.1 *Medicine Wheel, which honors the four directions of*
Native traditions
Source: Healthy Native Communities Partnership, 2008a, shows color version.

and materials. Coaching calls provide technical assistance to fellows in between retreats for implementing their new tools and skills; coaching involves use of the workstation to track progress, update learning plans, and discuss new postings on the various workstation features. During Fellow Space, fellows post their success stories, materials to share, and news items, and can chat on the *learning communities* feature.

Since its beginning the fellowship has supported a participatory evaluation learning team, which has monitored changes in fellows, teams, and communities in addition to evaluating curriculum and the HNCF Workstation. This effort has allowed a continuous evolution of both program and technology delivery. In the first year the staff and faculty were just one step ahead of the fellows in learning the best ways to use and adapt the workstation, yet each year new insights have led to a workstation that is more useful and easier to use.

During the first retreat in year one, the fellows were introduced to the learning communities and *introductions board* workstation features, where they posted their stories of who they were, where they came from, and what they wanted to gain from the fellowship. The workstation was used to supplement the curriculum (for assessments as well as documentation), yet fellows had insufficient time during the first-year retreats to gain adequate skills. Evaluation showed multiple early challenges:

- Participants had technical issues with computers at their own sites.
- Some participants had minimal experience with computers and with using the Internet.
- Participants displayed limited levels of access and control in the first year.
- Participants found it difficult to access files, documents, and pictures, owing to too many directory layers.
- Participants could attach only one document or picture at a time and could post only limited words in some features.
- Some participants did not offer success stories because they thought this was too "boastful" and their local cultures did not support placing one person above another.

During the second year of the fellowship the curriculum team made intentional decisions about ways to better employ the workstation for effective communication, better documentation, and better tracking of the fellows' community work. With workstation training by the coaches before the first session, the fellows were able to introduce themselves through the learning communities feature prior to week one. Hands-on training in workstation features was better integrated into each retreat. The *success stories* feature was promoted, and two-thirds of the teams posted success stories. Fellow capacity to manipulate the workstation also increased, with participants being able to add their own materials to the *materials to share* feature. Alumni could create their own online e-newsletter. A new *survey* feature allowed fellows to complete their end-of-week evaluations on line.

By year three the fellows were receiving the workstation training by teleconference prior to week one. Laptop computers were provided for each team to use during the weeklong retreats. Expectations were further clarified and communicated about how to use the workstation effectively. The results have been exciting: a doubling in postings of success stories; increased use of the *online documentation and support system* (ODSS) feature, more posting of fellows' own documents and pictures in their team folders in the materials to share feature; more immediate feedback on the survey feature; and a substantial increase in workstation use and viewing by all teams.

The learning team has sought to identify changes or outcomes at multiple levels: the fellows, their teams, their home teams, and their communities. (The evaluation logic model is available from the chapter authors.) Early on, it became clear that the fellows were acquiring new knowledge and skills, yet they also began to express deeper, *transformational* changes in relation to their views of themselves, their ability to work in teams, and their actions in their communities. At the individual level, fellows experienced increased confidence and self-awareness, self-reflection, and also self-efficacy for engaging in facilitation, planning, and actions. Most fellows have reported greater self-confidence in using such HNCF skills as deep listening, facilitating, using the personal medicine wheel, speaking in front of groups, and making personal changes related to exercise, diet, and taking time for their own healing.

As their use of the workstation has progressed into the third year, fellows have posted success stories of how they adapted many of the HNCF skills. For example, one team adapted the *gift inventory* into a summer camp curriculum. Another team used the medicine wheel with its marital couples group to help clients visualize their need to blend values and opportunities in their relationships. As a result of this sharing of adaptations, other teams reported that they felt empowered to make their own changes to tools and processes they had learned. The workstation evolved from a tool for keeping track of activities and actions into a shared learning space where teams could create tools and also adapt them to their unique situations.

Community changes have also increased as the curriculum has shifted over time to a greater emphasis on advocacy, strategic planning, community wellness and cultural actions, new partnerships, and policy change. Analyses of the workstation success stories from the third year teams have corroborated:

- High engagement with community footprints: for example, creating mission statements and planning documents
- Greater policy engagement: for example, one team's success at advocating for a new mental health policy to expedite more state support
- New cultural programs: for example, one team's success at applying for CDC tobacco grant money to translate materials into the Aleut language (which is being lost)
- Greater changes in community capacity, levels of participation, use of HNCF skills, and increased partnerships

In the fourth year the Web site continues to be transformed, with new blogs for community sharing, wiki tools for joint creation of documents, and easier access to training and documentation materials to support community capacity to develop community learning and for communities to be resources for each other.

CASE 2: JUST MOVE IT

The Internet has played a key role in the evolution of Just Move It (JMI), a national campaign to promote wellness through physical activity in American Indian and Alaska Native communities. JMI started in Navajo communities during 1993 as a series of local walking and running events, and expanded in 2003 to the national level as a partnership between the National Congress of American Indians, the National Indian Health Board, and the Shiprock Area Indian Health Service Health Promotion Program. JMI's goal has been to get over one million Native people moving, working through tribes, tribal communities, and organizations across the United States. By 2008, more than 300 Native communities had joined as Just Move It partners, representing over 50,000 participants from Alaska to Florida.

JMI partners receive several benefits from joining the campaign:

- The right to use the JMI national logo in their local activities
- Access to national corporate partners, including NIKE

▪ How-to support kits for community- and school-based physical activity promotion activities

▪ Support from other tribal communities and organizations that are also part of JMI

▪ Updates on wellness training opportunities in their area or region

The first visible Just Move It activity at the national level was the establishment of National Native American Health and Fitness Day as a yearly event, kicked off at the 2003 National Congress of American Indians (NCAI) conference. Native communities attending this NCAI event were urged to e-mail justmoveit@ihs.gov for information on how they could join JMI. Letters were sent to all tribal leaders from NCAI informing them about JMI and National Native American Health and Fitness Day. Tribal leaders from across the nation were recruited to provide overall direction to the program through the Indian Health Service Prevention Initiative Policy Advisory Committee.

Program development efforts initially focused on toolkits to support local events and campaigns, tracking tools, and incentives, all available to partners as they joined the campaign. Evaluation planning included tracking both the qualitative and the quantitative impacts of the campaign at the level of the communities by collecting stories; examining program and event descriptions; and counting the numbers of communities, schools, and worksites participating.

The Just Move It national Web site was launched in 2004 as a "front door" into the campaign, with the primary goal of improving access to JMI. Key elements of the Web site changed the entire focus of Just Move It national efforts. First, a national map with all the JMI partners gave an immediate visual representation of the growing national interest in the campaign, as well as a tool for communities to identify who was doing similar work in their region so they could make local connections. Second, the Web site increased the capacity of JMI to help local communities get started, share lessons learned, and use tracking mechanisms. This quickly led to a change in perspective for the entire Just Move It campaign as it shifted from an *expert-based model,* in which the Internet was seen as a dissemination mechanism for information and tools, to a community-based *network model,* in which the Internet was looked on as a tool for collaboration and the sharing of best and promising practices developed by the local partners themselves, and also as an opportunity to share struggles and challenges.

Rather than expend energy on promoting national best practice models, it quickly became clear to the JMI program staff that the local tools and materials being developed in many tribal communities were as good as or better than the tools being developed at the national level. The site was adapted to provide more sharing space for partners, and a special *tools* section was developed, using a "recipe-sharing" metaphor. A four directions model ("prepare it, promote it, do it, and keep track") was used to organize the tools (or recipes) developed by JMI partners. For example, Native programs that have developed culture-based posters promoting an event or logs for tracking individuals' physical activity can share their work with others to use or adapt.

The Just Move It Web site has become a virtual gathering place for partners in a national movement to reclaim the legacy of wellness for American Indian and Alaska Native peoples. For many smaller tribes and Native communities, in both rural and urban settings, it provides a means to be part of something bigger than themselves—to join together with other Native people to push back against the wave of chronic diseases, such as diabetes, obesity, and heart disease, that threatens to wash over their people. JMI partners feel that joining the program helps them assert control over their own physical health in a way that reconnects them to cultural, emotional, and spiritual wellness.

The Native identity of the program has been a key aspect of the Just Move It "brand" that attracts partners to join. Examples shared by JMI partners of the roles of tradition, culture, and Native identity in promoting physical activity include:

- The use of traditional materials, herbs, and plants as incentives
- The use of traditional language and teachings in promoting activity
- The connection of physical activities to Heritage Day celebrations
- The integration of traditional games and competitions
- The use of culturally relevant metaphors

In the latter regard, schoolchildren walking in a coastal tribal community were encouraged to keep track of their miles on a chart that visualized their class paddling virtual canoes all the way to Hawaii. In asserting their political identity, another group kept track of their miles on a virtual "walk to Washington, DC" to deliver a letter to the president about the strengths and challenges of its tribe.

The JMI project has identified almost four thousand communities around the country with significant Native populations, with a goal of reaching one million. The Web-based tools have already strengthened the movement at both local and national levels, assisted regional networking, and provided support, motivation, and recognition for local action.

SUMMARY

These case studies from health promotion efforts among Native Americans have illustrated how Internet-based tools can support collaboration between dispersed communities. From maintaining connections between HNCF Fellows between their quarterly retreat sessions and after their fellowship year to helping widely scattered Native communities to join together as part of a national movement to promote wellness through physical activity, Web-based tools have provided a means of shared learning, motivation, and networking.

While initially conceived of as a means to share centrally created tools and information with a dispersed public, the Web-based tools used in both cases quickly became a platform for distributed learning and support among participants who have shared interests but often live and work at great distances from each other. These online communities serve as virtual gathering places for an action-learning process—one in which members reflect on their experiences and develop their own learnings as they do so. In the four directions model used in both case studies (see Figure 10.1), the importance of this reflection process is that it generates the learnings that inform the next cycle of intention, planning, and action.

The experiences of partners and fellows provide important motivation for other participants. Success stories shared through the Web-based tools have led other partners and fellows to try new skills and approaches in their community work and to feel empowered to adapt and change the tools presented. Particularly in communities with little positive attention from the mainstream media, holding up examples of positive developments from similar communities can be an important step in motivating community change efforts.

These case studies also show how Web-based tools can go beyond the experiences of one community motivating another to a process of shared knowledge creation and capacity building. The tool box section of the JMI Web site and the new wiki tools on the HNCF WorkStation are examples of partner-created shared knowledge coming out of multiple communities. The immediate feedback and ability to reflect, question, and learn together that Web-based tools foster also allows these tools to be used for participatory evaluation. For example, data in the success stories sections of both the JMI and HNCF sites can be examined with qualitative analysis tools to identify patterns and lessons. Online documentation systems can be helpful to local CBPR research efforts at the same time that they enable national comparisons.

New opportunities for applying these kinds of Web-based tools to community health work are emerging as several trends come together. More and more young people, including those in isolated and marginalized communities, are becoming comfortable with a variety of Web-based tools, including social networking sites, blogs, and programs for sharing audio and video products they create, and are telling their own stories. Access to the Web for rural and isolated communities is improving. Tools for shared creation and recording of knowledge are now available for communal group processes across dispersed communities. The hope is that Internet resources will continue to become more accessible and user friendly in order to enhance the core work of communities in building their community and research capacity to enhance community health.

QUESTIONS FOR DISCUSSION

1. How do the case studies represent a changing environment in Internet use and the Internet's ability to foster participatory evaluation, CBPR knowledge creation, and community capacity building?

2. If you were participating in a CBPR project, what Internet methodologies might be helpful to you, and how would you enhance their use?

KEY TERMS

Internet use   Distributed knowledge networks   Participatory evaluation

REFERENCES

Agency for Healthcare Research and Quality. (2001). *Community-based participatory research: Conference summary.* Retrieved Apr. 24, 2008, from http://www.ahrq.gov/about/cpcr/cbpr/cbpr1.htm.

Agre, P., & Schuler, D. (1997). *Reinventing technology, rediscovering community: Critical explorations.* Greenwich, CT: Ablex.

Centers for Disease Control and Prevention. (2008). *Search results*. Retrieved April 24, 2008, from http://www.cdc. gov/search.do?queryText=CBPR&searchButton.x=0&searchButton.y=0&action=search.

Community-Based Collaboratives Research Consortium. (2008). [Home page.] Retrieved Apr. 24, 2008, from http:// www.cbcrc.org.

Community-based participatory research (CBPR) e-mail community. (2008). [Listserv.] Retrieved Apr. 24, 2008, from http://mailman1.u.washington.edu/mailman/listinfo/cbpr.

Community-Campus Partnerships for Health. (2008). [Home page.] Retrieved Apr. 24, 2008, from www.ccph.info.

Community Institutional Partnerships for Prevention Research Group. (2008). Developing and sustaining community-based participatory research partnerships: A skill-building curriculum. Retrieved May 20, 2008, from http://depts. washington.edu/ccph/cbpr/intro/intro.php.

Fawcett, S. B., Boothroyd, R., Schultz, J. A., Francisco, V., Carson, V., & Bremby, R. (2003). Building capacity for participatory evaluation within community initiatives. *Journal of Prevention and Intervention in the Community, 26*(2), 21–36.

Fawcett, S. B. Francisco, V. T., Schultz, J. A., Berkowitz, B., Wolff, T .J., & Nagy, G. (2000). The community tool box: A Web-based resource for building healthier communities. *Public Health Reports, 115,* 274–278.

Fawcett, S. B., Shultz, J. A., Carson, V. L., Renault, V. A., & Francisco, V. T. (2003). Using Internet-based tools to build capacity for community based participatory research and other efforts to promote community health and development. In M. Minkler & N. Wallerstein (Eds.), *Community-based participatory research for health* (pp. 155–178). San Francisco: Jossey-Bass.

Fetterman, D., & Wandersman, A. (Eds). (2004). *Empowerment evaluation principles in practice.* New York: Guilford Press.

Fetterman, D., & Wandersman, A. (2007). Empowerment education: Yesterday, today and tomorrow. *American Journal of Evaluation, 28*(2), 179–198.

Freire, P. (1973). *Education for critical consciousness.* New York: Continuum.

Green, L. W., George, M. A., Daniel, M., Frankish, C .J., Herbert, C. P., Bowie, W. R., et al. (1995). *Study of participatory research in health promotion: Review and recommendations for the development of participatory research in health promotion in Canada.* Vancouver, BC: Royal Society of Canada.

Healthy Native Communities Partnership. (2008a). *Healthy Native Communities Fellowship.* Retrieved May 20, 2008, from http://www.healthynativecommunities.org/initiatives.jsp.

Healthy Native Communities Partnership. (2008b). *Welcome to the workstation.* Retrieved May 20, 2008, from http://www.healthynativecommunities.org.

Heuertz, L., Gordon, A., Moore, E., & Gordon, M. (2002). *Public libraries and the digital divide: How libraries help.* Seattle: Public Access Computing Project, University of Washington.

Horton, M., & Freire, P. (1990). *We make the road by walking: Conversations on education and social change* (B. Bell, J. Gaventa, & J. Peters, Eds.). Philadelphia: Temple University Press.

Institute for Community Research. (2008). [Home page.] Retrieved Apr. 24, 2008, from http://www.incommunityresearch.org.

Jernigan, V. (2007). *The Native American diabetes self-management program.* Ann Arbor, MI: Proquest Dissertation Services, 69–99.

Johns Hopkins Urban Health Institute. (2008). *What is community-based participatory research?* Retrieved Apr. 24, 2008, from www.urbanhealthinstitute.jhu.edu/cbpr.html.

Living Knowledge. (2008). [Home page.] Retrieved Apr. 24, 2008, from http://www.scienceshops.org.

LOKA Institute. (2008). *CRN publications list.* Retrieved Apr. 24, 2008, from http://www.loka.org/ crnpublicationslist.html.

National Institutes of Health. (2008). *NIH search results.* Retrieved Apr. 24, 2008, from http://search2.google.cit.nih. gov/search?site=NIH_Master&client=NIH_frontend&proxystylesheet=NIH_frontend&output=xml_no_dtd&filter=0&getfields=&q=CBPR&btnG.x=0&btnG.y=0.

Norris, P. (2001). *Digital divide: Civic engagement, information poverty, and the Internet worldwide.* New York: Cambridge University Press.

Pew Trusts. Demographics, computers and the Internet. Retrieved May 20, 2008, from http://www.pewtrusts.org/ our_work_detail.aspx?id=52.

Schultz, J. A., Fawcett, S. B., Francisco, V. T., & Berkowitz, B. (2003). Using information systems to build capacity: The public health improvement tool box. In P. O'Carroll, W. A. Yasnoff, M. E. Ward, R. Rubin, & L. Ripp (Eds.), *Public health informatics and information systems: A contributed work* (pp. 644–660). New York: Springer-Verlag.

Southeast Community Resource Center. (2008). *CBPR.* Retrieved Apr. 24, 2008, from http://www.cbpr.org/index. php?option=com_content&task=view&id=87&Itemid=64.

Stanford University School of Medicine. (2008). *Stanford Patient Education Research Center.* Retrieved Apr. 24, 2008, from http://patienteducation.stanford.edu.

Wallerstein, N. (2000). A participatory evaluation model for healthier communities. Developing indicators for New Mexico. *Public Health Reports, 115,* 199–204.

Work Group for Community Health and Development. (2008a). *About us.* Retrieved Apr. 24, 2008, from http://communityhealth.ku.edu.

Work Group for Community Health and Development. (2008b). *The community tool box.* Retrieved Apr. 24, 2008, from http://ctb.ku.edu.

CHAPTER

11

USING PHOTOVOICE FOR PARTICIPATORY ASSESSMENT AND ISSUE SELECTION

LESSONS FROM A FAMILY, MATERNAL, AND CHILDHEALTH DEPARTMENT

CAROLINE C. WANG & CHERI A. PIES

Note: Portions of this chapter were adapted from "Family, Maternal and Child Health Through Photovoice," by Caroline C. Wang and Cheri A. Pies, 2004, *Maternal and Child Health Journal, 8*(2), pp. 95–102. Copyright 2004 by Plenum Publishing Company. Adapted with permission of Springer Science + Business Media. Picture This photovoice was supported in part by Contra Costa Health Services (CCHS). The authors are grateful to Wendel Brunner, public health director for CCHS, for providing ongoing support for this project, and Beth Tsoulos, Purnima Manghanani, and the staff of the Family, Maternal and Child Health Programs for valuable assistance. The authors are especially grateful to the participants in the Picture This project for their time and insight.

PHOTOVOICE INTEGRATES core tenets of health promotion, critical education, feminist theory, and community-based documentary photography in an innovative way, and is increasingly used in community-based participatory research (CBPR) (Wang & Burris, 1997). The process involves providing community people with cameras so that they can take pictures of their everyday health and work realities and use these pictures as the basis of group discussion and action. The photographs are then used to reach policymakers and others who can be mobilized to help bring about the desired changes.

This chapter focuses primarily on the use of photovoice as a tool that enables people in a community to identify that community's strengths and concerns as a basis for issue selection and action, in this case with a focus on family, maternal, and child health. We begin with an overview of the conceptual framework of photovoice and explain photovoice's advantages as an approach to community assessment. We then use a case study to illustrate the utility of this method as part of a county health department's efforts to better determine the needs of low-income mothers, children, and families (Wang & Pies, 2004). Both the strengths and the challenges and limitations of this approach are explored, as are the implications for its use with other populations and in other contexts.

BACKGROUND AND CONCEPTUAL FRAMEWORK

The photovoice concept and methodology were first developed and applied by Wang, Burris, and colleagues in the Ford Foundation–supported Women's Reproductive Health and Development Program in Yunnan, China (Wu et al., 1995; Wang, Burris, & Xiang, 1996). Since then, the approach has been used with young mothers and grandmothers who are establishing cross-generational linkages in Detroit (Killion & Wang, 2000); black and Latino youths in order to draw their attention to the AIDS epidemic in the San Francisco Bay area (May, 2001); people with mental illnesses in New Haven, Connecticut (Bowers, 1999); preadolescents wanting changes in their school environment in Richmond, California (Wilson et al., 2007); and homeless people in Ann Arbor, Michigan (Wang, Cash, & Powers, 2000), to name but a few. The theoretical underpinnings of photovoice, along with additional examples of its application, are described in detail elsewhere (Wang & Burris, 1997; Wang, Yuan, & Feng, 1996; Strack, Magill, & McDonagh, 2003; Wang, Morrel-Samuels, Hutchison, Bell, & Pestronk, 2004; Baker & Wang, 2006). An overview of the approach and its uses may also be found on the Web (Photovoice, 2008).

Photovoice adheres to the basic health promotion principles set forth in the Ottawa Charter for Health Promotion (World Health Organization, 1986) because it involves people at the grassroots level in community action. Moreover, it integrates Paulo Freire's (1970) approach to critical education, which stresses the importance of people's sharing and speaking from their own experience. Freire emphasizes that people need to identify the historical and social patterns that bind their individual lives together, so they can see how their situations are related to root causes and can develop solutions and strategies for change (Freire, 1970). Photovoice also reflects Freire's convictions on the power of the visual image as an aid to individuals trying to think critically about the forces and factors influencing their lives (Freire, 1970). Photovoice builds on a commitment to social and intellectual change through community members' critical production and analysis of the visual image.

The photovoice methodology also borrows from feminist theory, which suggests that power accrues to those who have voice, set language, make history, and participate in decisions (Smith, 1987). Photovoice participants work to change the way their public presence is defined: photovoice represents part of the attempt to disrupt and ultimately revise the views of gender, class, ethnicity, and other forces that contribute to oppression.

Finally, photovoice draws on participatory approaches to documentary photography developed by Wendy Ewald (1985 & 1996), Jim Hubbard (1991 &1994), Jo Spence (1995), and other activist photographers who suggest a grassroots approach to representation and demonstrate how women, children, homeless youths, and others can effectively use photographs as a personal voice. Using photography as community voice to reach policymakers, photovoice tries to go beyond the personal voice to the political.

Photovoice is designed to enable people to produce and discuss photographs as a means of catalyzing personal and community change. Using cameras, participants document the reality of their lives. By sharing and talking about their photographs, they use the power of the visual image to communicate their life experiences and perceptions. As they engage in a group process of critical reflection, participants may discuss individual change, community quality of life, and policy issues (Wallerstein, Sanchez, & Velarde, 2005). The immediacy of the visual image creates evidence and promotes a vivid participatory means of sharing expertise and knowledge.

COMMUNITY ASSESSMENT

Chapters Nine and Ten reviewed various community assessment tools and techniques that may be useful in community-based participatory research (see also Green & Kreuter, 1999; Israel, Cummings, Dignan, Heaney, & Perales, 1995; Hancock & Minkler, 2005; Sharpe, Greany, Lee, & Royce, 2000). Photovoice has several advantages over such familiar assessment and evaluation methods as community inventory, community assessment, and formative or process evaluation (Wang & Burris, 1997). These advantages are summarized briefly here in terms of program implementation and sustainability, the assessment process, and equity and community building.

Photovoice offers the perspective of what Freire (1970) calls *problem-posing education,* which helps participants to define both issues of concern and the most relevant social actions for tackling those concerns. Unlike conventional needs assessment, photovoice enables participants to advocate for themselves and their community. The process goes beyond assessment; it is a tool to reach, inform, and organize community members, thereby enabling them to prioritize their concerns and discuss problems and solutions.

The photovoice method can also sustain continuing community participation during the period between needs assessment and program implementation. The camera has unusual power and appeal for many people. Community pride is at the heart of photovoice. It can also provide a way to reaffirm or redefine program goals even while community needs are being assessed. Wang and Burris (1997) noted that in Yunnan, the village women were often asked by friends and neighbors why they were taking pictures. Their explanations served to focus attention on women's status and health, to teach the community about the goals of the project, and to solicit people's feedback about the process.

Photovoice provides powerful assessment opportunities for those engaged in community-based participatory research. As John Gaventa (1993) has noted, the participatory process implicitly legitimizes popular knowledge produced outside a formal scientific structure. In photovoice, knowledge put forth by people is given priority as a vital source of expertise, offering "the possibility of perceiving their world from the viewpoint of the people who live lives that are different from those traditionally in control of the means for imaging the world" (Ruby, 1991, p. 50). As an approach to needs assessment or appraisal, this method confronts disparities between what researchers think is important and what the community thinks is important. With its powerful use of visual images to capture and reflect a community context, photovoice satisfies the "descriptive mandate" of needs assessment (Wang & Burris, 1997). Photovoice also contributes a sampling of social and behavioral settings not available to health professionals or researchers. By allowing participants to bring the explanations, ideas, or stories of other community members to the assessment process, photovoice affords a flexible, accessible means of incorporating a wide array of perspectives (Baker & Wang, 2006).

When used for assessment, photovoice helps build community and equity. By focusing on long-term community relationships, it provides tangible and immediate benefits; returning photographs to neighbors and friends enables participants to express their appreciation, build ties, and pass along something of value that they have created. This can affirm the ingenuity of a society's most vulnerable populations. Wang and Burris (1997) describe Yunnan villages where there was little support from parents or the broader community for educating girls. Photovoice can be accessible to anyone, whether or not he or she is able to read and write, so photographs may capture the full context of a community, its assets as well as its needs. Kretzmann and McKnight (1993) note that a community's experience includes a variety of capacities, collective efforts, informal interactions, stories, celebrations, and, sometimes, tragedy. In Yunnan, the village women photographed moments of loss and grief as well as times of celebration and strength, and they elicited stories about the community's imagination, resources, and capabilities (Wang & Burris, 1997). In contrast, conventional methods of needs assessment, such as interviews or questionnaires, may inadvertently reinforce resentment by making people feel impotent and inferior. Photovoice can be a creative approach to enabling participants to identify, define, and enhance their community according to their own priorities.

We now turn to a study to illustrate the use of photovoice as a method of participatory community assessment (Wang & Pies, 2004; Wang, Cash, & Powers, 2000) as well as participatory evaluation (Wang, Yuan, & Feng, 1996).

A PHOTOVOICE CASE STUDY FROM A COUNTY HEALTH DEPARTMENT

Every five years, county maternal and child health (MCH) departments in the United States are required to conduct a needs assessment for the state in which they are located. The state MCH agency uses these assessments in drawing up its five-year plan and application for federal funding. Local MCH programs have historically relied on a range of data sources to meet this requirement; these sources tend to be epidemiological, focused on long-standing MCH categories for health status and outcomes. They do not tend to include first-hand accounts of the experience of low-income residents, non-English speakers, and others most likely to bear the greatest burden of poor family, maternal, and child health care.

Contra Costa is a large (719 square miles, about half the size of Rhode Island) and economically, geographically, and ethnically diverse county in California, with over 1.5 million residents. The poorest perinatal outcomes (for example, infant mortality, late or no entry into care, and births to teens) tend to be concentrated in five zip code areas where close to a quarter of the county's population resides. In these areas (including Richmond, Bay Point, and Pittsburg, where the photovoice project in this case study took place), the rates of teen births, for example, are 57.6 (Richmond) and 56.8 (Bay Point and Pittsburg) per 1,000 teens aged fifteen to nineteen, compared to the country rate of 23.8 births per 1,000 teens (Contra Costa County Public Health Division, 2007). To address such inequities, county MCH staff decided to initiate a photovoice project to gather qualitative data about family, maternal, and child concerns of community residents.

Participant Recruitment

To find participants who could describe issues requiring health department attention, an attractive flyer was developed and distributed throughout the five zip code areas, advertising the Picture This project. Public health nurses gave the flyers out at the county clinics and on home visits; community outreach workers posted flyers in community centers, WIC (Special Supplemental Nutrition Program for Women, Infants, and Children) and child care centers, children's health and social services locations, and community-based sites such as battered women's shelters, local preschools, and laundromats. Sixty participants were recruited for this project, which was facilitated by the chapter authors and a graduate student in social work. Participants ranged in age from thirteen to fifty, with an ethnic breakdown of close to 50 percent African American, 40 percent Caucasian, and 10 percent Hispanic. Most of the participants came from neighborhoods in the five zip code areas. Each participant signed a consent form saying that she or he would share the photographs and work in partnership with the county health department to improve the health of families, mothers, and children of the county. Each also received either a cash stipend or a gift certificate to local supermarkets, with incentives averaging $75 per participant.

Workshop Design and Implementation

Over a five-month period, two three-hour Picture This workshop sessions were held, one in West Contra Costa, the other in East County. To accommodate parenting and work schedules, workshops were held in the evening and included dinner and child care. After a slide presentation introducing photovoice and illustrating how it had been used effectively in other areas, participants were engaged in a discussion of the potential for using photovoice to promote better family, maternal, and child health in the county.

There were questions and dialogue about using a camera—including issues of power when taking photographs and the ethics of taking pictures of community people. Facilitators tried to extend such dialogue by asking, for example, What responsibilities does one have when using a camera? What is an acceptable way to approach someone when you want to take his or her picture? What types of situations or images would you want to avoid capturing in a photograph? This discussion was intended to lead participants to focus attention on ways to minimize risk—be it physical danger or loss of privacy to themselves and their community—when taking photographs (Wang & Redwood-Jones, 2001).

Participants each received a disposable camera and a stamped envelope addressed to the health department photovoice coordinator, and were asked to mail in their cameras by a particular date. Participants were taught some elementary rules of photography and asked to take pictures of people, places, and things that conveyed their perspectives on health issues in their community. In contrast to more traditional assessment methods that focus on problems, photovoice was presented as an approach based on strengths, one that lets community members explore the assets as well as the problems of their neighborhoods. Prior to taking photographs, therefore, participants brainstormed and discussed ways to photograph not only health issues but also ways to find and document community assets. Participants offered examples of how to tell a story to illustrate their concerns, such as children finding discarded needles where they play, gang members turf-marking with graffiti, and youth centers visibly lacking community support. They also discussed community resources that could address these issues. Thus photovoice was seen from the first as two-sided: a technique for participatory needs assessment and a tool to map assets and resources (Kretzmann & McKnight, 1993; see also Chapter Nine).

All who attended the first workshop returned their cameras within the allotted time, and health department staff had two sets of prints developed, one for themselves and the other for participants. At the next two workshops, participants were randomly divided into three discussion groups, each facilitated by a health department staff person. Each participant selected one or two photographs he or she found most meaningful (or simply liked best) and discussed them in the small group. To lead the discussion the facilitator used the mnemonic SHOWeD (Shaffer, 1983):

What do you **S**ee here?
What's really **H**appening here?
How does this relate to **O**ur Lives?
Why does this problem, concern, or strength exist?
What can we **D**o about it?

A few participants also used the SHOWeD mnemonic to do a *freewrite,* in which they wrote down their thoughts about their photographs. After the small-group discussions, participants and facilitators reconvened. Several participants from each group described one of their images to the entire large group. At the end of each workshop, participants completed written evaluations and received cash stipends and, at the final workshop, also received a certificate of appreciation from the county's director of family, maternal, and child health.

Learning from Pictures

Participants' definitions of maternal and child health and what would most improve that and family health differed from conventional health department views. Categorical funding by federal and state MCH sources has led health department staff to design interventions focused on improving the rate of entry into prenatal care and improving that care's quality, reducing low birth weight births and infant mortality, reducing family and domestic violence, preventing teen pregnancies, and addressing issues of tobacco and substance use during pregnancy. In contrast, participants of all ages said their principal concerns were safe recreation for children and improved living conditions in their neighborhoods.

The first theme, the concern with safe recreation for children, emerged when some participants photographed roadside crosses marking places where children had been killed; inadequate stop signs, specifically those near elementary schools; and a park sign that read, in English and Spanish, "This area is not maintained by the city of Antioch. Enter at your own risk." One woman who photographed her children and nephews playing at a park with such a sign explained that she worried about the children finding hypodermic needles in the sandbox area (Spears, 1999). Several of the parents photographed children at play in parks, in Little League activities, or in the house. An adult who took a picture of her nephew in his Little League uniform described with pride how happy he was to belong to a team and how important it was to the family that the child could participate in some kind of supervised recreational opportunity.

The second theme, the need to improve living conditions, emerged from residents' photographs of property neglected by landlords, graffiti, trash, filthy water sinks at a public elementary school, and a hospital closure that was a factor in inadequate health services for low-income people. Several adolescent participants shooting photographs in their schools exposed poorly maintained bathrooms, dangerous walkways, unusable basketball hoops, and abandoned playgrounds. One resident photographed oil refineries in his neighborhood and relayed his fears about the dangers they presented. Approximately one-quarter of the participants photographed trash, including several who, unknown to each other, photographed one particular site.

Residents also photographed neighborhood assets and resources, such as reclaimed parks, bright murals, and places where debris had been cleaned out. One participant wrote of his picture: "This is a beautiful site with lots of flowers. It used to be a dumping place, but people cleaned it up and grew flowers. The bars are there to protect the flowers and the murals, planted and created by youth. It used to be such a dirty place. If we keep the environment clean, we will have better health. We should use this place as an example. This place exists because there are people who care about their surroundings and are willing to clean up around them. The Iron Triangle neighborhood organized this."

Participants told powerful stories. A picture of a wheelchair and medical supplies belonging to an elderly person being cared for at home by her son (the photographer) had particular resonance for participants who either knew people caring for elderly relatives in the home or anticipated that they themselves would be doing so in the future. An adolescent shared a photograph of her best friend looking happy and contented, holding her new, calm, and healthy baby. The photographer explained that her friend, battered by the father of the baby, had had to move back into her parents' home. This led to talk about teenage pregnancy, and many expressed concern about the rise in the number of teen mothers, the battery and abuse experienced by some of these young women, and the welfare of the children.

Participants proved creative in choosing family, child, and maternal health issues they wished to photograph and in how they captured these issues. For example, one young woman used her photo of a tree silhouetted against the sky to depict neighbors' narrow attitudes toward children with disabilities: "You can see the isolation. Solitude. The neighbors are ignorant; they don't want the kids there. They see them as sick." A young man used his photograph of a steeple in his neighborhood to share his distinctive integration of church bells, time, and a sense of responsibility: "What you see is a church that is playing music. And, there's a big bell where the glass is. And what you are seeing is a cross at the top of the church that tells a story in itself. I don't go to this church, but it helps me out. When the bell chimes, it keeps me aware of the time. When I hear the bells, I know that I have to leave to catch the bus for school. This shows the positive side of our community. We can support the church even though it's not our church."

After taking self-portraits and pictures of family, friends, and pets, participants sometimes indicated that they did not intend to share or discuss these photographs with other group members, but many showed these images to a health department staff person as a way of sharing more about themselves and their lives.

Project Outcomes

The photographs and stories gathered through the Picture This project supplemented quantitative data used by the health department to determine MCH objectives for the five-year work plan. One new key objective, for example, involved after-school programs for youths, with a special focus on community service projects, and another involved better transportation linkages for pregnant and parenting women seeking services.

The Picture This project energized some residents to take action in their communities: some participants have started working to see that the parks are cleaned, others have mounted a campaign to keep a local recreation program open. Several participants have asked to be part of an MCH advisory committee to provide the health department with ideas, suggestions, and direction for future programs. The project helped to identify a cadre of community people who may contribute to the health department's outreach and program evaluation long after the formal project period has ended.

Following the two Picture This sessions, county health department staff displayed some of the photographs and stories at several venues; shows included a community health fair presentation, an exhibition at the health department, and an invited exhibition at a statewide maternal and child health conference at the state capitol. As Plummer (1983) notes, the stories shared by community members aren't just concrete illustrations of their reality but in their telling become a potent part of the political process. The photovoice methodology formalizes the making of stories, vivified with images and produced by community people to inform health planning. For its creativity, contribution to resource building, and overall impact, the Picture This project in California was recognized with a statewide MCH Special Achievement Award.

REFLECTING ON VALUE ADDED

The incorporation of a photovoice project appeared to contribute to family, maternal, and child health assessment and planning in ways not addressed by other approaches. First, photovoice served as a way of gaining community input from people directly affected by MCH programs, systems, and policies. The need for "real people" to participate in defining MCH questions, problems, assets, and solutions has been recognized broadly and institutionally at the county, state, and federal levels as well as among university researchers and practitioners. Indeed, the Public MCH Program Functions Framework notes that an essential public health service for promoting maternal and child health in the United States is to *"mobilize families and the general public,* in partnership with policy makers and providers, *to identify and solve maternal and child health problems"* (Grayson & Guyer, 1995, p. 28; emphasis added). Similarly, Wagner (1998) observes that "WHO has been working to correct the balance (in clinical and public health approaches) by expanding the body of knowledge in perinatology recognized as authoritative, opening it up to include, in addition to the viewpoint of clinicians, the viewpoint of midwives, scientific researchers, public health professionals, and women at large" (p. 29).

Photovoice offers MCH staff one strategy that can help agencies to realize these ideals—a novel way to tap the creativity, lore, and strengths of community people from diverse cultural subgroups, regardless of their formal educational background.

A second contribution relates to the mandate to perform needs assessments for MCH programs every five years; photovoice gives MCH staff a chance to complement or enhance quantitative assessment data with grassroots visual and narrative material. When they conducted interview or questionnaire surveys, MCH staff perceived that the questions were often framed in a way that limited responses, so the answers sometimes reflected not so much constituents' specific concerns as MCH staff's assumptions and judgments. Photovoice gave MCH staff an opportunity to learn about perceptions of family, maternal, and child health issues through constituent-produced information with a human face. By looking at the cumulative body of photographs and stories, MCH staff sought to use photovoice in conjunction with other survey and data gathering instruments to add to the overall community portrait.

Third, even the most experienced MCH staff person may learn from the body of images and stories generated through photovoice. Health department staff reported feeling invigorated by their new understanding of community issues as defined by the people they serve, and in fact, the project led staff to work on the design, maintenance, and promotion of recreational facilities and activities. MCH staff noted that recipients' thinking about health extended beyond typical maternal and child health categories. In other words, participants chose to define family, maternal, and child health in terms of the health of the community.

Fourth, photovoice may enhance MCH staff's ability as advocates by equipping them with narrative-driven policy and program recommendations. In this way, as Declercq (1998) notes, "Individuals still profoundly shape the policy-making process, particularly in the early stages, and, in health care, their personal experiences with the system matter" (p. 853). For example, one man photographed a closed community hospital, seeking to document the inadequacy of health services for low-income people. The photograph, along with other complaints, prompted the county to make improvements at its city clinic. Health department leaders Pierce and Blackburn (1998) have noted a "difficulty explaining to public officials and local officials what public health does." Photovoice can serve as a tool to educate participants and audiences alike about what public health does and, within the parameters of its emphasis on prevention and health promotion, what it ought to do. To inform local staff and state and local policymakers about participants' family, maternal, and child health concerns, Picture This exhibitions have been held at the county health department and the state capitol.

Fifth, photovoice may also serve to foster a sense of community and place among participants. Even though they did not know each other prior to the workshops, participants found that they could support one another by giving and getting advice about county health resources, that they sometimes photographed identical tangible community problems (like the piles of trash), and that concerns about local issues transcended generational, neighborhood, and ethnic differences.

Finally, MCH staff found the methodology an ideal way to identify a cadre of citizens willing to volunteer time, energy, and insights to initiatives supporting family, maternal, and child health programs; approximately two-thirds of the participants turned in information sheets asking to be contacted to collaborate on future MCH programs.

This case study also revealed several limitations of photovoice. Policy change is often slow and incremental, and policymakers use data of all kinds to inform a viewpoint and argue persuasively. This makes it somewhat difficult to demonstrate just how much a photovoice project has helped to improve a program or policy in a defined time period. In addition, information gleaned through photovoice, like all information, is subject to differences of interpretation and representation, and those who control or contribute to the public presentations of participants' photographs and stories can influence the ways they will be used.

Photovoice is not intended to produce a body of visual data for exhaustive analysis in the social science sense. For example, Collier and Collier's (1986) landmark text, *Visual Anthropology: Photography as a Research Method,* begins to explore how the *researcher* can systematically evaluate visual content. In contrast, photovoice offers a new framework and paradigm in which *participants* drive the analysis—from selecting photographs that they feel are most important or simply like best to the "decoding" or descriptive interpretation of the images (Wang & Burris, 1997; Wang, 1999). The authors and MCH staff have done their best to represent themes identified by participants in consensus-based group discussions.

The ideas presented have been those of individuals who chose to participate, take pictures, return to the second and third sessions, and share their photographs and stories. The issues might be different with different participants from other regions of the county. Like volunteers for clinical trials, photovoice participants, by definition, may not be representative of their broader cohort.

It seems reasonable to assume that participants are more likely to show concerns that can be easily photographed. However, as some of the examples given earlier illustrate, participants may use photovoice to create a visual language—defined by Horn (1998) as the integration of words, images, and shapes into a single communication unit—with inventive ways to convey meaning.

The circumscribed contact MCH staff had with participants made it difficult to understand the extent to which participants directly benefited from the project by gaining, for example, an increased sense of political efficacy or self-esteem. In addition, as with most photovoice projects, sample sizes might be too small for pre- and postworkshop surveys to lend themselves to statistical analyses. Finally, the health department found that with relatively few staff, it was challenged to follow up with participants who had self-identified as willing and available to assist county staff in planning and developing family, maternal, and child health programs and priorities.

RECOMMENDATIONS AND IMPLICATIONS

A number of themes emerged in the course of the Picture This project—concerning both the strengths of the photovoice approach and the challenges it presents—that in turn may have relevance for others interested in using this approach.

First, researchers will be better able to understand local assets and problems when community people are involved at a high level in the research process (Wang & Pies, 2004). Community members' perspectives may be unlike those held by "experts" in maternal and child health, homelessness, and other fields; the photovoice process can keep the community's interests central to both planning and evaluation. Photovoice can also be key to broadening outsiders' views as it supplements traditional epidemiological data. In southern California, Zebrack's work supported by the National Cancer Institute combines photovoice and quantitative approaches to focus on quality of life experiences for childhood cancer survivors and their families (B. J. Zebrack, personal communication, 2007). In Thailand, Brazil, and Texas, tuberculosis patients have used photovoice to advocate prevention and to reach policymakers and health care providers (Reid, 2007).

Second, experience gained from the Picture This projects as well as other efforts suggests that policymakers and community leaders should be recruited at the project's outset, in order to promote a political climate receptive to photovoice participants' potential policy and program recommendations (Wang, 2006; Gamboa et al., 2007). A *guidance committee* of policymakers and community leaders might serve this purpose.

In addition, photovoice facilitators need to be aware of participants' risks. Those who take part in photovoice projects tend to be among society's most vulnerable people: they often have low incomes; may be homeless or unemployed (or hold several jobs); cope with inordinate stigma; and may be accorded the lowest status by the community in which they live. Although researchers cannot fully protect all participants, they can minimize potential dangers by, among other things:

- Underscoring during group discussions that participants, when carrying a camera, must make a special effort to respect the privacy and rights of others
- Facilitating critical dialogue that yields specific suggestions on ways to manifest this respect
- Emphasizing that no picture is worth taking if it brings the photographer or subject harm or ill will

In the Picture This project, we obtained written consent from participants, and asked them, in turn, to obtain written consent in advance from people they photographed. This requirement might have made pictures less spontaneous—but it prevented misunderstandings. It also helped to build trust because it gave participants an opportunity to describe the project and to ask subjects for their views about the community. Furthermore, it established the possibility of a long-term relationship, allowing for future photographs and exchanges of knowledge, as well as the possibility of acquiring written consent to use the photographs for health promotion aims (Wang & Redwood-Jones, 2001).

The Picture This project offers an example of the important contributions photovoice can make to public health practice. These contributions synthesize the methodology's theoretical underpinnings: the production of knowledge and expertise that then influence personal and community action, the accrual of power to those who participate in promoting their own and their community's health, and the analytical use of a community-based approach to photography as personal voice.

Photovoice contributes to public health practice in several ways. First, health professionals can use photovoice as a tool to learn more about the people with whom they work, to build rapport, and to create productive settings for group discussion and problem solving. These advantages are substantial; many health professionals learn the hard way that people in the community view them with skepticism if not outright suspicion. Regardless of the individual CBPR worker's experience, skills, or commitment, he or she may initially be perceived as part of the problem—elitist; ignorant of people's everyday realities, priorities, and survival needs; and motivated by careerism (see Chapters Five and Six).

Second, photovoice offers a vehicle for understanding the health status, behavior, needs, strengths, and concerns of people belonging to often marginalized populations.

Third, CBPR workers can use photovoice as a tool for mapping personal and community assets that can in turn facilitate issue selection and action (Kretzmann & McKnight, 1993; see also Chapter Nine). Participants may find photovoice ideal for creatively documenting their environment and its resources and in the process may demonstrate their own ingenuity and imagination.

Fourth, participants may benefit from enhanced self-esteem and peer status as they are listened to—not talked at—and gain a sense of political efficacy.

Fifth, health promotion practitioners may find photovoice a creative and effective tool for fostering social support and productive long-term relationships among participants (Wang et al., 2004; Wang, 2006).

And finally, photovoice can bring willing, powerful members of a community together with marginalized and sometimes highly stigmatized people, enabling the former to assist the latter by first learning from them.

SUMMARY

Picture This participants are not unlike the many millions of Americans whose health is endangered by environmental conditions, lack of accessible health care, and the stressors in their lives. By allowing individuals and communities to speak from their own experience, photovoice can change the quality of their discussion both among themselves and with those committed to their well-being.

Whomever we researchers work for and with—mothers, children, and families; the homeless; or people with stigmatized conditions—our practice should be based on their concerns. Photovoice, an innovative and participatory method, can play a valuable role in achieving this larger vision.

QUESTIONS FOR DISCUSSION

1. Photovoice and documentary photography are both powerful tools for community and policymaker education and for social change. Photovoice, however, is much more frequently used as a CBPR approach. What are the differences between these two approaches, and why does photovoice better lend itself to CBPR?

2. You have just been asked to conduct a needs assessment for a local health department's health promotion unit, focusing on a low-income community with numerous problematic health and social indicators. You are interested in incorporating photovoice into the larger assessment process and focusing on community strengths as well as problems. However, you realize this project will be time consuming and costly at the front end. How might you justify undertaking such a project to your boss who will need to approve the staff time and money involved?

3. What are three strategies the chapter authors suggest for minimizing risks to participants when they are involved in a photovoice project? Can you think of any other strategies that should be added?

KEY TERMS

Documentary photography   Maternal and child health

REFERENCES

Baker, T . A., & Wang, C. C. (2006). Photovoice: Use of a participatory action research methodology to explore the chronic pain experience in older adults. *Qualitative Health Research, 16*(10), 1–9.

Bowers, A. A. (1999, November). *People with serious mental illnesses using photovoice: Implications for participatory research and community education.* Paper presented at the American Public Health Association annual meeting, Chicago.

Collier, J., & Collier, M. (1986.) *Visual anthropology: Photography as a research method.* Albuquerque: University of New Mexico.

Contra Costa County Public Health Division. (2007). *Community health indicators for Contra Costa County.* Retrieved Jan. 4, 2007, from http://cchealth.org/health_data/hospital_council_2007.

Declercq, E. (1998). "Changing childbirth" in the United Kingdom: Lessons for US health policy. *Journal of Health Politics, Policy and Law. 23*(5), 833–859.

Ewald, W. (1996). *I dreamed I had a girl in my pocket.* Durham, NC: DoubleTake Books/Center for Documentary Studies.

Ewald, W. (1985). *Portraits and dreams: Photographs and stories by children of the Appalachians.* New York: Writers & Readers.

Freire, P. (1970). *Pedagogy of the oppressed.* New York: Seabury Press.

Gamboa, C. E., Weir, S., Schulz, A. J., Ware., S., Shevrin, I., & Sand, S. (2007). *Youth photovoice: A community-based approach to engage youth in informing public health programming and policy.* Presentation to the annual meeting of the American Public Health Association, Washington, DC.

Gaventa, J. (1993). The powerful, the powerless, and the experts: Knowledge struggles in an information age. In P. Park, M. Brydon-Miller, B. L. Hall, & T. Jackson (Eds.), *Voices of change: Participatory research in the United States and Canada* (pp. 21–40). Westport, CT: Bergin & Garvey.

Grayson, H. A., & Guyer, B. (1995). Public MCH program functions framework: Essential public health services to promote maternal and child health in America: State applications. Baltimore: Johns Hopkins University, Child and Adolescent Health Policy Center.

Green, L. W., & Kreuter, M. W. (1999). *Health promotion planning: An educational and ecological approach* (3rd ed.). Mountain View, CA: Mayfield.

Hancock, T., and Minkler, M. (2005). Community health assessment or healthy community assessment: Whose community? Whose health? Whose assessment? In M. Minkler (Ed.), *Community Organizing and Community Building for Health* (pp. 138–158). New Brunswick, NJ: Rutgers University Press.

Horn, R. E. (1998). *Visual language.* Bainbridge Island, WA: MacroVU.

Hubbard, J. (1991). *Shooting back: A photographic view of life by homeless children.* San Francisco: Chronicle Books.

Hubbard, J. (1994). *Shooting back from the reservation: A photographic view of life by Native American youth.* New York: New Press.

Israel, B. A., Cummings, M., Dignan, M. B., Heaney, K., & Perales, D. P. (1995). Evaluation of health education programs: Current assessment and future directions. *Health Education Quarterly, 22,* 364–368.

Killion, C., & Wang, C. C. (2000). Linking African American mothers across life stage and station through photovoice. *Journal of Health Care for the Poor and Underserved, 11,* 310–325.

Kretzmann, J. P., & McKnight, J. L. (1993). *Building communities from the inside out: A path toward finding and mobilizing a community's assets.* Chicago: ACTA.

May, M. (2001, November 25). Sounding the alarm: East Bay's teenage "town criers" use cameras to bring new focus to AIDS. *San Francisco Chronicle.*

Photovoice. (2008). [Home page.] Retrieved Apr. 26, 2008, from http://www.photovoice.com.

Pierce, J. R., & Blackburn, C. P. (1998). The transformation of a local health department. *Public Health Reports, 113,* 152–159.

Plummer, K. *Documents of life: An introduction to the problems and literature of a humanistic method.* London: Allen and Unwin, 1983.

Reid, C. M. (2007). Wife's death inspires project: Photos honor wife, help others. The State.com. Retrieved Apr. 21, 2008, from www.cas.sc.edu/anth/PDF/RomelLacson.pdf.

Ruby, J. S. (1991). Speaking for, speaking about, speaking with, speaking alongside: An anthropological and documentary dilemma. *Visual Anthropology Review, 7*(2), 50–67.

Shaffer, R. (1983). *Beyond the dispensary.* Nairobi, Kenya: Amref.

Sharpe, P. A., Greany, M. L., Lee, P. R., & Royce, S. W. (2000). Assets-oriented community assessment. *Public Health Reports, 113,* 205–211.

Smith, D. E. (1987). *The everyday world as problematic.* Boston: Northeastern University Press.

Spears, L. (1999, Apr. 11). Picturing concerns: The idea is to take the message to policy makers and to produce change. *Contra Costa Times,* pp. A27, A32.

Spence, J. (1995). *Cultural sniping: The art of transgression.* New York: Routledge.

Strack, R. W., Magill, C., & McDonagh, K. (2003). Engaging youth through photovoice. *Health Promotion Practice, 5*(1), 49–58.

Wagner, M. (1998). The public health versus clinical approaches to maternity services: The emperor has no clothes. *Journal of Public Health Policy, 19*(1), 25–33.

Wallerstein, N., Sanchez, V., & Velarde, L. (2005). Freirian praxis in health education and community organizing: A case study of an adolescent prevention program. In M. Minkler (Ed.), *Community organizing and community building for health* (2nd ed., 218–236). New Brunswick, NJ: Rutgers University Press.

Wang, C. C. (1999). Photovoice: A participatory action research strategy applied to women's health. *Journal of Women's Health, 8,* 185–192.

Wang, C. C. (2006). Youth participation in photovoice as a strategy for community change. *Journal of Community Practice, 14*(2), 147–161.

Wang, C. C., & Burris, M. A. (1997). Photovoice: Concept, methodology, and use for participatory needs assessment. *Health Education & Behavior, 24,* 369–387.

Wang, C. C., Burris, M. A., & Xiang, Y. P. (1996). Chinese village women as visual anthropologists: A participatory approach to reaching policymakers. *Social Science & Medicine, 42,* 1391–1400.

Wang, C. C., Cash, J. L., & Powers, L. S. (2000). Who knows the streets as well as the homeless? Promoting personal and community action through photovoice. *Health Promotion Practice, 1,* 81–89.

Wang, C. C., Morrel-Samuels, S., Hutchison, P., Bell, L., & Pestronk, R. M. (2004). Flint photovoice: Community-building among youth, adults, and policy makers. *American Journal of Public Health, 94*(6), 911–913.

Wang, C. C., & Pies, C. A. (2004). Family, maternal, and child health through photovoice. *Maternal and Child Health Journal, 8*(2), 95–102.

Wang, C. C., & Redwood-Jones, Y. A. (2001). Photovoice ethics: Perspectives from Flint photovoice. *Health Education & Behavior, 28,* 560–572.

Wang, C. C., Yuan, Y. L., & Feng, M. L. (1996). Photovoice as a tool for participatory evaluation: The community's view of process and impact. *Journal of Contemporary Health, 4,* 47–49.

Wilson, N., Dasho, S., Martin, A. C., Wallerstein, N., Wang, C., & Minkler, M. (2007). Engaging young adolescents in social action through photovoice. *Journal of Early Adolescence, 27*(2), 241–261.

World Health Organization. (1986). *Ottawa charter for health promotion.* Copenhagen: Author.

Wu, K. Y., Burris, M., Li, V., Wang, Y., Zhan, W. T., Xiang, Y. P., et al. (Eds.). (1995). *Visual voices: 100 photographs of village China by the women of Yunnan Province.* Yunnan: Yunnan People's Publishing House.

CHAPTER

ISSUES IN PARTICIPATORY EVALUATION

JANE SPRINGETT & NINA WALLERSTEIN

THIS CHAPTER examines participatory evaluation and the specific challenges it faces in the context of community-based initiatives and community health promotion. The amount of literature on participatory evaluation in the evaluation field is increasing, reflecting the growing disillusion, at a number of levels, with approaches to evaluation derived from methodologies that originated in the natural sciences. This literature represents a continuing philosophical debate about the way knowledge is created and by whom. On a practical level, it is a response to the great divide between research and practice and the tendency for the results of a majority of evaluation studies to be ignored by the parties who commissioned them (Weiss, 1988). This chapter also presents a case study of a youth policy initiative in New Mexico as an illustration of both the opportunities and challenges of participatory evaluation.

Note: This chapter was adapted from "Participatory Approaches to Evaluation in Health Promotion," by Jane Springett, 2001, in *Evaluation in Health Promotion: Principles and Perspectives,* edited by I. Rootman et al., pp. 83–105. Copyright 2001 by the World Health Organization. Adapted by permission of the World Health Organization.

WHAT IS EVALUATION?

In recent years there has been much discussion in the field of community health promotion about the need for evidence-based practice and more evaluation. This debate has been driven in part by the increasing demand for accountability in the public sector (Henkel, 1991). It is also a sign of a maturing field seeking to establish its underlying theoretical base and philosophy and beginning to examine its effectiveness as a practice. Evaluation is something we do naturally all the time. It is essentially a process of reflection. It is also a process of learning from experience to inform future action. Kolb (1984), in his model of the adult experiential learning cycle, argues that for learning to take place, all elements of the cycle of thinking, deciding, doing, and reflecting must be accomplished. Thus evaluation must be seen as crucial for the development of the knowledge base of the field so that more is known about what works and, even more important, why and in what context.

Evaluation, however, is not the same as research. Although it uses the techniques and tools of research, it differs from research in a number of respects. A key difference lies in the word itself, in the notion of value and its assessment. Although it is widely recognized—in the social sciences, at least—that research is not value free, the conventions of science attempt to limit, through a variety of checks and balances, the degree of deviation from so-called objectivity. In contrast, value lies at the center of evaluation. It always has a political dimension and is intimately tied up with societal priorities, resource allocation, and power (Greene, 1994; House & Howe, 1999). For at the heart of evaluation lies the question of whose values are driving the evaluation and whose standards are being met by the activities being undertaken and assessed or whose standards are being measured against. For health promotion and community-based health interventions, this raises important issues, as quite often the values against which an intervention is being assessed are not those of the field but those of medicine and disease prevention (Springett, 2001).

In summary, evaluation is a process of reflection whereby the value of certain actions in relation to projects, programs, or policies is assessed. Moreover, evaluation can take many forms. Indeed, in the United States over one hundred different types have been recognized (Patton, 1997), with pluralistic approaches bringing many models together. Most important to choosing an evaluation methodology is the purpose of the evaluation and the question to be answered. Is the purpose to find out if client needs are being met, to improve the intervention or program, to assess its outcomes, to find out how it is operating, to assess efficiency, to assess its ability to facilitate empowerment, or to understand why a program of innovation works or does not work?

WHAT IS PARTICIPATORY EVALUATION?

Participatory approaches to evaluation attempt to involve in an evaluation all who have a stake in its outcomes, with a view to these individuals' and organizations' taking action and effecting change on the basis of the evaluation. If evaluation is going to change anything, it has to be useful and perceived as useful by everyone involved in a project or program, whether as a funder, a participant, or a project worker. The aim is to encourage every voice to be heard and at the very least taken into consideration when deciding on the focus and design (Fuerstein, 1988; Crishna, 2007a; Cousins & Whitmore, 1998; Wadsworth, 1991).

Participatory evaluation, however, goes beyond just being aware of stakeholder interests, in that there is a joint responsibility for the evaluation because the participants play an active role in the nuts and bolts of evaluation. By being involved, participants can see the value of the information they are collecting. Involvement also ensures that the indicators actually measure the right things in the right way—in other words, that the indicators are meaningful to all concerned (Macgillavray, 1998). However, the benefits of such an approach go beyond ownership and clarity. Involving a range of people in each stage often generates innovative ways of measuring process, impact, and outcomes. These innovations might, for example, include digital archiving, photovoice, collage, storytelling, and oral history (Springett & Young, 2002). To generate and maintain interest, a range of techniques, including celebration events, need to be employed (Springett & Dunkerton, 2001).

It could be argued that participatory evaluation is more a way of working based on a set of principles than an actual methodology. Indeed, the World Health Organization's (1998) recommendations to policymakers on the evaluation of health promotion specifically stipulate that evaluation should be participatory; this notion of participation at the center of health promotion evaluation was reinvoked in the Pan American Health Organization's principles issued in 2001 for the evaluation of healthy municipalities. Other names for participatory evaluation, reflecting some variations in practice, are empowerment evaluation (Fetterman, Kaftarian, & Wandersman, 1996; Fetterman & Wandersman, 2007), democratic evaluation (Floch'hay & Plottu, 1998), responsive evaluation (Abma, 2005), and stakeholder evaluation. Involving stakeholders in some way in evaluation is now generally considered to be a good practice (Robson, 2000). Key elements fundamental to all participatory evaluation are that involvement of marginalized groups is encouraged and dialogue and capacity for critical reflection are fostered (Weaver & Cousins, 2004; Diez, 2001; Themessl-Huber, 2003).

The philosophical and epistemological base of participatory evaluation lies in a hermeneutic tradition of knowledge creation (Dahlbom & Mathiassen, 1993). Its methodological and ideological roots lie in participatory action research. It is most commonly practiced at the community level in discrete localities and among disadvantaged groups with a tradition of grassroots activism (Jackson & Kassam, 1998; Aronson, Wallis, O'Campo, Whitehead, & Schafer, 2007; McKie, 2003; Standish, 1995). However, as more and more international aid agencies promote its use, there is an increasing if somewhat hesitant move toward a sustained use of participatory evaluation across multiple settings (Bradley, Mayfield, Mehta, & Rukonge, 2002).

Each of the three areas where participatory action research has been most commonly practiced—development research, management science, and education—has influenced the way participatory evaluation has developed. From its use in development work it has gained a close association with Freirian approaches to popular education (Kroeger & Franken, 1981). This means an emphasis in participatory evaluation on learning and capacity building. The increased use of such approaches stems from a widespread awareness of the inherent weaknesses of conventional evaluation methods (Rovers, 1986), especially when clear objectives have not been set at the outset of a project. However, the persistence of the idea of the project cycle in aid agency work, with its emphasis on relatively fixed procedures for the individual steps, is seen by some as a major constraint on full-scale adoption of participatory principles. Indeed, Mikkelsen (1995) argues that participatory evaluation in such a context is mostly a matter of adjusting a project while it is in progress to meet conditions set by the indigenous participants. Evaluation in this case is seen as a prerequisite to ensuring sustainability because of the focus on learning from experience. It serves, then, both as a management tool to enable people to improve their efficiency and effectiveness and as an educational process in which the participants increase their awareness and understanding of factors that affect their situation.

The influence of management science—a form of action learning that encourages the systematic collection of data and information for high-level organizational performance—supports the notion of using participatory evaluation to improve rather than evaluation to prove (Magerison, 1987). Thus participatory evaluation in organizational settings is geared to solving major problems on a group basis, with a focus on using decision makers as participants and moving from single-loop to double-loop learning (Argyris & Schön, 1978). Underpinning the rationale is the notion of learning and more particularly the notion of organizational learning. This reflects an increasing emphasis in management literature on the importance of participatory decision making in bringing about organizational change (Senge, 1990; Robinson & Cousins, 2004; Keast & Waterhouse, 2006).

Participatory evaluation in the context of organizations draws from this action research tradition, building on the notion of stakeholder involvement in evaluation. The approach is, however, distinguishable from the stakeholder tradition in evaluation practice (Fricke & Gill, 1989) in that it engages the primary users in all stages of the process. The other feature is that rather than being the principal investigator, the evaluator acts as a coordinator of the project, with responsibility for technical support training and quality control and joint responsibility for conducting the inquiry. The evaluator becomes a partner in an evaluation process where all involved have a commitment to change. The partnership is such that it may develop over a long period of time and not just for the duration of one project. It also means that the external evaluator is less likely to be co-opted or manipulated by managers in favor of their own agenda (Cousins & Earl, 1995; Mathison, 1994).

It is in the area of education that participatory evaluation has been used most extensively. Here it has also traditionally had an organizational focus, but a greater feature has been the emphasis on practitioners' becoming evaluators in order to become more reflexive and improve their practice (O'Hara & McNamara, 2001). The focus is on the systematic collection of evidence as well as collaborative inquiry, motivated by the quest to improve and understand the world by changing it. It focuses as well on learning how to improve practice from the effects of the changes made, particularly in the classroom but also in the whole school. This strand of influence is encapsulated in the notion of reflective practice, which has come to be adopted in a whole range of fields relevant to community health promotion, including policy analysis, social work, and urban planning.

In the research and evaluation literature, a subtle and perhaps semantic distinction is made between participatory research (PR) and participatory evaluation (PE). Some consider PE just one aspect of the PR cycle (Israel, Checkoway, Schulz, & Zimmerman, 1994); others see it as a distinctive approach to evaluation. PE shares with PR the key principle that the various parties are to be actively involved in the actual work and in decisions about the evaluation process, an involvement requiring the continuous exchange of knowledge, skills, and resources (Cousins & Earl, 1995). Some analysts, however, contend that there is no difference between the two if participation takes place throughout a project cycle (Mikkelsen, 1995). As PR does, participatory evaluation changes the relationship between the evaluated and the evaluator (Gustavsen, 1992; Hazen, 1994; Vanderplaat, 1995) and explicitly challenges the authority of the outside independent assessor. In essence participatory evaluation is about doing evaluation using participatory action research (PAR) methods.

This is important to emphasize because there are fundamental differences between participatory evaluation and conventional evaluation (see Table 12.1). Evaluation in

TABLE 12.1 **Differences Between Conventional Evaluation and Participatory Evaluation**

	Conventional evaluation	Participatory evaluation
Who	External experts	Community, project staff, expert as facilitator.
What	Predetermined indicators of success, primarily cost and health outcomes or gains	People identify their own indicators of success, which may include health outcomes and gains.
How	Focus on "scientific objectivity," distancing evaluators from other participants; uniform, complex procedures; delayed, limited access to results	Self-evaluation; simple methods adapted to local culture; open, immediate sharing of results through local involvement in evaluation processes.
When	Usually completion; sometimes also midterm	Merging of monitoring and evaluation; hence frequent small-scale evaluations.
Why	Accountability, usually summative, to determine if funding continues	To empower local people to initiate, control, and take corrective action.

Source: Adapted from PROWWESS/United Nations Development Program, 1990.

community health continues to be dominated by epidemiologists, demographers, and biomedical scientists with a positivist way of viewing the world that contrasts with the hermeneutic perspective that underpins action research. Moreover, there are some examples of so-called participatory research into health that bear little relationship to the underlying ideological, methodological, and epistemological bases of PAR, reflecting the reappropriation by positivist science of the terminology (Couto, 1987; Dockery, 1996; Lawell, Noriega, Martinez, & Villegars, 1992). Participation is more than just taking part; it is about engaging in a dialogue at all stages of the process of evaluation and shifting the power in favor of those who are being researched. It is, as Vanderplaat (1995) puts it, "evaluation for empowerment."

Participatory evaluation focuses on knowledge creation in the context of practice and the development of local theory (Greenwood, Whyte, & Harkavy, 1993). Such a perspective is based on a completely different conception of the relationship between science, evidence, learning, and action than is found in positivist methods in social science work (Peile, 1994; Wallerstein, 2007). It assumes that people can generate knowledge as partners in a systematic inquiry process based on their own categories and frameworks. This, it can be argued, enhances scientific validity, producing richer and more accurate data; creates active support for the results of the process of inquiry; and therefore creates greater commitment to change as well as a greater likelihood that ideas will be diffused and used. In traditional research the emphasis is on theory creation and testing, whereas in traditional practice the emphasis is on action. In participatory evaluation the production of knowledge results from collaboration between insider-practitioner and outsider-evaluator (or evaluator-researcher), producing reflection on both personal and collective engagement (Gatenby & Humphries, 2000). The aim is to encourage change and learning as a self-maintaining process that continues after the evaluator-researcher has left.

Although this approach is particularly appropriate to community-based projects, it also has value for the other end of the spectrum, policy development and implementation (Diez, Malagon, & Izquierdo, 2005). No longer is the production of knowledge retained in the hands of experts and the knowledge itself lodged on the shelves of libraries as interesting but not relevant to day-to-day practical and policy problems. Rather, by being involved in the evaluation process, practitioners and policymakers own both the ideas of the evaluation and its results. They thus can be ready to implement the appropriate action because the process of doing the evaluation has already begun to change the way they act and what they believe. Creating dialogue situations in which thoughts are exchanged begins to shape a new social reality (Habermas, 1984–1987; Schwandt, 2001). The role of the evaluator is to create those situations through various techniques, such as workshops, and allow the joint product, a more integrated and higher form of consciousness, to emerge from the interplay between the actors (Reason, 1988). A new set of social relations is created, and the new knowledge is the result of that process. The essence of this type of evaluation is that it is an emergent process controlled by local conditions (Wallerstein, 1999). It encourages innovation and change (Cranton, 1996). Traditional evaluation approaches can easily undermine innovation. As people become aware of being judged, instead of improving their capability they perform to satisfy the measurement chosen. The intrinsic motivation that drives learning and creates change is replaced by a desire to provide numbers for bureaucrats (Henkel, 1991; Seddon, 2000; Ackerman et al., 2007).

The strength of participatory evaluation is that it integrates evaluation into project work or an intervention, allowing a more natural emerging, empowering, and evolving approach to development (Springett & Leavey, 1995). It is equally process and outcome driven, rather than focusing on outcomes alone. Traditional evaluation can reinforce marginalization and social exclusion. Problems are often seen to be located in a particular community or ethnic group, and the evaluation often focuses exclusively on the individuals, rather than on the context in which that group operates (Goodman, Wheeler, & Lee, 1993). Little is done to probe the experience and assumptions of the organizations that are the source of disempowerment or to bring the two groups together in a dialogue concerning the problem, the program, and how its success or failure will be evaluated and against whose criteria. Similarly, little is done to change the power relationships so that excluded groups can have a say and take control of the factors that promote good health. The most appropriate type of evaluation, therefore, is one that involves enhancing this control (Vanderplaat, 1995). In other words, participatory evaluation is a health-promoting intervention in itself.

USE OF PE IN COMMUNITY HEALTH

In the last decade, following the report of the European Working Group on Health Promotion Evaluation of the World Health Organization (WHO, 1998) and subsequent initiatives in the Pan American Health Organization region, there has been a steady growth of participatory evaluation literature related to community health and community-based initiatives (Rice & Franceschini, 2007). This literature has evolved slowly due to the general lack of evaluation in the health promotion and community health development field and the paucity of outlets, until recently, for reporting this type of research. Another factor in this slow growth is the time required to complete this type of study and the time lag between completing an evaluation and the publication of the results, given the precedence of the demands from funding agencies for a report. The dominance and power of the randomized controlled trial and of the conventional scientific method are also major factors. Concerns about a lack of scientific rigor and generalizability, validity of the results, and replicability are put forward against the participatory approach; all still stem from a perceived failure to be objective, just as they originally did thirty years ago (Susman & Evered, 1978).

Concerns that do not stem from this perspective also have an impact on the amount of participatory evaluation that takes place. These concerns include the time it takes to undertake PE, the resources it involves, and the perceived messiness of the process. Even when the evaluation process has clear steps, PE's inherent messiness seems counter to the search for clarity and the need to control and be logical and plan. Furthermore, funders have difficulty funding such an unpredictable process and its indefinable outcomes (Maclure, 1990). Moreover, researchers often lack the skills required, and the community may fall short in critical thinking capacity (Fuerstein, 1988). In a policy context where multifaceted health promotion programs are involved, the potential complexity of the process to be handled can be problematic (Costongs & Springett, 1997). These barriers are reinforced by project evaluations being imposed from outside and often in ways that are inappropriate (Kennedy, 1995).

Nonetheless, the value of PAR and participatory approaches to research in health promotion is increasingly recognized, and the number of projects taking place using this approach is growing. The approach is increasing substantially in popularity in the areas of primary care and public health and health promotion in developing countries and in nursing research, particularly at the community level. It is the approach of choice in the growing number of community *arts for health* projects (Douglas, Warwick, Whitty, & Aggleton, 2000; Angus, 1999; Foster-Fisherman, Nowell, Deacon, Nievar, & McCann, 2005; South, 2005). In Canada the federal government has supported the participatory approach by, for example, funding a major report (Green et al., 1995) and providing a tool for project workers through a Web site. In the U.K. the National Assembly for Wales (2001) supported the use of PE to evaluate a five-year series of community-based initiatives, and in England and Scotland many *healthy living centres, health action zones,* and *sure start* projects have used this approach to evaluation (Cropper, Porter, Williams, Carlisle, Moore, O'Neill, et al., 2007; Reeves & Peerbhoy, 2006).

In the United States an increasing number of programs and projects are using participatory evaluation. Some of the major foundations, such as the W. K. Kellogg Foundation, have been instrumental in encouraging such an approach. An early adopter among programs with a specific community health focus is the Adolescent Social Action Program in New Mexico (Wallerstein & Bernstein, 1994), which has sought to empower youths from high-risk populations to make healthier choices using Freire's (1973) three-stage methodology of listening, dialogue, and action. Another was the Partners for Improved Nutrition and Health project, implemented in 1988 as a five-year collaborative program by Freedom from Hunger, the Mississippi State Department of Health, and the Mississippi Cooperative Extension Agency (Eng & Parker, 1994).

Participatory evaluation has also been used in evaluating health promotion programs in the workplace, especially those developed to deal with stress (Israel, Schurman, & House, 1989). Although the changing internal structures of organizations (owing to such things as layoffs and changes in product lines) may make randomized control trials difficult, these participatory evaluation studies have used statistical control techniques and time-series designs, demonstrating that participatory evaluation does not mean only qualitative approaches. Participation in the workplace setting, however, may become associated with co-optation and manipulation rather than true participation, depending on the culture of the workplace (Baker, Israel, & Schurman, 1993; Polanyi, McIntosh, & Kosny, 2005). Growth in the use of participatory methods is evolving more slowly in the area of policy development because of the inherent complexity of actors and levels of change. An excellent model was the development of an evaluation and monitoring framework and indicators for the City Health Plan in Liverpool (Springett, 1998). An attempt was made to satisfy a range of stakeholders while incorporating evaluation into the implementation process. The result was a pragmatic approach, which was the product of interplay between an ideal model and reality in a particular context. The cultural legacy resulted in the adoption of a participatory approach to evaluation in the subsequent Merseyside Health Action Zone, although local policymakers struggled to maintain the approach in the context of a central government wedded to top-down target setting (Springett, 2005).

PE ISSUES IN COMMUNITY HEALTH PROMOTION

It is the assumption of this chapter that participatory evaluation is a cyclical process, based on the action research cycle, that consists of a series of steps and decisions (which can be used as a checklist) in which all stakeholders participate (see Exhibit 12.1). Although it can be argued that participatory evaluation is a process, not a technique, there are methodological issues that concern how one engages in the process, ensures that it is systematic, adheres to basic principles, and creates opportunities for dialogue (Mathison, 1994). Many issues stem from the need to balance the requirements of participation; the use of appropriate, rigorous, verifiable, and valid tools and techniques; and the practical demands of the real world while retaining the values of social action (Crishna, 2007b). There is considerable variation in practice, though some differences are to be expected owing to the grounding in the local context.

EXHIBIT 12.1 Steps in Participatory Evaluation

1. All those involved in the program decide jointly to use a participatory approach.
2. They decide exactly what the objectives of the evaluation are. This can turn out to be far harder than originally thought.
3. When agreement on objectives is reached, a small group of evaluation coordinators is elected to plan and organize the details of the evaluation.
4. The methods that are best for attaining the evaluation objectives are now chosen. The choice of method will also be influenced by the capabilities of the people involved and the time and resources available.
5. As these decisions are made, the written evaluation plan is formed, showing why, how, when, and where the evaluation will take place and who will be involved.
6. Next, the methods are prepared and tested. Selected participants will need training in such matters as interviewing, and all participants will need explanations of objectives and methods. The more they understand, the more they will participate when asked.
7. The methods, having been tested, are now used to collect facts and information.
8. The information is analyzed by participants, the major part of the analysis being done by the coordinators.
9. The results are prepared in written, oral, or visual form.
10. Finally, program participants decide how the results will be used and how they can improve the effectiveness and performance of the program.

Source: Adapted from Fuerstein, 1988.

The first methodological issue concerns the level and nature of participation and the cyclical characteristics of that participation. It is a spiraling process rather than a series of static episodes. In practice, who participates is the product of the negotiated situation. Although the ideal is total participation by all, who participates will be a product of the existing distribution of power and resources among the potential stakeholders, the time available to undertake the evaluation, and the resources available. Inevitably, difficult decisions will have to be made, because who participates will have an impact on both the process and the results of the evaluation (Greenwood, Whyte, & Harkavy, 1993).

Couto (1987) notes that this balancing act can have different outcomes in different contexts and that often in the health context, because of the hegemony of medical science, it is likely that the balance will move in favor of traditional approaches (Reeves & Peerbhoy, 2006). The larger the reach of a project, the more difficult it is to ensure a democratic process. A great deal of creativity is required to succeed at this. Small-scale community-based programs are thus easier to manage. In all cases it is important to involve managers and funders in the process. Often managers will try to limit the extent of their participation, preferring to exercise control. And sometimes they fail to see the need to be involved in the process and send representatives to workshops and meetings or fail to attend at all. This means that they may not accept or even understand the results at the end of the process.

The development of an indicator tool for evaluating multisectoral collaboration in the U.K. provides a good example of the ways in which the characteristics of those involved in the process have an impact on the outcome. The research involved two hundred people and was conducted in three stages. Stage 1 consisted of a telephone survey, using the snowball technique, to gain an overview of "Healthy Alliance work." This was followed by six workshops, involving practitioner representatives from Healthy Communities networks, to generate definitions of characteristics and success for Healthy Alliances. The results were used to develop a process and outcome indicator pack. Stage 2 involved pilot-testing at three test sites to refine the indicator pack. Results were discussed in a workshop of twenty participants that included representatives of commissioners and purchasers of health and community services in addition to providers of services, after which the pack was modified again (Furnell, Oldfield, & Speller, 1995). The resulting final pack was therefore firmly grounded in experience (McKie, 2003).

There were several limitations, however. Opportunities for dialogue between the practitioner group and management resource holders only occurred to a limited extent at the end of the process, which meant that the pack did not include task and managerial indicators. Moreover, when tested in the three case study areas, the pack was found to be inappropriate for small-scale community-based projects, particularly those in the early stages of development, and was criticized by community participants. The pack's main advantage was that it provided a framework for discussion of more context-based and relevant indicators and suggested a process that could be replicated locally.

Another difficulty in this context can be the rapid turnover of project managers and other staff, both in government and the nonprofit sector. The facilitator of the evaluation needs to ensure that arenas for dialogue are created and there is feedback at each stage to involve new participants. The facilitator also needs to be aware of the inequalities in power between the participants and should take action to reduce it through the opportunities for dialogue.

A second methodological issue is the relationship between the evaluator and the evaluated and the balance between expert and lay involvement and particularly between insider and outsider evaluation. There are advantages and disadvantages on both sides (see Table 12.2). The use of an outside evaluator still carries the greatest credibility. At a minimum an external evaluator can serve as facilitator at workshops, writer of the report, and quality controller. However, the value of a participatory research approach is that it combines the technical expertise of the evaluator with the local knowledge of the lay participants so that the sum is greater than the parts. Tied up with this issue is the need to gain the commitment of busy professionals and the need to negotiate who owns the findings in the end. Even if the intention is for the findings to be used by the community, academics also face their own requirements to publish. There is little question that the process of cowriting with community participants is challenging, but joint writing legitimizes community knowledge and increases the potential for community use of the findings. Excluding community participants flies in the face of the ideology of participation and reinforces academic hegemony (Gaventa, 1993). These issues need to be negotiated at

TABLE 12.2 **Advantages and Disadvantages of External and Internal Evaluators**

External	Internal
Can take a fresh look at the program	Knows the program well
Not personally involved	Finds it harder to be objective
Is not part of the power structure	Is part of the power and authority structure
Gains nothing from the program but may gain prestige from the evaluation	May be motivated by hopes of personal gain
Trained in evaluation methods; may have experiences in other evaluations	May or may not be trained in evaluation methods
Is an outsider who may not understand the program or the people involved	Is familiar with and known by the program, so can interpret personal behavior and attitudes, and final recommendations may appear less threatening

Source: Adapted from Fuerstein, 1986.

the beginning and recorded in written agreements to ensure that roles and responsibilities are clear.

The role of the external evaluator can change (Cohen, 2001), and as in any development project, there is a skill in knowing when to take a leadership, facilitative, or back-seat role without disempowering participants. In one community-led participatory evaluation project in Salford, England, a researcher realized, during the reflection process, that in trying to allow the participants to drive the process and not to dominate the agenda herself, she had failed to realize that her expertise had an equal part to play in the process. Volunteers expressed frustration that she had not come forward in the early stages and filled a gap in their knowledge. Interestingly enough, in the same project, one participant withdrew from the process on the grounds that the decision makers would ignore the findings no matter how participatory the process (Young, 2001)!

Without a key facilitator, participants can sometimes get so carried away with the notion of having fun that evaluation can lack true critical reflection. Without a structure provided by an external facilitator, there is a tendency to lose sight of the bigger picture. In Netherton, a neighborhood in the Merseyside Health Action Zone in England, for example, project participants easily fell back into evaluating their own projects rather than looking for common themes across them (Springett & Dunkerton, 2001). Also, unless a special effort is made, there is no feedback loop into policy structures and decision making for policy change (Winje & Hewell, 1992).

Critical reflection also requires a safe environment, as well as a certain degree of skill and honesty (Mezirow, 1990). Looking at what is wrong is often challenging in organizations and communities that are experiencing difficulties, leading to defensive reactions that can undermine the participatory ethos (Levin, 1999). Ironically, the organizations that need to change most and could benefit from the approach are most often the most resistant. In these situations, people may refuse to participate at any stage of the process, and managers may refuse to engage directly with staff. To ignore the emotional response to evaluation and to see it only as a technical event is to ignore a fundamental element of the human experience (Smith, 2005). The emotional response to decision making is important and is beginning to be an acknowledged dimension in social science (Anderson & Smith, 2001; Dimasio, 1994).

Thus a third issue that needs to be faced is the inherent contradiction arising from participatory evaluation's dialectical nature. Different agendas are being overtly brought together. This inevitably results in conflict and power struggles, because it is the creation of knowledge on its own battleground (Rebien, 1996). Skills in conflict resolution therefore become as important for a good evaluator as knowledge of data collection and analysis techniques. Managing conflict includes the ability to be pragmatic while trying to keep to the participatory evaluation ethos and principles. Evaluators have competing and often contradictory tasks to fulfill. For example, to ensure the relevance of a policy evaluation, the evaluator should be involved with the policy initiative in order to collaborate effectively with local workers, but at the same time he or she must keep enough distance to be critical and ask the right questions (Quellet, Durand, & Forget, 1994). Also, the evaluator must find the balance between the public's right to know and the individual's right to privacy and discretion (Greene, 1994). Therefore a range of communication, negotiation, creativity, motivation, political, and facilitative skills is needed among evaluators. Long and Wilkinson (1984) have pointed out that evaluators must cope with complex social programs and personality conflicts in often difficult environments (Geva-May & Thorngate, 2003).

In addition, evaluators should play a more active role in the translation of evaluation results to policy processes (Greene, 1994). Simply publishing in journals is not enough. This is especially true with qualitative evaluations, which are often underread in comparison with the compact tables and summaries of quantitative work (Richardson, 1994). Ham (1991) remarks that communication and salesmanship with clarity in recommendations must go hand in hand with good academic techniques if the evaluator wants to influence policy.

A fourth issue is that the process is emergent, which can have a number of effects. First, there is a feeling among funders and evaluators of a lack of control (Van Eyk, Baum, & Blandford, 2001). Participatory evaluation does not always fit into a neat project cycle, and funds can be cut off at crucial moments with reports not yet finished. A committed project manager in the funding agency helps. Second, and particularly relevant to health promotion, is the fact that most projects are categorically funded, reflecting the disease and lifestyle model that still dominates health funding. Yet the community perspective is very different and reflects a more holistic approach to life. The aims and objectives that participants value, for example, better quality-of-life outcomes, may therefore be distinct from the funders' original aims and objectives. Moreover, with action and change being central, the whole project might move in a different direction. This again illustrates that it is vital that the funders and the initiators of the evaluation be part of the process, which ensures ongoing communication and feedback. Attempting to achieve all these goals while engaged in participatory evaluation in a complex environment of different interest groups and multiple causes is understandably difficult (Costongs & Springett, 1997).

A fifth methodological issue concerns funding. The participatory form of evaluation is funded relatively poorly compared to projects that adopt a more traditional paradigm. There is a general lack of expertise among funders, and their chief demand is for short-term task-oriented approaches to evaluation (Green et al., 1995). This is so despite the value added through the potential for change that participation produces because the evaluation results are actually implemented. The evaluator is dependent for effective follow-through on a sympathetic funding project officer who understands the unpredictability of the process and is willing to go along with it. So forming a good relationship at the beginning is crucial.

The evaluator's task is frequently made more difficult by the fact that health promotion project workers start to think about evaluation only when the end of a project is in sight. That is too late for adopting a truly participatory evaluation approach. Funding for evaluation needs to be allocated up front.

A sixth issue is common to all evaluation, that of choosing the appropriate tools and techniques for data collection and for dissemination of results. For participatory evaluation, in particular, tools should be simple but effective, and relevant for ongoing feedback cycles and for the specific context. The Yellow Creek Concerned Citizens, working with the Highlander Research and Education Center in Kentucky, for example, did a quantitative evaluation of the impact of waste dumping on health in order to be able to defend these findings before those trained in traditional epidemiology (Couto, 1987). The emphasis is on eclecticism and appropriateness (Baum, 1992; Everitt, 1996). Training will almost certainly be required and should be included in the budget. The aim is to create a process that is sustainable and that leaves added knowledge at the end of the process. As is discussed in Chapter Eleven, photovoice uses photographs as a form of data collection that provides a valuable and effective alternative to the statistical graphs often demanded by decision makers who want concrete measures. Often, however, the information gained from the evaluation process will have to be presented in more than one form. In both Nooralunga, Australia, and Drumchapel, Scotland, for example, a variety of methods, including artwork, were used for dissemination (Baum & Cook, 1990; Kennedy, 1995). Arts-based health projects abound with such examples (Angus, 1999).

The final issue is that of empowerment. The participatory evaluation process itself is seen to play a role in empowerment and can contribute to the elimination of social inequality, the intended outcome of many health promotion projects (Wallerstein, 2006). Participatory evaluation can openly address issues of power, can incorporate social action and community development methods, and can make explicit the values and interests inherent in evaluation, thereby enabling democratic dialogue as to whose values the evaluation serves and creating new social knowledge (Barnes, 1993; Keast & Waterhouse, 2006). If people are involved in decision making, the results of any evaluation are more likely to be used. This, according to Patton (1997), is the strongest argument for participation, alongside avoidance of orthodoxy and encouragement to use a range of methods and tools in data collection and analysis. Participation also creates in people a critical awareness of their problems, and this is seen as playing an important health promotion role in capacity building (Rahman, 1993).

There are benefits to be gained in the sharing of lay and expert knowledge, the pooling of resources, and the sharing of strengths. For example, if people are involved in decision making, they may even undertake the questionnaire survey themselves, thus reducing evaluation costs. Relevance is also important in bringing about sustainable behavioral and social change at the individual and community levels. As Pyle (1982) has suggested, "When long-term behavioral change, self-sustaining capacity and universal coverage is desired, community participation is essential" (p. 64).

The failure to ground evaluation indicators in the needs of local workers and their community led the people of Drumchapel to develop their own evaluation of their project. Disillusioned with the externally commissioned evaluation driven by the agenda of a university, they adopted a truly participatory approach, which enabled a whole range of innovative methods, including alternative ways of reporting the results through art and a video (Kennedy, 1995). The video made by the people explores the stories of the different community members and how the evaluation process enhanced their sense of self-worth and self-efficacy as well as their health.

There is great potential here. Just as participatory evaluation encourages empowerment within the community, which is one of the aims of health promotion, a collaborative problem-solving approach to evaluation in itself also encourages intersectoral collaboration. It forces those involved as project workers to make conscious choices on how to collaborate and reflect on practice (Clark, Baker, Chawla, & Maru, 1993).

YOUTH LINK CASE STUDY

This case study is used as an example of how the issues look in practice because it illustrates the opportunities and challenges of participatory evaluation. Youth Link, a multi-level youth empowerment project, was started over a decade ago in New Mexico to promote youths as public policy advocates to contribute to local and statewide youth policy development. Intergenerational community action teams (CATs) of youths, aged twelve to twenty-one, were started in twelve communities, though with a hiatus in funding in the fourth year, only four were maintained when funding resumed. Led by volunteer adult coordinators, the CATs researched their community's problems and met in regional trainings and statewide meetings to analyze policy issues that affected New Mexico youths. At the end of the second year, youth facilitators from the Albuquerque CAT prepared for and led a three-day residential *youth town hall,* which served for the next several years to frame statewide policy recommendations, with annual policy institutes to reinforce the youths' involvement.

In the first three years of Youth Link the Kellogg Foundation funded an intensive participatory evaluation, intended to provide both data on a unique statewide youth policy initiative and a model for participatory evaluation in small, nonprofit settings. In the first year a university evaluation team worked with Youth Link staff, the youth advisory council, and the CATs in developing a shared evaluation designed to (1) track the creation of a statewide youth policy logic model, including the barriers and facilitators to creating the model; (2) assess empowerment outcomes for participating youths; and (3) identify local or statewide policy outcomes.

A multimethods approach was used, including a pre-post questionnaire, at baseline and after year two (available from Wallerstein). This questionnaire was developed in collaboration with Youth Link staff and based on the youths' cognitive and behavioral empowerment constructs (that is, collective and political efficacy and policy actions). Qualitative data collection included annual CAT focus groups where the youths identified their own goals and objectives and their successes with them and also the barriers to reaching them; adult interviews; a review of CAT meeting minutes and documents; and the tracking of policy outcomes, that is, youths being invited to serve on local policy boards or actual public policy change through bill enactment or other institutional change. All trainings and the major event of the youth town hall were evaluated separately.

Analysis of the qualitative and quantitative data was triangulated to revise the logic model of change, identifying the characteristics and conditions of youth actions in the policy arena that facilitated their ability to affect policy change. The most important facilitator named was the youth town hall, which made policymaking concrete with important recommendations for youth-police relations, school policies to support youths, teen pregnancy prevention education, and prevention of gang violence and substance abuse (Blackwell, Minkler, & Thompson, 2005). Other facilitators were the role of supportive adults, the creation of a statewide group identity, and the learning of policy skills.

Additional Surdna Foundation funding in years four through seven enabled the evaluation to continue, though at a reduced level. Local achievements that were tracked included youths' succeeding at mobilizing the Los Cruces mayor's office to support a publicly funded skate park, as well as the introduction of bills in the state legislature related to appropriate sentencing and counseling for teen DWI offenders, teen access to tobacco products, resources for homeless youths, gun safety, suicide prevention, and school safety policies. Youth qualitative data triangulated with the evidence of policy efforts. As one youth said comparing Youth Link to other school groups at the legislature, "Most youth were just there to watch, but we were there to speak, to be heard."

As a multiyear participatory evaluation case study, the Youth Link project provides lessons for practitioners and researchers in the development of a viable youth policy model, in participatory evaluation strategies, and in the need for further research on the effects of youth empowerment and policy strategies on health. To systematically assess the Youth Link model, the evaluation embraced a practical approach that involved program stakeholders (both staff and youths) at each stage, with codevelopment of the questionnaire and focus group questions, opportunities for dialogue and reflection, and use of data to provide continuous feedback to the program and to garner additional funding.

Youth Link is typical of programs implemented by nonprofit community groups or clinics, which cannot afford randomized evaluation designs but need easily usable evaluation tools, such as logic models, to develop their own capacity to conduct evaluations. It was a strength of the Youth Link design that the evaluator was both an insider and outsider, involved from the beginning in the task force to develop the program yet also serving as a university evaluator, adopting the role of facilitator of a participatory evaluation process. Though there were strengths to this evaluation, the attrition of youths was problematic and meant there were insufficient pairs in the pre-post questionnaire design to assess significance in cognitive and behavioral changes. Despite the challenge in using a pre-post design, development of the questionnaire was helpful for the staff in redirecting program components and for reflection on program impacts. Triangulation of the pre-post results with focus group data and concrete policy actions was critical for validating and deepening understandings of the processes and impacts of change. With youths and staff participating in interpreting the evaluation, the validity of the change logic model was strengthened, with new understandings of the relationship between youth participation and policy change processes, and the findings could therefore be used directly by the program.

SUMMARY

The use of participatory action research methods in evaluation in community health development is increasing, but there is a long way to go before it is as widely accepted as it is in areas such as education, management, and development work. The dominance of medical science, with its methods rooted in the natural sciences, is a major factor in the slow adoption of this potentially fruitful approach to change. The irony is that participatory evaluation is the central feature, although it is not named as such, of clinical audit.

The review by Cornwall and Jewkes (1995) demonstrating the strong influence of development work on individuals working in primary health care and public health in developing countries, the Royal Society of Canada study (Green et al., 1995), the work of the Pan American Health Organization, and the work of the evaluators involved in health action zones in the U.K. and other community-based health initiatives in the United States should give a much needed impetus to the acceptance of this form of evaluation in the developed world.

For this to happen, there needs to be greater support for this type of approach through funding and more direct participation by policymakers themselves in evaluation. However, there is still a widespread need for skills training for researchers, practitioners, and policymakers. There needs to be recognition of the long-term and capability-building value of this type of approach and its contribution to knowledge development and effective change, rather than simply the completion of specific and often inappropriate short-term tasks. It is important, too, to accept that a participatory approach is inherently and overtly political. In it lies the potential to affect the broader social structures that are the source of disempowerment (Papineau & Kiely, 1996). Ensuring that evaluation is participatory is fundamental to addressing the real accountability issue, which is accountability to the community groups whose health any health-promoting intervention should serve.

At its best, participatory evaluation provides a solution to the practical problem of crossing the boundaries between theory and practice and the competing cultures of research and policymaking. As an approach, it can be a real catalyst for change (Charles, Schalm, & Seredek, 1994; Ledwith, 2005). At the same time, it is profoundly challenging in its execution.

QUESTIONS FOR DISCUSSION

1. What are the differences and similarities between CBPR (or other participatory research traditions), and participatory evaluation?

2. What is the rationale for participatory evaluation? In answering also discuss these questions: What are the differences between participatory evaluation and conventional evaluation? Between external and internal evaluators? As an external evaluator, when would you choose a participatory approach and when a conventional approach?

3. How does the Youth Link case study illustrate the issues embedded in participatory evaluation? What steps would you take as a participatory evaluator to create an effective evaluation that acknowledges the various issues?

KEY TERMS

Participatory evaluation   Empowerment evaluation

REFERENCES

Abma, T. A. (2005). Responsive evaluation in health promotion: Its value for ambiguous contexts. *Health Promotion International, 20*(4), 391–397.

Ackerman, M., Arroyo, H., Jones, C. M., O'Neil, M., Roca, A., & Wallerstein, N. (2007). Evaluation of health promotion effectiveness: A political debate and/or a technical exercise? *Promotion & Education* (Suppl. 1), 13–15.

Anderson, K., & Smith, S. J. (2001). Emotional geographies. *Transactions of the Institute of British Geographers, New Series, 26*(1), 7–10.

Angus, J. (1999). *An enquiry concerning possible methods for evaluating art for health projects.* Durham, U.K.: University of Durham, Centre for Arts and Humanities in Health and Medicine.

Argyris, C., & Schön, D. (1978). *Organizational learning: Vol. 1. A theory of action perspective.* Reading, MA: Addison-Wesley.

Aronson, R., Wallis, A., O'Campo, P., Whitehead, T., & Schafer, P. (2007). Ethnographically informed community evaluation: A framework and approach for evaluating community-based initiatives. *Maternal and Child Health Journal, 11*(2), 97–109.

Baker, E. A., Israel, B. A., & Schurman, S. J. (1993). A participatory approach to worksite health promotion. *Journal of Ambulatory Care Management, 17*(2), 68–81.

Barnes, M. (1993). Introducing new stakeholders: User and researcher interests in evaluative research. *Policy and Politics, 21,* 47–58.

Baum, F. (1992). Research for Healthy Cities: Some experiences from Down Under. In E. de Leeuw, M. O'Neill, M. Goumans, & F. de Bruijn (Eds.), *Healthy Cities research agenda: Proceedings of an expert panel* (RHC Monograph Series No. 2, pp. 45–54). Maastricht, The Netherlands: University of Maastricht.

Baum, F., & Cook, D. (1990). *Healthy Cities Nooralunga Project evaluation.* Adelaide: South Australian Community Health Research Unit.

Blackwell, A. G., Minkler, M., & Thompson, M. (2005). Using community organizing and community building to influence policy. In M. Minkler (Ed.), *Community organizing and community building for health* (2nd ed., pp. 405–418). New Brunswick, NJ: Rutgers University Press.

Bradley, J. E., Mayfield, M. V., Mehta, M. P., & Rukonge, A. (2002). Participatory evaluation of reproductive health care quality in developing countries. *Social Science & Medicine, 55*(2), 269–287.

Charles, C., Schalm, C., & Seredek, J. (1994). Involving stakeholders in health services research: Developing Alberta's resident classification system for long-term care facilities. *International Journal of Health Services, 24,* 749–761.

Clark, N. M., Baker, E. A., Chawla, A., & Maru, M. (1993). Sustaining collaborative problem solving: Strategies from a study of six Asian countries. *Health Education Research: Theory and Practice, 8,* 385–402.

Cohen, R. (2001, December 6). *Call in a doctor or a plumber? Participatory empowerment evaluation in a South London food project.* Paper presented at the annual meeting of the UK Evaluation Society, London.

Cornwall, A., & Jewkes, R. (1995). What is participatory research? *Social Science & Medicine, 41,* 1667–1676.

Costongs, C., & Springett, J. (1997). Toward a framework for the evaluation of health related policies in cities. *Evaluation, 3,* 345–362.

Cousins, J. B., & Earl, L. M. (Eds.). (1995). *Participatory evaluation in education: Studies in evaluation use and organizational learning.* Washington, DC: Falmer.

Cousins, J. B., & Whitmore, E. (1998). Framing participatory evaluation. In E. Whitmore (Ed.), *Understanding and practicing participatory evaluation* (pp. 5–24). San Francisco: Jossey-Bass.

Couto, R. A. (1987). Participatory research: Methodology and critique. *Clinical Sociology Review, 5,* 83–90.

Cranton, P. (1996). *Professional development as transformative learning: New perspectives for teachers of adults.* San Francisco: Jossey-Bass.

Crishna, B. (2007a). Participatory evaluation (I): Sharing lessons from fieldwork in Asia. *Child: Care, Health and Development, 33,* 217–223.

Crishna, B, (2007b), Participatory evaluation (II): Translating concepts of reliability and validity in fieldwork. *Child: Care, Health and Development, 33,* 224–229.

Cropper, S., Porter, A., Williams, G., Carlisle, S., Moore, R., O'Neill, M., Roberts, C., & Snooks, H. (eds). (2007). *Community health and well-being: Action research on health inequalities.* Bristol, U.K.: Policy Press.

Dahlbom, B., & Mathiassen, L. (1993). *Computers in context: The philosophy and practice of systems design.* Malden, MA: Blackwell.

Diez, M. A. (2001). The evaluation of regional innovation and cluster policies: Towards a participatory approach. *European Planning Studies, 9*(7), 907–923.

Diez, M. A., Malagon, E., & Izquierdo, B. (2005). *Using evaluation for collective learning and improving regional policies: A case study in the Basque Country.* Paper presented at "Regional Growth Agendas," the international conference of the Regional Growth Association, Aalborg, Denmark.

Dimasio, A. R. (1994). *Descartes' error: Emotion, reason, and the human brain.* New York: Putnam.

Dockery, G. (1996). Rhetoric or reality? Participatory research in the National Health Service, UK. In K. De Koning & M. Martin (Eds.), *Participatory research in health: Issues and experiences* (2nd ed., pp. 164–175). London: Zed Books.

Douglas, N., Warwick, I., Whitty, G., & Aggleton, P. (2000). Vital youth evaluating a Theatre in Education project. *Health Education, 100,* 207–215.

Eng, E., & Parker, E. A. (1994). Measuring community competence in the Mississippi Delta: The interface between program evaluation and empowerment. *Health Education Quarterly, 21,* 199–220.

Everitt, A. (1996). Values and evidence in evaluating community health. *Critical Public Health, 6*(3), 56–65.

Fetterman, D. M., Kaftarian, S. J., & Wandersman, A. (Eds.). (1996). *Empowerment evaluation: Knowledge and tools for self-assessment and accountability.* Thousand Oaks, CA: Sage.

Fetterman, D. M., & Wandersman, A. (2007). Empowerment evaluation: Yesterday, today, and tomorrow. *American Journal of Evaluation, 28*(2), 179–198.

Floch'hay, B., & Plottu, E. (1998). Democratic evaluation: From empowerment evaluation to public decision making. *Evaluation, 4,* 261–277.

Foster-Fisherman, P., Nowell, B., Deacon, Z., Nievar, A., & McCann, P. N, (2005). Using methods that matter: The impact of reflection, dialogue and voice. *American Journal of Community Psychology, 36*(3/4), 275–291.

Freire, P. (1973). *Education for critical consciousness.* New York: Seabury Press.

Fricke, J. G., & Gill, R. (1989). Participative evaluation. *Canadian Journal of Program Evaluation, 4,* 11–25.

Fuerstein, M. T. (1986). *Partners in evaluation.* London: Macmillan.

Fuerstein, M. T. (1988). Finding methods to fit the people: Training for participatory evaluation. *Community Development Journal, 23,* 16–25.

Furnell, R., Oldfield, K., & Speller, V. (1995). *Toward healthier alliances: A tool for planning, evaluating, and developing healthier alliances.* London: Health Education Authority/Wessex Institute of Public Health Medicine.

Gatenby, B., & Humphries, M. (2000). Feminist participatory action research: Methodological and ethical issues. *Women's International Forum, 23,* 89–105.

Gaventa, J. (1993). The powerful, the powerless, and the experts: Knowledge struggles in an information age. In P. Park, M. Brydon-Miller, B. L. Hall, & T. Jackson (Eds.), *Voices of change: Participatory research in the United States and Canada* (pp. 21–40). Westport, CT: Bergin & Garvey.

Geva-May, I., & Thorngate, W. (2003). Reducing anxiety and resistance in policy and programme evaluations: A socio-psychological analysis. *Evaluation, 9*(2), 205–227.

Goodman, R. M., Wheeler, F. C., & Lee, P. R. (1993). Evaluation of the Heart to Heart project: Lessons from a community-based chronic disease prevention program. *American Journal of Health Promotion, 9,* 443–455.

Green, L. W., George, M. A., Daniel, M., Frankish, C. J., Herbert, C. P., Bowie, W. R., et al. (1995). *Study of participatory research in health promotion: Review and recommendations for the development of participatory research in health promotion in Canada.* Vancouver, BC: Royal Society of Canada.

Greene, J. C. (1994). Qualitative program evaluation, practice, and promise. In N. K. Denzin & Y. S. Lincoln (Eds.), *Handbook of qualitative research* (pp. 530–544). Thousand Oaks, CA: Sage.

Greenwood, D., Whyte, W. F., & Harkavy, I. (1993). Participatory action research as a process and as a goal. *Human Relations, 46,* 171–191.

Gustavsen, B. (1992). *Dialogue and development: Theory of communication, action research and the restructuring of working life.* Assen, The Netherlands: Van Gorcum.

Habermas, J. (1984–1987). *The theory of communicative action* (T. McCarthy, Trans., Vols. 1 & 2). Boston: Beacon Press.

Ham, C. (1991). Analysis of health policy: Principles and practice. *Scandinavian Journal of Social Medicine, 46*(Suppl.), 62–66.

Hazen, M. A. (1994). A radical humanist perspective of interorganizational relationships. *Human Relations, 47,* 393–415.

Henkel, M. (1991). The new evaluative state. *Public Administration, 69,* 121–136.

House, E. R., & Howe, K. R. (1999). *Values in evaluation and social research.* Thousand Oaks, CA: Sage.

Israel, B. A., Checkoway, B., Schulz, A. J., & Zimmerman, M. A. (1994). Health education and community empowerment: Conceptualizing and measuring perceptions of individual, organizational, and community control. *Health Education Quarterly, 21,* 149–170.

Israel, B. A., Schurman, S. J., & House, J. S. (1989). Action research in occupational stress: Involving workers and researchers. *International Journal of Health Services, 19,* 135–155.

Jackson, E. T., & Kassam, Y. (1998). *Knowledge shared: Participatory evaluation in development cooperation.* Bloomfield, CT: Kumarian Press.

Keast, R., & Waterhouse, J. (2006). Participatory evaluation: A missing component in the sustainable social change equation for public services. *Strategic Change, 15*(1), 23–35.

Kennedy, A. (1995). Measuring health for all: A feasibility study of a Glasgow community. In N. Bruce, J. Springett, J. Hodgkiss, & A. Scott Samuel (Eds.), *Research and change in urban community health* (pp. 199–217). Aldershot, U.K.: Avebury.

Kolb, D. A. (1984). *Experiential learning: Experience as a source of learning and development.* Upper Saddle River, NJ: Prentice Hall.

Kroeger, A., & Franken, H. P. (1981). The educational value of participatory evaluation of primary health care programmes: An experience with four indigenous populations in Ecuador. *Social Science & Medicine, 15B,* 535–539.

Lawell, A. C., Noriega, M., Martinez, S., & Villegars, J. (1992). Participatory research on worker health. *Social Science & Medicine, 34,* 603–613.

Ledwith, M. (2005). *Community development: A critical approach.* Bristol, U.K.: Policy Press.

Levin, R. (1999). Participatory evaluation researchers and service providers as collaborators versus adversaries. *Violence Against Women, 5,* 1213–1227.

Long, R. J., & Wilkinson, W. E. (1984, May). A theoretical framework for occupational health program evaluation. *Occupational Health Nursing,* pp. 257–259.

Maclure, R. (1990). The challenge of participatory research and its implications for funding agencies. *International Journal of Sociology and Social Policy, 10,* 1–21.

Macgillavray, A. (1998). Turning the sustainable corner: How to indicate right. In D. Warburton (Ed.), *Community and sustainable development: Participation in the future* (pp. 81–95). London: Earthscan.

Magerison, C. J. (1987). Integrating action research and action learning in organisational development. *Organisational Development,* pp. 88–91.

Mathison, S. (1994). Rethinking the evaluator role: Partnerships between organizations and evaluators. *Evaluation and Planning, 17,* 299–304.

McKie, L. (2003). Rhetorical spaces: Participation and pragmatism in the evaluation of community health work. *Evaluation, 9*(3), 307–324.

Mezirow, J. (Ed.). (1990). *Fostering critical reflection in adulthood: A guide to transformative and emancipatory learning.* San Francisco: Jossey-Bass.

Mikkelsen, B. (1995). *Methods for development work and research: A guide for practitioners.* Thousand Oaks, CA: Sage.

National Assembly for Wales. (2001). *Sustainable health action research programme.* Retrieved May 22, 2008, from http://new.wales.gov.uk/topics/health/ocmo/research/sharp/?lang=en.

O'Hara, J., & McNamara, G. (2001). Process and product issues in the evaluation of school development planning. *Evaluation, 7,* 99–109.

Pan American Health Organization. (2001). *Report of the Healthy Municipalities meeting, Antigua, Guatemala.* Washington, DC: Author.

Papineau, D., & Kiely, M. (1996). Participatory evaluation in a community organization: Fostering stakeholder empowerment and utilization. *Evaluation and Program Planning, 19,* 79–93.

Patton, M. Q. (1997). *Utilization-focused evaluation* (3rd ed). Thousand Oaks, CA: Sage.

Peile, C. (1994). Theory, practice, research: Casual acquaintances or a seamless whole? *Australian Social Work, 47*(2), 17–23.

Polanyi, M., McIntosh, T., & Kosny, A. (2005). Understanding and improving the health of workers in the new economy: A call for a participatory dialogue-based approach to work-health research. *Critical Public Health, 15*(2), 103–119.

PROWWESS/United Nations Development Program. (1990). *Taking the pulse for community management in water and sanitation.* New York: Author.

Pyle, D. F. (1982). *Framework for the evaluation of health sector activities by private voluntary organizations receiving matching grants.* Washington, DC: Agency for International Development.

Quellet, F., Durand, D., & Forget, G. (1994). Preliminary results of an evaluation of three Healthy Cities initiatives in the Montreal area. *Health Promotion International, 9,* 153–159.

Rahman, M. A. (1993). *People's self-development: Perspectives on participatory action research.* London: Zed Books.

Reason, P. (Ed.). (1988). *Human inquiry in action: Developments in new paradigm research.* Thousand Oaks, CA: Sage.

Rebien, C. (1996). Participatory evaluation of development assistance. *Evaluation, 2,* 151–171.

Reeves, J., & Peerbhoy, D. (2006). Evaluating the evaluation: Understanding utility and limitations of evaluation as an organizational learning tool. *Health Education Journal, 66*(2), 120–131.

Rice, M., & Franceschini, M. C. (2007). Lessons learned from the application of a participatory evaluation methodology to Healthy Municipalities, Cities and Communities initiatives in selected countries of the Americas. *Promotion & Education, 14*(2), 68–73.

Richardson, L. (1994). Writing: A method of inquiry. In N. K. Denzin & Y. S. Lincoln (Eds.), *Handbook of qualitative research* (pp. 516–529). Thousand Oaks, CA: Sage.

Robinson, T. T., & Cousins, J. B. (2004). Internal participatory evaluation as an organizational learning system: A longitudinal case study. *Studies in Educational Evaluation, 30*(1), 1–22.

Robson, C. (2000). *Small-scale evaluation: Principles and practice.* Thousand Oaks, CA: Sage.

Rovers, R. (1986). The merging of participatory and analytical approaches to evaluation: Implications for nurses in primary health care programs. *Nursing Studies, 23,* 211–219.

Schwandt, T. A. (2001). Understanding dialogue as a practice. *Evaluation, 7*(2), 228–237.

Seddon, J. (2000, August 27). On target to nothing. *Observer,* p. 36.

Senge, P. M. (1990). *The fifth discipline: The art and practice of organizational learning.* New York: Doubleday.

Smith, P. (2005). Participatory evaluation: Navigating the emotions of partnerships. *Journal of Social Work Practice, 19*(2), 195–209.

South, J. (2006). Community Arts for Health: An evaluation of a district project. *Health Education, 106,* 155–167.

Springett, J. (1998). Quality and effectiveness in evaluation of healthy cities. In J. K. Davies & G. MacDonald (Eds.), *Quality, evidence, and effectiveness in health promotion: Striving for certainties* (pp. 167–193). New York: Routledge.

Springett, J. (2001). Appropriate approaches for the evaluation of health promotion. *Critical Public Health, 11,* 139–151.

Springett, J. (2005). Geographical approaches to the integration of health promotion in health systems: A comparative study of two health action zones in the UK. *Promotion & Education* (Suppl. 3), 39–45.

Springett, J., & Dunkerton, L. (2001). *Working together: A report on the evaluation of the Netherton Partnership Health Action Zone/Urban Projects:.* Liverpool, U.K.: John Moores University, Institute for Health.

Springett, J., & Leavey, C. (1995). Participatory action research: The development of a paradigm; dilemmas and prospects. In N. Bruce, J. Springett, J. Hodgkiss, & A. Scott Samuel (Eds.), *Research and change in urban community health* (pp. 57–66). Aldershot, U.K.: Avebury.

Springett, J., & Young, A. (2002). Comparing theories of change and participatory approaches to the evaluation of projects within health action zones: Two views from the North West on engaging community level projects in evaluation. In L. Baud & K. Judge (Eds.), *Learning from health action zones* (pp. 149–159). London: Aeneas Press.

Standish, M. (1995). A view from the tightrope: A working attempt to integrate research & evaluation with community development. In N. Bruce, J. Springett, J. Hodgkiss, & A. Scott Samuel (Eds.), *Research and change in urban community health* (pp. 259–262). Aldershot, U.K.: Avebury.

Susman, G. I., & Evered, R. D. (1978). An assessment of the scientific merits of action research. *Administrative Science Quarterly, 23,* 582–602.

Themessl-Huber, M. T. (2003). The shifting locus of control in participatory evaluations. *Evaluation, 9*(1), 92–111.

Van Eyk, H., Baum, F., & Blandford, J. (2001). Evaluating healthcare reform: The challenge of evaluating changing policy. *Evaluation, 7*(4), 487–503.

Vanderplaat, M. (1995). Beyond technique: Issues in evaluating for empowerment. *Evaluation, 1*(1), 81–96.

Wadsworth, Y. (1991). *Everyday evaluation on the run.* Melbourne: Action Research Issues.

Wallerstein, N. (1999). Power between evaluator and the community: Research relationships within New Mexico's healthier communities. *Social Science & Medicine, 49,* 39–54.

Wallerstein, N. (2006). *What is the effectiveness of empowerment to improve health?* Copenhagen: World Health Organization, Health Evidence Network. Retrieved May 20, 2008, from http://www.euro.who.int/HEN/Syntheses/empowerment/20060119_10.

Wallerstein, N. (2007). Making traces: Evidence for practice and evaluation. In J. Green & R. Labonté (Eds.), *Critical perspectives in public health* (pp. 80–92). New York: Routledge.

Wallerstein, N., & Bernstein, E. (1994). Empowerment education: Freire's ideas adapted to health education. *Health Education Quarterly, 15,* 379–394.

Weaver, L., & Cousins, J. B. (2004). Unpacking the participatory process. *Journal of Multidisciplinary Evaluation, 1,* 19–40.

Weiss, C. H. (1988). Evaluation for decisions: Is there anybody there? Does anybody care? *Education Practice, 9,* 15–20.

Winje, G., & Hewell, H. (1992). Influencing public health policy through action research. *Journal of Drug Issues, 22,* 169–178.

World Health Organization. (1998). *Health promotion evaluation: Recommendations to policymakers.* Copenhagen: Author.

Young, A. (2001). *The PEG report.* Salford, U.K.: Institute for Public Health Research and Policy/Salford University Press.

PART

4

METHODOLOGICAL AND ETHICAL CONSIDERATIONS IN PLANNING AND CONDUCTING CBPR

A frequent criticism of participatory research is that it pays little attention to concepts such as validity and rigor and is indeed long on stories and short on discussion of the knotty methodological issues involved in its implementation. In Part Four, we address these issues head on, as well as some ethical and practical concerns, beginning with Hilary Bradbury and Peter Reason's exploration of the issues of quality and validity in the family of participatory and action-oriented approaches to inquiry that they term action research. *Arguing that in such research, "knowledge is a verb rather than a noun," these authors help us move from the language of validity criteria popular in traditional social science research to the language of choice points for improving quality along multiple dimensions. From this broader perspective, they engage us in addressing such questions as whether our work is useful, helpful, and capable of making a difference; whether it is conceptually clear to all involved; to what degree it is experientially grounded; and whether it can be sustained over the long haul once the original initiator has gone. As their chapter powerfully suggests, and McTaggart (1998) and Buchanan and his colleagues (Buchanan, Miller, & Wallerstein, 2007) also have noted, rather than skirting issues of validity and quality, action research and other participatory approaches to inquiry by definition urge us to substantially "broaden" the conversation in this realm. In so doing, we carefully consider such issues throughout the research process and not merely in relation to a narrowly defined discussion of "research methods."*

As Phil Brown (1992, p. 272) suggests with respect to his own field of popular epidemiology, "Lay involvement is not merely 'good politics.' It is also 'good science,' since it changes the nature of scientific inquiry." Yet as earlier chapters have demonstrated, the high level of community involvement sought in CBPR also raises difficult questions, related to the tensions that frequently exist between using data gathering and analysis methods in ways that help empower rather than intimidate community members and ensure that solid and credible research is in fact being conducted. In Chapter Fourteen, Meredith Minkler and Andrea Corage Baden draw on recent literature reviews and interviews with CBPR partners in the field of environmental justice to explore these and other issues in more depth. They consider in particular perceived contributions and controversies raised by CBPR in areas including data methodology and quality, dissemination and use of findings, and power dynamics in the relationships between outside researchers and their community partners.

In Chapter Fifteen, Stephanie Farquhar and Steve Wing further illustrate many of these issues through two CBPR partnership efforts designed to document and expose health problems and related social and environmental realities in rural North Carolina. Exploring respectively patterns of environmental racism in the placement of industrialized hog factories and discriminatory practice and inadequate emergency policies in the aftermath of a major hurricane, these case studies illustrate that even when high-quality data collection and analysis are undertaken, potential charges of bias may be leveled when powerful corporate or political interest groups are crossed.

As noted in earlier chapters, although CBPR strives to "equitably" involve community partners in all stages of the research process (Israel, Eng, Schulz, & Parker, 2005), in reality, time constraints and other barriers frequently result in little or no community involvement in data analysis. In Chapter Sixteen, Suzanne Cashman and her colleagues use four short case studies to illustrate the value added—and the challenges faced—when expanding community partner involvement in analyzing data and interpreting findings. The cases involve, respectively, mixed methods research, survey methods, focus groups, and community mapping. Together they make a strong case for expanding our efforts to involve community partners, as appropriate and desired, in both these phases of the research process.

REFERENCES

Buchanan, D. R., Miller, F. G., & Wallerstein, N. (2007). Ethical issues in community-based participatory research: Balancing rigorous research with community participation in community intervention studies. *Progress in Community Health Partnerships: Research, Education, and Action, 1*(2), 153–160.

Brown, P. (1992). Popular epidemiology and toxic waste contamination: Lay and professional ways of knowing. *Journal of Health and Social Behavior, 33,* 267–281.

Israel, B. A., Eng, E., Schulz, A. J., & Parker, E. A. (2005). Introduction to methods in community-based participatory research. In B. A. Israel, E. Eng, A. J. Schulz, & E. A. Parker (Eds.), *Methods in community-based participatory research for health* (pp. 3–26). San Francisco: Jossey-Bass.

McTaggart, R. (1998). Is validity really an issue for participatory action research? *Studies in Organization, Culture and Societies, 4,* 211–236.

CHAPTER

13

ISSUES AND CHOICE POINTS FOR IMPROVING THE QUALITY OF ACTION RESEARCH

HILARY BRADBURY & PETER REASON

We cannot regard truth as a goal of inquiry. The purpose of inquiry is to achieve agreement among human beings about what to do, to bring about consensus on the ends to be achieved and the means used to achieve those ends. Inquiry that does not achieve coordination of behavior is not inquiry but simply wordplay.

RICHARD RORTY (2000, P. XXV)

We must keep on trying to understand better, change and reenchant our plural world.

ORLANDO FALS-BORDA (1997)

Note: The authors are listed alphabetically. This chapter was adapted from the Introduction and Conclusion they wrote for *The Handbook of Action Research: Participative Inquiry and Practice,* by P. Reason and H. Bradbury (Eds.), 2001. Copyright 2001 by P. Reason and H. Bradbury. Adapted by permission of the authors and of Sage Publications Ltd. For some of the more detailed arguments and illustrations, the reader is invited to refer to the original and to the second edition of this handbook (Reason and Bradbury, 2008).

THERE IS NO short answer to the question, What is action research? But let us say, as a working definition, that *action research* is a participatory, democratic process concerned with developing practical knowing in the pursuit of worthwhile human purposes and grounded in a participatory worldview. It seeks to reconnect action and reflection, theory and practice, in participation with others, in the pursuit of practical solutions to issues of pressing concern to people. More generally, it grows out of a concern for the flourishing of individuals and their communities.

We therefore see action research practitioners as necessarily concerned with three important purposes. The first purpose is to bring an action dimension back to the overly quietist tradition of knowledge generation that has developed in the modern era. The second is to loosen the grip over knowledge creation held traditionally by universities and other institutions of "higher learning." The third is to contribute to the ongoing revision of the Western disposition—to add impetus to the movement away from a modernist worldview based on a positivist philosophy and a value system dominated by crude notions of economic progress in a universe devoid of transcendent meaning, and to move toward an emerging participatory perspective.

Thus for us action research is a practice for the systematic development of knowing and knowledge, but arising in a rather different form than that of traditional academic research. It has different purposes and is based in different relationships; it has different ways of conceiving of knowledge and its relation to practice. Though the field of action research is hugely varied and there are countless choices to be made in practice, there are five broadly shared features that characterize action research, as shown in Figure 13.1.

A significant purpose of action research is to produce practical knowledge that is useful to people in the everyday conduct of their lives. A wider purpose of action research is to contribute through this practical knowledge to the increased well-being—economic, political, psychological, and spiritual—of persons and communities and to a more equitable

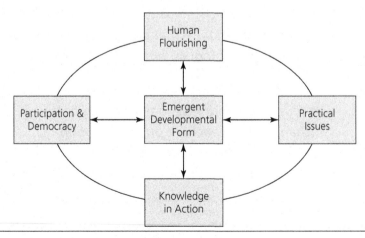

FIGURE 13.1   *Characteristics of Action Research*

and sustainable relationship with the wider ecology of the planet of which all involved in action research are an intrinsic part.

So action research is about working toward practical outcomes and also about creating new forms of understanding, because action without reflection and understanding is blind, just as theory without action is meaningless. And more broadly, theories that contribute to human emancipation, to the flourishing of community, that help people reflect on their place in the ecology of the planet and contemplate their spiritual purposes, can lead people to different ways of being together as well as provide important guidance and inspiration for practice (a feminist perspective, for example, would invite people to consider whether an emphasis on action without a balancing consideration of ways of being is rather too heroic).

As researchers search for practical knowledge and liberating ways of knowing, working with people in their everyday lives, they can also see that action research is participative research, and all participative research must be action research. People are agents who act in the world on the basis of their own sense making; human community involves mutual sense making and collective action. Action research is only possible with, for, and by individuals and communities, ideally involving all stakeholders both in the questioning and sense making that informs the research and in the action that is its focus.

Because action research starts with everyday experience and is concerned with the development of living knowledge, in many ways the process of inquiry is as important as specific outcomes. Good action research emerges over time in an evolutionary and developmental process as individuals develop skills of inquiry and as communities of inquiry develop within communities of practice. Action research is emancipatory; it leads not just to new practical knowledge but also to new abilities to create knowledge. Action research is a living, evolving process of coming-to-know rooted in everyday experience; it involves *knowing,* the verb, more than *knowledge,* the noun. This means that action research cannot be programmatic and cannot be defined in terms of hard-and-fast methods but is, in Lyotard's (1984) sense, a work of art.

These five interdependent characteristics of action research shown in Figure 13.1 emerge from our reflections on practice in this developing field. Together they imply an *action turn* in research practice that both harks back to the antique classical sense of holistic inquiry (Eikeland, 2001) and also builds on and takes researchers beyond the *language turn* of recent years (the language turn drew our attention to the ways in which knowledge is a social construction). In some ways this awakening to the ability to create one's world anew is simultaneously paralyzed by the deep interdependence of self and language. Hilary Putnam (1992) points out that language and mind penetrate so deeply into reality that any project of representing ourselves as language-independent is fatally compromised. Action research offers a fresh path from this quandary: the action turn draws our attention to how people can act in intelligent and informed ways in a world that they understand is not independent of their coconstruction.

We start from these assertions—which may seem contentious to some of the academic community and at the same time obvious to those of a more activist orientation—because the purpose of knowledge making is so rarely debated. The institutions of conventional science and academia, which have created such a monopoly on the knowledge-making process, place a primary value on pure research, the creation of knowledge unencumbered by practical questions, driven simply by intellectual curiosity. In contrast, the primary purpose of action research is not to produce academic theories based on action, nor is it to produce theories about action, nor is it to produce theoretical or empirical knowledge that can be applied in action; it is to reweave knowing and doing so as to liberate the human body, mind, and spirit in the search for a better, freer world.

These characteristics of action research are not simply questions of methodology. To be sure, one can argue that they lead to "better" research because the practical and theoretical outcomes of the research process are grounded in the perspective and interests of those immediately concerned and not filtered through an outside researcher's preconceptions and interests. But far more than that, when we assert the practical purposes of action research and the importance of human interests, when we join knower with known in a participative relationship, and as people move away from operational measurement into a science of experiential qualities (Reason & Goodwin, 1999), they undercut the foundations of the empirical-positivist worldview that has been the foundation of Western inquiry since the Enlightenment (Toulmin, 1990) and start exploring the possibility that new worldviews are emerging. This in turn draws our attention to a broader bandwidth of choices that action research practitioners need to make in the course of their work, choices that have implications for the quality and validity of their inquiries.

BROADENING THE BANDWIDTH OF VALIDITY

Our reflections on the practices of action research and a participatory worldview lead us to ask different questions about the nature of high-quality practice in action research. How do action researchers, both individually and together with coresearchers, address the questions, Am I doing good work? and, Are we doing good work? We can use the five dimensions of the participatory worldview to interrogate our inquiry practice, and the questions and the subsequent choice points posed allow us to consider issues of validity and quality in action research work. We hope to build a bridge between academic concerns about validity and more reflexively practical questions about the work of action research.

For the academic community, we see our writing on the issue of quality as initiating and sustaining an engaging conversation among action researchers and between action researchers and other researchers. For although the issues and questions that provoke choice points in our work obviously inform the work of action research, we believe that they may also be extended to a conversation about validity in other types of research work. We hereby join the lively debate that has been referred to as the "fertile obsession" with validity (Lather, 1993). In joining this debate to add voices from action research, we hope to broaden the bandwidth of concerns associated with the question of what constitutes good knowledge research and practice.

We are aware that even the possibility of having standards or criteria of validity has been questioned in this era of postmodern loss of legitimacy (Lyotard, 1984). Kvale (1989) has questioned the validity of the very question of validity, that is to say, raised a question as to whether it is foolish to try to fit the qualities of action research into a traditional discourse about validity whose concerns have little to do with those of action research. Wolcott (1990) has argued for dismissing validity altogether precisely because the discourse is inextricably bound to the ideals of positivism. Schwandt (1996) has also bid a "farewell to criteriology," where criteriology has meant a uniform set of measures. In light of those important concerns, we say that our purpose in this chapter is with continuing the discourse about validity predicated on our concern for continuing an ongoing and important dialogue. We hope that a shared and no doubt growing vocabulary that clarifies common ground and disagreement can only improve both the quality of the work and the collegial relationships in action research. To some measure, we hereby also stand on the shoulders of the scholars who have preceded us in their concern for continuing but shifting the dialogue about validity from a concern with idealist questions in search of Truth to concern for engagement, dialogue, pragmatic outcomes, and an emergent, reflexive sense of what is important.

Lincoln (1995), in calling for a profusion of validities that emerge from the context of a given study, began a shift in the discourse from examining what the criteria for validity are (the criteriology) to investigating the function of the criteria. Lather (2001) has continued this trajectory as "a rehearsal for a new social imaginary out from under scientism." She writes, "Our framing is shifting validity from a discourse about quality as normative to a discourse of relational practices" (p. 2). Habermas (1979; see also Kemmis, 2001) posits that truth results from an emancipatory process that emerges as people strive toward conscious and reflexive emancipation, speaking, reasoning, and coordinating action together, unconstrained and uncoerced. And so we follow a number of scholars by taking up a point well made by Gustavsen (2001): our concern is not with getting the labels of the criteria "very right" but with drawing attention to important choices that an action researcher must make and thus with extending a useful conversation about getting valuable work done well.

A new set of validity criteria—we refer to them as choice points—is related to the participatory disposition that we believe is replacing the modernist worldview.

TOWARD A PARTICIPATORY WORLDVIEW

Many writers and commentators are suggesting that the modernist worldview or paradigm of Western civilization is reaching the end of its useful life. It is suggested that a fundamental shift is occurring in the Western understanding of the universe and the human place in it, that new patterns of thought and belief are emerging that will transform experience, thinking, and action. People in the West have, since the Reformation, the beginning of the era of modern science, and the industrial revolution, made enormous strides in material welfare and control of their lives. Yet the costs of this progress in ecological devastation, human and social fragmentation, and spiritual impoverishment is increasingly apparent. So if we fail to make a transition to new ways of thinking, our civilization will decline and decay. Gregory Bateson (1972/2000), one of the great original thinkers of our time, argued that the most important task we face is learning to think in new ways; he was deeply concerned with what he called the "epistemological errors" of our time, the errors built into our ways of thinking, and their consequences for justice and ecological sustainability. So the challenge of changing our worldview is central to our times.

The emergent worldview has been described as systemic, holistic, relational, feminine, and experiential, but its defining characteristic is that it is participatory: our world does not consist of separate things but of relationships that we coinvent. We participate in our world in such a way that the "reality" we experience is a mutual creation that involves the primal givenness of the cosmos and human feeling and construing. (For an extended reflection on the qualities of participation, see Reason & Torbert, 2001; Reason, 2005.) The participative metaphor is particularly apt for action research because as we participate in creating our world, we are already embodied and breathing beings who are necessarily acting—and this draws us to consider how to assess the quality of our acting.

A participatory worldview places persons and communities as part of their world—both human and more-than-human—embodied in their world, cocreating their world. A participatory perspective asks us to be both situated and reflexive, to be explicit about the perspective from which knowledge is created, to see inquiry as a process of coming to know, a process serving the democratic, practical ethos of action research.

A participatory view competes with both the positivism of modern times and the deconstructive postmodern alternative—and this chapter holds this view to be the more adequate and creative paradigm for our times. However, this view can also be said to draw on and integrate both paradigms: it follows positivism in arguing that there is a "real" reality, a primeval givenness of being (of which we partake), and it draws on the constructionist perspective in acknowledging that as soon as we attempt to articulate this, we enter a world of human language and cultural expression. Any account of the given cosmos in the spoken or written word is culturally framed, yet if we approach our inquiry with appropriate critical skills and discipline, our account may provide some perspective on what is universal and on the knowledge-creating process that frames this account.

The dimensions of a participatory worldview (shown in Figure 13.2) echo the characteristics of action research identified earlier in Figure 13.1.

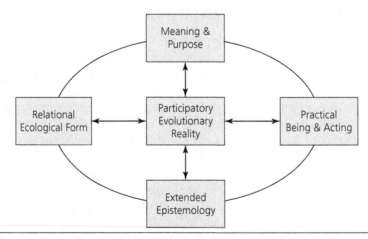

FIGURE 13.2 *Dimensions of a Participatory Worldview*

On the Nature of the Given Cosmos

At the center of a participatory worldview lie our intimations of the participatory nature of the cosmos that we both inhabit and cocreate, whose form is relational and ecological. We live in a participatory world. There is a primordial givenness of being in which the human body and mind actively participate in a cocreative dance that gives rise to the reality we experience. Subject and object are interdependent. Thus participation is fundamental to the nature of our being, an ontological given (Heron, 1996a; Heron & Reason, 1997). Because we are a part of the whole, we are necessarily actors within it, which leads us to consider the fundamental importance of the practical.

On Practical Being and Acting

Given this fundamental participation in the whole, we humans are already engaged and thus are already acting (Skolimowski, 1994). Thus for the action researcher, practical knowing is the purpose, the consummation, the fulfillment of the knowledge quest (Heron, 1996b). All ways of knowing serve to support our skillful being-in-the-world from moment to moment to moment, our ability to act intelligently in the pursuit of worthwhile purposes. Human inquiry is necessarily practical, and a participatory form of inquiry is an action science.

On the Nature of Knowing

A participative worldview, with its notion of reality as both subjective and objective, involves an extended epistemology: we draw on diverse forms of knowing as we encounter and act in our world. Heron and Reason (2001; Heron, 1996a) argue that a knower participates in the known, articulating the world in at least four interdependent ways. *Experiential knowing* is acquired through direct, face-to-face encounters with a person, place, or thing; it is knowing through empathy and resonance, that kind of in-depth knowing that is almost impossible to put into words. *Presentational knowing* grows out of experiential knowing and provides the first form of expression through story, drawing, sculpture, movement, and dance, drawing on aesthetic imagery (Seeley, 2006; Seeley and Reason, 2008). *Propositional knowing* draws on concepts and ideas, and *practical knowing* consummates the other forms of knowing in action in the world. Other theorists, writing from pragmatic, constructionist, critical, feminist, and developmental perspectives, have articulated different ways of framing an extended epistemology (Belenky, Clinchy, Goldberger, & Tarule, 1986; Greenwood & Levin, 1998; Park, 2001; Torbert, 1991).

On Relational Ecological Form

A participatory worldview is a political statement as well as a theory of knowledge. Just as the classical Cartesian worldview emerged in part from the political situation of the time (Toulmin, 1990) and found its expression not only in science and technology but also in our political structures and organizational forms, so a participatory worldview implies democratic peer relationships as the political form of inquiry.

This political dimension of participation affirms people's right and ability to have a say in decisions that affect them and that claim to generate knowledge about them. It asserts the importance of liberating the muted voices of those held down by class structures and neocolonialism, by poverty, sexism, racism, and homophobia. Action research practitioners from all perspectives have argued strongly that there are deep connections between power and knowledge.

Relationships do not exist only with other humans; we also have relationships with the more-than-human world. As we become increasingly aware that the damage being done to the planet's ecosystems and the resultant sustainability crisis (Brown, 1999) are in part the result of our failure to understand the systemic nature of the planet's ecosystems and humanity's role in the course of natural processes, we can also see that participation is an ecological imperative.

On Purpose and Meaning: Spirit and Beauty

Action research practitioners may suggest slightly different emphases in describing the purpose of their work—they write of the "quest for life," of "making the world better" or "more loving" or "freer"—but they broadly agree that the purpose of human inquiry is the flourishing of life, the life of persons, of human communities, and increasingly of the more-than-human world of which we are a part. A participative worldview invites us to inquire into what we mean by "flourishing" and into the meaning and purpose of our endeavors, and this, as this chapter will argue, is a key dimension of quality in inquiry. As Berry (1999) asks us, what is the "great work" of humanity in our time, and how are our individual human projects aligned with it? Participative consciousness is part of a resacralization of the world, a kind of reenchantment (Berman, 1981; Berry, 1988; Skolimowski, 1993). Sacred experience is based in reverence, in awe and love for creation, valuing it for its own sake, in its own right as a living presence. To deny participation not only offends against human justice, not only leads to errors in epistemology, not only strains the limits of the natural world, but is also troublesome for human souls and for the anima mundi.

So a participatory worldview places the practical response to human problems in a necessarily wider spiritual context—human practical inquiry is a spiritual expression, a celebration of the flowering of humanity and of the cocreating cosmos, and as part of a sacred science, it is an expression of the beauty and joy of active existence.

CHOICE POINTS FOR ACTION RESEARCH

In offering a new set of criteria (*choice points*), this chapter make no pretense of being comprehensive—indeed, to do so would be to fall into the totalizing and essentialist trap of seeking to provide a new set of firm criteria for validity. Instead, it brings action researchers' attention to a smorgasbord of important issues and asks that they choose wisely and in conversation with other inquirers when deciding what is important in their research. Offering a perfect set of criteria is neither possible nor desirable because each piece of inquiry or practice is its own work of art articulating its own standards. The goal is to sketch out the basis for some of the choices and questions that need to be faced by an individual action researcher and by action research communities (see also Reason, 2006; Bradbury, 2007).

Each theory of the way the world is gives rise to particular ways of seeing the world. This chapter has argued that action research emerges within a participative way of seeing or acting in the world in which we find ourselves always in relationship. At the start, then, we need to be concerned with both the quality of our theory and our holistic, everyday, lived experience. Gustavsen (1996, p. 94) writes that "both our theoretical worlds and our life world [or lived experience] are necessary and cannot be substituted. More theory cannot fill the vacuum of a lack of experience, and more experience cannot bring more order into an uninterpreted world." Such concerns lead into the following five broad issues, already discussed at the start of this chapter, within which choice points for good action research may be articulated.

A participative worldview draws our attention to the qualities of the participative and relational practices in our work. Issues of interdependence, politics, power, and empowerment must be addressed at both micro and macro levels—that is, in inquiring relationships in face-to-face and small-group interaction and in determining how the research is situated in its wider political context. In particular, we must pay attention to the congruence between qualities of participation that we espouse and the actual work we accomplish, especially as our work involves us in networks of power dynamics that both limit and enable our work (Gaventa & Cornwall, 2001). A mark of quality in an action research project is that people will get energized and empowered by being involved, leading them to develop newly useful, reflexive insights as a result of a growing critical consciousness. They may, ideally, say, "That was our own research, and it helped us see ourselves and our context through new eyes and taught us to act in all sorts of new ways." We may therefore say that as action researchers, we must ask questions that inquire into and seek to ensure quality of participation and relationship in the work.

As we participate with people, oriented by our shared concerns and interests, the practical outcome of our work is important. Thus a series of pragmatic questions must be asked of action research work, such as, Is the work useful or helpful? and, Do people whose reputations and livelihoods are affected act differently as a result of the inquiry? We acknowledge that what is considered "helpful" or "useful" is itself not at all a straightforward issue—as Stephen Kemmis (2001) shows us by distinguishing between technical, practical, and emancipatory outcomes—and must be explored reflexively by those who are participating, and this reflection in turn informs the relational process. Ideally, people's response to action research work is "That worked" or "That was helpful." We may therefore say that as action researchers, we must ask pragmatic questions about outcome and practice in our work and consistently strive to be reflexive about this. So even though we may begin in a mode of *single-loop inquiry,* seeking merely to get things accomplished, we must proceed appropriately to *double-loop inquiry* (Argyris & Schön, 1996), in which we ask questions about the value of the very things we are seeking to accomplish.

As we participate, our knowledge of the world includes—but is never limited to—conceptual or intellectualized forms of knowledge, the forms most often associated with academic enterprise. Action research recognizes the importance of conceptual knowledge while also consciously engaging in extended epistemologies. We may ask how different ways of knowing, be they aesthetic or presentational, representational, experiential, or more theoretical or conceptual, have been drawn on or allowed to surface in our work. How have they informed the ways in which the work itself is represented? Each particular way of knowing raises questions concerning quality in its own right. How well is an inquiry experientially grounded? How is it embodied in sensuous knowing? What is the appropriate form of presentation for this particular audience? Is it aesthetically elegant? Is it conceptually clear to all involved? Does it promote further knowing by raising new questions or by allowing us to "see through" old conceptual frameworks so that they are newly experienced as more limiting than enabling? By drawing on and integrating diverse ways of knowing, people will, ideally, say of action research work, "That is true," "That is right," "That is interesting, engaging, thought-provoking." And as action researchers, we must ask how the palette of extended ways of knowing is acknowledged in and by our work.

Inquiry methods may be seen as an outgrowth of epistemology in service to the research question. We must therefore ask why certain methods are chosen, how well they have been pursued, and whether they are indeed congruent with the participative orientation of the action research work. As Hall (2001) points out, participatory research is an attitude, a way of creating knowing in action, possibly even a way of life, not simply a method. So a question for action researchers is whether they have drawn on the different methodological traditions appropriately and creatively in the context of their own work.

Because our work together includes the commingled aspects of reflecting and acting, we must take time to ask questions about the value and worthiness of our work. It is not enough to do good work if the work itself is not of real importance—indeed, it seems essential that researchers take the risk of asking big questions, even if that turns out to be as simple as stopping with one's colleagues to inquire, Why are we doing this work? and, Why are we doing it this way? Sometimes it will be obvious what is important—preventing children from being poisoned or an ecology from being damaged, for example—at other times it will be far more complex—for example, in a holistic medical cooperative inquiry (Reason, 1988), participants continually debated the relative significance of power sharing with patients, developing a complementary range of clinical treatments and bringing spiritual disciplines into medical practice, for there was not time to attend to everything.

We may ask as action researchers how our work calls forth a world worthy of human aspiration, so that, ideally, people will say, "That work is inspiring; it helps make me live a better life."

The last broad issue concerns thinking through the developmental quality of our work, through its history and into the future. Developing self-reflective practice, which, as described later, this chapter calls *first-person research practice* (Marshall, 1999, 2001; Torbert, 2001; Marshall & Mead, 2005), is a lifetime project. Second-person collaborative inquiry is something that has to be grown over time, moving from a tentative beginning to full cooperation (McArdle, 2008). Participatory action research is emergent and evolutionary: you cannot just go to a village or an organization or a professional group and "do it"; the work either evolves or does not evolve as a result of mutual engagement and influence. Further, because we are participating in work of enduring consequences, we must attend to the question of viability in the longer term. We must therefore ask whether the ground on which the work proceeded was seeded in such a way that participation can be sustained in the absence of the initiating researcher. We must create a living interest in the work.

Action research is a potent orientation to change and transformation. Before intentional change can be fostered, however, it helps to realize, at the individual, group, and community levels, that the reality we have cocreated, however unintentionally, can be repatterned in participative inquiry. In thinking of our institutions as emergent in our activities and therefore continuously changing, we suggest that the human world as we know it is produced and reproduced by the innumerable acts and conversations that we undertake daily. This is not to conflate large systems with aggregates of individual actors acting consciously; we must recognize that systems have their own logic. However, a *structurationist* view (Bourdieu, 1977; Giddens, 1984) offers a logic from which to commence the work of change by implicitly asserting that systems are not totalizing and that conscious, action-oriented people, especially those working and reasoning together, can indeed achieve systematic and systemic change over time. What seems important in action research, which leaves new institutional patterns in its wake, is its ability to integrate the three manifestations of work: work for oneself (*first-person research practice*), work for partners (*second-person research practice*), and work for people within the wider context (*third-person research practice*). The integration of these three approaches to action research suggests a logic of continuous change, which supports the work of radical transformation of those patterns of behavior that do not foster a world worthy of human aspiration. Ideally, people involved in emerging and enduring work will say, "This work continues to develop and help us," and other people will say, "Can we use your work to help develop our own?" We may say that as action researchers, we must ask questions about how our work has emerged and developed over time, whether it is sustainable into the future, and how it will influence related work.

These five issues, about relationships, practical outcomes, extended ways of knowing, purpose, and enduring consequences, are quite demanding of action researchers. Before paralysis or emotional overload strikes, it is important to remember that action research is emergent and along the way is probably concerned with one broad issue more than another.

We can also say that in a pluralist community of inquiry—whether it be a face-to-face inquiry group, an organization, or a community—different individual members are likely to have different questions and different degrees of interest. Some will be most concerned with relationships, some with action, some with understanding, and some with raising awareness. The more that dialogue is encouraged regarding these different perspectives, the greater the quality of the inquiry will be. Therefore, it is likely important for the action research team or community of inquiry as a whole to take time regularly for reflection on the choice points encountered along the way and the possible need for reorientation from time to time.

Some action researchers (for example, Heron, 1996b) have argued for the primacy of one issue above all others—Heron, for instance suggests the "primacy of the practical." This chapter takes the position that the issues are choice points and that the action researcher is therefore partial as a result of the material circumstances of each given situation.

In summary, the following five sets of questions broaden the bandwidth of issues to take into account in exploring the quality of action research.

Quality as Relational Praxis

A fundamental claim to quality in action research practice is that it is participative, fully involving others in the inquiry project. That means that in our research, we must endeavor to meet the others as subjects, equal to ourselves, in what Martin Buber (1958) famously called an *I-Thou* relationship. In this relational stance, we move away from the *I-It* relationship of traditional science, which asks that a researcher not contaminate the relationship with the research objects by coming in "too close." This is not to say that distance is unimportant; distance can help with seeing what is hard to see close up. But such distancing is not exercised in the relationship with the co-inquirers. We must therefore generally ask ourselves whether the action research group is set up for (eventual) maximal participation; whether opportunities are used to allow all to feel free to be fully involved; whether when push comes to shove, serious decisions are made on the principle that the best decision is one that maximizes participation; and especially whether less powerful people are helped by their experience of participation in inquiry.

Quality as a Reflexive or Practical Outcome

Action research claims to make a difference in people's lives and practices. We are led to ask whether, in principle, our work has pragmatic consequences. Greenwood and Levin (1998) write of Dewey's "warranted assumptions": Are people with real material issues at stake (jobs, reputations, livelihoods) willing to act on what has been learned in the course of their research? An important question to ask, therefore, is whether the research is "validated" by participants' new ways of acting in light of the work. In the simplest sense, people should be able to say, "That was useful—I am using it!"

Quality as Plurality of Knowing

Here we discuss different forms of knowing in an effort to embrace more than the traditional focus on propositional, theoretical knowledge.

Quality Through Conceptual and Theoretical Integrity Without theory, practice is impoverished. Action research practitioners are concerned that propositional and conceptual integrity exist and also that the efforts at theorizing be anchored in people's experience. Theory is used to bring order to complex phenomena, with a goal of parsimonious description so that the theorizing is of use to the community of inquiry. And bringing this order may require iterative cycles in which the researcher steps back from co-inquirers in order to be a spectator and theorize but then discusses the developing theory with those whose experience is its basis. It was Kurt Lewin, in many respects the contemporary era's father of action research, who said that theory is practical—not that it should be practical, merely that it is practical! In developing conceptual and theoretical integrity, we may wish to draw on current qualitative and ethnographic practices of making sense of data (Denzin & Lincoln, 2000). We might also ask if our new theory allows us to resee the world or to see past taken-for-granted conceptual categories that are oppressive or no longer helpful.

Quality Through Extending Our Ways of Knowing Action research respects and works with many epistemologies. This discussion has drawn on John Heron's fourfold distinction, but the range of ways of knowing can also be expressed in more vernacular form. "Ordinary women's talk" can hold an important place in inquiry (Barrett, 2001; Barrett & Taylor, 2002), song and dance are artful ways of expressing and continuing knowledge

(Lewis, 2001), and traditional forms can bring power to hitherto poorly educated people in that these forms allow them to successfully question the practices of the powerful. Heron (1998, 2001) describes the primary outcomes of his spiritual inquiries not as descriptions or theories or pragmatic consequences but as transformations of personal being and associated skills brought about by the inquiry. In this view, practical knowing is the fulfillment and consummation of the knowledge quest.

In seeing that the outcome of inquiry can be a shift in ways of being in the world and in the development of new skills, we are liberated from the tyranny of having to "write up" everything. And in asking how our work responds to the aesthetic representation, we are offered a chance to be creative and to liberate the creative impulses of those we work with. Conversation and writing on paper are valuable tools, but the worlds of theater, dance, video, poetry, and photography invite us to be inspired in the service of better theory and practice.

Quality Through Methodological Appropriateness In action research the quality of inquiry practice lies far less in impersonal methodology and far more in the emergence of a self-aware, critical community of inquiry nested within a community of practice. However, this does not mean that a judicious choice of method from the large range available is not important, even though method is there to support the community of inquiry rather than to supplant it. If we are animated by a worldview of participation and seek to have congruence between our theory of reality and our practice, then our selected methods must also be relational and be able to describe a relational worldview (Bradbury & Lichtenstein, 2000). They will provide a systematic way of engaging people on issues of importance, drawing on many ways of knowing in an iterative fashion.

Quality as Engaging in Significant Work

This chapter has argued that action research is a form of inquiry in pursuit of worthwhile human purposes, issues of significance.

It can of course also be argued that any participative form of inquiry, well grounded in the everyday concerns of people, will necessarily be worthwhile. This is particularly so if the inquiry moves beyond addressing simple, technically oriented questions toward emancipatory questions—in which case, people's capacity for asking questions of deeper significance is developed. It is arguable that as inquiry groups cycle between action and reflection over time, they move from surface concerns to more fundamental issues. And so critical attention to these questions should be applauded. Because the action research community as a whole is committed to bringing an attitude of inquiry to questions of fundamental importance, we would do well to find ways to address the question of what purposes are worthy of attention more directly.

In our own reviews of action research projects, we are struck that although most practitioners are concerned to address questions they believe to have significant worth, few pay explicit attention to inquiring into what is worthy of attention, how people choose where to put their efforts. Significant exceptions are the action inquiry of Torbert (1999, 2001), the "appreciative" orientation of Cooperrider and his colleagues (Cooperrider, Sorensen, Whitney, & Yaeger, 2000; Ludema, Cooperrider, & Barrett, 2001), and the community systems approach of Senge (Senge & Scharmer, 2001).

EMERGENT INQUIRY TOWARD ENDURING CONSEQUENCE

Action research is best seen as an emergent, evolutionary, and educational process of engaging with self, others, and communities that needs to be sustained for a significant period of time. For example, Marja-Liisa Swantz (Swantz, Ndedya, & Masaiganah, 2001) refers to participatory research in Tanzania over three decades, involving people in their communities, academia, and government; she emphasizes the importance of a long-term commitment from these different parties. More modestly, many projects continue over several months of developing engagement in which the quality and focus of engagement deepens over time. Action research in all its forms is a long-term, evolutionary, emergent form of inquiry.

As Peter Park (2001) argues, in addition to creating objective knowledge of social conditions, action research also strengthens community ties and heightens transformative potential through critical consciousness. The simultaneous pursuit of these three goals makes action research a holistic activity addressing key human social needs, making it unique among social change activities. Seeing social change as a research activity forces us to think of community ties and critical awareness as forms of knowledge.

Action research practitioners repeatedly criticize institutional structures, especially universities, as being inappropriate vehicles for the kinds of inquiry practices advocated here, noting that good action research, in a way that truly differentiates it from traditional research, seems to leave repatterned institutional infrastructures in its wake, some of them embryonic but others surprisingly robust over the years.

SUMMARY

No action research project can address all issues equally, and choices must be made about what is important in the emergent and messy work of each action research project. As we have suggested in this chapter, making explicit the questions of what is important to attend to is itself often part of good action research. This might be done by reviewing the issues and the questions that they raise and deciding where to put the weight of attention. This may be the task of an individual action researcher acting alone; certainly we would expect a PhD thesis based on action research to contain a review of the strengths and weaknesses of the work in relation to these issues. In contrast, a facilitator of an action research project will wish to share this work with his or her inquiry colleagues; the role here is educative, to explore the issues with them so they can together decide which are most relevant. Of course, in a participative inquiry that has emerged in its fullest sense as research conducted not on people but with people, responsibility for exploring these issues will rest with the community as a whole.

We believe that it is helpful to address all questions of how to create quality in participative research, if only to elucidate why one is more important than another. Doing so supports the quality of participative research during a new phase of high adoption rates traceable to its ability to solve what have been intractable challenges. "Actionable" approaches to knowledge (see Bradbury, 2007) offer more than merely better insights and leave those involved literally better off. Thus when next asked how big one's sample was or what to do about the fact that one's data must be considered contaminated by interests or that the co-inquirers were all self-selected, the action research may refer to the differing axiomatic assumptions in action research, which arise from a participatory worldview and the lived experience of participation. We suggest that the action researcher seek to expand the conversation about validity to include the broader bandwidth of considerations that inhere in research and practice in search of a world worthy of human aspiration.

We have stated that there are five interrelated issues that together call forth seven choice points in action research. Questions of quality and validity in research involve encouraging debate and reflection about these issues among all participants. The following list is intended as a checklist for action researchers starting and continuing to develop a world worthy of human aspiration. These six questions will, we hope, provoke many others appropriate to the needs and desired outcomes of the action research work undertaken.

Issues as Choice Points and Questions in Action Research

- Is the action research explicit in developing a praxis of relational participation?
- Is it guided by reflexive concern for pragmatic outcomes?
- Does it ensure conceptual and theoretical integrity?
- Does it include extended ways of knowing?
- Can it be considered significant?
- Does it lead toward a new and enduring infrastructure?

QUESTIONS FOR DISCUSSION

1. The authors state that action research "involves *knowing,* the verb, more than *knowledge,* the noun." What do they mean by this, and how does this statement fit with your own sense of action research or CBPR?

2. What do the authors mean by "broadening the bandwidth of validity"? Do you agree with their perspective? Are there ways beyond those discussed here in which action research or CBPR may increase validity?

3. Bradbury and Reason use the term "self-reflexive practice." Thinking back over previous chapters or other examples of action research or CBPR with which you are familiar, think of a case in which self-reflexive practice was well illustrated. What did this quality add to the process or outcomes? Did this chapter give you any new ideas about ways of being more reflexive in your own practice? If so, what were these ideas?

KEY TERMS

Validity   Action research
Self-reflexive practice   Praxis

REFERENCES

Argyris, C., & Schön, D. A. (1996). *Organizational learning: Vol. 2. Theory, method, and practice.* Reading, MA: Addison-Wesley.

Barrett, P. A. (2001). The Early Mothering project: What happened when the words "action research" came to life for a group of midwives. In P. Reason & H. Bradbury (Eds.), *Handbook of action research: Participative inquiry and practice* (pp. 294–300). Thousand Oaks, CA: Sage.

Barrett, P. A., & Taylor, B. J. (2002). Beyond reflection: Cake and cooperative inquiry. *Systemic Practice and Action Research, 15,* 237–248.

Bateson, G. (2000). Form, substance and difference. In G. Bateson, *Steps to an ecology of mind* (pp. 454–471). (Original work published 1972)

Belenky, M., Clinchy, B. M., Goldberger, N., & Tarule, J. (1986). *Women's ways of knowing: The development of self, voice, and mind.* New York: Basic Books.

Berman, M. (1981). *The reenchantment of the world.* Ithaca, NY: Cornell University Press.

Berry, T. (1988). *The dream of the earth.* San Francisco: Sierra Club.

Berry, T. (1999). *The great work: Our way into the future.* New York: Bell Tower.

Bourdieu, P. (1977). *Outline of a theory of practice.* Cambridge, U.K.: Cambridge University Press.

Bradbury, H. (2007). Quality and "actionability": What action researchers offer from the tradition of pragmatism. In A. B. (Rami) Shani, S. A. Mohrman, W. Pasmore, B. Stymne, & N. Adler (Eds.), *Handbook of collaborative management research* (pp. 583–600). Thousand Oaks, CA: Sage.

Bradbury, H., & Lichtenstein, B. M. (2000). The space between: Operationalizing relationality in organizational research. *Organizational Science, 11,* 551–564.

Brown, L. (Ed.). (1999). *State of the world, 1999: A Worldwatch Institute report on progress towards a sustainable society.* London: Earthscan.

Buber, M. (1958). *I and thou* (R. G. Smith, Trans.). New York: Scribner.

Cooperrider, D. L., Sorensen, P. F., Whitney, D., & Yaeger, T. F. (2000). *Appreciative inquiry: Rethinking human organization toward a positive theory of change.* Champaign, IL: Stipes.

Denzin, N. K., & Lincoln, Y. S. (Eds.). (2000). *Handbook of qualitative research* (2nd ed.). Thousand Oaks, CA: Sage.

Eikeland, O. (2001). Action research as the hidden curriculum of the Western tradition. In P. Reason & H. Bradbury (Eds.), *Handbook of action research: Participative inquiry and practice* (pp. 145–155). Thousand Oaks, CA: Sage.

Fals-Borda, O. (1997). Concluding remarks at the eighth participatory action research world conference, Cartagena, Colombia.

Gaventa, J., & Cornwall, A. (2001). Power and knowledge. In P. Reason & H. Bradbury (Eds.), *Handbook of action research: Participative inquiry and practice* (pp. 70–80). Thousand Oaks, CA: Sage.

Giddens, A. (1984). *The constitution of society: Outline of the theory of structuration.* Berkeley: University of California Press.

Greenwood, D. J., & Levin, M. (1998). *Introduction to action research: Social research for social change.* Thousand Oaks, CA: Sage.

Gustavsen, B. (1996). Development and the social sciences: An uneasy relationship. In S. Toulmin & B. Gustavsen (Eds.), *Beyond theory: Changing organizations through participation* (pp. 5–30). Amsterdam: Benjamins.

Gustavsen, B. (2001). Theory and practice: The mediating discourse. In P. Reason & H. Bradbury (Eds.), *Handbook of action research: Participative inquiry and practice* (pp. 17–26). Thousand Oaks, CA: Sage.

Habermas, J. (1979). *Communication and the evolution of society* (T. McCarthy, Trans.). Boston: Beacon Press.

Hall, B. L. (2001). I wish this were a poem of practices of participatory research. In P. Reason & H. Bradbury (Eds.), *Handbook of action research: Participative inquiry and practice* (pp. 171–178). Thousand Oaks, CA: Sage.

Heron, J. (1996a). *Cooperative inquiry: Research into the human condition.* Thousand Oaks, CA: Sage.

Heron, J. (1996b). Quality as primacy of the practical. *Qualitative Inquiry, 2,* 41–56.

Heron, J. (1998). *Sacred science: Person-centred inquiry into the spiritual and the subtle.* Ross-on-Wye, U.K.: PCCS Books.

Heron, J. (2001). Transpersonal cooperative inquiry. In P. Reason & H. Bradbury (Eds.), *Handbook of action research: Participative inquiry and practice* (pp. 333–339). Thousand Oaks, CA: Sage.

Heron, J., & Reason, P. (1997). A participatory inquiry paradigm. *Qualitative Inquiry, 3,* 274–294.

Heron, J., & Reason, P. (2001). The practice of cooperative inquiry: Research with rather than on people. In P. Reason & H. Bradbury (Eds.), *Handbook of action research: Participative inquiry and practice* (pp. 179–188). Thousand Oaks, CA: Sage.

Kemmis, S. (2001). Exploring the relevance of critical theory for action research: Emancipatory action research in the footsteps of Jürgen Habermas. In P. Reason & H. Bradbury (Eds.), *Handbook of action research: Participative inquiry and practice* (pp. 91–102). Thousand Oaks, CA: Sage.

Kvale, S. (1989). To validate is to question. In S. Kvale (Ed.), *Issues of validity in qualitative research* (pp. 73–92). Stockholm: Studentliteratur.

Lather, P. A. (1993). Fertile obsession: Validity after poststructuralism. *Sociological Quarterly, 34,* 673–693.

Lather, P. A. (2001). Validity as an incitement to discourse: Qualitative research and the crisis of legitimation. In V. Richardson (Ed.), *Handbook of research on teaching* (4th ed., pp. 241–250). Washington, DC: American Education Research Association.

Lewis, H. M. (2001). Participatory research and education for social change: Highlander Research and Education Center. In P. Reason & H. Bradbury (Eds.), *Handbook of action research: Participative inquiry and practice* (pp. 356–362). Thousand Oaks, CA: Sage.

Lincoln, Y. S. (1995). Emerging criteria for quality in qualitative and interpretive research. *Qualitative Inquiry, 1,* 275–289.

Ludema, J. D., Cooperrider, D. L., & Barrett, F. J. (2001). Appreciative inquiry: The power of the unconditional positive question. In P. Reason & H. Bradbury (Eds.), *Handbook of action research: Participative inquiry and practice* (pp. 189–199). Thousand Oaks, CA: Sage.

Lyotard, J.-F. (1984). *The postmodern condition: A report on knowledge* (J. Bennington & B. Massumi, Trans.). Minneapolis: University of Minnesota Press.

Marshall, J. (1999). Living life as inquiry. *Systematic Practice and Action Research, 12,* 155–171.

Marshall, J. (2001). Self-reflective inquiry practices. In P. Reason & H. Bradbury (Eds.), *Handbook of action research: Participative inquiry and practice* (pp. 433–439). Thousand Oaks, CA: Sage.

Marshall, J., & Mead, G. (2005). Self-reflective practice and first-person action research. *Action Research, 3*(3, special issue), 233–332.

McArdle, K. L. (2008). Getting in, getting on, getting out: On working with second-person inquiry groups. In P. Reason & H. Bradbury (Eds.), *Handbook of action research: Participative inquiry and practice* (2nd ed., pp. 602–614). Thousand Oaks, CA: Sage.

Park, P. (2001). Knowledge and participatory research. In P. Reason & H. Bradbury (Eds.), *Handbook of action research: Participative inquiry and practice* (pp. 81–90). Thousand Oaks, CA: Sage.

Putnam, H. (1992). *Renewing philosophy.* Cambridge, MA: Harvard University Press.

Reason, P. (1988). Whole person medical practice. In P. Reason (Ed.), *Human inquiry in action: Developments in new paradigm research* (pp. 102–126). Thousand Oaks, CA: Sage.

Reason, P. (2005). Living as part of the whole. *Journal of Curriculum and Pedagogy, 2*(2), 35–41.

Reason, P. (2006). Choice and quality in action research practice. *Journal of Management Inquiry, 15*(2), 187–203.

Reason, P., & Bradbury, H. (Eds.). (2001). *Handbook of Action Research: Participative inquiry and practice.* Thousand Oaks, CA: Sage.

Reason, P., & Bradbury, H. (Eds.). (2008). *Handbook of action research: Participative inquiry and practice* (2nd ed.). Thousand Oaks, CA: Sage.

Reason, P., & Goodwin, B. C. (1999). Toward a science of qualities in organizations: Lessons from complexity theory and postmodern biology. *Concepts and Transformations, 4,* 281–317.

Reason, P., & Torbert, W. R. (2001). Toward a participatory worldview: Part 2. *ReVision, 24*(2), 1–48.

Rorty, R. (2000). *Philosophy and social hope.* New York: Penguin.

Schwandt, T. A. (1996). Farewell to criteriology. *Qualitative Inquiry, 2,* 58–72.

Seeley, C. (2006). *Wild margins: Playing at work and life.* Unpublished doctoral dissertation, University of Bath, Centre for Action Research in Professional Practice, Bath, U.K.

Seeley, C., & Reason, P. (2008). Expressions of energy: An epistemology of presentational knowing. In P. Liamputtong & J. Rumbold (Eds.), *Knowing differently: Arts-based and collaborative research methods.* New York: Nova Science.

Senge, S., & Scharmer, O. (2001). Community action research: Learning as a community of practitioners, consultants, and researchers. In P. Reason & H. Bradbury (Eds.), *Handbook of action research: Participatory inquiry and practice* (pp. 238–249). Thousand Oaks, CA: Sage.

Skolimowski, H. (1993). *A sacred place to dwell.* Rockport, MA: Element.

Skolimowski, H. (1994). *The participatory mind.* London: Arkana.

Swantz, M.-L., Ndedya, E., & Masaiganah, M. S. (2001). Participatory action research in southern Tanzania, with special reference to women. In P. Reason & H. Bradbury (Eds.), *Handbook of action research: Participatory inquiry and practice* (pp. 386–395). Thousand Oaks, CA: Sage.

Torbert, W. R. (1991). *The power of balance: Transforming self, society, and scientific inquiry.* Thousand Oaks, CA: Sage.

Torbert, W. R. (1999). The distinctive questions developmental action inquiry asks. *Management Learning, 30,* 189–206.

Torbert, W. R. (2001). The practice of action inquiry. In P. Reason & H. Bradbury (Eds.), *Handbook of action research: Participative inquiry and practice* (pp. 250–260). Thousand Oaks, CA: Sage.

Toulmin, S. (1990). *Cosmopolis: The hidden agenda of modernity.* New York: Free Press.

Wolcott, H. (1990). On seeking—and rejecting—validity in qualitative research. In E. Eisner & A. Peshkin (Eds.), *Qualitative inquiry in education: The continuing debate* (pp. 121–152). New York: Teachers College Press.

CHAPTER

14

IMPACTS OF CBPR ON ACADEMIC RESEARCHERS, RESEARCH QUALITY AND METHODOLOGY, AND POWER RELATIONS

MEREDITH MINKLER & ANDREA CORAGE BADEN

THE CONTINUUM of research orientations known as community-based participatory research is distinct, in part, not in the *methods* used—which span a wide range of quantitative and qualitative approaches—but in the *ways* they are used and "the methodological contexts of their application" (Cornwall & Jewkes, 1995, p. 1667). As Cornwall and Jewkes point out, what is new is "the attitudes of researchers, which in turn determine how, by and for whom the research is conceptualized and conducted" and "the corresponding location of power at every stage in the research process" (p. 1667).

Governmental and philanthropic support for community-based participatory research (CBPR) and related traditions in many parts of the world has helped confer increasing legitimacy on this approach (Braine, 2005; Flicker, Travers, Guta, McDonald, & Meagher, 2007; Gebbie, Rosenstock, & Hernandez, 2003; Green et al., 1995; Jones & Wells, 2007). In the United States, as noted in Chapter One, the prestigious Institute of Medicine even named CBPR one of eight new content areas in which all schools of public health should offer training (Gebbie et al., 2003).

Despite such optimistic assessments, however, considerable skepticism about the scientific legitimacy and feasibility of this approach to research remains. CBPR's critical, social constructionist, and action orientation is seen by some as antithetical to the theoretical tenets and approaches of public health science with their moorings in a positivist tradition that privileges expert technical knowledge, objectivity (methodological and sociopolitical), and universal truths as essential and superior in making sense of the world (Wright & Treacher, 1982; see also Chapter Two). Further, power in the health and medical sciences is hierarchically distributed according to elite status, with academic and leadership positions in prestigious research institutions disproportionately held by individuals who are already more privileged in terms of race and ethnicity, social class, gender, and other dimensions (Israel, Eng, Schulz, & Parker, 2005; Wallerstein & Duran, 2006). Although addressing these power dynamics head on has been increasingly recognized as part of the CBPR endeavor (Flicker et al., 2007; Minkler, 2004; Wallerstein, 1999; see also Chapters Five, Fifteen, and Twenty-One), traditional research protocols tend to maintain such hierarchies (Flicker et al., 2007; see also Appendix G).

Another set of tensions exists between public health's premiere mode of action—peer-reviewed publication—and that of community groups. The latter often are more concerned with the translation of research results into action on the community and policy levels and may tend to be more politically outspoken in their orientation (Corburn, 2005; Minkler, 2004; see also Chapter Seventeen).

Given these substantial differences between CBPR and more traditional research approaches, several questions are frequently raised: Does CBPR add value to health research, or is the very premise of involving communities in the conduct of research contradictory to the tenets of "science," defined traditionally as expert based and objective? Does CBPR truly shift the power relations between the observer and observed? And if so, does this serve the public health agenda of improving the science on which that agenda is based?

In addressing these questions we draw on the social science and public health literature as well as on in-depth interviews with epidemiologists and other public health researchers involved in a recent cross-site analysis of the impacts of CBPR on health-related public policy in the United States (Minkler, Breckwich Vásquez, Chang, Blackwell, et al., 2008a; Minkler, Breckwich Vásquez, Tajik, & Petersen, 2008b; Minkler and Breckwich Vásquez, 2004).

We examine in particular the perceptions of public health researchers concerning their involvement in a scientific approach that engages communities of interest in the production of the research itself. Specifically addressed are issues of scientific rigor and methodology and of the changing social dynamics between researcher and community.

We conclude by suggesting that CBPR, with its valuing of lay knowledge and its emphasis on community involvement in the research process itself, may add substantial value to public health scholarship as well as to the democratization of the scientific process itself. This appears particularly salient when addressing health issues strongly linked to power differentials, including much of the research on health disparities (Israel et al., 2005; Wallerstein & Duran, 2006; Wells & Norris, 2006).

METHODS

This chapter is based in part on primary and secondary reviews of the peer-reviewed literature; we used both social science (for example, SocAbstracts) and medical (for example, PubMed) search engines to identify health-oriented community-researcher collaborations, with special attention to CBPR. An Internet call for articles and reports on CBPR projects focused specifically on policy was delivered through twenty-four relevant list serves (for example, the Community-Campus Partnerships for Health listserv), and was helpful in identifying international publications and reports as well as several in-press publications not uncovered through more traditional search engines and processes.

In addition to our own literature reviews, and a detailed analysis of sixty CBPR studies in North America (Viswanathan et al., 2004), data from a recent national study, "Documenting the Impacts of CBPR on Healthy Public Policy" (DICPP) were used (Minkler et al., 2008a, 2008b; Minkler & Breckwich Vásquez, 2004). This W. K. Kellogg Foundation–funded study incorporated a qualitative multimethod case study approach and in-depth analysis within and across ten partnerships. The cases were identified through purposeful sampling (Patton, 2002) of a sampling frame compiled from key CBPR resources, including literature reviews and the Internet call noted above.

Although the DICPP study did not set out explicitly to study the attitudes of health researchers about the impacts of community involvement on scientists and their approaches to research, much rich data emerged in the course of data collection that was salient to the current investigation. Of particular relevance were the perspectives of epidemiologists and other public health researchers in four case study sites focused on environmental justice (Minkler et al., 2008a, 2008b; Petersen, Minkler, Breckwich Vásquez & Baden, 2006; see also Table 14.1).

Drawing on these diverse sources, we now examine and illustrate the ways in which CBPR appears to add value to the scientific enterprise in public health, along with some of the pitfalls involved. We focus in particular on the impact of CBPR on research methodology and processes, on research quality and rigor, and on power relations in public health research.

TABLE 14.1 DICPP CBPR Partnerships Focused on Environmental Justice

Partnership name	Dates	Primary partners	Research aim
West Harlem Environmental Action (WE ACT) Partnership	1996–present	Staff and youth interns at WE ACT; epidemiology staff at Center for Children's Environmental Health at Columbia University	To study community-level exposure to diesel exhaust emissions and related air pollution
The Southern California Environmental Justice Collaborative (LA Collaborative)	1998–present	Communities for a Better Environment; Liberty Hill Foundation; researchers at University of California, Santa Cruz, Occidental College, and Brown University	To determine if there is environmental inequality (in air quality and toxic exposure levels) in southern CA and, if so, who bears the burden
Tribal Efforts Against Lead (TEAL)	1996–present	TEAL clan mothers and fathers from 8 local tribes; researchers from University of Oklahoma, University of New Mexico, Emory University, and Ottawa County Health Department	To assess lead exposure levels among local children; to evaluate lay health worker model
Concerned Citizens of Tillery (CTT) Partnership	1995–present	Concerned Citizens of Tillery; epidemiology faculty and students at University of North Carolina, Chapel Hill School of Public Health; (initially) selected county health department staff	To systematically quantify extent to which industrial hog operations are disproportionately located in low-income and African American communities in the state and how they affect communities' health

Source: Minkler et al., 2008a, 2008b.

IMPACTS OF CBPR ON METHODOLOGY AND PROCESSES

A predominant theme in the literature addressed CBPR's influence on study methodology and specifically community involvement in various stages of the research process. As discussed later, these stages are identifying the initial problem or research question, formulating the research design, defining the study population, conducting an ethical review and obtaining informed consent, designing research instruments and measures, recruiting the study sample, administering the research instruments, analyzing and interpreting data, disseminating results, and articulating subsequent action steps (Petersen et al., 2006; Corburn, 2005; Israel, Schulz, Parker, & Becker, 1998; Torres-Harding, Herrell, & Howard, 2004; Lynn, 2000; O'Fallon & Dearry, 2002).

Research Question Selection

Nyden and Wiewel (1992) argue that in traditional academic inquiries, research questions are derived from internal disciplinary debates, typically without concern for the needs of those outside the discipline, including those communities and individuals who constitute the populations studied. Shifting who determines the research question inevitably alters the traditional power dynamics of academic research. As Arcury and colleagues (1999) explain, "[t]he most powerful aspect of community participation in health intervention projects is that it forces the projects to address the health concerns of community members rather the concerns of health professionals" (p. 564).

Several of the projects reviewed began their collaboration by engaging communities in the identification of research problems, rather than imposing research agendas from the outside (Morello-Frosch, Pastor, Porras, & Sadd, 2005; Schulz et al., 1998; Jordan, Lee, & Shapiro, 2000; see Chapter Fifteen). For example, Schulz and colleagues (1998, 2005) described the initial efforts of the East Side Village Health Worker Partnership in identifying community health concerns through survey methodology. Committed to building on community strengths, the collaborative not only articulated health problems but also explored the community's history of collective actions, the community's current resources, and those protective factors perceived by community members to influence health. Focusing on community concerns from the start increased the possibilities that the research would be grounded in community realities and that the community would benefit in the process (Schulz et al., 1998, 2005).

Outside researchers who began by defining the initial research questions themselves also sometimes reported modifying their initial problem statement in response to community feedback. In South Africa, for example, high rates of cervical cancer in the black and colored populations led Mosavel and his colleagues (Mosavel, Simon, van Stade, & Buchbinder, 2005) to propose a study on this subject. In response to community partner feedback, however, they broadened their topic to "cervical health," a concept that "acknowledges the fact that women's health in South Africa extends well beyond the risk of developing cervical cancer, and includes HIV and STDs, sexual violence, and multiple other social problems" (p. 2577).

Public health researchers interviewed in the DICPP study frequently reported feeling that the research benefited from community involvement because that involvement made sure that the research questions being asked were in fact the right questions. As a researcher with the Southern California Environmental Justice Collaborative commented, "We adopted a policy wherein we decided that [the community partner] would really have the final say on what should be the research priorities . . . we felt that they had their finger on the pulse best of all" (Minkler & Breckwich Vásquez, 2004).

As O'Fallon and Dearry (2002) state, "Without a mutually beneficial research question, the potential impact of the project on public health will be lessened," and community participation at this stage in the research process can therefore play a critical role (p. 158).

Instrument and Research Design

Many of the CBPR studies reviewed reported community involvement in developing or selecting study instruments, with some also noting that community partners had a substantial impact on the research design itself. In the former regard, community members in the Minneapolis-based lead-exposure project, DREAMS, assisted with selecting and developing cognitive assessment tools that were more culturally appropriate for their study population (that is, low-income, minority youths) than were "gold standards" such as the Weschler IQ test, which were seen by some as biased toward middle- and upper-class students (Jordan et al., 2000).

In the West Harlem Environmental Action (WE ACT) partnership in New York, an academic partner similarly pointed out the value of the community's input in helping him to put aside preconceived ideas concerning appropriate research design and methods. In his words: "Sometimes as scientists we make assumptions and don't rethink assumptions to see how they fit in a natural situation. I think community people, because they are looking at it from a fresh perspective, will question the assumptions in a way that actually improves the science. It may tailor things to the situation in a way we would not have thought of" (Minkler & Breckwich Vásquez, 2004; see also Chapter Eighteen).

In the Healthy Homes Project in Seattle-King County, Washington, which was aimed at assessing exposure to indoor asthma triggers, community health workers' observations that the questions they were asking about smoking were not sensitive enough to pick up whether or not others in the home were smoking led to some revisions in question wording. As Kreiger and his colleagues (Kreiger, Allen, Roberts, Ross, & Takaro, 2005) pointed out, "Any loss in the ability to make 'pure' baseline and exit comparisons may be outweighed by the higher quality of the exit data" (pp. 242–243).

Researchers also reported, however, that their partnerships occasionally pursued research designs that in traditional academic circles would be seen as less than ideal in order to meet specific community objectives (Jordan et al., 2000; Schulz et al., 1998; Petersen et al., 2007). For example, Schulz et al. (1998, 2005) noted that the East Side Village Health Worker Partnership chose not to include a comparison community in its study for ethical reasons (since the comparison community would not receive intervention). Instead the collaborative channeled those funds into extended research on the primary intervention community. Similarly, in the Tribal Efforts Against Lead (TEAL) study in Tar Creek, Oklahoma, the academic researchers had originally planned to conduct their lay health worker intervention and collect before and after blood lead samples and other data only among Native American children, using their white peers as controls. Native American community members objected, however, arguing that white children were also affected by the lead problem and that race-based exclusion from a potentially useful intervention was wrong. As stated by an academic partner, "They wanted us to do [things] that contaminated our control group, but we had to work with them. We couldn't impose the exclusiveness when they really wanted to do some things that were across cultures or across what we had initially intended to be separate networks." In point of fact, baseline screenings conducted by TEAL contradicted earlier Indian Health Service data and demonstrated that blood lead levels were, indeed, elevated for both Native American and white populations. This finding made it easier for the academic partners to justify altering their design (contaminating their control group), because withholding the intervention from the white population could be considered unethical (Minkler & Breckwich Vásquez, 2004; Petersen et al., 2007).

Ethical Review and Informed Consent

As the previous example illustrates, community participation has been credited by some researchers with raising ethical issues that otherwise may not have been addressed (see also Buchanan, Miller, & Wallerstein, 2007; Flicker et al., 2007). In a Tibetan study that included a randomized controlled trial of an indigenous medicine to prevent maternal hemorrhaging (Bell, 2004), midwives and other community partners were instrumental in working with an ethnographer and the public health researchers to help facilitate true informed consent. As the author pointed out, "risk disclosure" was an unacceptable term, since such disclosure was believed to disturb the wind elements responsible for emotions and to have the potential to lead to adverse mental health outcomes. By reframing risk disclosure as "safety issues," needed information could be conveyed in a culturally acceptable manner (Bell, 2004).

As Buchanan and his colleagues (2007), Khanlou and Peter (2005), and Flicker and her colleagues (2007) have noted, many traditional ethical review and informed consent processes are ill-suited to participatory research collaborations. The failure of most institutional review boards (IRBs) to extend their purview to community-level, as well as individual-level, benefits and risks also has been suggested, and Flicker et al. (2007), in Toronto, have developed an online workshop to address this and other such ethical challenges (wellesleyinstitute.com). They and others also have developed alternative ethical review principles for IRBs (Flicker et al., 2007; see also Appendixes G and H). Green et al.'s (1995) guidelines for appraising participatory research projects in health promotion further include a number of Likert scale items with direct relevance for grappling with difficult ethical challenges before the fact and revisiting them throughout the research process. (Green and colleagues' new reliability-tested guidelines appear as Appendix C in this volume.)

Data Collection

The East Side Village Health Worker Partnership in Detroit (Schulz et al., 1998, 2005) exemplified the data collection experience of many CBPR partnerships, wherein community members successfully identified respondent sites (for example, hard-to-locate housing units) and administered data collection instruments in a culturally competent manner. In this case, such activities contributed to a higher than predicted response rate (81 percent achieved versus 70 percent anticipated). Similarly, a marked increase in recruitment was observed in a participatory epidemiology project on diabetes in an urban Aboriginal community in Melbourne, Australia, following the hiring of a community codirector with insider knowledge and standing in the community, factors seen by the outside researcher as making a major contribution (Thompson, 2000).

In Southeast Halifax County, North Carolina, where historical and contemporary racial discrimination has left an indelible mark, university-based researchers involved in a survey research study reported the benefits of having academics who would be conducting the actual survey introduced by African Americans from a nearby community who would go with them door-to-door. Such introductions were seen as essential to help break down barriers of distrust in the community. But having outsiders conduct the research itself also was seen as critical to avoid accusations of bias on the politically loaded subject of industrialized hog operations and their potential health impacts in this community (see Chapter Fifteen; Tajik & Minkler, 2007; Minkler & Breckwich Vásquez, 2004).

Data Analysis and Interpretation

With few exceptions (Fadem et al., 2003; Wallerstein et al., 2003; see also Chapter Sixteen), the studies reviewed suggest that communities tend not to be involved with the actual data analysis phase of CBPR projects. Sometimes, as Wing (2005) observes, this reflects the nature of the data analysis (for example, computer modeling or multivariate analysis) or the fact that community members are less interested in this stage of the work (see also Chapter Fifteen). In some instances, however, community partner involvement in data analysis has been undertaken with good results, particularly with qualitative inquiry (see Chapter Sixteen). Epidemiologist Chuck McKetney with the Healthy Neighborhoods Project in West Contra Costa County, California, for example, reported that following their interviews with 500 local residents, trained *neighborhood health advocates* took the lead in sorting and analyzing open-ended responses to questions such as, "What do you like best about living in this neighborhood?" and "What would you most like to see changed?" As the project evaluator, McKetney commented that at first some of the categorizations made little sense from an epidemiological perspective. Yet as residents described the logic behind their sorting, it became clear that their analyses were based on a sophisticated knowledge of the communities in which they lived (Minkler, 2000).

Community partners also played a key role in analysis of air sampling and geographic information system (GIS) data on exposure to air pollutants in Brooklyn, New York (Corburn, 2005). The community partners' expert knowledge of neighborhood practices (for example, routes being used illegally by truckers to avoid traffic congestion on a major thoroughfare) helped to explain the unexpectedly high exposure readings found on particular streets and further suggested an important avenue for more study (see also Chapter Sixteen). Finally, in a study by and with people with disabilities on the contentious topic of attitudes in their community toward physician-assisted suicide legislation (Fadem et al., 2003), a subgroup of the community advisory committee was trained in qualitative data analysis and used redacted transcripts to identify codes and themes in the interview data. After doing their independent coding, they met on alternate Saturdays over two to three months to compare and reconcile findings. As one of the trained researchers (and the only member of the team who did not have a disability) later commented, this process enabled a more nuanced understanding of the root causes of the ambivalence seen among many study participants, including the fact that perceived discrimination by health care providers was viewed as symptomatic of broader and more pervasive discrimination on the societal level (Fadem et al., 2003).

Far more frequently, community members participate in the interpretation of preliminary research findings (Israel et al., 1998; Torres-Harding et al., 2004; Wing, 2005), often attending community forums, town hall meetings, or small-group sessions where early results are presented and community members' feedback is sought. Although the great majority of studies that spoke to the role of community involvement in data collection and analysis were positive in their assessments, some cautionary notes were also sounded. Some partnerships restricted either data analysis or data presentation at the request of community partners in order to avoid casting the community in a negative light (Jordan et al., 2000). In the Oakland-based Grandparent Caregiver Study, for example, a single (and fortunately very minor) research finding was perceived by study participants at a presentation of preliminary results to be potentially damaging if it "got into the wrong hands." At the women's request, the researchers refrained from publishing this particular finding (Roe, Minkler, & Saunders, 1995). In subsequent studies, however, memoranda of understanding (MOUs) were put in place to prevent such after-the-fact decision making, which can lead to questions about study integrity.

Finally, and as noted in earlier chapters, the time required for a systematic data analysis process may end up frustrating some community partners for whom the imperative to get to action may result in a desire to skip or foreshorten important steps in the process.

Dissemination and Use of Findings

Dissemination of study results is a critical component of an action-oriented CBPR process (O'Fallon & Dearry, 2002; Israel et al., 1998; 2005) and an increasingly common requirement of funding agencies. Whereas traditional academic research focuses primarily on academic journal publication, CBPR pursues multiple venues to get its messages out. In an innovative HIV/AIDS study in Gujarat, India, CBPR partners learned that men who engaged in unprotected sex sometimes did so out of erroneous beliefs about the long-term consequences of noncoital sexual behaviors, which were believed to cause "thinning of the semen," sexual dysfunction, and fatigue. To correct this misinformation, the partners designed culturally relevant interventions, such as street theater pieces performed separately for men and for women at *melas,* or street fairs, by locally recruited youth. They also disseminated the study findings through fifteen local credit unions, which had previously proven effective platforms for the discussion of reproductive health information (Shah, 2004). Although involvement of community members in determining appropriate venues for local dissemination of research findings is not unique to CBPR, the ongoing partnerships and trust levels developed through CBPR may increase the likelihood of incorporating useful insider knowledge in this stage of the research process.

In their North Carolina disaster relief efforts after a flood, Farquhar and her community partners (Chapter Fifteen) also felt the need to have their results communicated quickly and effectively, and they targeted the media and policymakers. Anticipating that these audiences would require different types of data, the partners designed their study to capture both quantitative and qualitative descriptions. The mass dissemination of results through press releases, policy meetings, and media interviews successfully forced the state emergency management director to address the special needs of low-income and predominately African American flood survivors (with, for example, extended access to temporary housing), survivors who had previously received treatment inferior to that of their wealthier white counterparts.

Although academic researchers frequently describe feelings of satisfaction in seeing the results of their efforts used in a timely manner to help bring about change (see, for example, Morello-Frosch et al., 2005; Petersen et al., 2006), the dissemination phase of CBPR projects can also engender tensions between academic researchers and community partners. Although community members are often motivated by the desire to get credible data that can be used quickly to bring about changes in programs or policies, academics may have different goals and priorities. As an epidemiologist in the WE ACT partnership recalled when discussing the policy focus of his community partners, "My motivation for doing these studies is not framed that way. It is more framed in terms of trying to fill scientific gaps." This individual was clearly committed to helping his community partners in their efforts to address environmental justice objectives, and he noted that "what makes scientific gaps interesting . . . [is that] there is a policy need." However, as a WE ACT staff member pointed out with respect to her university collaborators, "It is not natural for [researchers], based on their training, to come out and want to be advocates. There are times when we need their weight and credibility as scientific researchers, to say something. That has been, in some instances, a tug and a pull" (Minkler & Breckwich Vásquez, 2004; Minkler et al., 2008a; see also Chapter Eighteen).

The length of time between completing study findings and their publication in peer-reviewed journals was also frequently cited as a source of tension in the dissemination phase of CBPR projects, particularly when academic partners were concerned about having findings used prior to their own publication of them (Minkler, 2004; Minkler & Breckwich Vásquez, 2004; Israel et al., 1998). Finally, for academics whose research is funded by the National Institutes of Health (NIH) or other sources seen as precluding active involvement in efforts to have an impact on policy, there may be an understandable reluctance to engage in policy-related activities during a CBPR project's action phase. As an academic partner with TEAL put it, she and other project staff had to "steer clear because of lobbying restrictions." As a result: "When our [Native American community partners] went to the City Council events they went as citizens as opposed to [representatives of TEAL]. When they wrote letters to congressmen, they did so as a citizen. We had to be very clear about drawing this distinction because of the federal funding issue" (Minkler et al., 2008b; Petersen et al., 2007).

Partners in the Concerned Citizens of Tillery/UNC collaboration in North Carolina, whose project also was funded through the NIH, expressed similar concerns, with one partner frequently reiterating in interviews that "we don't do policy—we just educate legislators" (Tajik & Minkler, 2007). This partnership had been very successful in using its research outcomes to inform change in state and local policy regulating the expansion of industrial hog operations, and a community partner had appeared twice on the popular television program *60 Minutes,* strongly advocating for the community's position. Yet he and others demonstrated a real reluctance to discuss their role in the action phase of this CBPR project beyond that of "educating policy makers" (Minkler et al., 2008a; Tajik & Minkler, 2007).

IMPACTS ON RESEARCH QUALITY

Overall, scientifically trained research partners claimed that CBPR enhanced study relevance because the inquiry was grounded in the lived experience of community members (Israel et al., 1998, 2005; Altman, 1995; Corburn, 2005; Lynn, 2000). Not only were research questions more likely to address important community health concerns but the study findings led to potentially more acceptable and effective interventions based on these concerns (Israel et al., 1998, 2005; Altman, 1995; O'Fallon & Dearry, 2002).

For example, study validity was described by a number of academically trained researchers as having been enhanced by CBPR. As Green and Mercer (2001) suggested, "Engaging communities and practitioners will not invariably improve the internal validity of research, but almost certainly will improve its external validity—that is, its applicability and usability in the settings in which the research occurs" (p. 1928).

Other scientifically trained researchers spoke more directly to the contributions of CBPR to internal validity. As Jordan and her colleagues (2000) asserted, "research . . . benefits [accrued] through improved recruitment rates, lower attrition, increased compliance, improved accuracy of reported information, and fewer cultural and language barriers. . . . [Additionally,] participants may share more personal information with peers, which is vital to the collection of accurate data on confounding variables" (pp. 735–736).

All these factors strengthened the quality of data and statistical power of analysis. CBPR was not without challenges for the scientists, however. As mentioned earlier, eliminating or mixing control groups and withholding data from the analysis or dissemination phase because these data were perceived as potentially harmful to the community's reputation were reported by various researchers. From a pure science perspective these challenges may be viewed as shortfalls of CBPR. Yet from the vantage point of public health practice, many of these concerns can be recast as ethical issues typically associated with human research. If the goal, for instance, is improving health status and reducing disparities, it is critical to frame the data in a way that avoids just focusing on the negative, so that the community continues to stay involved to address the issues. Here, however, the unit of concern becomes the community, rather than the individual as in clinical research.

IMPACTS ON POWER RELATIONS

A key differentiation between CBPR and more traditional public health research is that whereas the latter promotes a lay-expert dichotomy, CBPR strives to acknowledge expertise among all participants. Communities thus are seen as contributing local knowledge about the ways in which their communities work, along with the constraints, obstacles, and resources that influence community behavior (Dressler, 1993; Jones & Wells, 2007). Scientists, in contrast, are seen as contributing technical knowledge, skills, and access to various resources such as study personnel, scientific equipment, and funding (Altman, 1995; Israel et al., 1998, 2005). Because knowledge is both intrinsically linked to power (Foucault, 1993) and a core element of science, incorporating community knowledge claims into scientific processes can radically shift not only the shape and direction of the research but, more fundamentally, the power dynamics of science production itself.

Although many articles and other sources reviewed suggested a generalized appreciation of the role of CBPR in shifting power relations between scientists and community residents, the public health literature offered little explicit discussion of the ways in which such shifts actually occurred. In one notable exception, Wallerstein (1999) described in detail the power that rested in what her community partners saw as the "weight of authority" she carried as a university professor, a member of the dominant white culture, and the recipient of a large grant from the state (p. 48). Israel et al. (1998; see also Chapter Three) have further articulated how power differentials manifest among partners as differences in time availability, resource access, knowledge, and skills, reflecting larger structural patterning based on race, ethnicity, class, and gender. As these authors (1998, p. 183) explain, "[t]hese inequalities affect who attends, who participates, whose opinions are considered to be valid, and who has influence over decisions made."

More typically, the literature addressed power dynamics implicitly by illustrating for example how community involvement in the various stages of the research process reshaped the scientific inquiry to encompass a community perspective. Through such community engagement, CBPR was seen by academics as contributing to the democratization of the science (Gaventa, 1993; Reason & Bradbury, 2006, 2008; see Chapter One). Community participation thus was described as influencing both the form and direction of inquiry, with study questions helping to reflect a community agenda and action steps generated to create change.

Some investigators argued further that CBPR was not simply useful in improving public health research but was in fact essential in pursuing certain types of research. As Schulz et al. (1998, p. 22) explain, "community research and intervention that seeks to address social inequalities that are fundamental to differentials in health should explicitly work to establish more equitable power relationships among participants." By engaging the community in the research process, CBPR can interrupt the reproduction of hierarchical power relations inherent in traditional academic research practices.

This shift in relations is clearly illustrated in the decision-making process developed by the Southern California Environmental Justice Collaborative (Morello-Frosch et al., 2005). As explained by one of the partnership's researchers: "We came up with a decision-making structure [that said that] any of the three partners: [the community-based organization, the funder, or the researchers] could bring a research project to the table and suggest it, argue for it, etc., but that ultimately the decision about which research project would roll forward would rest with [the community organization]. They would have veto power, really" (Minkler & Breckwich Vásquez, 2004; see also Petersen et al., 2006).

For researchers Nyden and Wiewel (1992), the community was seen as providing "a human quality" to the otherwise positivist and technically rational domain of science. In the case of an environmental health risk assessment, for example, the scientific approach emphasized probabilities and objectivity whereas the community underscored issues of "fairness, distributions, voluntariness, reasonability, control, trust, reversibility and identifiable victims" (Corburn, 2002, p. 457). As one researcher suggested, if they made choices without considering the value-based judgments of affected communities, risk assessment scientists were essentially imposing their risk selections on someone else's community (Corburn, 2002, 2005).

An additional shift in the research enterprise with CBPR involves the actual sites in which the research occurs. Whereas in traditional academic research, much of the investigative activity takes place at university-affiliated sites, in CBPR many key activities (for example, planning, data collection, results dissemination) physically occur in the community (Schulz et al., 1998; Jordan et al., 2000; Israel et al., 2005). Regular travel to the community then becomes part of the academic researchers' collaborative responsibilities.

The influence of race, ethnicity, and class on science is of particular interest in reconstructing power relations in science, and several of the studies reviewed made reference to this dynamic. For example, Torres-Harding and colleagues (2004) challenged a presumption, derived from clinical population studies, that chronic fatigue syndrome (CFS) was primarily a disease of white, middle- to upper-class, Caucasian women. By shifting to a community sampling design, these investigators demonstrated that CFS prevalence was in fact highest among Latinos, African Americans, and those individuals with middle to low socioeconomic status, suggesting that earlier clinical studies were biased toward populations that had access to and used health care services.

In a critique of environmental risk assessment, Corburn (2002) exposed foundational assumptions that appeared prejudiced toward dominant group characteristics (such as being white, male, and of middle income). For example, dose-response predictions relied on a default *reference man*—a Caucasian male weighing 70 kilograms—for their determinations. Corburn argued that traditional risk calculations typically ignore important "background" risks (such as low income, poor access to health care, and multiple exposures) commonly experienced by disadvantaged minority communities. He further has illustrated ways in which a New York community helped remedy such research biases—for example, by identifying various indoor and outdoor environmental risks (such as lead exposure and contaminated fish consumption) not originally acknowledged within a traditional risk assessment frame.

Although documentation of the ways in which CBPR alters power relations within the conduct of research is limited, the actual processes in which researchers and communities engage are even more elusive in the extant literature. Among the notable exceptions, Israel and colleagues (1998, 2005), Jordan et al. (2000), Fadem et al. (2003), and Wallerstein (1999) each articulate obstacles and strategies in addressing power imbalances. To create more equitable, productive partnerships, for example, Israel et al. (1998) recommend that academics and communities jointly develop operating norms that emphasize mutual respect, quality communication systems, and a democratic process of collaboration. Wallerstein (1999) adds a personal account of the difficulties in reshaping power dynamics between researcher and community when traditional hierarchical structures remain deeply entrenched.

DISCUSSION

Our review and analysis of the influence of CBPR on academic researchers, research quality and methodology, and power relations focused on three thematic areas: (1) the engagement of communities in the research process, from study question definition to results dissemination; (2) the ways in which this participation shapes both the research process and its products, including impacts on scientific rigor and quality; and (3) the changing social relations between academic researchers and communities pursuing CBPR, particularly in regard to decision making, roles in the conduct of the research, and tackling larger structural issues related to such factors as race and ethnicity, gender, and social class.

The examples of community participation in research activities examined in this chapter clearly demonstrate a shift in research processes relative to more traditional academic approaches. Most notable among these were the ongoing negotiation processes between academically trained researchers and community partners to address not only the research objectives but, equally important, the specific relationships among CBPR partners (Israel et al., 2005; Kreiger et al., 2005; Wallerstein, 1999; Jordan et al., 2000; see also Chapter Twenty-One). In the latter regard, such negotiations are critical given community histories of academic exploitation by previous researchers who used these groups for study without giving back to the community (Flicker et al., 2007; Israel et al., 1998; Hall, 1992; Fisher & Ball, 2003). Moreover, class and status differences between academics and the community require continual navigation. For a partnership to succeed, such issues of power and control must be carefully attended to through ongoing negotiation (Flicker et al., 2007; Wallerstein & Duran, 2006). Although in many of the case studies explored, CBPR was seen to contribute importantly to research processes and outcomes, this approach involved inherent challenges as well. A detailed examination of these challenges is beyond the scope of this chapter and is provided elsewhere (Buchanan et al., 2007; Flicker et al., 2007; Israel et al., 2005; Minkler, 2004; Sullivan et al., 2003; Wallerstein, 1999); see also Chapter Twenty-One). Key among them, however, was the large amount of time required to negotiate the collaborative's research process and partner relationships, which can lead to project delays, missed funding opportunities, and burnout. Relatedly, as Price and Behrens (2003) have noted, there is often a tension between "the necessary skepticism of science" and "the action imperative of communities" that can play out, for example, in frustrations over the timely release of findings to advance an action agenda. The fact that partnerships sometimes compromised conventional research designs to address community concerns in ways that may have reduced the value of a study from an academic perspective also was presented as a challenge (Jordan et al., 2000; Minkler, 2004; Petersen et al., 2007; Schulz et al., 1998), though one that often resulted in beneficial outcomes from a community standpoint.

As this review suggests, the methodological challenges of CBPR to the scientific endeavor can be viewed as primarily ethical and value based. In CBPR the community becomes the ethical unit of concern and must be addressed as such. Particularly among marginalized populations, which frequently are stigmatized by Western racialized and class-based ideologies, maintenance of a protective stance against research that may further add to this oppression is both common and understandable. In developing ethical guidelines for CBPR, Flicker et al. (2007) recommend that ethical review processes—including questions of this sort, "Are there built-in mechanisms for how unflattering results will be dealt with?"—be built in at the front end of CBPR projects (see Appendix G). Similarly, Green and colleagues' (1995) detailed guidelines for appraising participatory research in health promotion and the reliability-tested guidelines that followed (see Appendix C) can be a valuable aid in such endeavors.

SUMMARY

Drawing on several literature reviews and in-depth interviews with public health researchers engaged in CBPR projects, we have identified several important themes related to the impacts of CBPR on researchers and the research itself. These themes address the *research stages* in which communities participate, the *alternative venues* for the dissemination of findings, the unique CBPR research *processes,* and the *benefits and limits of CBPR approaches* in regard to the production of the research. From a sociological perspective, the literature also offers insights into CBPR's *impacts on the power relations and hegemonic practices* that support expert knowledge and the racialization of science.

The findings of this review suggest that CBPR can indeed add value to health research by helping to (1) ensure that the topic under investigation has meaning and importance to the community, (2) enhance validity in the interpretation of results by reflecting, in part, community understanding, and (3) enhance the study's utility if the results are seen as practical and feasible and if they lead to education and action for change as part of the research process.

This review, however, also clearly underscores the need for a more focused look at the impacts of CBPR on academic researchers and on the research itself. First, the role of academic researchers in CBPR partnerships is currently not well articulated. A deeper look at their engagement in scientific activities as well as collaborative and political activities within the CBPR context clearly is needed to help address this gap (see Chapter Twenty-One). Additionally, more attention should be focused on articulating the tensions between critical constructionist and positivist models of inquiry, determining in particular which elements of the positivist approach are malleable and thus open to change and which are not. Finally, and building on important recent efforts (Wells & Norris, 2006), much more research is needed that will further current dialogues addressing the influence of race, ethnicity, and class on research methods and outcomes.

Despite the substantial continuing challenges, however, a growing number of traditionally trained epidemiologists and other public health researchers clearly are finding in CBPR a way to increase the relevance, rigor, and utility of their scholarship, while sharing power with communities in the process (Schwab & Syme, 1997; Wells & Norris, 2006). In the words of Ann Macaulay and Paul Nutting (2006): "community members will bring new perspectives and new research questions, gain new skills in the process, and use their expertise to be active participants in the generation and application of new knowledge. Unforeseen solutions will begin to emerge to many of the problems in health and health care that currently seem insurmountable" (p. 7).

QUESTIONS FOR DISCUSSION

1. You have been asked by a skeptical student or colleague how CBPR can possibly be considered "good science" when community members without advanced training (and sometimes without even a high school education) are involved as coresearchers. Using examples from this or other chapters, how might you make the case for the ways in which CBPR can in fact strengthen the quality of research?

2. The authors cite community psychologists Price and Beherns as pointing to the tension between the "necessary skepticism of science" and the "action imperative of communities." With a class member or a small group of colleagues, role-play the different arguments you might make as, respectively, a community member convinced that early findings of your CBPR study should immediately be put to use in promoting the community's agenda, and an outside researcher for whom this activity seems premature. What arguments of the "other side" were most and least convincing to you? Is there a compromise position with which you would be comfortable?

3. Thinking about some of the challenges presented in this chapter, review the guidelines presented in Appendix C for appraising participatory research in health promotion. Can you envision using these guidelines in working with a community or other CBPR collaborator? Were issues raised in this chapter for which no relevant guideline was developed? If so, give an example of such an issue, and describe what a new Likert scale item to help partnerships better address this issue might look like.

KEY TERMS

Academic researchers

Power relations

Community-academic partnerships

Ethical and methodological challenges

REFERENCES

Altman, D. G. (1995). Sustaining interventions in community systems: On the relationships between researchers and communities. *Health Psychology, 14,* 526–536.

Arcury, T., Austin, C., Quandt, S., & Saavedra, R. (1999). Enhancing community participation in intervention research: Farmworkers and agricultural chemicals in North Carolina. *Health Education & Behavior, 25*(4), 563–578.

Bell, C. (2004). *One Heart (Health Education and Research in Tibet): Community-based participatory research on top of the world.* Unpublished manuscript, University of California, Berkeley, School of Public Health.

Braine, T. (2005). Brazil and Peru pool view of their people to set health agenda. *Bulletin of the World Health Organization*. Retrieved Oct. 17, 2007, from www.who.int/bulletin/volumes/83/7/infocus0705.

Buchanan, D. R., Miller, F. G., & Wallerstein, N. (2007). Ethical issues in community-based participatory research: Balancing rigorous research with community participation in community intervention studies. *Progress in Community Health Partnerships: Research, Education, and Action, 1*(2), 153–160.

Corburn, J. (2002). Environmental justice, local knowledge, and risk: The discourse of a community-based exposure assessment. *Environmental Management, 29*(4), 451–466.

Corburn, J. (2005). *Street science: Community knowledge and environmental health justice*. Cambridge, MA: MIT Press.

Cornwall, A., & Jewkes, R. (1995). What is participatory research? *Social Science & Medicine, 41*(12), 1667–1676.

Dressler, W. (1993). Commentary on community research: Partnership in black communities. *American Journal of Preventive Medicine, 9*(Suppl.), 32–34.

Fadem, P., Minkler, M., Perry, M., Blum, K., Moore, L., Rogers, J., et al. (2003). Attitudes of people with disabilities toward physician-assisted suicide legislation: Broadening the dialogue. *Journal of Health Politics, Policy and Law, 28,* 977–1002.

Fisher, P. A., & Ball, T. J. (2003). Tribal participatory research: Mechanisms of a collaborative model. *American Journal of Community Psychology. 32*(3–4), 207–216.

Flicker, S., Travers, R., Guta, A., McDonald, S., & Meagher, A. (2007). Ethical dilemmas in community-based participatory research: Recommendations for institutional review boards. *Journal of Urban Health, 84*(4), 478–493.

Foucault, M. (1993). Power as knowledge. In C. Lemert (Ed.), *Social theory: The multicultural and classic readings* (pp. 475–481). Boulder, CO: Westview Press.

Gaventa, J. (1993). The powerful, the powerless and the experts: Knowledge struggles in an information age. In P. Park, M. Brydon-Miller, B. L. Hall, & T. Jackson (Eds.), *Voices of change: Participatory research in the United States and Canada* (pp. 21–40). Westport, CT: Bergin & Garvey.

Gebbie, K., Rosenstock, L., & Hernandez, L. M. (2003). *Who will keep the public healthy? Educating public health professionals for the 21st century*. Washington, DC: Institute of Medicine.

Green, L. W., George, M. A., Daniel, M., Frankish, C. J., Herbert, C. P., Bowie, W. R., et al. (1995). *Study of participatory research in health promotion: Review and recommendations for the development of participatory research in health promotion in Canada*. Vancouver, BC: Royal Society of Canada.

Green, L. W., & Mercer, S. L. (2001). Can public health researchers and agencies reconcile the push from funding bodies and the pull from communities? *American Journal of Public Health. 91,* 1926–1929.

Hall, B. (1992). From margins to center? The development and purpose of participatory research. *American Sociologist, 23*(4), 15–28.

Israel, B. A., Eng, E., Schulz, A. J., & Parker, E. A. (2005). Introduction to methods in community-based participatory research. In B. A. Israel, E. Eng, A. J. Schulz, & E. A. Parker (Eds.), *Methods in community-based participatory research for health* (pp. 3–26). San Francisco: Jossey-Bass.

Israel, B. A., Schulz, A. J., Parker, E. A., & Becker, A. B. (1998). Review of community-based research: Assessing partnership approaches to improve public health. *Annual Review of Public Health, 19,* 173–202.

Jones, L., & Wells, K. (2007). Strategies for academic and clinician engagement in community-partnered participatory research. *Journal of the American Medical Association, 297,* 407–410.

Jordan, C., Lee, P., & Shapiro, E. (2000). Measuring developmental outcomes of lead exposure in an urban neighborhood: The challenges of community-based research. *Journal of Exposure Analysis and Environmental Epidemiology, 10,* 732–742.

Khanlou, N., & Peter, E. (2005). Participatory action research: Considerations for ethical review. *Social Science & Medicine, 60*(10), 2333–2340.

Krieger, J., Allen, C. A., Roberts, J. W., Ross, L. C., & Takaro, T. K. (2005). What's with the wheezing? Methods used by the Seattle-King County Healthy Homes Project to assess exposure to indoor asthma triggers. In B. A. Israel, E. Eng, A. J. Schulz,, & E. A. Parker (Eds.), *Methods in community-based participatory research for health* (pp. 230–250). San Francisco: Jossey-Bass.

Lynn, F. M. (2000). Community-scientist collaboration in environmental research. *American Behavioral Scientist, 44*(4), 649–663.

Macaulay, A. C., & Nutting, P. A. (2006). Moving the frontiers forward: Incorporating community-based participatory research into practice-based research networks. *Annals of Family Medicine, 4,* 4–7.

Maguire, P. (2006). Uneven ground: Feminisms and action research. In P. Reason & H. Bradbury (Eds.), *Handbook of action research: Participatory inquiry and practice* (Concise edition, pp. 60–70). Thousand Oaks, CA: Sage.

Minkler, M. (2000). Participatory action research and healthy communities. *Public Health Reports, 115,* 191–197.

Minkler, M. (2004). Ethical challenges for the "outside" researcher in community-based participatory research. *Health Education & Behavior, 31*(6), 684–697.

Minkler, M., & Breckwich Vásquez, V. (2004). Documenting the impacts of CBPR on healthy public policy. Unpublished raw data.

Minkler, M., Breckwich Vásquez, V., Chang, C., Blackwell, A. G., Thompson, M., and Rubin, V. (2008a). *Promoting healthy public policy through community-based participatory research.* Oakland, CA: PolicyLink.

Minkler, M., Breckwich Vásquez, V., Tajik, M., & Petersen, D. (2008b). Promoting environmental justice through community-based participatory research: The role of community and partnership capacity. *Health Education & Behavior, 35*(1), 119–137.

Morello-Frosch, R., Pastor, M., Porras, C., & Sadd, J. (2005). Environmental justice and regional inequality in Southern California: Implications for future research. In D. Brugge & H. P. Hynes (Eds.), *Community research in environmental health: Studies in science, advocacy and ethics* (pp. 205–218). Burlington, VT: Ashgate.

Mosavel, M., Simon, C., van Stade, D., & Buchbinder, M. (2005). Community-based participatory research (CBPR) in South Africa: Engaging multiple constituents to shape the research question. *Social Science & Medicine, 61,* 2577–2587.

Nyden, P., & Wiewel, W. (1992). Collaborative research: Harnessing the tensions between researcher and practitioner. *American Sociologist, 23*(4), 43–55.

O'Fallon, L. R., & Dearry, A. (2002). Community-based participatory research as a tool to advance environmental health sciences. *Environmental Health Perspectives, 110*(Suppl. 2), 155–159.

Patton, M. (2002). *Qualitative research and evaluation methods* (3rd ed.). Thousand Oaks, CA: Sage.

Petersen, D., Minkler, M., Breckwich Vásquez, V., & Baden, A. C. (2006). Community-based participatory research as a tool for policy change: A case study of the Southern California Environmental Justice Collaborative. *Review of Policy Research, 23*(2), 339–353.

Petersen, D., Minkler, M., Breckwich Vásquez, V., Kegler, M., Malcoe, L. H., & Whitecrow, S. (2007). Shaping policy to prevent lead exposure among Native American children: A case study in community-based participatory research. *Progress in Community Partnerships, 1*(3), 249–256.

Price, R. H., & Behrens, T. (2003). Working Pasteur's quadrant: Harnessing science and action for community change. *American Journal of Community Psychology, 31*(3–4), 219–223.

Reason, P., & Bradbury, H. (Eds.). (2006). *Handbook of action research: Participatory inquiry and practice* (Concise ed.). Thousand Oaks, CA: Sage.

Reason, P., & Bradbury, H. (Eds.). (2008). The SAGE *handbook of action research: Participatory inquiry and practice* (2nd ed.). Thousand Oaks, CA: Sage.

Roe, K. M., Minkler, M., & Saunders, F. F. (1995). Combining research, advocacy and education: The methods of the Grandparent Caregiver Study. *Health Education Quarterly, 22*(4), 458–475.

Schulz, A. J., Parker, E. A., Israel, B. A., Becker, A. B., Maciak, B. J., & Hollis, R. (1998). Conducting a participatory community-based survey for a community health intervention on Detroit's East Side. *Journal of Public Health Management and Practice, 4*(2), 10–24.

Schulz, A. J., Zenk, S. N., Kannan, S., Israel, B. A., Koch, M. A., & Stokes, C. A. (2005). CBPR approach to survey design and implementation. In B. A. Israel, E. Eng, A. J. Schulz, & E. A. Parker (Eds.), *Methods in community-based participatory research for health* (pp. 107–127). San Francisco: Jossey-Bass.

Schwab, M., & Syme, S. L. (1997). On paradigms, community participation, and the future of public health. *American Journal of Public Health, 87*(12), 2049–2052.

Shah, R. (2004). *A retrospective analysis of an HIV prevention program for men in Gujarat, India.* Unpublished manuscript, University of California, Berkeley, School of Public Health.

Sullivan, M., Chao, S. S., Allen, C. A., Koné, A., Pierre-Louis, M., & Krieger, J. (2003). Community-researcher partnerships: Perspectives from the field. In M. Minkler & N. Wallerstein (Eds.), *Community-based participatory research for health* (pp. 113–130). San Francisco: Jossey-Bass.

Tajik, M., & Minkler, M. (2007). Environmental justice research and action: A case study in political economy and community-academic collaboration. *International Quarterly of Community Health Education, 26*(3), 215–232.

Thompson, S. J. (2000). Participatory epidemiology: Methods of the Living with Diabetes Project. *International Quarterly of Community Health Education, 19*(1), 3–18.

Torres-Harding, S., Herrell, R., & Howard, C. (2004). Epidemiological research: Science and community participation. In L. Jason, C. B. Keys, Y. Suarez-Balcazar, R. R. Taylor, & M. I. Davis (Eds.), *Participatory community research: Theories and methods in action* (pp. 53–69).Washington, DC: American Psychological Association.

Viswanathan, M., Ammerman, A., Eng, E., Gartlehner, G., Lohr, K. N., Griffth, D., et al. (2004). *Community-based participatory research: Assessing the evidence* (Evidence Report/Technology Assessment No. 99; Prepared by RTI International-University of North Carolina). Rockville, MD: Agency for Healthcare Research and Quality.

Wallerstein, N. (1999). Power between evaluator and community: Research relationships within New Mexico's healthier communities. *Social Science & Medicine, 49*, 39–53.

Wallerstein, N., & Duran, B. (2006). Using community based participatory research to address health disparities. *Health Promotion Practice, 7*(3), 312–323.

Wallerstein, N., Duran, B., Aguilar, J., Belone Joe, L., Loretto, F., Padilla, R., et al. (2003). Jemez Pueblo: Built and social-cultural environments and health within a rural American Indian community in the Southwest. *American Journal of Public Health, 93*(9), 1517–1518.

Wells, K., & Norris, K. C. (Eds.). (2006). The Community Health Improvement Collaboration: Building community-academic partnerships to reduce disparities [entire issue]. *Ethnicity & Disease, 16*(1, Suppl. 1).

Wing, S. (2005). Social responsibility and research ethics in community-driven studies of industrialized hog production. In D. Brugge & H. P. Hynes (Eds.), *Community research in environmental health: Studies in science, advocacy and ethics* (pp. 245–261). Burlington, VT: Ashgate.

Wright, P., & Treacher, A. (1982). Introduction. In P. Wright & A. Treacher (Eds.), *The problem of medical knowledge: Examining the social construction of medicine* (pp. 1–22). Edinburgh: Edinburgh University Press.

15

METHODOLOGICAL AND ETHICAL CONSIDERATIONS IN COMMUNITY-DRIVEN ENVIRONMENTAL JUSTICE RESEARCH

TWO CASE STUDIES FROM RURAL NORTH CAROLINA

STEPHANIE ANN FARQUHAR & STEVE WING

INEQUALITIES IN HEALTH among gender, race, and class groups are generated by social institutions that create disparities in exposure to adequate nutrition, hazardous agents, safe living and working conditions, educational opportunities, and personal medical services. Because governments and corporations cannot be expected to eliminate these disparities without pressure from those who are adversely affected, environmental justice is not only about avoidance of harmful agents and access to basic services; it is also about the right of all people to participate as equal partners in policy and decision making, regardless of class, race, ethnicity, or national origin (Kuehn, 1996; U.S. Environmental Protection Agency, 1998). However, participation in democracy requires access to knowledge, including research, and most environmental health research has been conducted to investigate problems identified by governments, industries, health professionals, and the scientific community. In contrast, the communities that are most exposed to environmental hazards, especially low-income communities and communities of color, seldom have access to environmental researchers and have been underrepresented in the public health research professions (Corburn, 2004, 2005; Lynn, 2000; St. George, Schoenbach, Reynolds, Nwangwu, & Adams-Campbell, 1997).

Public health researchers and practitioners can play a critical role in ensuring meaningful participation of communities in research that informs environmental health decision making. During the past two decades, some environmental health research has united communities and researchers to challenge some of the basic assumptions of traditional research. Environmental studies informed by community-based principles of research can arise from mutually beneficial partnerships that define and address environmental health problems (Bhatia, 2007; Lynn, 2000; Israel, Schulz, Parker, & Becker, 1998). However, the actual application of the methods and principles of community-based participatory research (CBPR), as well as the definition of community participation, can vary among different researchers and public health disciplines (Israel et al., 1998). CBPR projects can also differ in terms of the roles of researchers and community residents (see Chapters Six and Fourteen), the goals and "products" of the research, the research methodology and data sources, and the targets of change (for example, pollution prevention and cleanup versus screening and self-protection).

Faber and McCarthy (2000) argue that researchers need to make visible the connections between environmental inequity, economic inequality, racism, and the lack of democracy. Research has the greatest potential to contribute to improved conditions for exposed populations when it is driven by community needs. Collaborative studies in Love Canal, New York, and Woburn, Massachusetts, are examples of community-academic partnerships that raised awareness and contributed to changes in public environmental policy (Brown & Mikkelsen, 1990; Levine, 1982; Shepard, 2000; Corburn, 2005).

However, it can be difficult for community members to become involved in the research process, especially where a community has a history of disempowerment and community members must expend most of their available time and energy on work and meeting basic needs. Moreover, involvement in efforts that challenge the status quo can inflict an emotional burden and fear for jobs, especially when local employers and politicians are the focus of the research. Participating in the research process can leave community partners feeling vulnerable, exposed, and open to criticism from neighbors and family members who do not support their efforts. This is especially true of those employees who are labeled *whistleblowers* for exposing improper practices or noncompliance with environmental regulations (Cwikel, 2006). Despite these challenges, it is important to consider the central and valuable role of community members in defining the research questions, informing data collection protocols, influencing the application of study results, and creating change (Bhatia, 2007; Cornwall & Jewkes, 1995; Gaventa, 1993).

This chapter explores these and other issues of CBPR through an examination of two community-based, participatory, public health projects initiated by residents of rural eastern North Carolina. Both projects provide examples of the collective efforts of community-academic partnerships that were organized to challenge environmental, social, and health disparities. The case studies involved different community members and researchers and used varying research methods, yet they faced similar obstacles and methodological dilemmas. Both depended on a history of effective community organizing and the existence of powerful community assets. The chapter concludes with a discussion of the similarities and differences of the projects, highlighting some of the universal challenges that many CBPR projects must address.

EASTERN NORTH CAROLINA SNAPSHOT

The eastern region of North Carolina is located in the "Black Belt," the area where most of this nation's rural African Americans reside. At the time the studies discussed here were conducted, approximately one out of four residents lived in poverty, and 44 percent were not served by a public sewer system (Eastern North Carolina Housing Summit, 1999). This area remains heavily affected by poverty, discrimination, and joblessness. With the rise of industrialized agriculture and the decline of independent family farmers, jobs in agriculture have declined dramatically and been replaced by low-paying factory jobs. These factories are notorious for unfair labor policies and antiunion sentiments (Le Duff, 1999). At the same time, land ownership, a significant building block for economically and socially stable African American communities, is diminishing, due in part to the growth of large agribusinesses (Edwards & Ladd, 2000; Tajik & Minkler, 2007) and discrimination in U.S. Department of Agriculture loan programs. One result of this lack of desirable jobs has been a sizable out-migration of working-age adults, leaving behind a large senior population.

In the face of these challenges, eastern rural North Carolina has for several decades successfully initiated local self-improvement efforts, including a farmers' cooperative, the region's first NAACP chapter, free health care clinics, and a nationally recognized prolabor union association (Minkler, 2000). The two case studies presented in this chapter describe the process and results that occurred when these community building blocks partnered with researchers from a public university to define and address community issues.

CASE 1: INDUSTRIALIZED HOG PRODUCTION

This case study was first recounted in Wing (2002).

Demographic Analysis of Disproportionate Exposure

Between the mid-1980s and the late 1990s, as the hog population of North Carolina expanded from under three million to approximately ten million, the number of hog-raising operations decreased as smaller independent family farmers were replaced by industrial-style operations (Furuseth, 1997). Expansion of industrial operations occurred under regulatory controls that were influenced by hog producers and other agribusiness interests in the North Carolina general assembly. State legislation was enacted to prevent local and county governments from rezoning agricultural land, and state universities closely allied with agribusiness concerns provided research support (Cecelski & Kerr, 1992; Tajik & Minkler, 2007).

As rural residents learned about industrialized hog production, many became deeply concerned about the impact of the industry on their communities. They worried about air pollution and noxious odors associated with the confinement of thousands of hogs and liquid waste management systems that included open fecal waste pits and spray fields. Noxious odors prevented some hog operation neighbors from enjoying their homes and the outdoors. Because odorant chemicals can penetrate clothing, curtains, and upholstery, they can affect people long after plumes of emissions pass, and may subject them to ostracism at school or in public. Hog operation neighbors, most of whom depended on groundwater, feared that their wells could be contaminated in an area with sandy soils and high water tables and that surface water pollution from spray-field runoff and lagoon failures would contaminate creeks and rivers. They were concerned about the loss of independent family farmers and the land that they had farmed and also about the vitality of their churches, schools, and communities. Residents also felt that they had been targeted for this kind of "economic development" because their primarily African American, low-income communities lacked political power (Wing, 2002; Wing, Grant, Green, & Stewart, 1996).

The Concerned Citizens of Tillery (CCT), a grassroots organization in southeastern Halifax County in eastern North Carolina, worked with county officials to develop an intensive livestock ordinance that would impose stricter environmental controls than state regulations. In that effort, and in the course of providing assistance to other communities in the path of corporate pork production, CCT sought support from environmentalists, social activists, and researchers who could help CCT to document economic, social, environmental, and public health issues affecting communities living near industrialized hog operations. Although university scientists had conducted many studies related to agricultural technologies, veterinary health, and the health of agricultural workers, relatively little research had addressed environmental, social, and health concerns of communities affected by industrial hog production. One of the studies that had been conducted suggested that hog odors affect the mental health of nearby residents (Schiffman, Miller, Suggs, & Graham, 1995). Another suggested that neighbors experience respiratory effects similar to those seen among workers (Thu et al., 1997). Consistent with the latter findings, mothers in eastern North Carolina reported that their asthmatic children experienced episodes of wheezing in the presence of strong plumes from nearby hog operations.

In 1996, a partnership formed by CCT with the Halifax County Health Department and the University of North Carolina (UNC) School of Public Health received funding from a National Institute of Environmental Health Sciences (NIEHS) program: Environmental Justice: Partnerships for Communication (Thu et al., 1997). Along with environmental justice education and outreach to communities and medical providers, the partnership was funded to conduct research that could quantify systematically, using official records, the extent to which hog operations were located disproportionately in low-income areas and communities of color (primarily African American) in North Carolina. Aims of the project were to evaluate data for local communities, to consider possible alternative explanations for observed patterns, and to examine data on household water sources and potential groundwater contamination. The partnership, originally known as Southeast Halifax Environmental Reawakening, was later renamed Community Health and Environmental Reawakening (CHER), to reflect its statewide work (Wing, 2002).

In 1998, the CHER partnership obtained a list of all industrial livestock operations permitted by the North Carolina Division of Water Quality. Following intensive efforts to evaluate errors in these data and make corrections, the partnership's epidemiologist members linked information on the locations and sizes of industrial hog operations to data for U.S. Census Bureau block groups, areas that average about five hundred households. They compared the prevalence of operations in whiter and wealthier communities with the prevalence in poorer and more nonwhite areas. Because rural areas are often poor and nonwhite, and agricultural operations by definition take place in rural areas, the investigators recognized that findings of disparate impact might be dismissed by industry and government as reflecting merely the demographics of rural areas. They therefore developed a statistical model to adjust for population density in their comparisons of areas with different racial and income characteristics (Wing, Cole, & Grant, 2000).

Although the data analysis was undertaken at the university, the study questions originated in the exposed communities. Community members participated in evaluating data quality through their knowledge of local hog operations. Decisions about how to define the study population and data sources, choose and define variables for the analysis, and interpret results were made in consultation with community partners; researchers and community members became both teachers and learners (Israel, Checkoway, Schulz, & Zimmerman, 1994). The university-based researchers augmented their statistical analyses with maps and charts. They found that hog operations were far more common in low-income communities and communities of color, that this concentration was more extreme for hog operations owned or operated by large corporations than for independent operations, and that the pattern was only partly explained by differences in population density. Furthermore, they found that hog operations were concentrated in areas where most people depend on household wells for drinking water (Wing et al., 2000).

University and community partners issued a press release about the research findings, in conjunction with a presentation they made at a national meeting. The release was coordinated by the UNC News Service, which routinely prepares stories about topical research, and several major state newspapers ran stories on the findings, some including interviews with community members. The CHER partnership was invited to present the findings before the North Carolina general assembly's agriculture committee, and the study was considered in a policy paper prepared by the governor's office on the future of the hog industry.

The Quantification of Health Effects

In addition to the environmental justice study, the CHER partnership conducted more traditional health effects research. In the fall of 1998, with support from the North Carolina State Health Department, the partnership initiated a survey of rural residents in eastern North Carolina. Reports of odor problems and respiratory effects had been coming in from hog operation neighbors across eastern North Carolina, and the health department was interested in obtaining more information. In consultation with community members and staff from the health department, the CHER partnership designed a survey to compare the health and quality of life among residents of three communities, one in the neighborhood of a hog operation, one in the neighborhood of a cattle operation, and one with no intensive livestock production.

A number of challenges arose in designing the study. The earlier environmental justice analyses had confirmed the observations made by community members that industrial hog operations were disproportionately located in low-income and African American communities. Members of the research partnership would need to ask for the participation of people whose previous experiences of discrimination led them to distrust health departments, medical providers, universities, and researchers. Strong relationships with community-based organizations established through the CHER partnership would be essential for collecting reliable data and establishing a high response rate from defined populations in the three areas. At the same time, the research partnership knew the potential biases that could be introduced in areas divided between those with negative feelings about the hog industry and those whose livelihood depended on the industry. To collect valid data, they would need to insulate the data collection process from peer pressure or leading questioning. As in all environmental epidemiology, the power of the study to detect real effects would be weakened by lack of good measurements of exposures and outcomes. Members of the partnership debated whether it would be ethical to conduct a study if they could not measure exposures and outcomes sufficiently well to detect a health effect if one existed, recognizing that the study design would be constrained by the level of funding that the state health department could provide. The decision to proceed was influenced by the evidence from previous studies and by community members and state officials who felt there was an urgent need for respiratory health data from North Carolina (Wing, 2002).

Health Survey Design and Administration

CHER partners developed a structured symptom questionnaire, basing their work on previous studies and input from eastern North Carolina residents, who helped them develop a culturally appropriate survey instrument. The study used the same questions in each of the three communities; there were no questions about odor, hogs, or livestock because one community had no livestock. The three communities were chosen so that they had similar demographic characteristics according to Census data. In each community, occupied dwellings were enumerated on a map and assigned a random identifying number (Wing & Wolf, 2000).

The partnership collaborated with a community-based organization in each area. Community members helped researchers locate roads and houses, and they served as community consultants during the data collection. Trained interviewers from UNC visited households in each area accompanied by a community consultant who made the initial introduction of the interviewer. Interviews were conducted without the presence of the community consultant unless the participant requested that the consultant remain. The interviewer provided each study participant with a copy of an "agreement to participate" that explained that the study was about environmental exposures and the health of rural residents, and the interviewer also read the agreement aloud. Participants were assured that their responses would be kept confidential and that their names would not be written on their questionnaires, although a link would be maintained between their address and their responses. UNC's institutional review board gave permission to obtain only oral consent because there were no interventions or sensitive questions involved.

Households nearest to the livestock operations were visited first. The interviewing teams then visited households in order, moving away from the livestock operations until the target sample size of fifty was reached. One adult in each household was interviewed in January and February 1999. Over 150 interviews were completed, with a refusal rate of just 14 percent. Respondents were 92 percent African American, 65 percent female, and 27 percent aged sixty-five or over (Wing & Wolf, 2000).

In keeping with a core principle of CBPR—returning research findings to the community (Cornwall & Jewkes, 1995; Gaventa, 1993; see also Chapter Three), the CHER team invited members of the three community-based organizations to a meeting to discuss the initial findings of the research prior to submitting the report to the state health department. Input from community members was obtained, and the university partners responded to community members' concerns about excesses of respiratory and digestive symptoms that had been reported by hog operation neighbors compared to residents of the other communities. Community members decided at this meeting that they did not want the names of their communities to be included in the report. Respecting and responding to this feedback, researchers removed from the report data on numbers of households, population size, race, and income characteristics of the census block groups in the study, along with information about the exact size of the hog and cattle operations.

State Reaction to Survey Results

A draft report was submitted to the state health department, presenting analyses that showed that the frequency of miscellaneous symptoms such as muscle aches and vision and hearing problems was similar in the three communities. In contrast, residents near the hog operations reported increased numbers of headaches, runny noses, and sore throats and increased incidence of excessive coughing, diarrhea, and burning eyes. These residents also reported many more occasions when they could not open windows or go outside, even in nice weather. The report was reviewed by health department staff, the chief statistician for the State Center for Health Statistics, the chair of the UNC Department of Epidemiology, and others, and the final report incorporated their comments.

The state health department issued a press statement releasing the study's report to the public on May 7, 1999. Later that day, attorneys for the North Carolina Pork Council wrote to the university members of the research partnership, demanding that they "make available for copying by this office any and all documentation in your possession (or that you are aware of in the possession of other State agencies or State personnel) that contain, represent, record, document, discuss, or otherwise reflect or memorialize the results of the Study."

The Pork Council request raised a number of ethical concerns, including the protection of the confidentiality of participants. In order to evaluate the quality, internal consistency, and analytical methods in the study, the industry would need to be able to conduct an independent reanalysis. However, although participants' names were not recorded, maps of the locations of their homes were linked to their responses. Even without the maps the information about participants—including age, race, sex, occupation, industry, number in household, water source, and health status—was sufficient to deductively disclose which individuals in these sparsely populated rural communities were in the study.

Breach of confidentiality was a concern not only from a legal and ethical standpoint. The community trust on which the CHER partnership depended would be seriously compromised, potentially destroying valued professional and personal relationships and threatening the continuation of research into the exposures and health of neighbors of industrial swine operations. In addition, the need for protection of confidentiality would have to be considered in relation to a scientific culture in which reanalysis is essential and in relation to power inequalities between industry and the exposed communities.

The state's public records statute required release of the research documents, which were the property of the university, not of the researchers who conducted the study. After much consultation and legal deliberation, the university and CHER researchers released records to the Pork Council, including computerized files of individual responses, interviewer training instructions, draft copies of the report, other statistical tabulations, and study-related correspondence, including electronic mail messages of project staff. To protect confidentiality of the participants and the communities, however, information that could lead to disclosure of where the study was done—including maps, driving instructions, phone records, travel records, and names of persons that would identify locations in the study—were withheld from the Pork Council. This was done under the assumption that individuals could not be identified from information in the survey unless the locations of the survey were known (Wing, 2002).

In the years since the Pork Council took legal action to acquire analytical data sets, CHER investigators have not learned of any published refutations or reanalyses of the health survey data. During the same time period, community members and researchers have used the study to help draw attention to public health concerns associated with industrial hog production. Results of the health survey have been considered by health departments, the U.S. Environmental Protection Agency's National Environmental Justice Advisory Council, and the U.S. Department of Agriculture and have supported applications for the funding of additional research on environmental exposures resulting from industrial hog operations and the biological effects of these exposures. In addition, plaintiffs in civil suits against industrial hog operations have cited the health study as evidence of the impact of these facilities on the health and quality of life of neighbors.

In 2007, the North Carolina Environmental Justice Network (NCEJN), which CCT had played a key role in organizing, in turn helped form a coalition of grassroots environmental justice groups and progressive environmental organizations to advocate for a ban on the lagoon and spray-field technology, as the first step toward complete elimination of this form of waste management. To support public education and organizing, NCEJN also produced a digital video, "The Rest of the Story: Corporate Hog Farming in NC," in which community members powerfully tell the stories of the impact that living near the hog factories has had on their lives (Muhammad, 2007, p. 13). Copies were distributed to the state legislators, who also witnessed a hog rally and a fifty-one-hour vigil held at the state capitol in June 2007. Model hog operations were erected, complete with ceramic pigs and two pools filled with forty gallons of hog waste. Together with the rigorous research described above, the work of the coalition helped get a bill passed and signed by the governor in late summer 2007, banning any new hog factories.

Yet the struggle is far from over. Thousands of industrial hog operations in North Carolina continue to threaten the health, quality of life, and independence of low-income rural communities in the eastern part of the state. Between 1997 and 2007, hundreds of thousands of hogs were added to the herd under permits that were approved before the "moratorium" on new facilities that was first adopted in 1997. Despite the permanent ban on new waste lagoons adopted in 2007, the struggle to reduce pollution and malodor from industrial hog production in North Carolina continues.

As this case study and its continuing legacy suggest, the role of community members in defining the research questions and informing data collection and application is a vital component of CBPR. However, as this case also illustrates, ethical, legal, and personal dilemmas may arise for both the researchers and the community members engaged in community-academic research partnerships.

CASE 2: DISCRIMINATION IN DISASTER RELIEF

The context of this second case study—Hurricane Floyd, which hit North Carolina in 1999—quickly brings to mind another, more recent social, environmental, and public health disaster, to which it offers some important parallels: Hurricane Katrina and its aftermath of human suffering, social and environmental devastation, and government neglect and mismanagement. The impact of Hurricane Katrina on Gulf Coast communities in August of 2005 and well beyond is indeed emblematic of the destructive effects of environmental devastation on communities already burdened with social, economic, and environmental challenges (Quinn, 2006). Natural disasters such as Hurricane Katrina exacerbate existing conditions of poverty and threaten health; such disasters also tend to exclude the most marginalized and heavily affected populations from any research and decision making around the recovery and revitalization of their communities (Brodie, Weltzien, Altman, Blendon, & Benson, 2006). Predominantly African American residents of New Orleans were abandoned and even attacked by government authorities as they struggled to survive and escape the flooding of their city. Post-Katrina movements for popular democracy, environmental protection, and human rights in New Orleans are characteristic of the role that community-led coalitions can play in improving public health (Quinn, 2006). As noted in the case study that follows, community-based participatory research also can play a useful role in such efforts, enabling some of those most affected by a natural disaster and its aftermath to help shape and determine the questions that are asked, share in the data gathering and interpretation, and disseminate and use the findings to bring about change.

Hurricane Floyd and Intensified Community Challenges

On September 16, 1999, Hurricane Floyd hit rural eastern North Carolina. In its destructive path it left 7,000 homes destroyed, 17,000 homes uninhabitable, and more than 47,000 residents in public shelters (Segrest, 1999). This area of North Carolina, suffering from racial discrimination, poverty, unemployment, and inadequate housing (Segrest, 1999), is also highly segregated, with the communities most affected by Floyd and the ensuing floodwaters being predominantly African American. The historic town of Princeville, for example, one of the most heavily damaged communities, is the oldest incorporated all-black town in the United States and was founded by former slaves after the Civil War.

The flooding forced thousands of rural eastern North Carolina residents out of their homes and into temporary housing sites located in several counties. These sites, consisting largely of trailers and mobile homes, were established and maintained by the Federal Emergency Management Agency (FEMA) and state and local government agencies and organizations. Despite the initial response and assistance from citizens and charitable organizations, the long-term recovery efforts carried out by local, state, and federal governments were inadequate. Two years after the flooding, more than one thousand citizens were still without permanent housing. Nearly all these displaced citizens were African American residents who had been turned down for financial assistance, had received misinformation about opportunities for recovery aid, and had been unable to secure affordable and decent housing due to a dearth of rental units (Lindenfeld, 2001). Like the survivors of Hurricane Katrina in 2005, the survivors of Hurricane Floyd were largely excluded from influencing local and state decisions about community recovery efforts and the allocation of recovery funds. This exclusion intensified their feelings of being vulnerable, discriminated against, and disempowered. A similar analysis by Fothergill, Maestas, and Darlington DeRouen (1999) documented differences in disaster experiences between racial and ethnic groups and found that compared to majority populations, communities of color typically endure longer recoveries from natural disasters, have more limited access to insurance, and use aid and relief organizations differently.

In an effort to create conditions in which the survivors of Hurricane Floyd could be empowered and to unify the survivors in the struggle for social and environmental equity, a coalition of local organizations was formed. The Workers and Community Relief and Aid Project (RAP) comprised flood survivors and partners from its member organizations, which included Black Workers for Justice (BWFJ), North Carolina Fair Share, North Carolina Low Income Housing, Concerned Citizens of Tillery, and the North Carolina Student Rural Health Coalition. From its inception, RAP conducted meetings at the temporary housing sites and encouraged survivors to contribute to the development and implementation of RAP's mandate and action plan. Although the process of mobilizing the survivors and partner organizations was not without its challenges, the usually slow and laborious process of developing a partnership of multiple individuals and organizations was accelerated. RAP was focused on the survivors' immediate and urgent recovery needs—such as dealing with health threats and substandard housing—which demanded swift organizing and decision making. As noted earlier, the process of issue selection provides an opportunity for the participatory action research team to reflect and make decisions as a group. Throughout the process, the partnership attempted to balance the more immediate concerns (for example, pushing back FEMA deadlines) with the more fundamental issues of discrimination and inequity.

RAP benefited from the long history of successful community-academic partnerships formed through CHER. Because of CHER, a new public health researcher, Stephanie Ann Farquhar, from the University of North Carolina, was relatively quickly embraced by RAP. As discussed in earlier chapters, all CBPR projects must establish trust and address any past injustices between university and community to create successful partnerships. The extensive history of community organizing in eastern North Carolina helped RAP member organizations to bring together disparate groups, including university researchers, to address a common goal of disaster recovery in the context of larger struggles for social justice.

RAP collaborated with university researchers on two projects. One uncovered state records showing that hundreds of African American flood survivors had been relocated, without their knowledge, on an industrial coal ash landfill. The second documented experiences and needs of hundreds of survivors, highlighting cases of discrimination by local and state agency representatives. Both projects were initiated based on input from the flood survivors. These projects followed the fundamental CBPR principle that says "start where the people are" (Nyswander, 1967), thus ensuring greater participation, project success, and the sustainability of the partnership.

Unearthing State Landfill Data

In March 2000, Saladin Muhammad, a member of RAP and BWFJ, spoke about environmental injustice and the 1999 floods in North Carolina in a new environmental justice class initiated by students at the UNC School of Public Health (Wing, 2000). He described a broad range of problems in disaster response in an area with a history of racial discrimination and economic underdevelopment, including deplorable environmental conditions and dehumanizing treatment at Fountain Industrial Park, a temporary housing site in Edgecombe County established by local, state, and federal officials. At the time, the Fountain site, nicknamed Camp Depression, included 207 travel trailers and 64 mobile homes, inhabited largely by residents of Princeville. Muhammad reported that residents and other community members were concerned that the temporary housing facility had been constructed on top of a landfill. Sooty material was evident around some of the trailers and mobile homes, and large mounds of material, some covered with grass and others looking like fresh ash, were near a playground and a pond where some residents fished.

A student in the class took on the task of finding documentation on the history of the site and the site's potential risks. Despite his access to telephones, libraries, the Internet, and other university resources that were not available to Camp Depression residents, this student had difficulty obtaining information from county and state officials. After initially being denied copies of public documents by the North Carolina Division of Emergency Management (in violation of the same state public records act invoked by the North Carolina Pork Council in the previous case study), he obtained site records and reports with the assistance of UNC faculty and state officials. These documents confirmed that the flood survivors had been relocated on an industrial coal ash landfill that had been in use up to the day of the hurricane and had not been tested or closed according to EPA standards required for coal ash to be used as fill material for housing. The student summarized the published information on health hazards present in coal ash, including arsenic, chromium 6, lead, mercury, cadmium, barium, and thallium. Following a presentation of his findings at Camp Depression, RAP held a press conference that was covered by local media, the North Carolina State Health Department arranged for soil testing and coverage of exposed coal ash with a layer of soil, and the pace of finding alternative housing for site residents was accelerated.

This was a mixed victory. Even though environmental sample results indicated that contaminants were not above actionable levels, officials had clearly failed to inform survivors about the landfill prior to relocation, denying survivors the "human right to make a conscious decision about placing their lives in another potentially dangerous situation" ("Environmental Racism," 2000). Moreover, despite the fact that the residents were all African American, state officials denied that any issue of environmental racism was involved. Finally, the new site where many residents were offered housing presented other hazards: it was an area that had flooded badly in the rains following Hurricane Floyd, and the only entrance required passing over a railroad crossing with no protections.

Although the victory was a partial one, it was very important, and achieving it clearly required the collaboration and shared resources of the community and the university. The university partners had contacts in state government and were knowledgeable about the public records statute and citizens' rights to view government documents. More important, and unlike recipients of agency assistance, university partners did not have to be concerned that their research would jeopardize their own financial or housing aid. Equally critical, however, the survivors and members of local organizations possessed important historical knowledge of the area, were familiar with local key players, and provided poignant accounts of the offensive and potentially harmful dust and odors. Working in partnership, the coalition successfully collected and applied the data necessary to raise awareness and demand action.

Combining Strengths to Document Discrimination and Need

One year after Hurricane Floyd, many flood survivors were still without permanent housing and unhappy with the flood recovery process. Through CHER, RAP organizations enlisted the help of Farquhar, who began attending bimonthly RAP meetings convened at a temporary housing site. During the meetings, survivors voiced their concerns and shared individual stories of discriminatory treatment by local and state government agencies, unmet needs, and great frustration with the recovery process to date. At the next several meetings, RAP members and their university partner discussed and reached consensus on the benefits of collecting and releasing survey data and survey objectives. Their shared goals were (1) to systematically document the survivors' experiences of relocation, living conditions, and potential threats to health and loss of community as a result of the flooding; (2) to begin to mobilize the survivors for action; and (3) to give the survivors a voice. The group also reached agreement on the content of and intended audience for a final report that would be released at a flood survivor summit.

A few participating community members, however, expressed some concern about their involvement with RAP. Some survivors worried that their financial or medical benefits might be reduced or discontinued by agencies whose recovery efforts were identified as substandard. Others were concerned about being labeled "moles" by fellow survivors who were suspicious of their involvement with RAP's community organizations and its university partner. RAP was mostly successful in assuring flood survivors that their affiliation with RAP would not threaten their benefits, as they would not be identified in the report or in RAP's organizational records. Further, since RAP was composed largely of local grassroots organizations and was established on the basis of survivors' expressed needs for organization and representation, few survivors perceived RAP as a threatening or exclusive organization. This accurate perception of RAP as "for the survivors and of the survivors" reduced concerns that affiliation would lead to ostracism by others.

RAP committed several meetings to focusing on the primary objectives of the flood survivor survey report. During these meetings, flood survivors struggled with research concepts such as statistics, scientific validity, confidentiality, and data analysis methods. The university partner shared knowledge and skills through discussion, interviewer training, and examples of past research projects. Similarly, community members shared information about their social norms, vernacular (such as use of the term *FEMAvilles* in reference to temporary housing sites set up in the aftermath of Hurricane Floyd), and past experiences with researchers and health agencies that were especially useful when thinking through the details of the survey instrument and protocol. Valuing and using community expertise early in the project clearly contributed to a more successful partnership (Northridge et al., 2000; see also Chapter Fourteen).

Yet attending to community issues and concerns can slow any process (Green & Mercer, 2001), and all members of the research team must have the patience to enable needed dialogue about areas of conflict. There were several instances, for example, in which the university partner and other members of RAP disagreed with regard to survey design and administration. For example, some community members were reluctant to ask interviewers to read the informed consent paragraphs and to require interviewers to read questions exactly as written. Some RAP members considered these procedures too formal and "scientific" and felt that they distracted from the community orientation of the survey. During numerous discussions the university partner talked about the need to be prepared to defend the data from those who would question their scientific validity. In each of these instances, the challenge for the researcher was to work with community members to frame questions and to design procedures that respected community concerns while at the same time investigating them with the best technical approaches possible. The university partner explained that such investigations are useful to communities burdened by environmental problems because they can address topics that cannot be examined without the technical resources of institutions, and that the investigation findings can be used in situations where community observations are not highly valued. Rather than facing a conflict between standard academic research procedures and alternatives that are acceptable to the community but viewed as *unscientific* by scientists, both researchers and community members can benefit from negotiating the use of rigorous methods. A healthy partnership should encourage discussion of concerns and alternative points of view (Northridge et al., 2000). Furthermore, as discussed in Chapter Three, the processes and products of CBPR develop through the mutual engagement and influence of all members (academics, community partners, health department personnel, service agency staff) of a partnership. Such collaborative and engaged efforts are more likely to contribute to the sustained viability of an empowered and capable community than are traditional research approaches (Israel et al., 1998).

Survey Design and Administration

Flood survivors and members of RAP visited temporary housing sites to describe the purpose of the survey and ask survivors for their ideas on questions to include in the survey. Survey items generated during this process were categorized under the following general headings: flooding experience, housing situation, health status, children's well-being, finances and employment, environmental threats, interactions with agencies, and hopes for the future. For example, survivors were asked, "Has the flood affected your children's health?" and, "Do you think community citizens should participate in decision making during an emergency situation such as this?" RAP's university partner formatted the survey according to general category themes and used the survivors' language. Only a few survey items had to be reworded, as they were either leading or double-barreled. For example, one item was originally worded, "Are you unhappy living here and would you move to a house permanently?" Following dialogue about the importance of asking only one question per survey item, the question was reworded, "Would you like to move into permanent housing?" Members of RAP reviewed the revised survey, and after minor modifications, the instrument was approved. A draft of the survey and a description of the survey protocol were submitted to and approved by UNC's institutional review board (IRB). The IRB process presented an ideal opportunity for helping community members and survivors to better understand the research process and for again emphasizing the importance of confidentiality, informed consent, and voluntary participation.

Several RAP partners agreed to serve on a survey subcommittee that was responsible for designing and conducting the survey interviewer training. Two survivors from each site were invited to participate in all-day interviewer training. The training included a module that described survey methodology and issues of data reliability and validity. In an effort to increase the proportion of completed surveys, the trained interviewers surveyed survivors residing at the interviewers' own sites, where they were familiar with the survivors and their daily schedules.

Despite such training, some obstacles to data collection remained. One challenging aspect of participatory research, for example, is the difficulty in tracking attempted versus completed interviews. The survey interviewers did not consistently record refusals, not-at-homes, passive refusals, and so on, making it difficult to calculate an overall response rate.

Survey data collection lasted approximately three weeks, during which 270 surveys were completed from ten temporary housing sites located in six counties. The partnership determined that RAP's university partner would analyze the data, as she had the time and experience to conduct a quick turnaround and produce a summary report. Survey items had required the respondent to answer yes or no, after which the interviewer invited the survivor to elaborate, using his or her own words. This format required both qualitative and quantitative methods of analysis, allowing data to be presented either in words or in numbers, as appropriate (Denzin & Lincoln, 1994). Early in the survey meetings, RAP partners recognized that different audiences respond to different forms of information delivery. For example, the media and emergency service representatives might be more affected by the survivors' words, and those who are writing policy might require numbers and percentages. Furthermore, the use of multiple methods can also increase the validity of the study's conclusions and the range of information collected (Livingood, Goldhagen, Little, Gornto, & Hou, 2007; Cook & Reichardt, 1979; Steckler, McLeroy, Goodman, Bird, & McCormick, 1992).

Survey results were tested for validity through a series of member checks (Patton, 1990), during which survey data were summarized and shared with more than seventy survivors. As noted earlier, bringing the data back to the community is an important step in the CBPR process and one that encourages community ownership and control of the data. Although the overall feedback was positive, a few flood survivors said that they felt "lumped together" with all the other survivors and that this process of data summary ignored individual experiences. A final survey report and subsequent presentations were modified to acknowledge that the flood survivors are not a homogeneous group but rather many unique individuals. The next section presents some of the findings included in the survey report.

Preliminary Survey Results

Immediately after the flooding, many of the survivors were forced to seek shelter in motels, with relatives, or in local schools. Survivors who spent anywhere from one day to several weeks in a shelter were dissatisfied with the accommodations, describing them as "overcrowded," "hectic," and lacking privacy. Some survivors felt that the first cases of discriminatory relief and aid occurred at the shelters. As one survivor reported, "My family stayed [in the shelter] for three days. Blacks stayed at school on floors and blankets that they brought in the carts. Whites stayed in Hope House Plantation, a historical site."

Survey results indicated that almost 50 percent ($n = 119$) of the survivors were unable to find affordable housing in their communities or neighborhoods and that 110 survivors were turned down for housing loans or rentals because of poor credit histories or low income. Many survivors described the cost of housing and rentals as a major barrier to finding permanent housing, noting that "since the flood, all the realtors and landlords have been allowed to raise their rent," and, "I don't make enough to afford these high-price apartments." Survivors also reported encountering multiple structural and administrative barriers to finding housing, such as complicated paperwork and restrictive eligibility criteria.

After the flooding, over one-third ($n = 96$) of the survivors reported that their health declined. Health problems associated with stress and living conditions included a decrease in appetite, depression, crying spells, loss of sleep, nightmares, worry, panic attacks, arthritis, chest pains, headaches, and stomachaches. Many survivors reported suffering from serious respiratory, sinus, and breathing problems related to exposure to mold, mildew, and wetness.

Eighty-six of the survivors reported that the flooding damaged their community's church or school. "Both the church and the school [were destroyed]. The church is being rebuilt. The school is operating. It's torn apart our neighbors." The collapse of pivotal community structures, such as schools and churches, is devastating beyond the physical and structural loss. As Eng (1993) has noted, for example, the church is a unit of identity, affirmation, and solution in African American communities, so the loss of a church structure may consequently be experienced on several levels. The loss of meeting places and familiar sites can similarly result in a loss of personal identity and a decreased sense of community cohesion (Chavis & Wandersman, 1990). Familiarity and community were also frequently cited as reasons why survivors chose not to relocate outside of their communities.

Dissemination of Survey Report

These and other findings were included in a ten-page report that communicated the experiences and perspectives of the flood survivors. RAP partners spent several meetings discussing how to apply these findings to create broader structural and systemic change at the local and state levels. It was agreed that the data should be presented in several different formats and to a variety of audiences. RAP members, including flood survivors, attended rallies and visited North Carolina legislators to advocate for the fair treatment of all flood survivors as they struggled to restore their lives. RAP members also met with the North Carolina budget director and the senior policy adviser of the North Carolina Department of Commerce and with representatives of North Carolina Low Income Housing, North Carolina Fair Share, and other organizations to argue for the rebuilding of affordable low-income housing. Results from the survey were useful during these meetings to inform state-level decision makers of the flood survivors' needs and the inadequacies of the state's response. The experiences that survivors had gained by participating in research helped them better communicate their own concerns and needs and tell the stories of other survivors.

Survey results were also presented, using slides and interview excerpts, to an audience of flood survivors, grassroots organizations, and agency representatives at the Hurricane Floyd Survivors' Summit. RAP organized and sponsored the summit at a local conference center with the goals of uniting the voices of the hundreds of flood survivors throughout North Carolina and planning a common agenda for unity and empowerment. To encourage coverage by the local news and print media, RAP partners worked together to create and widely circulate a press release. Several local newspapers and television and radio stations covered the summit. As a result of this coverage the director of the state emergency management division was pushed to respond publicly and to grant survivors six additional months beyond the original deadline to remain at the temporary sites and to locate permanent housing.

Some academics are reluctant to interact with the media. Researchers may feel that their findings will be misrepresented and misunderstood, and interviews take considerable time and have little potential to influence scientific publications or grant funding, the criteria that matter most for career advancement. However, researchers working in partnership with communities have responsibilities in this area: making scientific findings public in appropriate ways and participating in processes involving the media and policymakers (Sandman, 1991). Mass media campaigns and targeted media advocacy have the potential to reframe health and social issues, set policy agendas, and influence funding priorities (Wallack, 2005; Dorfman & Wallack, 2007). Environmental health findings presented via mainstream media channels can protect exposed community members, motivate participation in democratic processes, and influence public opinion and policymakers.

Progress and Continued Problems

In the eight years since this second case study took place, several longer-term outcomes and by-products have emerged. RAP did not sustain as an organization, but some of its members transferred skills that they refined during these projects to other community-building and community-organizing efforts. For example, one woman who was an effective community leader and organizer prior to joining RAP applied the research skills she developed through the project to her work with other environmental justice efforts in North Carolina. The academic partner gained a deeper appreciation for the importance of scientific rigor and its potential to inform policymaking during her work with RAP. The skills gained during this experience continue to inform her work as a researcher with indigenous migrant farmworkers in Oregon, a population that is burdened with pesticide exposures and other occupational hazards. Finally, despite efforts to gain the support of some of the state's black legislators, at least one all-black community that sustained extensive water damage during the flooding never received adequate financial assistance.

SUMMARY

The two case studies presented in this chapter differ from each other in several important respects. Although both cases involved community-driven research partnerships, the industrial hog operation studies were more quantitative and used multivariate statistical analyses and principles of experimental design in order to compare exposed and unexposed groups. Trained university interviewers were employed in the rural health survey in order to standardize comparisons between communities. In contrast, the RAP study relied more heavily on narratives and qualitative methods to create a portrait of the flood survivors' situation. RAP determined that those individuals who were most affected by Hurricane Floyd—the flood survivors themselves—would be the most appropriate persons to collect and help analyze the data. Finally, whereas the rural health survey examined, more specifically, health and quality of life in relation to livestock operations, the RAP study examined, more broadly, the consequences of the displacement and mistreatment of people and people's associated basic needs.

Despite these differences, however, each case study illustrates the vulnerability of both researchers and communities to the agendas of politicians and decision makers. The research partnerships provide examples of the potential power such collaborative endeavors have to influence political decision making and practice related to the public's health and well-being. Furthermore, both research partnerships faced ethical dilemmas and worked with their communities to identify potential solutions.

Of central importance to both studies was what Randy Stoecker (in Chapter Six) describes as "the haunting question of how I, as an academic, can become relevant." Public health researchers have the opportunity, and the social responsibility, to be relevant by using their skills, wherever possible, to promote public health through democracy and social justice. Although many scientists remain unaware of or disinterested in the social construction of science, no research question, method, or result can be separated from its social context. Meaningful and influential community involvement in research studies can help public health researchers to address the structural and power issues that perpetuate inequity (Wing, 2001; Farquhar, Patel, & Chidsey, 2007). More objective research—whether in support of democratic social change or commercial interests—can be achieved by relentlessly analyzing and revealing a study's policy and advocacy dimensions (Wing, 1998).

QUESTIONS FOR DISCUSSION

1. This chapter presents some of the ethical considerations that may arise in doing research with communities. Can you identify additional ethical considerations in CBPR that were not mentioned?

2. Sometimes a researcher is asked by a community group to help determine the presence of environmental exposure or of an elevated rate of disease when she or he strongly suspects that none exists. If you were in this position, how might you proceed? And how might your decision harm or benefit the community?

3. Discuss one of the two case studies presented, and consider additional policy implications of the research results. How could the CBPR participants apply the study findings to broader social and policy change?

REFERENCES

Bhatia, R. (2007). Protecting health using an environmental impact assessment: A case study of San Francisco land use decision making. *American Journal of Public Health, 97*(3), 406–413.

Brodie, M., Weltzien, E., Altman, D., Blendon, R. J., & Benson, J. M. (2006). Experiences of Hurricane Katrina evacuees in Houston shelters: Implications for future planning. *American Journal of Public Health, 96*(8), 1402–1408.

Brown, P., & Mikkelsen, E. J. (1990). *No safe place: Toxic waste, leukemia, and community action.* Berkeley: University of California Press.

Cecelski, D., & Kerr, M. L. (1992, February). Hog wild. *Southern Exposure,* pp. 9–15.

Chavis, D. M., & Wandersman, A. (1990). Sense of community in the urban environment: A catalyst for participation and community development. *American Journal of Community Psychology, 18,* 55–81.

Cook, T. D., & Reichardt, C. S. (Eds.). (1979). *Qualitative and quantitative methods in evaluation research.* Thousand Oaks, CA: Sage.

Corburn, J. (2004). Confronting the challenges in reconnecting urban planning and public health. *American Journal of Public Health, 94*(4), 541–546.

Corburn, J. (2005). *Street science: Community knowledge and environmental health justice.* Cambridge, MA: MIT Press.

Cornwall, A., & Jewkes, R. (1995). What is participatory research? *Social Science & Medicine, 41,* 1667–1676.

Cwikel, J. (2006). *Social epidemiology: Strategies for public health activism.* New York: Columbia University Press.

Denzin, N. K., & Lincoln, Y. S. (Eds.). (1994). *Handbook of qualitative research.* Thousand Oaks, CA: Sage.

Dorfman, L., & Wallack, L. (2007). Moving nutrition upstream: The case for reframing obesity. *Journal of Nutrition Education and Behavior, 39*(2, Suppl.), S45–S50.

Eastern North Carolina Housing Summit. (1999, April). *The state of housing in eastern North Carolina: Final report.* New Bern: Eastern North Carolina Sustainable Community Economic Development Center.

Edwards, B., & Ladd, A. (2000). Environmental justice, swine production and farm loss in North Carolina. *Sociological Spectrum, 20,* 263–290.

Eng, E. (1993). The Save Our Sisters project. A social network strategy for reaching rural black women. *Cancer, 72*(3, Suppl.), 1071–1077.

Environmental racism at FEMA camp. (2000, August-September). *Justice Speaks,* p. 6.

Faber, D. R., & McCarthy, D. (2000). *A different shade of green: A report on philanthropy and the environmental justice movement in the United States.* Washington, DC: Aspen Institute.

Farquhar, S., Patel, N., & Chidsey, M. (2007). Preventing injustices in environmental health and exposures. In L. Cohen, V. Chávez, & S. Chehimi (Eds.), Prevention is primary: *Strategies for community well-being* (pp. 235–256). San Francisco: Jossey-Bass.

Fothergill, A., Maestas, E., & Darlington DeRouen, J. (1999). Race, ethnicity and disasters in the United States: A review of the literature. *Disasters, 23*(2), 156–173.

Furuseth, O. (1997). Restructuring of hog farming in North Carolina: Explosion and implosion. *Professional Geographer, 49,* 391–403.

Gaventa, J. (1993). The powerful, the powerless, and the experts: Knowledge struggles in an information age. In P. Park, M. Brydon-Miller, B. L. Hall, & T. Jackson (Eds.), *Voices of change: Participatory research in the United States and Canada* (pp. 21–40). Westport, CT: Bergin & Garvey.

Green, L. W., & Mercer, S. L. (2001). Can public health researchers and agencies reconcile the push from funding bodies and the pull from communities? *American Journal of Public Health, 91,* 1926–1929.

Israel, B. A, Checkoway, B., Schulz, A. J., & Zimmerman, M. A. (1994). Health education and community empowerment: Conceptualizing and measuring perceptions of individual, organizational, and community control. *Health Education Quarterly, 21,* 149–170.

Israel, B. A., Schulz, A. J., Parker, E. A., & Becker, A. B. (1998). Review of community-based research: Assessing partnership approaches to improve public health. *Annual Review of Public Health, 19,* 173–202.

Kuehn, R. (1996). The environmental justice implications of quantitative risk assessment. *University of Illinois Law Review, 103,* 103–172.

Le Duff, C. (1999, July 16). At a slaughterhouse, some things never die: Who kills, who cuts, who bosses can depend on race. *New York Times.*

Levine, A. G. (1982). *Love Canal: Science, politics, and people.* Lexington, MA: Heath.

Lindenfeld, S. (2001, February 13). Floyd recovery in their own hands: Survivors "stand up." *Raleigh News and Observer,* p. 1B.

Livingood, W. C., Goldhagen, J., Little, W. L., Gornto, J., & Hou, T. (2007). Assessing the status of partnerships between academic institutions and public health agencies. *American Journal of Public Health, 97*(4), 659–666.

Lynn, F. M. (2000). Community-scientist collaboration in environmental research. *American Behavioral Scientist, 44*(4), 649–663.

Minkler, M. (2000). Participatory action research and healthy communities. *Public Health Reports, 115,* 191–197.

Muhammad, N. (2007). ". . .and the struggle continues." *CCT Notes, 8*(2), 13–15.

Northridge, M. E., Vallone, D., Merzel, C., Greene, D., Shepard, P., Cohall, A. T., et al. (2000). The adolescent years: An academic-community partnership in Harlem comes of age. *Journal of Public Health Management and Practice, 6*(1), 53–60.

Nyswander, D. (1967). The open society: Its implications for health educators. *Health Education Monographs, 1,* 3–13.

Patton, M. Q. (1990). Qualitative evaluation and research methods (2nd ed.). Thousand Oaks, CA: Sage.

Quinn, S. C. (2006). Hurricane Katrina: A social and public health disaster. *American Journal of Public Health, 96*(2), 204.

St. George, D. M., Schoenbach, V. J., Reynolds, G. H., Nwangwu, J., & Adams-Campbell, L. (1997). Recruitment of minority students to U.S. epidemiology degree programs. *Annals of Epidemiology, 7,* 304–310.

Sandman, P. M. (1991). Emerging communication responsibilities of epidemiologists. *Journal of Clinical Epidemiology, 44*(Suppl. 1), 41S–50S.

Schiffman, S. S., Miller, E. A., Suggs, M. S., & Graham, B. G. (1995). The effect of environmental odors emanating from commercial swine operations on the mood of nearby residents. *Brain Research Bulletin, 37,* 369–375.

Segrest, M. (1999). *Looking for higher ground: Disaster and response in North Carolina after Hurricane Floyd.* Durham, NC: Urban-Rural Mission USA.

Shepard, P. M. (2000). Achieving environmental objectives and reducing health disparities through community-based participatory research and interventions. In L. R. O'Fallon, F. L. Tyson, & A. Dearry (Eds.), *Successful models of community-based participatory research. Final report* (pp. 30–34). Research Triangle Park, NC: National Institute for Environmental Health Science.

Steckler, A., McLeroy, K. R., Goodman, R. M., Bird, S. T., & McCormick, L. (1992). Toward integrating qualitative and quantitative methods: An introduction. *Health Education Quarterly, 19,* 1–8.

Tajik, M., & Minkler, M. (2007). Environmental justice research and action: A case study in political economy and community-academic collaboration. *International Quarterly of Community Health Education 26*(3), 215–232.

Thu, K., Donham, K., Ziegenhorn, R., Reynolds, S., Thorne, P. S., Subramanian, P., et al. (1997). A control study of the physical and mental health of residents living near a large-scale swine operation. *Journal of Agricultural Safety and Health, 3,* 13–26.

U.S. Environmental Protection Agency. (1998). *Final guidance for incorporating environmental justice concerns in EPA's NEPA compliance analyses.* Washington, DC: Government Printing Office.

Wallack, L. (2005). Media advocacy: A strategy for empowering people and communities. In M. Minkler (Ed.), *Community organizing and community building for health* (2nd ed., pp. 419–432). New Brunswick, NJ: Rutgers University Press.

Wing, S. (1998). Whose epidemiology, whose health? *International Journal of Health Services, 28,* 241–252.

Wing, S. (2000). Community-driven epidemiology and environmental justice: A course at the University of North Carolina. *Networker, 5*(5). Retrieved Dec. 19, 2000, from http://www.sehn.org/Volume_5–5_4.html.

Wing, S. (2001). Review: Challenging inequalities in health: From ethics to action. *New England Journal of Medicine, 345,* 1857–1858.

Wing, S. (2002). Social responsibility and research ethics in community-driven studies of industrialized hog production. *Environmental Health Perspectives, 110,* 437–444.

Wing, S., Cole, D., & Grant, G. (2000). Environmental injustice in North Carolina's hog industry. *Environmental Health Perspectives, 108,* 225–231.

Wing, S., Grant, G., Green, M., & Stewart, C. (1996). Community-based collaboration for environmental justice: Southeast Halifax environmental reawakening. *Environment and Urbanization, 8,* 129–140.

Wing, S., & Wolf, S. (2000). Intensive livestock operations, health, and quality of life among eastern North Carolina residents. *Environmental Health Perspectives, 108,* 233–238.

CHAPTER

16

ANALYZING AND INTERPRETING DATA WITH COMMUNITIES

SUZANNE B. CASHMAN, ALEX J. ALLEN III, JASON CORBURN,
BARBARA A. ISRAEL, JAIME MONTAÑO, SCOTT D. RHODES,
SAMARA F. SWANSTON, & EUGENIA ENG

IN 2001, THE AGENCY for Healthcare Research and Quality (AHRQ) commissioned a systematic review of published work describing community-based participatory research (CBPR) approaches to improving health. In this review, CBPR is defined as a "collaborative research approach that is designed to ensure and establish structures for participation by communities affected by the issue being studied, representatives of organizations, and researchers in all aspects of the research process to improve health and well-being through taking action, including social change" (Viswanathan, Ammerman, Eng, et al., 2004).

Note: This chapter was adapted from an article by S. Cashman, S. Adeky, J. Corburn, B. Israel, J. Montaño, A. Rafelito, S. D. Rhodes, S. Swanston, N. Wallerstein, & E. Eng, (in press) *American Journal of Public Health.* Copyright American Public Health Association. Adapted with permission. Partial funding for the Latino men's health study came from the W. K. Kellogg Foundation Community Health Scholars Program. The East Side Village Health Worker Partnership (ESVHWP) was conducted in conjunction with the Detroit Community-Academic Urban Research Center, funded through a cooperative agreement with the Centers for Disease Control and Prevention (grant U48/CCU515775). The New York project was partially funded by CDC Prevention grant U50/CCU272296–03).

As reported in the sixty studies reviewed, community involvement extended through all areas of research, and many study authors argued that involvement of community partners encouraged greater participation rates, strengthened external validity, decreased loss to follow-up, and increased individual and community capacity (Viswanathan et al., 2004). These positive attributes not withstanding, however, the strongest and most common engagement occurred in recruiting study participants and designing and implementing the research and interventions; less common was community participation in data analysis and interpretation of findings.

It is unclear whether community partner involvement in these latter phases of research has simply been reported less frequently in peer-reviewed publications or whether community partners have actually been less engaged in data analysis and interpretation. It has been suggested that diverting community expertise, time, and attention to acquiring analytical skills, both quantitative and qualitative, may be misplaced, particularly when balanced against (1) the efficiencies of drawing on analytical skills and resources that academic partners bring to the research enterprise, and (2) the priorities focused on enhancing existing community expertise (Steckler, Orville, Eng, & Dawson, 1992). It also has been asserted that both the community and academic partners for a single study could be overwhelmed by the commitment of time and resources necessary to prepare for equitable engagement in all phases of the research, especially data analysis and interpretation (MacLeod, 1997; Wang, Burris, & Ping, 1996). Some community partners have argued that their involvement—particularly in data analysis—is not always the best use of their time. Nevertheless, most academic partners engaged in CBPR stress the fundamental value of having the community-academic partnership decide upon specific roles and responsibilities. Although these may be fluid as people and organizations adjust to a project's unique needs, the critical role of community partners in interpreting and synthesizing findings—even if they are not involved fully in data analysis—remains a hallmark of CBPR. Through the participatory process of jointly interpreting data, differing perspectives are articulated and integrated, thereby enriching insights and discoveries (Centers for Disease Control and Prevention, 1998; Israel, Eng, Schulz, & Parker, 2005; Minkler & Wallerstein, 2003).

With little empirical evidence on the implications of engaging community partners in data analysis and interpretation, we are at the beginning stages of understanding the benefits and challenges of bringing these partners into these phases of research. We may find that working in partnership during data analysis and interpretation could require skills—yet to be articulated fully—from community partners that are different from but complementary to the skills of the academic partners, thereby increasing the credibility of outcomes and likelihood of translation into action.

To contribute to the current limited evidence on community and academic partners' roles in and contributions to data analysis and interpretation, as well as to synthesis of findings, this chapter presents three case examples from the authors' own CBPR studies. The cases represent a range of methods for data analysis or interpretation of findings. The purposes of this chapter are to (1) review the collaborative processes used; (2) identify challenges and impacts in each case example for data analysis or interpretation of findings, or both; (3) discuss how community-academic collaboration added value to the analytical and interpretive phases of research; and (4) highlight lessons learned across the three cases.

The first case describes the role of community partners in interpreting results from a community survey aimed at examining and addressing social determinants of health. The partnership, described in Chapter Three and focused on Detroit's east side, involved participants from community-based organizations; the local health department; an integrated care system; and faculty, students, and staff from the University of Michigan School of Public Health. In the second case, a partnership between a North Carolina Latino men's soccer league, other community-based organizations, and faculty at the University of North Carolina School of Public Health used focus group methodology to understand issues related to sexually transmitted infections, particularly HIV. The final case reports on mapping as a methodology for documenting environmental health and its use by a partnership between neighborhood organizations in Brooklyn, New York, and faculty from Hunter College, Queens College, and City University of New York. Table 16.1, at the end of the chapter, provides a descriptive summary of the cases with accompanying challenges and impact.[1]

CASE 1: SURVEY DATA FROM THE EAST SIDE VILLAGE HEALTH WORKER PARTNERSHIP

The East Side Village Health Worker Partnership (ESVHWP) represents a CBPR effort that involved a lay health adviser intervention to examine and address the social determinants of health on the east side of Detroit, Michigan (Parker, Schulz, Israel, & Hollis, 1998; Schulz et al., 2002, 2003). Established in 1995 with funding from the Centers for Disease Control and Prevention (CDC), the partnership was initially an affiliated project of the Detroit Community-Academic Urban Research Center. It was guided by a twelve-member steering committee (SC) that met monthly and was composed of representatives from the local health department, six community-based organizations, a managed care entity, and an academic institution (see Chapter Three). The SC partner organizations were selected based on their history of involvement and credibility in the community, interest in the health and quality of life of community residents, and prior relationship with the academic institution or the local health department (Parker, Shulz, et al., 1998; Schulz et al., 2002, 2003). Since the termination of its CDC funding in 2003, the partnership has been a citywide effort based at the local health department. In accordance with the CBPR principles the partnership adopted (Parker, Shulz, et al., 1998), the SC guided all aspects of the research and intervention (see Chapter Three for a discussion of the partnership's establishment of working relationships, operating norms, and CBPR principles.)

The steering committee decided to conduct a random sample survey in the community for the purposes of: assessing community needs and assets to guide interventions, gathering baseline data to evaluate the impacts and outcomes of interventions, and testing a stress process model that links stressors and protective factors to enduring health outcomes in the context of Detroit's east side (Parker, Shulz, et al., 1998; Schulz et al., 1998). Through a series of group discussions and in-depth interviews, the SC was instrumental in creating a conceptual framework of stress and health, identifying key variables to examine, selecting and modifying the measures for the survey questionnaire, developing procedures for survey administration, interpreting survey results, applying the findings to guide interventions, and disseminating the results (Parker, Shulz, et al., 1998; Schulz et al., 1998). For example, the SC engaged in a focused group discussion that produced a stress process model that featured numerous stressors and protective factors that the university researchers had not considered; questionnaire items were developed to assess these factors and were included in the survey (Becker, Israel, Schulz, Parker, & Klem, 2005; Israel et al., 2001; Schulz et al., 2003). The SC made several key decisions, including designating the eligibility criteria for survey respondents, delineating the intervention area boundaries within which households were randomly selected, and hiring and training neighborhood residents to conduct the interviews (Schulz et al., 2003). The SC's contributions helped to ensure questionnaire content validity. (The ability to generalize to other community settings was not an aim of the survey.) A total of 700 women were interviewed, giving the survey a response rate of 81 percent (Israel et al., 2001).

Participatory Data Analysis and Interpretation of Findings

Given the time and skills required, the steering committee decided that the survey data would be analyzed initially by the University of Michigan School of Public Health partners and that the SC and the village health workers would be actively engaged in determining the meaning of the results and their implications for action. As the survey was fielded, the intervention component of the partnership was being implemented and the village health workers (VHWs) were selected and trained and began meeting regularly (Parker, Shulz, et al., 1998; Schulz et al., 2002). Over a six-month period, a series of separate SC and VHW monthly meetings were held, culminating in a half-day retreat with both SC members and VHWs, to carry out this collaborative, interpretive process. Approximately twelve SC members and twenty-five VHWs participated in this series of meetings in which basic descriptive results were shared and discussed to determine meaning and to identify priority areas to address, along with potential strategies for working on these areas. Initially, the data were shared by distributing a copy of the survey questionnaire with the number of responses and the corresponding percentages for each item inserted (for example, the percentage of respondents experiencing each of the stressors). At these meetings, SC members and VHWs were asked to discuss several questions, including these: In reviewing results from the survey, what do you think they mean? What is your interpretation? Are there any surprises, that is, findings that you would not have expected, and if so, how do you make sense of them? In order to foster further dissemination of the survey results, the SC developed a report on key survey findings, which was distributed widely throughout the community. Using bar charts and pie graphs, and shaped by considerable review and revision by the SC, this report displayed results in an accessible, visually appealing format.

Subsequently, the university partners conducted correlation analyses between a number of key variables (for example, stressors and health outcomes) and regression analyses to examine the SC's major research questions. In all instances, results were brought to the

SC with the university partners presenting findings and community partners providing their interpretations of the results. As necessary, university partners provided information on the statistical methods used and how to read the data presented in the tables; no formal workshops or training were necessary, and community members were readily able to make sense of the results, using their knowledge of the community. Through a series of meetings, using experiential learning methods such as nominal group process and force field analysis (Becker et al., 2005), the SC engaged in a process of setting priorities on issues and strategies for addressing the problems identified in the survey.

Benefits and Outcomes

Several benefits were associated with involving all partners in the process of interpreting survey findings. First, the community partners were able to provide an in-depth understanding of the broader community context and how that should shape the meaning of the quantitative results. For example, the academic researchers were surprised by the finding that community members were generally satisfied with their access to health care providers. The community partners explained that the issue of concern in the community was quality of health care, not access per se, which had implications for the selection of appropriate action strategies. Second, the community partners were able to enhance their own understanding of the strengths and limitations of survey data, and the data themselves often helped to validate these partners' assessment of what was happening in their community. Third, community partner involvement ensured community input into the translation of strategies to address issues raised in the survey. For example, through the priority-setting process described earlier, the SC members and VHWs initially decided on four priority action areas (strengthen relations with police precincts, improve physical safety for children, reduce financial vulnerability, and support adults with responsibility for children) that were based not only on the survey results but also on their understanding of the neighborhood context.

CASE 2: FOCUS GROUP DATA FROM A LATINO MEN'S SOCCER LEAGUE

Since 1991, Chatham Communities in Action (CCIA), a community-based, health-focused coalition in rural central North Carolina, has been conducting health promotion projects that follow CBPR principles. Following the coalition's initial successes in African American, church-based diabetes prevention and management programs (Margolis et al., 2000; Parker, Eng, et al., 1998), CCIA partners expanded Latino community representation in CCIA through a process of recruitment and self-appointment. Representatives from several key Latino organizations joined CCIA, including a Latino soccer league of over 1,800 adult Latino men, a farmworker advocacy group, a statewide coalition established to promote Mexican leadership, a local *tienda* (Latino grocer), and a local Latino-serving, community-based organization (CBO). The expanded CCIA decided to undertake a focus group study to (1) explore sociocultural determinants of sexual risk among the non-English-speaking, less acculturated Latino men living in North Carolina, a region experiencing rapidly growing Latino populations and disproportionate HIV and sexually transmitted disease rates; and (2) identify potentially effective intervention approaches that would be context sensitive and gender relevant. Together, the partners created, reviewed, revised, and approved a focus group moderator's guide. This process was rapid, taking about one month. CCIA then completed seven focus groups. The league president recruited focus group participants; a CCIA partner served as the focus group moderator, and a university researcher proficient in Spanish served as note taker. A Latino-serving CBO, one of the new CCIA partners, hosted the focus groups.

Participatory Data Analysis and Interpretation of Findings

Using an inductive approach to data analysis (Glaser & Strauss, 1967), the partnership focused its analysis on a wide array of experiences and on building understanding grounded in real-world patterns. Participants used a systematic multistage process to analyze and interpret the data. All audio recordings of the focus groups were professionally transcribed, verbatim, and then translated into English. A CCIA community partner and an academic partner listened to each tape while reviewing both the Spanish and English language transcripts, to ensure that the recordings had been accurately transcribed and to evaluate the translation of the transcripts from Spanish to English to ensure that meaning was not lost.

An ad hoc committee of the CCIA membership ($n = 9$) was formed to serve as the data analysis team. This team included one to three representatives from each of the following groups: the lay Latino community, the Latino soccer league, the Latino-serving CBO, the local health department, an AIDS service organization, and the university. Because some analysis team members were not bilingual, each member read and coded transcripts in his or her concordant language.

The goal of the analysis was to identify common themes through coding text. Conducting their analyses separately, analysis team members read and reread the transcripts to identify potential codes, convened to create a common coding system and data dictionary, and then separately assigned agreed-upon codes to relevant text. The academic partner used NVivo (second edition, from QSR International), an analytical software program, to electronically code and retrieve text. Analysis took about eight months due to the competing demands experienced by the members, including the academic partner. Similarities and differences across transcripts were examined and codes and themes revised accordingly. Analysis team members met to compare and revise themes. An example is found in the "traditional" notions of masculinity that are often identified as having negative influences on health among men. The partnership approach teased out positive aspects of masculinity, such as respecting oneself and taking care of one's family, which are linked to immigrating to the United States. After team members had refined their themes, the themes and accompanying interpretations were presented to research partners in both English and Spanish; this permitted verification of validity (Strauss & Corburn, 1998) and helped ensure high-quality, accurate findings (Lukens, Thorning, & Lohrer, 2004; MacQueen, McLellan, Kay, & Milstein, 1998; Shibusawa & Lukens, 2004).

The data analysis process was completed by writing draft themes on flip charts so that representatives from the CCIA partnership could review, discuss, revise, and interpret them during four iterative discussions. During each step of the process, information generated was combined with partners' cultural knowledge as well as previous research to inform theme development and derive interpretations. This approach yielded five themes, which the partnership subsequently used for action.

Benefits and Outcomes

This study was successful in large part because of early efforts to develop trust among all partners. Owing to early successes in establishing the research questions, developing the study design, and creating the focus group moderator's guide (Rhodes et al., 2007), partners were engaged and thus willing to participate in subsequent phases. Although conflicts occurred, anticipating and accommodating disagreements led to an improved and more informed understanding of sexual health among Latino men. As a Latino community partner noted, "What we are doing is comparing what we think and know to what others think and know. We [then] walk away knowing more."

The partnership has used the focus group findings as background data for organizational and agency service grants. It also received funding to support a three-year quasi-experimental study to develop, implement, evaluate, and revise an intervention to promote sexual health among immigrant Latino men living in rural North Carolina. The intervention is designed to build on results of the CBPR study through bolstering existing community strengths and assets while affirming positive social norms through maintaining well-being and healthy relationships.

CASE 3: MAPPING DATA IN THE WATCHPERSON PROJECT AND EL PUENTE

In the Greenpoint/Williamsburg (G/W) neighborhood of Brooklyn, New York, community groups and professionals have engaged in research partnerships and map making to address environmental health disparities. Mapping is increasingly understood as a central component of epidemiological research and as a key resource for moving community knowledge from research to action (Cromley & McLafferty, 2002; Diez-Roux, 1998; Elliott & Wartenberg, 2004; Maantay, 2002; Nuckols, Ward, & Jarup, 2004; Schorr & Auspos, 2003). Less well documented is the role maps and map making can play in organizing community members and their expertise and in reframing academic research to better reflect community needs.

The G/W neighborhood is a low-income community in which several ethnic groups and polluting industries coexist. Latino, Hasidic (Jewish), Polish immigrant, and African American families, along with young white families, live in a neighborhood where over 35 percent of residents have incomes below the poverty line. Within less than five square miles, the neighborhood houses over thirty waste transfer stations, the city's largest sewage treatment facility, and seventeen Toxics Release Inventory (TRI) sites identified by the U.S. Environmental Protection Agency (Corburn, 2002).

Participatory Data Analysis and Interpretation of Findings

A community mapping project began after residents learned that the New York State Department of Environmental Conservation had scheduled a public hearing to review the operating permit of Radiac, a low-level radioactive waste transfer and storage facility in the G/W neighborhood. In preparation for the hearing, students at El Puente Academy, a high school run by a community-based organization of the same name, organized a group called El Puente Toxic Avengers to research and document existing environmental health burdens. After walking the neighborhood with professionals and gathering existing environmental and health data, including information from the city's department of environmental protection about facility location and pollutant emissions, and also demographic information from the U.S. Census, the students produced a map depicting how they viewed their community (Figure 16.1).

The student effort showed skulls describing numerous local hazards against a background map made to look like an X-ray, all aimed at portraying a sense of urgency about local pollution that is compromising residents' health. Pictures of local facilities were included on the map to ensure viewer recognition of polluters by sight, not just by name, and each image was accompanied by brief text about the facility's environmental performance. Copies of this map were placed around the community to alert residents about the upcoming hearing.

The Toxic Avengers' map helped organize over 200 residents to attend the Radiac hearing, but not necessarily to challenge existing data or how it was being interpreted for policymaking. Instead, El Puente (2007), the community-based organization, used the student-generated map as evidence and argued that the cumulative exposures depicted on the map ought to be the focus of regulatory efforts, not the reviewing and permitting of one facility at a time. Of equal importance, the Toxic Avengers' map encouraged the formation of the first multiethnic environmental health coalition in the neighborhood, the Community Alliance for the Environment (CAFE), whose members included three membership-based organizations in the neighborhood that represented thousands of residents: El Puente, the Polish-Slavic Center, and United Jewish Organizations (Corburn, 2005).

The CAFE alliance provided the political support behind a second project, which was aimed at measuring street-level exposures to hazardous air pollutants and volatile organic compounds (VOCs). For this project a research partnership was formed among four research scientists at City University of New York's Hunter College, El Puente, and the Watchperson Project, a community-based organization established to monitor local pollution. Created in 1990, the Watchperson Project was established to develop community capacity for monitoring neighborhood environmental health hazards and holding private and public sector polluters accountable. An early step in this process involved the four Hunter College scientists meeting with over twenty community members to identify and map local polluting facilities, using geographic information system (GIS) technology. Because there were potentially hundreds of small polluters in this industrialized neighborhood that were not tracked or monitored by any city, state, or federal agency, the research team organized neighborhood-based staff and volunteers to walk the streets to document on paper maps the locations of polluting facilities and the type of each operation. These community field surveys revealed hundreds of facilities not found in the phone book or in any agency database, including a number of dry cleaners, nail salons, and offset printers located in residential buildings, where they represented potentially dangerous situations. These field survey data were entered into a GIS and joined with demographic and other land-use data, such as school and day-care facility locations.

After reviewing the maps the research team found that over fifty residential buildings had a printer, dry cleaner, or nail salon on the ground floor, so the team members decided

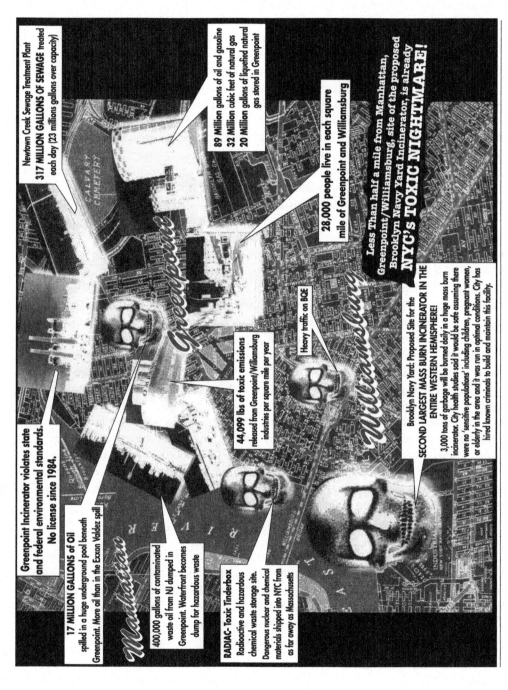

FIGURE 16.1 *Toxic Avengers' Skulls Map*

Source: El Puente Toxic Avengers

to target air sampling in and around these buildings. The samples revealed elevated concentrations of perchloroethylene (perc), toluene, and xylene outside of homes and elevated VOC concentrations inside apartments located in buildings with a targeted facility operating on the ground floor. During community meetings for sharing initial results, residents noted that some of the elevated readings were also being found along streets they had observed being used illegally by trucks trying to avoid traffic on the Brooklyn-Queens Expressway. This suggestion altered the project in a new way, expanding the research effort to include pollutant sampling along streets designated as truck routes and those suspected of being used by trucks illegally. Map making provided a mechanism for real-time, collaborative spatial data analysis, with university researchers generating maps while community members continually checked map validity and interpreted results according to their own lived experience. Maps gave community members and researchers a common medium for communicating about technical issues that were sometimes difficult to convey through words. Maps also provided those members of the research team who spoke only English, Spanish, Polish, or Yiddish with a common "language" to facilitate interpreting and assigning meaning to results.

Benefits and Outcomes

The community mapping efforts helped activists in Brooklyn convince the U.S. Environmental Protection Agency (EPA) to pilot its first community-based Community Exposure Project (CEP) in this neighborhood (U.S. EPA, 1999). According to the EPA's Office of Policy and Planning, the agency selected G/W for the CEP because community members were engaged in assessing multiple hazards in their neighborhood and had uncovered exposures that regulators had overlooked (U.S. EPA, 1999). The mapping projects also helped community groups extend their own research capacity. El Puente partnered with the nonprofit consulting firm Centro de Investigacion de Enfermedades Tropicales to design and complete a series of asthma-focused health surveys, establish a community health worker program, publish the survey results (Ledogar, Penchaszadeh, Garden, & Iglesias, 2000), and direct this partnership's own NIEHS-funded research (Acosta, 2005). The Watchperson Project has continued to use the air sampling results to educate and enroll local businesses in pollution prevention programs and to expand GIS mapping and analytical capacity in the community.

LESSONS LEARNED

Exhibit 16.1 summarizes major lessons the community and academic partners learned from involving all partners in data analysis or interpretation of findings to arrive at outcomes that led to concrete actions. Achieved through reviews of project documentation, self-reflection, discussion, and distillation, these emergent lessons address the following questions on engaging all partners in data analysis or interpretation of findings:

1. What are the complementary roles and skills for academic and for community partners?

2. How can academic and community partners anticipate the time and the iterative processes required?

3. Is engaging all partners in data analysis or interpretation of findings worth doing and doable?

These lessons underscore the importance of an approach that creates space for both community and university partners to draw on their different, yet complementary, experiences and skills and to determine the respective analytical roles and responsibilities for each research phase (Israel, Schulz, Parker, & Becker, et al., 1998). For example, the North Carolina practice sessions on coding and the Detroit procedure for conceptualizing issues were not carried out so that community partners could acquire the expertise of university partners. Rather, these workshops, practice sessions, and procedures were attended by community and university partners alike to achieve consensus decision making about the ways the partnership would address the iterative nature of data analysis, the time required to complete that analysis, conceptualization of key research concepts, and the implications of taking shortcuts to adhere to timelines and funding agencies' expectations. To sustain community-university engagement, therefore, the research teams in all three case examples relied on experiential learning methods to review summarized data and worked closely with community and university partners to solicit their commitment to the time and iterative process required to engage their respective constituents in arriving at outcomes. Finally, the university partners made time to reassure community members about the benefits of the iterative process and presented intermediate stages of data so participants could see progress.

In addition, a thread that ran throughout the three cases was the time and iterative processes necessary for achieving common ground and an understanding of data analysis and interpretation. University partners were challenged to avoid using jargon, particularly terminology related to data analysis, and to recognize that significant research findings were not a replacement for their community partners' vision for developing and implementing interventions. In the New York mapping case example, the search for common language challenged the neighborhood residents to translate their knowledge into terms that professional partners could understand and manipulate.

SUMMARY

The case examples in this chapter point to the value of combining academic partners' expertise in data reduction, through statistical packages or thematic categorization, with community partners' expertise in increasing face and construct validity through language and cultural insight. Delineation of complementary roles and skills can move the research forward with regard to identifying additional analyses and future research questions or ensuring that interpretation of the findings has meaning for the local community, or both. Capacity building in research skills can then be encouraged through short-term training (possibly provided by the university partner or a third party), and through creating a long-term pipeline that increases the number of racially and ethnically diverse health researchers with a career commitment to CBPR and the elimination of health disparities.

As attested to by the cases highlighted in this article, given adequate time and using relevant modalities, engaging all partners in data analysis or interpretation of findings is both doable and worth doing. Building on the foundation of trust and respect established through the earlier research phases of problem identification, study design, and data collection,

EXHIBIT 16.1 **Lessons Learned from Working with Communities to Analyze and Interpret Findings**

What Are the Complementary Roles and Skills for Academic and Community Partners?

■ *Academic and community partners' respective roles in data analysis or interpretation of findings should be determined collaboratively.* Decisions regarding partners' specific roles and where their respective energies can be best applied need to be made through open dialogue and consensus. There are times when academic and community partners work collaboratively on data analysis and interpretation of findings. At other times, community partners' roles figure prominently in the data interpretation and not in the analysis phase. In the cases presented here, when the research methodology called for collecting quantitative data, trained academics took the first steps in structuring data collection and analysis. Community partners were able to contribute ideas for analyses and to offer insights into the reality reflected by the raw numbers. In addition, they refined questions that the data would explore and then made significant contributions to interpreting and synthesizing results. Community members unaccustomed to working with data were able to interpret results when these were presented as percentages or in graphic form. Their contributions to data interpretation often resulted in shared insights that significantly shaped subsequent interventions.

■ *Community partners' roles and skills in relation to data analysis and interpretation can be influenced by these partners' prior experiences in research endeavors.* Contained in the power and the promise of using a CBPR approach is the potential for building community capacity. In some cases, engaging community members in iterative experiences and projects resulted in their becoming sufficiently familiar with research to entertain the idea of gaining formal academic credentials. At a minimum, academic partners were able to build on community members' prior experiences; additionally, experienced community members helped to mentor community participants who were new to the process.

How Can Academic and Community Partners Anticipate the Time and Iterative Processes Required?

■ *Data analysis and interpretation of findings are iterative processes.* The iterative process of analyzing and interpreting data needs to be made explicit. The process is well served when academic partners prepare community partners (who are less experienced in research) for the iterative effort and then provide reminders throughout about the ways in which prior efforts are shaping current and future decisions. This should not be assumed to be understood but made explicit. Although all the academic partners in the cases understood the value of using an iterative process to digest data, the community partners generally needed reassurance that recurring efforts at understanding were an accepted part of data analysis and interpretation.

■ *Obtaining commitment from community partners reduces analysis fatigue and the temptation to take shortcuts.* Although both academic and community partners are often anxious to get to outcomes, retaining community partners' commitment to the data analysis and interpretation processes that precede interventions and outcomes can be particularly challenging. The desire for action over analysis can result in shortcuts that fail to consider important information. As demonstrated by these three cases, commitment of community partners can be critical to ensuring that the data analysis and interpretation phases are carried out to completion. The process can be well served by ensuring that partners who have an understanding of the need for balance in analysis and action make these issues explicit for all. Simultaneously, they might highlight gains in understanding that are likely to enhance the effectiveness of subsequent interventions.

- *Simplifying data can aid understanding but may also obscure complex relationships.* Although it is critical to present data in a format easily understood by all partners involved, caution is warranted to avoid oversimplifying complex relationships. When using mapping methodology, for example, it is important to consistently remind partners that the aggregation process can obscure complex interactions. This can be done by continually raising questions about what is known and still unknown when interpreting the meaning of mapped data.

- *Time required is lengthened considerably and a given.* There are no shortcuts to including both community and academic partners in data analysis or interpretation, or both. Although equitable involvement lengthens project time considerably, the insights gained from juxtaposing different viewpoints should be viewed as milestone accomplishments along the way to outcomes. Methodologies such as visioning workshops and practice sessions on coding or mapping often lend themselves to brief action interventions while overall research processes continue to be carried out simultaneously. This duality of research and action can encourage and support continued community, academic, and funding partner engagement.

Is Engaging All Partners in Data Analysis and Interpretation of Findings Worth Doing and Doable?

- *Experiential learning approaches are effective in engaging community partners.* Although all adult learners can benefit from experiential learning approaches, each case study highlighted the benefits for community partners of interacting with the data beyond just hearing and talking about them. When they could see data displayed in an easily understood, visual format such as a map or coded transcript, community partners contributed to discussions that reinforced mutual participation and reflection. Through visioning the application of data during facilitated discussions, community partners were able to incorporate information they saw into their lived context and contribute to decisions on an initiative's future direction.

- *Including the community in data analysis or interpretation, or both, can increase authenticity of findings.* Ensuring data validity and accuracy and then communicating findings effectively is a concern that underlies all research. Although partners in each of the cases had concluded that their research data were accurate, those in the Latino soccer league case found that through multiple revisions of the focus group codes, the partners produced and interpreted themes that were trustworthy representations of the local Latino community and not just of the coalition itself. Time spent using an analysis and interpretation process that involved multiple steps meant that a wide variety of perspectives could be incorporated; this resulted in findings that reflected the broader community rather than simply those individuals who were confident in expressing their views in public forums.

TABLE 16.1   **Summary of Case Examples**

Case	Composition	Structure	Co-learning methodology	Type of data	Community partner role	Academic partner role	Time required to analyze or interpret data	Techniques to make data accessible	Challenges	Impact
East Side Village Health Worker Partnership	Representatives from local health department, CBOs, integrated care system, and academia made up steering committee. Local lay health advisers, village health workers (VHWs).	Steering committee met monthly, followed adopted CBPR principles and operating procedures. VHWs met monthly.	Discussed and interpreted data feedback materials and results. Identified priorities and action strategies. Shared descriptive results. Selected research questions.	Quantitative: derived from random sample household survey.	Defined scope of work. Developed conceptual framework. Identified key variables. Selected or modified measures for questionnaire. Interpreted, disseminated data. Applied data to guide intervention. Reviewed pie charts and bar graphs for wider community distribution.	Facilitated SC meetings. Provided data. Helped revise questionnaire. Hired, trained, and supervised interviewers. Analyzed data. Developed feedback materials.	Over a six-month period, monthly meetings of SC and VHWs and a half-day retreat.	Placed frequencies on questionnaire. Used pie charts and bar graphs to present results. Engaged in experiential learning activities to examine and prioritize results.	Time. Determining community and academic partner roles. Identifying mechanisms for data sharing.	Neighborhood residents hired and trained to conduct interviews. Increased knowledge of community strengths and stressors. Enhanced understanding of social determinants of health. Village health worker project implemented. Built capacity.*
Latino Men	People from Hispanic soccer league, Latino grocery store,	CCIA met monthly and followed adopted CBPR principles.	Partner in all phases of data analysis and interpretation.	Qualitative: derived from focus groups.	Set priorities. Moderated and hosted focus groups. Read transcripts.	Provided leadership and expertise in data analysis.	Eight months.	Systematic, multistage process. Data analysis teams had lay and	Time. Racial tensions in larger community being reflected in	HIV and STD prevention initiative developed. Built capacity.*

	leadership development coalition, farmworker advocacy group, and Latino-serving CBOs.				With academic partners, developed coding system and data dictionary; assigned codes to text; refined and interpreted themes. Provided cultural knowledge.	Used NVivo to code and retrieve text.		professional members. Flip charts were used throughout the process for review, revision, and final presentation of approved themes.	community partners. Addressing concern about suitability of topic selected. Dealing with tension between process and action.	
Greenpoint/ Williamsburg, Brooklyn, NY	Local students. Latino, Polish immigrant, and Hasidic (Jewish) community members.	Participants partnered with academic scientists. Map making was done by both community members and professionals.	Partner in all phases of data gathering and analysis.	Qualitative and quantitative: mapping; air pollution samples.	Introduced professionals to neighborhood. Contributed knowledge about local environmental hazards. Produced visuals on map depicting polluters. Distributed maps in neighborhood. Galvanized community to action.	Provided means, namely GIS, to help local people map what was important to them. Learned from community about existence of specific hazardous locations that professionals routinely overlooked. Participated in public action for reduction in pollutants.	Six to nine months.	Maps acted to provide "common language" for all participants. Visuals allowed the non-technically trained to participate in technical data analysis and interpretation.	Time. Retaining complexity while simplifying. Recognizing maps as provisional products that complement other sources of information. Capturing community knowledge in quantitative format.	Neighborhood residents activated. Project aim altered to focus on pollution. EPA's decision affected regarding pilot community exposure project. New pollution prevention programs developed. Built capacity.*

* See the chapter text for discussions of capacity building.

CBPR partners are uniquely positioned to take lead roles in data analysis and interpretation of findings to get to outcomes. In each of the cases discussed here, involving all members of the partnership in data analysis or interpretation, or both, strengthened community capacity building and increased community members' ability to understand complex issues that affected their health. Simultaneously, the presence of the community voice expanded the academic researchers' understanding of the issues. With partners contributing unique strengths and sharing responsibility for enhancing understanding of a given phenomenon, these brief cases demonstrate that there is no one correct approach to incorporating the community voice in data analysis and interpretation.

In sum, we have articulated the skills and processes used in three CBPR efforts by community and university representatives who worked in partnership during data analysis and interpretation of findings. The roles and skills of community partners were found to be different from but complementary to those of the academic partners. Moreover, these efforts generated outcomes that informed larger studies or interventions and led to externally funded actions. These observations reaffirm the premise that the issue is not *who* has the requisite knowledge and skills for data analysis and interpretation. Rather, the issue is *how* such knowledge and skills can be generated, shared, and applied. The next generation of CBPR studies can benefit from placing continued emphasis on specifying evolving roles and responsibilities for all partners in research. In particular, future work needs to build on the lessons identified in this chapter in order to further facilitate engagement of community partners with university partners in data analysis and interpretation.

QUESTIONS FOR DISCUSSION

1. The authors state that working in partnership with communities to analyze and interpret data can increase the credibility of outcomes and the likelihood of translating the work into action. Given that community partners do not have scientific research expertise, do you agree with the authors? Why? Why not? Develop arguments for and against this assertion.

2. Select a research project with which you are familiar and describe the community's role and contributions. If the community was included as a partner in data analysis or interpretation, or both, what processes were used to ensure its contribution? What was the outcome of including the community partner? How might the community partner's role have been expanded? What would the likely result of this expansion have been? If the community partner was not included in data analysis or interpretation, how could it have been included? In what ways might the results have been altered?

3. The definition of CBPR describes an approach whereby communities affected by the issue being studied are included in "all aspects of the research process." Do you think community partners must be included in either data analysis or interpretation for the approach to be truly CBPR? Why? Why not?

KEY TERMS

Participatory data analysis

Participatory data interpretation

Survey data

Focus groups

Mapping

Geographic information systems (GIS)

NOTE

1. For an illustration of community partner involvement in the analysis phase of CBPR with tribes program, a Ramah Navajo, New Mexico case study is described in Cashman et al. (in press) and English et al. (2004).

REFERENCES

Acosta, L. G. (2005). *Williamsburg Brooklyn Asthma and Environment Consortium.* Retrieved Nov. 11, 2006, from http://www.niehs.nih.gov/translat/envjust/projects/acosta.htm.

Becker, A. B., Israel, B. A., Schulz, A. J., Parker, E. A., & Klem, L. (2005). Age differences in health effects of stressors and perceived control among urban African American women. *Journal of Urban Health, 82*(1), 122–141.

Cashman, S., Adeky, S., Corburn, J., Eng, E., Israel, B., Montaño, J., et al. (in press). *American Journal of Public Health.*

Centers for Disease Control and Prevention. (1998). *Building community partnership in research: Recommendations and strategies.* Washington, DC: National Institutes of Health.

Corburn, J. (2002). Combining community-based research and local knowledge to confront asthma and subsistence-fishing hazards in Greenpoint/Williamsburg, Brooklyn, New York. *Environmental Health Perspectives, 110*(Suppl. 2), 241–248.

Corburn, J. (2005). *Street science: Community knowledge and environmental health justice.* Cambridge, MA: MIT Press.

Cromley, E., & McLafferty, S. (2002). *GIS and public health.* New York: Guilford Press.

Diez-Roux, A. V. (1998). Bringing context back into epidemiology: Variables and fallacies in multilevel analysis. *American Journal of Public Health, 88*(2), 216–222.

El Puente. (2007). *El Puente: Inspiring and nurturing leadership for peace and justice.* Retrieved Sept. 5, 2007, from http://www.elpuente.us/homepage.htm.

Elliott, P., & Wartenberg, D. (2004). Spatial epidemiology: Current approaches and future challenges. *Environmental Health Perspectives, 112*(9), 998–1006.

English, K. C., Wallerstein, N., Chino, M., Finster, C. E., Rafelito, A., Adeky, S., et al. (2004). Intermediate outcomes of a tribal community public health infrastructure assessment. *Ethnicity & Disease, 14*(3, Suppl. 1), S61–S69.

Glaser, B. G., & Strauss, A. L. (1967). *The discovery of grounded theory: Strategies for qualitative research.* Chicago: Aldine.

Israel, B. A., Eng, E., Schulz, A. J., & Parker, E. A. (Eds.). (2005). *Methods in community based participatory research for health.* San Francisco: Jossey-Bass.

Israel, B. A., Lichtenstein, R., Lantz, P. M., McGranaghan, R. J., Allen, A., Guzman, J. R., et al. (2001). The Detroit Community-Academic Urban Research Center: Development, implementation, and evaluation. *Journal of Public Health Management and Practice, 7*(5), 1–19.

Israel, B. A., Schulz, A. J., Parker, E. A., & Becker, A. B. (1998). Review of community-based research: Assessing partnership approaches to improve public health. *Annual Review of Public Health, 19*, 173–202.

Ledogar, R. J., Penchaszadeh, A., Garden, C. C., & Iglesias, G. (2000). Asthma and Latino cultures: Different prevalence reported among groups sharing the same environment. *American Journal of Public Health, 90*(6), 929–935.

Lukens, E. P., Thorning, H., & Lohrer, S. (2004). Sibling perspectives on severe mental illness: Reflections on self and family. *American Journal of Orthopsychiatry, 74*(4), 489–501.

Maantay, J. (2002). Mapping environmental injustices: Pitfalls and potential of geographic information systems in assessing environmental health and equity. *Environmental Health Perspectives, 110*(Suppl. 2), 161–171.

MacLeod, C. (1997). Research as intervention within community mental health. *Curationis, 20*(2), 53–56.

MacQueen, K. M., McLellan, E., Kay, K., & Milstein, B. (1998). Codebook development for team-based qualitative analysis. *Cultural Anthropology Methods, 10*(2), 31–36.

Margolis, L. H., Stevens, R., Laraia, B., Ammerman, A., Dodds, J., Eng, E., et al. (2000). Educating students for community-based partnerships. *Journal of Community Practice, 7*(4), 21–34.

Minkler, M., & Wallerstein, N. (2003). *Community-based participatory research for health.* San Francisco: Jossey-Bass.

Nuckols, J. R., Ward, M. H., & Jarup, L. (2004). Using geographic information systems for exposure assessment in environmental epidemiology studies. *Environmental Health Perspectives, 112*(9), 1007–1015.

Parker, E. A., Eng, E., Laraia, B., Ammerman, A., Dodds, J., Margolis, L., et al. (1998). Coalition building for prevention: Lessons learned from the North Carolina community-based public health initiative. *Journal of Public Health Management and Practice, 4*(2), 25–36.

Parker, E. A., Schulz, A. J., Israel, B. A., & Hollis, R. (1998). Detroit's East Side Village Health Worker Partnership: Community-based lay health advisor intervention in an urban area. *Health Education & Behavior, 25*(1), 24–45.

Rhodes, S., Eng, E., Hergenrather, K. C., Remnitz, I. M., Arceo, R., Montaño, J., et al. (2007). Exploring Latino men's HIV risk using community-based participatory research. *American Journal of Health Behavior, 31*(2), 146–158.

Schorr, L., & Auspos, P. (2003). Usable information about what works: Building a broader and deeper knowledge base. *Journal of Policy Analysis and Management, 22*(4), 669–676.

Schulz, A. J., Israel, B. A., Parker, E. A., Lockett, M., Hill, Y., & Wills, R. (2003). Engaging women in community-based participatory research for health: The East Side Village Health Worker Partnership. In M. Minkler & N. Wallerstein (Eds.), *Community-based participatory research for health* (pp. 293–315). San Francisco: Jossey-Bass.

Schulz, A. J., Parker, E. A., Israel, B. A., Allen, A., DeCarlo, M., & Lockett, M. (2002). Addressing social determinants of health through community-based participatory research: The East Side Village Health Worker Partnership. *Health Education & Behavior, 29*(3), 326–341.

Schulz, A. J., Parker, E. A., Israel, B. A., Becker, A. B., Maciak, B. J., & Hollis, R. (1998). Conducting a participatory community-based survey for a community health intervention on Detroit's east side. *Journal of Public Health Management and Practice, 4*(2), 10–24.

Shibusawa, T., & Lukens, E. (2004). *Analyzing qualitative data in a cross-language context: A collaborative model.* Belmont, CA: Wadsworth/Thomson Learning.

Steckler, A., Orville, K., Eng, E., & Dawson, L. (1992). A summary of a formative evaluation of PATCH. *Journal of Health Education, 23*(3), 174–178.

Strauss, A., & Corburn, J. (1998). *Basics of qualitative research* (2nd ed.). Thousand Oaks, CA: Sage.

U.S. Environmental Protection Agency. (1999, Apr. 19). *Cumulative exposure project.* Retrieved May 22, 2008, from http://www.greenlink.org/assess/pdfs/cumulativeexposure.pdf.

Viswanathan, M., Ammerman, A., Eng, E., Garlehner, G., Lohr, K. N., Griffith, D., et al. (2004). *Community-based participatory research: Assessing the evidence* (Evidence Report/Technology Assessment No. 99; Prepared by RTI International-University of North Carolina). Rockville, MD: Agency for Healthcare Research and Quality.

Wang, C. C., Burris, M. A., & Ping, X. Y. (1996). Chinese village women as visual anthropologists: A participatory approach to reaching policymakers. *Social Science & Medicine, 42*(10), 1391–1400.

USING CBPR TO PROMOTE SOCIAL CHANGE AND HEALTHY PUBLIC POLICY

Almost three decades ago, in one of the most celebrated examples of community-driven participatory research in the United States, Anne Anderson and her neighbors in Woburn, Massachusetts, worried about the high rates of childhood leukemia in their community, gathered data that led them to suspect a link with the community's water supply. Unsuccessful in their efforts to get local government authorities to test the water, they approached researchers at Harvard University's School of Public Health, who then worked collaboratively with community members, and also conducted their own analyses, to document what the community residents had long suspected. As Jason Corburn (2005) points out, "What this case revealed was that residents with no prior scientific training could not only competently engage in complex science, but that they had unique information about exposure to health outcomes that, when combined with traditional epidemiologic inquiry, could improve scientific inquiry" (p. 35). Yet the case also demonstrated another key tenet of CBPR, namely the importance of using the knowledge created through community-academic collaborations to help effect change. In this case, a subsequent civil suit against corporations that had for years dumped toxic chemicals into the town's water supply won a multimillion-dollar, out-of-court settlement for victims and their families. Moreover, the community-driven partnership's work was also credited with having been a major catalyst for the reauthorization of federal Superfund legislation designed to force the cleanup of one of the worst toxic waste sites in the nation (Sclove, 1997).

The Woburn case is a dramatic and admittedly atypical one in the nature and magnitude of its policy-related outcome. Yet it is also a vivid reminder that CBPR's commitment to action need not shy away from action that takes the form of influencing public and private sector policy. Part Five of this book explores the important yet often neglected role that CBPR can play in influencing policy decisions on multiple levels. Makani Themba-Nixon, Meredith Minkler, and Nicholas Freudenberg begin this exploration, in Chapter Seventeen, by summarizing two conceptual frameworks for understanding the policy-making process in the United States and also a third framework more directly tailored to policy advocacy through CBPR. Using as examples the efforts of varied CBPR partnerships and community coalitions around the country to influence policy, they illustrate diverse roles and entry points for such policy-focused work and set the stage for more detailed case examples in the remainder of this section.

In Chapter Eighteen, Peggy Shepard and her colleagues describe a now-classic example of the potential of CBPR for studying and addressing environmental injustice. The original study described in this chapter, in which youth interns with West Harlem Environmental Action (WE ACT) worked with epidemiologists at Columbia University to study diesel bus emissions exposure in their neighborhood, took place well over a decade ago. Yet the effectiveness of the partnership in translating and using the findings to effect policy change and its continued work today in this and related research and policy arenas powerfully attest to both the short-term and the longer-term impacts of such work.

Although we tend to think of policy in broad public policy terms, CBPR can also play a role in influencing private sector policies in the workplace and other nongovernmental arenas. In Chapter Nineteen, Pam Tau Lee and her colleagues examine two union-supported CBPR projects undertaken by university partners and hotel room cleaners, most of them immigrant women, in San Francisco and Las Vegas. They document the key role of the room cleaners in each stage of the research, with a special emphasis on how increasing individual and community capacity building through this project eventually played out in part in the women's strong policy advocacy and in their contributions to bringing about contract changes to improve working conditions.

In the final chapter in this section, Victoria Breckwich Vásquez and her colleagues describe a partnership between a youth environmental justice organization and a local health department to promote voluntary agreements to address lack of access to fresh fruits and vegetables in a low-income neighborhood in San Francisco. The chapter highlights the partnership's use of store shelf diagramming and other data collection methods and demonstrates how the findings were used to work with city policymakers and other players to mount a major new program that gave local stores incentives to become "good neighbors." The impacts of this work on both the local situation and broader state policy efforts are described, as are lessons for other policy-focused CBPR efforts involving youths.

In her examination of feminist research aimed at social change, Michelle Fine (1994) suggests that "the raison d'etre for such research is to unsettle questions, texts, and collective struggles; to challenge what is, incite what could be, and help imagine a world that is not yet imagined." The aim of the chapters in Part Five is to demonstrate yet again the particular potency of CBPR for helping all of us imagine and realize a more just and equitable society, one in which individuals and communities have a genuine voice in influencing the factors that determine their health.

REFERENCES

Corburn, J. (2005). *Street science: Community knowledge and environmental health justice.* Cambridge, MA.: MIT Press.

Fine, M. (1994). Dis-stance and other stances: Negotiation of power inside feminist research. In A. Gitlin (Ed.), *Power and method: Political activism and educational research* (pp. 13–35). New York: Routledge.

Sclove, R. E. (1997). Research by people, for people. *Futures, 29,* 541–549.

CHAPTER

17

THE ROLE OF
CBPR IN POLICY
ADVOCACY

MAKANI THEMBA-NIXON, MEREDITH MINKLER,
& NICHOLAS FREUDENBERG

UNLIKE MORE TRADITIONAL approaches to scientific inquiry, community-based participatory research (CBPR) is defined in part by its belief that action and the fostering of social change are an integral part of the research process (Cornwall & Jewkes, 1995; Hall, 1992; Israel, Eng, Schulz, & Parker, 2005). As the case studies throughout this book illustrate, action may take many forms, from promoting community dialogue about a difficult health topic to changing health-related practices at a local school or hospital.

Note: The authors gratefully acknowledge the helpful comments of Sonja Herbert on an earlier version of this manuscript. We are grateful as well to Lawrence Wallack and Lori Dorfman for their contributions to our thinking about the ability of community residents and their academic and professional partners to harness the power of the media to promote healthy public policy.

Although such outcomes are important, if public health efforts are to influence the lives of large numbers of people, action aimed at changing policy is often essential. In this chapter we consider how the CBPR process can be applied to efforts to change policy, suggest some frameworks that can guide policy-oriented CBPR, and assess some of the challenges that face policy researchers using a CBPR approach.

As Toby Citrin (2000, p. 84) has noted, "For grassroots community-based organizations, the term 'policy' is an abstract concept not clearly related to the quality of life of the community, even though many community residents do, in fact, engage in activities to address 'policy issues.'" Similarly, academics engaged in CBPR, like those involved in more traditional research approaches, have often shied away from policy-level activity, partly because they tend to think of policy and policy processes as occurring on the national and state levels, far removed from the local contexts of a CBPR project. As Rist (1994) has argued, although research may influence policy at this level, in most cases it is only one of many often competing and contradictory forces that influence the final form of a policy.

However, as we shall discuss later in this chapter, in recent years some researchers and activists have challenged this belief and have asked whether emerging networks might be able to apply CBPR methods to national and global policy change (World Social Forum, 2008).

To date, most CBPR policy work has attempted to change policy on the local level, the arena most accessible to community-based participants. Much of the best work in local policy development translates existing community concerns into concrete action. As CBPR begins with community selection of an issue, the bridge to policy advocacy should be a logical one. Yet even though people, particularly in low-income communities, may be used to having outsiders come in to "mobilize" them around predetermined issues (Minkler & Pies, 2005), they have often had little experience in getting a hearing for their own issues in the corridors of power—and having power listen. On the one hand, as the examples here suggest, at best such local involvement can make a critical difference in the local policy environment and can sometimes also build momentum for related policy changes on the state or national levels.

On the other hand, given the deep roots of individualism in American culture, CBPR participants often have to confront the same pressures that other activists and reformers face and that ask them to focus their efforts on changing individuals rather than changing policies. To succeed in convincing communities that it is possible and desirable to focus attention on the upstream causes of ill health is often the first step in a CBPR-initiated community dialogue.

As public health researchers call for greater emphasis on the social as well as the individual determinants of health, CBPR policy initiatives might be a useful tool for improving understanding of the opportunities for intervention at the intersections of the individual, the community, and policy levels (Krieger et al., 2002; Bryant, Raphael, & Travers, 2007).

Nancy Milio (1998) has defined public policy as "a guide to government action at any jurisdictional level to alter what would otherwise occur. The intent is to achieve a more acceptable state of affairs and, from a public health perspective, a more health-promoting society" (p. 15). She goes on to suggest that organizational policy typically involves a single agency or type of organization (for example, a health department or public school system) whereas broader policies tend to operate across multiple organizations and affect large populations. Policy change can occur both as a result of regulatory, legislative, or other formal actions, and also as a result of changes in the informal norms or expectations that govern people's actions.

Recently, the influence of private organizations on health and health policy has drawn increasing attention as well. For example, the decisions that tobacco, food, alcohol, and firearms companies make about advertising, pricing, and retail distribution contribute to patterns of illness, health, and disparities (Freudenberg, 2005), and business groups also shape the political environment in which local, state, and national governments make decisions about health. By identifying opportunities for influencing these policies at the local and higher levels, CBPR researchers may be able to make new contributions to health.

This chapter defines a *policy initiative* as a planned set of activities, with clear goals and objectives, intended to change informal or formal practices or rules of organizations and institutions that affect people's lives. Many models of policy processes that are relevant for CBPR exist in public health and related fields (see, for example, Brownson, Newschaffer, & Ali-Abarghoul, 1997; Kingdon, 1995; Longest, 2006; Milio, 1998; Steckler, Dawson, Goodman, & Epstein, 1987). Such models tend to have in common an emphasis on the various stages of policy development, from initiation through adoption, implementation, evaluation or assessment, and reformulation or repeal (Milio, 1998). They also frequently place a heavy emphasis on the sociopolitical environments in which policymaking takes place, recognizing that developing good policy requires a careful examination of the larger context in which the issue is embedded. Finally, models of the policy process typically stress the often circuitous processes involved in policy development. In Milio's words, policy processes "are not linear, and are often punctuated by legal and social challenges, retrenchment or rescissions. They are always embedded in historical and current social contexts. Policymaking processes shape content as interested parties attempt to direct the course and pace of policy development to their own needs and priorities" (1998, p. 17).

This chapter briefly reviews two conceptual frameworks for understanding the public policy process and the steps involved in policy formulation and enactment. It then examines a third framework (developed by chapter author Makani Themba-Nixon) that is more heavily focused on policy advocacy and has relevance for influencing both public policy and policies made outside the public policy arena. Examples and illustrations of opportunities for CBPR involvement at each stage of the policy process are provided. As this chapter demonstrates, although not all CBPR lends itself to policy change, CBPR practitioners often report that finding opportunities for policy-level action adds a powerful tool to their repertoire and enables deeper and more sustainable improvements in health.

THE POLICYMAKING PROCESS

In 1995, political scientist John Kingdon proposed an influential model for policy development that posited that in order to get the attention of policymakers, those seeking to bring about change have to address three processes: convincing decision makers that a problem exists; proposing feasible, politically attractive proposals to solve the problem; and negotiating the politics that influence whether a proposal succeeds in the political arena. The first stage, moving a policy issue onto the political agenda, is often the starting point for CBPR projects, and several researchers have used Kingdon's model to analyze opportunities for agenda setting on issues such as gun control, food security, and tobacco control (Wallack, Winnett, & Lee, 2005; Breckwich Vásquez et al., 2007; Blackman, 2005; see also Chapters Nineteen and Twenty-One).

According to Kingdon, a *policy window* opens when favorable developments occur in at least two of the three processes (problems, proposals, and politics). Identifying opening policy windows and being able to jump through them are important skills for policy advocates. Thus, monitoring developments in all three processes is an important task for CBPR policy researchers. Then, as new opportunities arise, CBPR participants can be ready to move in any of the three arenas.

Beauford B. Longest Jr., a health policy researcher, describes a second model of the policymaking process, one that builds on Kingdon's work (Longest, 2006). Figure 17.1 illustrates this model, which finds the following features in the process:

- It is a "distinctly cyclical" process, with a circular flow of interactions and influences among the various stages.
- It is an open system, defined as "one in which the process interacts with and is affected by events and circumstances in its external environment."
- It emphasizes several distinct process components but also stresses their intimate interdependence.
- It is a highly political process, reflecting a mix of influences on both public and individual interests and rarely proceeding on the basis of rational or empirical decision making.

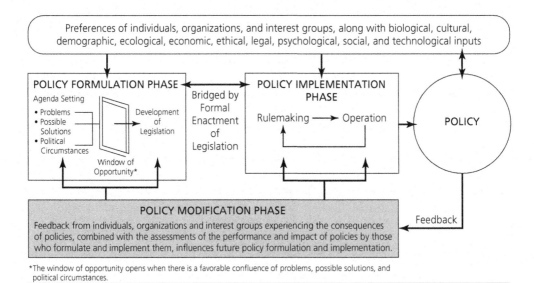

FIGURE 17.1 *Model of the Public Policymaking Process in the United States: Policy Modification Phase*
Source: Longest, 2006. Reprinted with permission.

The three interconnected phases of the public policymaking process identified in Longest's model are

- *Policy formulation:* all activities involved in setting the policy agenda and later in the actual development of legislation
- *Policy implementation:* all activities connected with rule making to guide the actual implementing and operationalizing of a policy
- *Policy modification:* all activities included in the revisiting and possible alteration of all previous decisions and compromises made during the policymaking process

As Longest's model suggests, the formal enactment of legislation is the bridge between the policy formulation process and the subsequent implementation phase (see Figure 17.1). The subsequent policy modification phase comes into play in turn as a feedback loop through which minor tweaking of the legislation or a major revisiting of the agenda-setting process may take place. Both the political nature of policymaking and the dynamic nature of the external environment in which policymaking occurs underscore the likelihood of policy modification—and in extreme cases, even repeal—during this phase.

DEFINING AND FRAMING A POLICY GOAL

As Citrin (2000) has pointed out, "While academics and practitioners are inclined to look first at policymaking and then at its impacts on constituent groups, community residents usually reverse this process, looking first at their daily needs and then at the way these are affected by policy decisions" (p. 84). The general policy goal for a CBPR project flows, by definition, from the community's identification of the problem and the outcomes of the dialogical processes in which it has engaged in order to better explore this issue or problem. As always, reconciling different perspectives on the problem within various community constituencies is an essential task and often a formidable challenge.

Although the community's perception of a problem is one major influence on planned action, a wide variety of additional factors influence policy outcomes. Ensuring that these other contextual factors are considered in formulating a policy goal is a vital step in setting goals. A good policy goal requires cutting or shaping the issue into effective or doable action that engages broader community interest and support. Framing the problem in ways that will attract a wide and diverse constituency whose members care enough about the issue to become actively involved is critical at this stage. Moreover, because CBPR is always concerned about both process and outcome (consistent with the principles of CBPR, delineated in Chapter Three), the chosen policy goals and activities should help a community or community-based organization or coalition to achieve such goals as the following:

- Building community and organizational capacity by expanding the leadership base and creating more involved community members
- Solving real problems, ideally through policy results that can be concisely stated in twenty-five words or less
- Contributing to a sense of community, bringing more people together and giving them a sense of their own power and leadership

- Laying the foundation for later policy, serving as an incremental step on the path toward the community partners' larger goals, and placing this specific policy goal within a longer-term community strategic action plan
- Bringing the community closer to its vision of a healthy community and a better world

An additional frequently cited feature of a good policy goal in this era of cost containment is that it pays for itself. CBPR efforts to reduce the plethora of alcohol and tobacco outlets in low-income communities of color might thus craft a policy goal of establishing local permit fees for the selling of these products or conditional use permits for such environmental land uses as billboards (Themba, 1999). Whatever the ultimate goal selected, however, CBPR partners should be guided in their thinking by coherent principles so that the selected goal has a good likelihood for success and for contributing to subsequent community building in the process.

SELECTING A POLICY APPROACH

After selecting a policy goal, CBPR partners will need to determine who has the power to make the change, whether that be an elected official, a planning commission, or a business. As noted earlier, although the focus of this chapter is primarily on efforts to influence local public policy (for example, through initiatives and ordinances), efforts to bring about similar policy changes at higher levels or in relevant private sector arenas should also be considered, especially in partnership with other CBPR or advocacy groups in other jurisdictions. Let us look at a range of possible policy-related strategies.

Voluntary Agreements

Voluntary agreements are "pacts between a community and one or more institutions that outline conditions, expectations, or obligations without the force of law" (Themba, 1999, p. 91). Such agreements provide a useful alternative to more formal regulations when support for enacting such regulations is not quite sufficient. In some cases a voluntary agreement can be an interim step toward more meaningful changes in policy, either because the voluntary agreements do not succeed in solving the problem or because some large organizations prefer public policy change to negotiating many agreements with many communities. Ideally, a written memorandum of understanding should be developed that clearly spells out the conditions of each agreement, and care must be taken to ensure that the terms of the agreement are being honored.

In Chapter Twenty, Vásquez and her colleagues describe a campaign to persuade grocery stores in low-income neighborhoods in San Francisco to sign voluntary agreements to stock healthier foods. These agreements led to improvements in nutritional choices for local residents and also contributed to efforts, still under way, to pass a state assembly bill supporting similar ventures elsewhere in California (Breckwich Vásquez et al., 2007).

Legal Actions

Well-framed legal actions, such as lawsuits and other court actions, can also accomplish significant long- and short-term goals, even if they simply result in getting the other party to the table. Yet such actions can be tedious and expensive, as well as a major distraction if not integrated into a broader community agenda (Themba, 1999). Further, failure to identify the right defendants (for example, the parent company of a major local polluter) can lead to embarrassing and demoralizing defeats. In lieu of (or in addition to) bringing a lawsuit, simply filing complaints about bad or illegal practices with the appropriate regulatory agency can be an effective policy approach. In recent years community and advocacy groups have used legal action against the food, pharmaceutical, and tobacco industries (Freudenberg, 2005; Jacobson & Soliman, 2002) and against local governments. In Chapter Eighteen, Peggy Shepard and her colleagues describe their co-filing of a legal complaint under the Civil Rights Act as one of many strategies used to get a public agency to act to reduce air pollution from diesel buses.

Studies and Moratoriums

Mandated studies and moratoriums pending data collection can be helpful under certain circumstances. Although CBPR can uncover valuable information about an unhealthy or unlawful institutional practice, far more extensive study may be necessary to collect the hard data needed to support a policy change. In such instances, CBPR partners may identify a policy goal of getting a mandated study or other data collection activity performed (or protecting what is currently being collected, such as data on racial or ethnic disparities in health). When a Los Angeles coalition's preliminary investigation led it to fight for and get a mandated city study on wage levels, the resulting information was so disconcerting that it laid an important basis for subsequent work toward a living-wage law (Themba, 1999).

Another useful policy approach may involve calling for a moratorium on continued enactment of existing policy until more data are available. For example, during conflicts about local and state laws that would dictate the process for locating polluting facilities, environmental justice activists in West Harlem called for a moratorium on siting new facilities in their neighborhood, both to protect their community and to set a precedent that could guide future action. The breathing time allowed by a moratorium may also permit CBPR partners to organize neighborhood hearings or town hall meetings and forums with legislators in attendance. Such events, particularly if well publicized and offering a blend of the numbers and stories needed to influence public opinion (Wallack, Woodruff, Dorfman, & Diaz, 1999), can mobilize support for a policy change.

Electoral Strategies

Electoral strategies, like legal approaches to policy change, tend to be extremely time consuming and labor intensive. Yet such approaches, including ballot initiatives, referendums, and even support of candidates, can have a considerable payoff over the longer term. As Steckler and Dawson (1982) suggest, "States which offer the possibility of a referendum or initiative enable citizens themselves to become policy makers" (p. 289). There may be short-term payoffs as well. Electoral campaigns can raise the profile of an issue, attract volunteers, and pull an issue out of the purview of nonsupportive policymakers and place it directly before a more supportive public. Whether helping to craft an initiative or becoming involved in an effort to react to an existing policy through a referendum, CBPR partners can facilitate bringing an issue to public attention.

Each of these policy-related approaches—voluntary agreements, legal actions, mandated studies and moratoriums, and electoral strategies—has both advantages and disadvantages that must be carefully weighed by CBPR partners in their efforts to select the alternative most likely to succeed. This chapter next describes some of the key considerations and advocacy steps that are relevant in the use of a variety of alternative approaches to policy change and that complement and expand on the policy process stages in the conceptual models just described.

IDENTIFYING A TARGET

As noted earlier, decisions about the particular policy approach best suited to a given CBPR effort should be driven in part by a careful analysis of the most appropriate change target or decision-making body with the power to bring about the changes sought. Several key questions may be helpful to community members and their outside research partners as they choose an appropriate target, including these (Themba, 1999):

- Who or what institutions have the power to solve or ameliorate the problem and grant the community's demands?
- Are there key actors who must be approached first as gatekeepers to the people with real power?
- What would motivate key actors to take the actions you want to see (for example, would a politician who is up for reelection be aided by your cause)?
- Which targets are appointed? Which are elected?
- Are there relevant bodies (such as commissions or subcommittees) that are open to community participation and that one or more of your members might join?
- What are the most powerful and strategic influences on the targets (for example, voters, consumers, faith-based organizations, taxpayers, investors, neighborhood organizations)?
- What are each target's self-interests where this issue is concerned?
- Who would have jurisdiction if you redefined the issue (for example, if you turned a tobacco advertising issue into a question of fair business practices)? Would this increase your likelihood of success?

As some of these questions suggest, each decision-making body or target selected will require different organizing strategies to move it to action. A critical part of the CBPR process will therefore be conducting strategic analysis to narrow down potential targets and researching each target's self-interests, strengths, and vulnerabilities. Not infrequently, such research will reveal the existence of a more vulnerable target with whom the possibility of success is greater. This target is often referred to as the primary target, the one on whom pressure can be focused. Recent community organizing and CBPR around billboard advertising of alcohol and tobacco provides a good case in point. Participants have found it more effective, for example, to target local and in some cases state governments to restrict the placement and content of ads than to pressure the billboard industry itself to give up a sizable portion of its revenue from such advertisements (Themba, 1999). In other instances, CBPR partners may need to identify additional, secondary targets to bring about the desired change.

Finally, CBPR participants need to ask about the relative importance of short-term victories versus consciousness raising and longer-term political mobilization. Ideally, both are possible, but in the real world, groups often need to choose between the more achievable but superficial victories and the more time-consuming but critical changes in power relationships. With experience, some groups find it helpful to have a portfolio of activities and campaigns that balance these two policy objectives.

SUPPORT, POWER, AND OPPOSITION

Building support for a CBPR policy goal or approach often requires building a coalition of organizations that come together temporarily for a specific reason (Berkowitz & Wolff, 2000; Wandersman, Goodman, & Butterfoss, 2005). As PolicyLink (2005) has pointed out, "Building a strong coalition will show community-wide concern and demonstrate to agency officials, the media, and the public at large that there is a serious problem that must be addressed, and a consensus about what needs to be done." Coalitions oriented toward policy change can work at diverse jurisdictional levels, depending on the level of the government or private policymaking group that has decision-making authority for the changes being sought (Sofaer, 2001). In deciding whether to put together such a coalition, CBPR partners should consider the kinds of support needed to win, which groups are most likely to support the policy goal or initiative, and which groups can influence the target or decision maker. Community members of the CBPR team can be particularly helpful at this stage in sharing their knowledge of key community players and the potential interests of each. Both informal groups (for example, parents of children with asthma) and formal community organizations should be considered potential allies. Each potential ally's commitment to the issue and self-interests, as well as the resources and the risks and liabilities this ally's involvement might entail, need to be considered in building a base of support for the policy action being proposed.

At the same time that CBPR partners work to build their own power base, they need to think strategically about the interests and potential power base of the opposition (see also Appendix K). Community interests in lead abatement, improved air quality, and the like may translate into policy initiatives whose implementation would hurt a powerful industry or a local employer's bottom line. Because these likely opponents may also have powerful lobbies or make substantial contributions to the coffers of elected decision makers, the importance of their opposition should not be minimized. CBPR partners need to consider such matters as whose interests might be adversely affected by a policy initiative, in what ways these interests might be affected, and whether the proposed initiative will cost money or raise fees or taxes. As in other forms of community-based research and organizing, doing one's homework, understanding in detail who will pay for a proposed policy, and being able to justify the policy to the decision makers being targeted are critical to success.

POLICY PROCESS STAGES AND CBPR OPPORTUNITIES

The discussion in this section assesses the unique opportunities for CBPR involvement at each stage of the policy process, using the stages developed by one of the chapter authors (Themba, 1999) as a guide for policy advocates.

Assessing the Policy Environment

As Milio (1998) suggests, "Organized activity surrounding the policymaking process in any given issue is set in a historical context derived from past experience with similar issues and current constraining circumstances that affect all interested parties" (p. 20). Thus demographic, epidemiological, political, economic, and other factors are all likely to influence the reception a given policy initiative will receive and its chances for success. Monitoring the policy environment must therefore begin as a key component of the data gathering that will inform what a potential policy initiative might look like.

At the same time that they are assessing the environment, CBPR partners may "try on," or test, a number of potential approaches to addressing their issue. Broad community support, legality, and the likelihood of success are among the criteria that should be considered at this early stage.

Reframing the Issue and Defining the Initiative

A critical step in the action phase of CBPR for policy change involves helping community partners refine the issue they have collectively identified and collaboratively examined so that it becomes a clear policy initiative. In the context of CBPR, the best policy initiatives often come from having community partners articulate their ideal policy, and then looking for the best mechanism to bring that vision to reality (Themba, 1999). Reframing the issue may be needed at this point so that the policy initiative that is crafted clearly reflects the community's interests while also showing sensitivity to broader environmental issues (Milio, 1998) and the concerns of existing or potential allies and other stakeholders. A CBPR project focused on preventing youth violence, for example, and targeting a local city council with the goal of limiting handgun availability and increasing youth employment opportunities might reframe its initial initiative to emphasize the social and economic aspects of youth violence (Wallack, 1994). By tapping into the aspects of the issue of greatest concern to local council members and reframing the issue to reflect these concerns, the CBPR partners may substantially increase their chances for success.

Part of reframing may also involve defining issues nationally and internationally as well as locally. Many environmental groups, for example, have researched the practices of companies seeking to build new plants in order to assess the companies' record on environmental issues in other states or countries. When unethical or dubious practices are uncovered, this information can be used in legal or educational campaigns. Similarly, local CBPR groups attempting to mobilize against the tobacco industry have sometimes studied and publicized that industry's increased targeting of people of color in Third World countries and Eastern European nations (World Health Organization, 1996). Revealing such practices overseas may have value at home in delegitimizing the image of multinational parent companies that allow or encourage such practices. It can also serve as a starting point for global alliances that can better contest the power of these multinational companies.

Strategic Power Analysis

Once the initiative has been identified, the CBPR partners should conduct a strategic *power analysis* to identify the targets, allies, opponents, and other factors that will be important in the campaign (Ritas, 2003; see Appendix K). Kurt Lewin's (1947) classic *force field analysis* may be used at this stage, as participants lay out the driving forces in support of the initiative and the likely resisting or restraining forces that may work against its success (Appendix K). Methods for removing or weakening the resisting forces and both adding new driving forces and strengthening the power of those already operative are then considered. Often the initiative is refined further in the light of this new information.

This approach figured prominently in the decision by tobacco control organizations working in African American communities to mount a campaign to shut down X brand cigarettes. Typically, the focus in tobacco control is on further regulation, because the industry is both very powerful and well funded. However, Duffy Distributors, the packager and distributor of X brand, was a small, family-operated business in predominantly white Charlestown, Massachusetts, not far from Boston.

Activists seeking to persuade the company to withdraw the brand for health reasons and for its appropriation of the cultural image of Malcolm X were not making headway. However, the power analysis and strategic planning process revealed that concerted media pressure would likely force the small company to discontinue the brand. They were right. After just two weeks the company could not withstand the barrage of media coverage, protests, and bad publicity and decided to drop the brand altogether. Without research and power analysis to guide the group's strategy, it might have settled for far less (Themba, 1996).

Although the X brand action was a clear success story, strategic analysis and related processes can also be helpful when victory may be less likely or incomplete. As Rochefort and Cobb (1993) suggest, the feasibility analysis conducted during this stage of the policy process may well suggest possible compromise positions, which can be explored in advance but then held in reserve to be used only if a compromise appears necessary.

Organizing Support for the Initiative

Informed by the power analysis and strategic planning, organizing for the proposed policy change begins. A variety of strategies may be useful at this stage, including town hall meetings, door-to-door canvassing, outreach to additional organizational partners, and media advocacy. Defined as the strategic use of mass media to advance a social or public policy initiative (U.S. Department of Health and Human Services, 1989), *media advocacy* has increasingly been used by local community groups and CBPR partners to deliver their message and create pressure for change (Dorfman, Wallack, & Woodruff, 2005; Wallack et al., 1999).

Media advocacy is critical to policy advocacy. Important political debates are carried out in fifteen-second sound bites, and a single news story can be the catalyst for new legislation. For better or worse, the media are clearly central to setting the public agenda, with news media playing a particularly important role as the public's source of the "official story." It is now nearly axiomatic that what story is chosen for coverage and how it is covered largely determines public sentiment—especially among public officials.

Given the importance of the media's agenda-setting and legitimizing functions, data and research play critical roles in establishing the credibility of community policy initiatives with policymakers and the public at large. CBPR findings have been particularly important to efforts that were unpopular or focused on communities with few resources. For example, welfare rights groups partnered with Virginia Polytechnic University researcher Susan Gooden to disseminate research on discrimination in workfare programs. Gooden's work documented what many organizers knew anecdotally—that women of color did not receive equal access to training, placement, and employment services. Groups leveraged the data in an intensive media campaign to pressure the federal government to enact civil rights protections for program participants. The media campaign helped raise awareness about problems with the administration of workfare programs and put pressure on state and federal agencies to make changes (Themba, Delgado, Vribe, & Calpotura, 2000).

In the Belly of the Beast

Once the initiative is on the table and support is made clear, groups should work closely with decision makers to ensure that the policy is actually enacted. Often further research and expertise are needed as community groups and researchers make their case. It is at this stage that CBPR partnerships are at greatest risk, as decision makers will often look to researchers and other traditional "experts" for input and will sometimes act to exclude community-based groups that they perceive are less "professional." These classic divide-and-conquer tactics have hurt a wide variety of movements.

To address this problem, environmental justice advocates (groups working to address dimensions of racism in environmental policy) have developed protocols for community work with researchers in order to avoid further conflicts. Similar protocols have been developed by other groups working to foster more effective community-researcher partnerships (see Chapter Three and Appendix A), and sample memorandums of understanding have been published and widely disseminated (Fawcett, Francisco, Paine-Andrews, & Schultz, 2000; see also Appendix H).

Victory and Defense

In the case of progressive policies, winning enactment can mean that a corporate court challenge is soon to follow (Themba, 1999). CBPR practitioners taking the roles of advocates must prepare for the possibility of litigation at the beginning of the initiative and be ready to play an active role in any legal action, even if the local government (and not their group) is the defendant. CBPR partners have played an important role in this stage of the policy process by working with communities to craft public testimony with an eye toward building a strong public record as a defense against any future litigation. For example, Baltimore's Citywide Liquor Coalition made sure that its attorney worked closely with the city attorney throughout an initiative process. The objective of the city and the coalition was to carefully craft testimony that would be part of a strong public record in preparation for the litigation that would follow passage of the policy they were supporting (Themba, 1999). In sum, and although celebrating a victory is always in order (Staples, 2005), preparing for challenges to a controversial new policy is also a critical part of the action in which CBPR partners may usefully engage.

Enforcement and Evaluation

After the policy is enacted and has cleared any legal challenges, the work to get the new law enforced begins. For initiatives with powerful opposition, negotiation continues around issues such as the timeline for implementing the policy, the interpretation of particular clauses, and fitting the new policy in with other staffing priorities. Researchers and community-based groups working together have helped agencies identify existing enforcement models and propose new enforcement procedures that meet community needs. In addition, research partners have helped community groups design processes for evaluating new policies, with an eye toward strengthening these policies and their enforcement. One example of such a partnership was the work of South Carolina Fair Share with University of South Carolina researchers on the enforcement and effectiveness of new child health insurance policies. Research partners were able to develop a participatory evaluation process that provided accessible information on how well the program was working and why. Armed with good data, community groups could take an active, informed, and ongoing part in the implementation process (Themba et al., 2000).

From Local to Global and Back

Although much of the action on the CBPR policy front has been at the local level, some emerging networks are creating opportunities for national and global CBPR alliances. The World Social Forum, for example, brings together activists from around the world to discuss strategies and analyze opportunities to weave local struggles together into a more powerful force. Similarly, the Framework Convention on Tobacco Control Alliance (2008) brings together hundreds of nongovernmental organizations from around the world to develop strategies to counter the work of the multinational tobacco companies. In the coming decade these global networks might offer local CBPR groups powerful new allies.

SUMMARY

Community-based participatory research has been an important asset in community-based policy development. CBPR partners have identified, made visible, and legitimized issues so that they are placed on the public's agenda. It has also helped community advocates to attract media attention for long-standing but long-ignored issues when there are newsworthy findings. The best initiatives use research as a means of documenting and elucidating problems that are already of concern to communities, and they do so in ways that build confidence in community-based knowledge and ways of knowing (Ansley & Gaventa, 1997).

In policy arenas, CBPR can be an agent for the democratization of information through bringing about the active involvement of communities in data gathering and by giving community-based groups equal access to the kinds of data that drive policymaking. It can help communities influence the policy process in ways that can benefit the groups of which they are a part. CBPR partnerships are of course only one influence on policy; yet as the examples in this and several other chapters illustrate, community groups and academic researchers who are intentional about policy outcomes from the beginning can build CBPR projects that result in lasting, formal policy changes that promote health and reduce inequities.

QUESTIONS FOR DISCUSSION

1. Although its action orientation would seem to make policy work a natural for CBPR, both community and academic partners may be reluctant to move into this area. What are some of the reasons for this reluctance? As a partnership member who sees the potential for engaging in a policy-related action, what arguments might you make to encourage those you are working with to consider becoming engaged in this way?

2. To take insights from this chapter and Appendix K further, divide into groups around common areas of interest (for example, reproductive rights or health care access for the uninsured). Think of a real or hypothetical policy you would like to see enacted, and do a policy-mapping exercise, modified according to your time constraints (see the options in Appendix K). At a minimum, after deciding on the policy you want to support, list the policy targets (people or institutions with the power to make the change) and the key stakeholders who are likely to be for or against the policy. Following the instructions and the diagram for Figure K.1 (in Appendix K), use circles to indicate the relative power of these stakeholders and where they stand on the issue and in relation to each other. Finally, brainstorm some steps your partnership (or individual members) could take to weaken the opposition forces, strengthen your allies, and in other ways help bring about the change you seek. Be sure to leave time to reflect on this exercise and its utility, as well as on any "nuggets" you may have picked up about policy advocacy in the course of taking part.

KEY TERMS

Policy advocacy   Community participation
Policymaking process   Power analysis

REFERENCES

Ansley, F., & Gaventa, J. (1997, January-February). Researching for democracy and democratizing research. *Change,* pp. 46–53.

Berkowitz, B., & Wolff, T. (2000). *The spirit of the coalition.* Washington, DC: American Public Health Association.

Blackman, V. S. (2005). Putting policy theory to work: Tobacco control in California. *Policy, Politics & Nursing Practice, 6*(2), 148–155.

Breckwich Vásquez, V., Lanza, D., Hennessey Lavery, S., Facente, S., Halpin, H. A., & Minkler, M. (2007). Addressing food security through public policy action in a community-based participatory research partnership. *Health Promotion Practice, 8*(4), 342–349.

Brownson, R. C., Newschaffer, C. J., & Ali-Abarghoul, F. (1997). Policy research for disease prevention: Challenges and practical recommendations. *American Journal of Public Health, 87,* 735–739.

Bryant, T., Raphael, D., & Travers, R. (2007). Identifying and strengthening the structural roots of urban health in Canada: Participatory policy research and the urban health agenda. *Promotion & Education, 14*(1), 6–11.

Citrin, T. (2000). Policy issues in a community-based approach. In T. A. Bruce & S. Uranga McKane (Eds.), *Community-based public health: A partnership model* (pp. 83–90). Washington, DC: American Public Health Association.

Cornwall, A., & Jewkes, R. (1995). What is participatory research? *Social Science & Medicine, 41,* 1667–1676.

Dorfman, L., Wallack, L., & Woodruff, K. (2005). More than a message: Framing public health advocacy to change corporate practices. *Health Education & Behavior, 32*(3), 320–336.

Fawcett, S. B., Francisco, V. T., Paine-Andrews, A., & Schultz, J. A. (2000). A model memorandum of collaboration: A proposal. *Public Health Reports, 115,* 174–179.

Framework Convention on Tobacco Control Alliance. (2008). *The WHO Framework Convention on Tobacco Control: A Public Health Movement.* Retrieved May 4, 2008, from http://www.fctc.org.

Freudenberg, N. (2005). Public health advocacy to change corporate practices: Implications for health education practice and research. *Health Education & Behavior, 32*(3), 298–319.

Hall, B. L. (1992). From margins to center? The development and purpose of participatory research. *American Sociologist, 23*(4), 15–28.

Israel, B. A., Eng, E., Schulz, A. J., & Parker, E. A. (Eds.). (2005). *Methods in community-based participatory research for health.* San Francisco: Jossey-Bass.

Jacobson, P. D., & Soliman, S. (2002). Litigation as public health policy: Theory or reality? *Journal of Law, Medicine & Ethics, 30*(2), 224–238.

Kingdon, J. W. (1995). *Agendas, alternatives, and public policies* (2nd ed.). Reading, MA: Addison-Wesley.

Krieger, J., Allen, C., Cheadle, A., Ciske, S., Schier, J. K., Senturia, K., et al. (2002). Using community-based participatory research to address social determinants of health: Lessons learned from Seattle Partners for Healthy Communities. *Health Education & Behavior, 29*(3), 361–382.

Lewin, K. (1947). Quasi-stationary social equilibria and the problem of social change. In T. Newcomb & E. Hartley (Eds.), *Readings in social psychology* (pp. 340–344). Austin, TX: Holt, Rinehart and Winston.

Longest, B. B., Jr. (2006). *Health policymaking in the United States* (4th ed.). Chicago: Health Administration Press/ Washington, DC: AUPHA Press.

Milio, N. (1998). Priorities and strategies for promoting community-based prevention policies. *Journal of Public Health Management and Practice, 4*(3), 14–28.

Minkler, M., & Pies, C. (2005). Ethical issues and practical dilemmas in community organizing and community participation. In M. Minkler (Ed.), *Community organizing and community building for health* (2nd ed., pp. 116–133). New Brunswick, NJ: Rutgers University Press.

PolicyLink. (2005). *Advocating for change: Administrative petitioning; Making stronger rules.* Retrieved Jan. 15, 2008, from http://www.policylink.org/AdvocatingForChange/AdminPetitions.pdf.

Rist, C. (1994). Influencing the policy process with qualitative research. In N. K. Denzin & Y. S. Lincoln (Eds.), *Handbook of qualitative research* (pp. 545–557). Thousand Oaks, CA: Sage.

Ritas, C. (2003). *Speaking truth, creating power: A guide to policy work for community-based participatory research practitioners.* Retrieved Jan. 15, 2008, from http://futurehealth.ucsf.edu/pdf_files/Ritas.pdf.

Rochefort, D., & Cobb, R. (1993). Definition, agenda, access, and policy choice. *Policy Studies Journal, 21,* 56–71.

Sofaer, S. (2001). *Working together, moving ahead: A manual to support effective community health coalitions.* New York: Baruch College, School of Public Affairs.

Staples, L. (2005). Selecting and cutting the issue. In M. Minkler (Ed.), *Community organizing and community building for health* (2nd ed., pp. 173–192). New Brunswick, NJ: Rutgers University Press.

Steckler, A., & Dawson, L. (1982). The role of health education in public policy development. *Health Education Quarterly, 9,* 275–292.

Steckler, A., Dawson, L., Goodman, R. M., & Epstein, N. (1987). Policy advocacy: Three emerging roles for health education. *Advances in Health Education and Promotion, 2,* 5–27.

Themba, M. N. (1996). *Chalk one up for David: The African American Tobacco Education Network and the fight to stop X brand.* Sacramento, CA: African American Tobacco Education Network.

Themba, M. N. (1999). *Making policy, making change: How communities are taking law into their own hands.* San Francisco: Jossey-Bass.

Themba, M. N., Delgado, G., Vribe, J., & Calpotura, F. (2000). *Grassroots innovative policy program.* Oakland, CA: Applied Research Center.

U.S. Department of Health and Human Services. (1989). *Media strategies for smoking control: Guidelines.* Washington, DC: U.S. Government Printing Office.

Wallack, L. (1994). Media advocacy: A strategy for empowering people and communities. *Journal of Public Health Policy, 15,* 420–436.

Wallack, L., Winett, L., & Lee, A. (2005). Successful public policy change in California: Firearms and youth resources. *Journal of Public Health Policy, 26*(2), 206–226.

Wallack, L., Woodruff, K., Dorfman, L., & Diaz, I. (1999). *News for a change: An advocate's guide to working with the media.* Thousand Oaks, CA: Sage.

Wandersman, A., Goodman, R. M., & Butterfoss, F. D. (2005). Understanding coalitions and how they operate: An "open systems" organizational framework. In M. Minkler (Ed.), *Community organizing and community building for health* (2nd ed., pp. 368–385). New Brunswick, NJ: Rutgers University Press.

World Health Organization. (1996). The tobacco epidemic: A global public health emergency. *Tobacco alert* (Special issue: World No Tobacco Day).

World Social Forum. (2008). [Homepage.] Retrieved May 4, 2008, from http://www.forumsocialmundial.org.br/index.php?cd_language=2.

CHAPTER

18

USING CBPR TO PROMOTE ENVIRONMENTAL JUSTICE POLICY

A CASE STUDY FROM HARLEM, NEW YORK

PEGGY SHEPARD, VICTORIA BRECKWICH VÁSQUEZ, & MEREDITH MINKLER

Note: This chapter is adapted from Promoting environmental health policy through community-based participatory research: A case study from Harlem, New York, by V. Breckwich Vásquez, M. Minkler, and P. Shepard, 2006. *Journal of Urban Health, 83*(1), pp. 101–110. Adapted with permission of the New York Academy of Sciences. The study on which this chapter is based was made possible by a grant from the W. K. Kellogg Foundation, and we gratefully acknowledge the foundation and particularly Barbara Sabol and Tamra Fountaine-Jones for their belief in and support of this project. We acknowledge as well the assistance of researcher Shelley Facente, consultant Angela Glover Blackwell and her team at PolicyLink, and members of the study's community advisory board for the board's many contributions. Finally, our deepest appreciation is extended to the community and academic partners and policymakers whose insights greatly enriched this study.

WITH ITS ACCENT on partnering with communities and on carrying out action to effect change as part of the research process itself (Israel, Schulz, Parker, & Becker, 1998), community-based participatory research (CBPR) has demonstrated special relevance in the area of environmental justice (Brugge & Hynes, 2005; Minkler, Breckwich Vásquez, Tajik, & Petersen, 2008; O'Fallon & Dearry, 2002; Shepard, Northridge, Prakash, & Stover, 2002). As Morello-Frosch, Pastor, Sadd, Porras, and Prichard (2005) point out, "Despite the inherent challenges in bridging the academic and activist worlds to collect and interpret scientific data [in CBPR], the involvement of communities who directly experience exposures and diseases of concern can promote new avenues of research" and further aid in the dissemination of findings and their use to impact on policy (p. 376). To date, however, and with some important exceptions (cf. Brugge & Hynes, 2005; Morello-Frosch et al., 2005; Petersen, Minkler, Breckwich Vásquez, & Baden, 2006; see also Chapters Nineteen and Twenty), little attention has been focused on the impacts of CBPR on the policy level.

This chapter helps to address this gap in the literature by examining the partnership in Northern Manhattan between West Harlem Environmental Action, Inc. (WE ACT), and Columbia University's Center for Children's Environmental Health to study and address diesel bus pollution and related air quality issues in this low-income community. The partnership's research and WE ACT's follow-up public education and policy advocacy have been widely credited with helping to bring about environmental health policy changes on the municipal and state levels (Kinney, Aggarwal, Northridge, Janssen, & Shepard, 2000; Perera et al., 2002; O'Fallon & Dearry, 2002; Blackwell, Minkler. & Thompson, 2005).

Drawing in part on the results of a detailed, multimethod case study analysis (Yin, 2003) of the WE ACT partnership conducted by two of the chapter authors and described in detail elsewhere (Breckwich Vásquez et al., 2006), we begin by providing some background on the partnership, the setting in which that partnership took place, and also the problem of poor air quality and asthma morbidity and morality. We then discuss the evolution, research, and policy processes and outcomes of this partnership and its multilevel impacts on health policy concerning diesel bus emissions and related environmental justice issues.

CASE BACKGROUND

WE ACT was founded in 1988 as a nonprofit organization that used community-based action (and later CBPR) to advance environmental health policy, public health, and quality of life (Shepard et al., 2002). The organization contributes to community capacity building through special activities, such as its youth programs and environmental justice leadership training institutes, and also plays a pivotal role in building coalitions around environmental justice issues. With a few notable exceptions, however (for example, the Earth Crew study described in this chapter), the CBPR projects in which WE ACT has participated have involved principally WE ACT staff as the community partners, with other community members mobilized to participate in special follow-up community events and advocacy-related activities.

WE ACT serves Northern Manhattan (comprising East, West, and Central Harlem and Washington Heights), a 7.4-square-mile area in which over 1.5 million mostly low- to middle-income African Americans and Latinos reside. Known for its richly diverse population and cultural history, the area also bears disproportionate rates of disability and premature death. Morbidity and mortality rates from asthma in Harlem are among the highest in the nation, with one recent study finding that over one in four children in central Harlem suffers from this disease (Nicholas et al., 2005).

Contributing to this problem is the poor air quality that results from the diesel buses and related polluting facilities that are disproportionately located in the area. Six of the eight Manhattan diesel bus depots, housing one-third of New York City's bus fleet, were sited in Northern Manhattan, and at the time of the project described in this case study, the Metropolitan Transit Authority was purchasing land for parking lots for additional buses.

Diesel engines emit thirty to one hundred times more particles than gasoline engines that have emission control devices (McCellan, 1987), and research has demonstrated a significant association between high levels of diesel exhaust and elevated rates of respiratory ailments and asthma (Diaz-Sanchez, 1997; Northridge, Meyer, & Dunn, 2002). These studies also have supported Harlem residents' concerns about the deleterious effects of diesel buses, documenting that the largest contributor to area pollution is excessive bus idling in lots and in the streets around the depots. As a WE ACT press release put it, "The City-wide benefit of public transportation services is Northern Manhattan's burden."

The formal partnership between WE ACT and the Columbia Children's Center for Environmental Health (CCCEH) began in the mid-1990s, with the goals of (1) studying the relationship between community-level environmental exposures and environmental health outcomes and (2) translating those findings into policy changes that create equity in environmental decision making and environmental protection. Of the several CBPR efforts the WE ACT partnership has undertaken, its Earth Crew study has been particularly useful from a policy perspective, and that study is the focus of this chapter.

RESEARCH METHODS, ROLES, AND FINDINGS

In July 1996, seventeen Earth Crew youths, under the supervision of epidemiologists from Columbia University, undertook a study to measure sidewalk concentrations of diesel exhaust particles in order to determine whether particular areas in Harlem were disproportionately affected by higher diesel exhaust emissions. The topic for this study came from the community partner, and the study itself was designed largely by the academic partners. The Earth Crew youths, who were paid community interns aged fourteen to eighteen, were trained to operate and calibrate backpack air monitors and to conduct traffic counts (using digital counters to track the numbers of diesel buses, diesel trucks, cars, and pedestrians) on selected streets for five weekdays, eight hours per day (Kinney et al., 2000). The four sites chosen for the study had been designated by the U.S. Environmental Protection Agency (EPA) as *hot spots* that had particularly heavy foot and vehicular traffic and were near bus depots. Largely in response to WE ACT's urging, the EPA agreed to conduct ambient monitoring in these same locations, providing an important source of comparative data.

Researchers from Columbia were assigned to each site, providing training, general study oversight, and mentoring for the youths in the field. Air monitors measured particulate matter small enough to have potentially harmful health effects ($PM_{2.5}$) and also elemental carbon (EC) concentrations; EC is a key component of diesel exhaust particles.

Data were analyzed primarily by the researchers, using two-way analysis of variance (ANOVA). Findings indicated that variations in $PM_{2.5}$ and EC appeared to be related to the magnitude of local diesel sources, and this reinforced community concerns about the disproportionate burden of diesel traffic and bus depots in Harlem. Results also showed that $PM_{2.5}$ concentrations ranged from 22 to 69 $\mu g/m^3$ in eight hours (Kinney et al., 2000), compared to the annual fine particle standard (15.1 $\mu g/m^3$) proposed by the U.S. Environmental Protection Agency (EPA). WE ACT's finding closely mirrored the EPA's own findings using ambient monitors, a fact that further increased the credibility of the Earth Crew study.

The genuine co-learning involved in WE ACT's partnership research was frequently pointed up in our interviews. An academic researcher thus described how in one instance, input from community members caused him to rethink the placement of ambient monitors. Community members thus questioned the outside researchers' decision to place air monitors solely on school rooftops, suggesting that they be placed instead outside the windows, nearer where the children breathe. As this academic partner commented: "Sometimes as scientists we make assumptions and don't rethink assumptions to see how they fit in a natural situation. I think community people, because they are looking at it from a fresh perspective, will question the assumptions in a way that actually improves the science. It may tailor things to the situation in a way we would not have thought of."

In sum, the participation of community partners in identifying research questions and offering advice on study design and the extensive involvement of WE ACT Earth Crew youths in implementing the study appeared to contribute substantially to the research component of this CBPR project.

From Research to Policy Action

A hallmark of CBPR is its commitment to combining research with action to effect change (Israel et al., 1998; see also Chapter Seventeen), and for WE ACT, policy-level change has been a particularly important avenue for working to improve urban environmental health. Although differences in partner timetables and sense of urgency led to some frustration (for example, over a long delay in the publication of findings), WE ACT, sometimes aided by the lead academic partner, moved ahead to undertake a number of policy-related steps and activities to effect change. As Milio (1998) points out, policymaking proceeds nonlinearly and is embedded within changing sociohistorical contexts. Yet policy steps and activities like those described in the following paragraphs nonetheless shape the content, course, pace, and development of policy.

Identifying and Defining the Problem WE ACT had identified air pollution and its link to respiratory health as a key problem and policy issue well prior to the initiation of its collaboration with Columbia University researchers. By demonstrating that exposure to fine particulate matter and elemental carbon appeared related to the magnitude of local diesel sources, the Earth Crew study played an important role in providing credible evidence during the problem identification phase of the policy process.

Setting an Agenda and Creating Awareness Kingdon (1995) describes *agendas* as lists of issue areas to which government officials are paying attention. Through its focus on the relationship between the environment and asthma, the partnership played a leadership role in highlighting a health issue that has become a national priority and invites policy action.

The community partners, researchers, and policymakers interviewed all agreed that WE ACT helped to educate community residents and policymakers through broad-based public awareness campaigns, including a signature effort titled If You Live Uptown, Breathe at Your Own Risk. Graphically illustrated with a picture of two children in gas masks on a busy street corner, this slogan appeared in seventy-five bus shelter ads as well as on buttons, posters, and widely distributed brochures describing the problem. From the perspectives of those we interviewed, WE ACT's cosponsorship of conferences such as the Alternative Fuel Summit, its testimony at public meetings, its briefing of elected officials, and its press conferences further contributed to agenda setting and creating awareness. The hosting of *toxics and treasures tours,* which acquainted policymakers and others with both the adverse exposure sources in the community and the historic landmarks that make this neighborhood unique, also helped in this awareness-generating stage of the process.

Although WE ACT was front and center in such activities, the lead academic partner noted that he too had testified, attended meetings at city hall, and in other ways helped in the partnership's efforts to bring attention to the issue. Academic partners also participated in WE ACT–led environmental health workshops and informal discussions as a means of creating awareness and interest in environmental justice issues in the broader community.

Constructing the Policy Alternatives WE ACT went through a deliberate process of policy-oriented research to identify targets, allies, opponents, and other forces and factors likely to be important in addressing partnership issues. As one community partner remarked: "we will literally unfold charts of paper and start mapping the key actors: who is responsible for decision making, who is making policy and what is the policy. . . . What are the impacts on these types of policies coming out of this particular agency? How does it play out in terms of impacting our community, our organization, and our allies?"

Through this process, three government entities with the power to make the relevant policy change were identified—the Metropolitan Transit Authority (MTA), the state governor, and a state legislative oversight committee. Alternative policy scenarios involving these targets were also considered by WE ACT, with the academic partner sometimes called in to provide advice and engage in discussions of the pros and cons of policy alternatives being considered.

Deciding on the Policy to Pursue Policy advocates and community organizers emphasize the importance of developing a policy goal that is specific, winnable, and easy to articulate (see Chapter Nine). Through conducting both formal and informal strategic planning processes to consider policy options, WE ACT identified as its primary policy goals for the period from 2000 to 2004: (1) obtaining 300 new buses powered by compressed natural gas, and (2) having all new MTA depots converted to using compressed natural gas.

Although the lead academic partner sometimes participated in discussions with WE ACT staff, he noted that for researchers like himself, the motivation for involvement did not lie in identifying policy goals but rather in "trying to fill scientific gaps." He added, however, that "what makes scientific gaps interesting [is that] there is a policy need."

Engaging in Policy Advocacy WE ACT staff engaged in a variety of activities to achieve their goals. For example, after repeated efforts to meet and negotiate with the MTA were unsuccessful, WE ACT launched a campaign through which 10,000 postcards signed by residents were sent to the state governor and the chair of the MTA. Then in 2000, after failing to get the desired results and carefully examining a range of legal tools and tactics, WE ACT took the risky but important step of joining in the filing of an administrative complaint against the federal Department of Transportation under Title VI of the Civil Rights Act. Charging the MTA with siting diesel bus depots and parking lots disproportionately in minority neighborhoods in Northern Manhattan, WE ACT and some of its collaborators (not including the public health academic partners) invoked Title VI's prohibition of racial discrimination on the part of any agency receiving federal financing. As a WE ACT leader noted, the filing was one of many avenues pursued, and although the participants did not expect to win, this legal approach was felt to be useful as a pressure strategy and one that would offer needed political visibility.

The public health academic partners' role in the policy advocacy phase of the project was quite limited, because, in the words of a community partner, "It is not natural for [researchers], based on their training, to come out and be advocates." Yet, she added, "There are times when we need their weight and credibility as scientific researchers to say something," and this sometimes has involved "a tug and a pull." As noted earlier, the lead academic partner in the Earth Crew study did participate in hearings and meetings with policymakers and community groups and also presented study findings at scientific meetings. The goal of such activity, in his words, was to "spread the word around in different settings about the partnership, the products, and the policies" and to better integrate environmental health and justice into conversations among researchers and policymakers.

Policy Implementation and Outcomes

Credible research and follow-up actions by WE ACT and its academic partners were described by policymakers and others as having had a substantial impact on the capital plan of the MTA, particularly in relation to the conversion of its entire bus fleet from "dirty" diesel to "clean" (ultra-low sulfur) diesel. Although not what the partnership had hoped for (conversion to compressed natural gas, or CNG, technology), this change was nevertheless an important step forward. A senior EPA official further commented that both the Earth Crew study findings and the community's strong advocacy played a key role in getting the government to undertake regular air monitoring in Harlem and other previously unmonitored and high-risk locations in Northern Manhattan and in other urban areas nationwide. In his words, "They [came] to us and . . . provided us with health information and local health studies that convinced us that there was a real problem here [and] that we ought to devote the time and energy to help this community."

WE ACT and its partners were not successful in getting a favorable judgment on their legal complaint against the U.S. Department of Transportation. However, some of that agency's findings in this case closely mirrored WE ACT and its partners' statements and concerns. And as a community partner pointed out, the process itself "served as a point of entry for community residents," who could potentially use this potent tool in future advocacy work. Finally, and in an effort to promote more effective future collaboration, WE ACT presented a memorandum of understanding to the MTA on a number of issues, which they have since been discussing through mediation.

Broader Outcomes and Policy Considerations

Although this chapter has focused primarily on the neighborhood- and municipal-level outcomes of the WE ACT partnership's early Earth Crew study and its policy-level activities, WE ACT and its CBPR partnership both went on to make progress on broader public policy fronts as well (WE ACT for Environmental Justice, 2008; Corburn, 2005; Blackwell et al., 2005). On the state level, for example, WE ACT played a catalytic role by working with other groups to call for a New York State environmental justice program, a program that was finally begun in 1999. Four years later, WE ACT again played a leadership role in the development of a statewide environmental justice policy that lays the foundation for new legislation and enhanced regulations in the environmental permit review and approval process. WE ACT currently is involved in the state implementation plan fostering state conformity to federal air quality regulations, and further is working to help develop ways in which Manhattan can come into compliance with the federal Clean Air Act.

Both WE ACT as an organization and the partnership's collaborative research also contributed to federal-level policy concerning environmental justice. WE ACT's executive director served for several years as both a member and the chair of the EPA's National Environmental Justice Advisory Council (NEJAC), providing independent advice and recommendations to the administrator of the EPA on matters related to environmental justice. And the partnership's Earth Crew study remains a frequently cited source, used by the EPA and others in advocating for tighter emissions standards.

Finally, both WE ACT and its partnership with the CCCEH have moved in several important new directions. Through its membership on the steering committee of a new citywide coalition, the Campaign for New York's Future, for example, WE ACT is working to help ensure a sustainable "greener" New York for all residents. And the WE ACT partnership is collaborating on a citywide campaign (Our Housing Is Our Health) focused on indoor air quality. Together with nearly thirty organizational members, including tenant associations, housing groups, and community-based organizations, the partnership is particularly focused on influencing city policy on mold. Critical in this regard was its securing of an agreement with the Public Advocate to copublish a report on mold, with recommendations for action. WE ACT and its partners now are working to change the city building construction code, banning building materials that promote the growth of mold, and potentially even making mold a housing violation.

Through such multilevel collaborations, the WE ACT partnership continues to demonstrate the power of CBPR and subsequent policy advocacy for working to study and address environmental health problems.

DISCUSSION

The partnership between WE ACT and the Columbia Center for Children's Environmental Health offers a useful example of a CBPR effort that appears to have both produced credible scientific research and helped to bring about environmental health policy change. From a research perspective, as noted earlier, the 1996 Earth Crew study and the WE ACT partnership's careful look at the relationship between bus diesel emissions and asthma are still widely cited more than a decade later (Blackwell et al., 2005; Brown et al., 2003; Corburn, 2005). Similarly, from a policy perspective, the conversion of New York City's bus fleet to clean diesel, the EPA's initiation of permanent, community-based air monitoring in Northern Manhattan and other hot spots, and New York's adoption of a state environmental justice policy all were described in media accounts, in scholarly articles, and by policymakers and others interviewed as having been substantially related to the work of WE ACT and its research partnership. As an academic partner commented, "There weren't many community-based studies that showed exposure to diesel particles at that time. From a scientific perspective I think it played a role in [getting] the diesel exhaust controls." Several factors appeared to have played a key role in the partnership's success, among them WE ACT's strong community base, the scientific credibility of the partnership's research, strong policy alliances, and the careful background work and strategic planning in which WE ACT engaged. The relationship of mutual trust and respect between partners and the community partner's effective use of the mass media also appeared to have contributed to the visibility and impact of the WE ACT partnership and its policy change efforts.

At the same time, this case study illustrated the tension between the "necessary skepticism of science" and the "action imperative of communities" (Price & Behrens, 2003). Given such tensions (for example, over the slow pace of publication of study findings), the importance of taking seriously CBPR's commitment to genuine co-learning is underscored. Through both structured workshops and informal conversations joining together academics, community partners, and residents, the WE ACT partnership attempted to address this commitment and to meet the demands of both strong and credible science and community partners' need to move at a reasonable pace into the action phase of the work.

A second lesson pointed up by this case study, and one widely discussed in the CBPR literature (Israel et al., 1998; Wallerstein, Duran, Minkler, & Foley, 2005; see also Chapters Three and Twenty-One), involves the importance of devoting sufficient time up front to developing the partnership and coming to agreement on a host of research and policy issues and strategies. As an academic partner commented: "[CBPR] requires a lot of effort and energy. If you are going to do it, do it fully. . . . If you honestly approach it with genuine interest and commitment, then it can be a very effective way to study environmental health issues that are important for disadvantaged communities."

The need for clarity on partnership goals and timetables was also stressed both in the present case study and in other CBPR endeavors (Wallerstein et al., 2005; see Chapters Three and Fourteen). Further, because community partner participation in the policy arena requires a substantial time commitment over a long period, the importance of equitable sharing of resources is also underscored. The "differential reward structure" for CBPR partners, wherein outside researchers receive the lion's share of the budgetary resources, has been described elsewhere (Israel et al., 1998; Minkler, 2004; see also Chapter Fourteen) as a major cause of insider-outsider tensions in this work that must be carefully addressed. The WE ACT partners reported negotiating such issues, particularly as their partnership matured, and the eventual awarding of a federal grant on which WE ACT was the primary grantee represented an important step forward. Yet as a community partner suggested, tensions sometimes still surfaced, for example, when budget cuts were announced that hit the community partner harder because of its far smaller initial allocation.

Still another lesson emerging from the WE ACT partnership case study, and one particularly well articulated by the policymakers interviewed, was how critical it is for partnership members to "do their homework," particularly in determining which government agencies or individuals are likely to have decision-making authority and what evidence and arguments are likely to appeal to them.

Finally, lessons were learned in relation to the policy outcomes of this project. As Themba-Nixon and her colleagues noted in Chapter Seventeen, well-framed legal actions such as lawsuits and complaints remain important policy strategies, even though they carry significant risks. The complaint filed against the U.S. Department of Transportation by WE ACT and others achieved increased political visibility for the community's issue. Further, it was an important contributing factor to discussions with the MTA, which occurred over the last two years and resulted in a number of positive actions, including environmental controls at the depots and quarterly meetings with the diesel leadership teams of residents WE ACT had organized at all six depots.

The outcomes of the WE ACT partnership's policy work also demonstrated the utility of incremental change as a precursor to the broader policy goals being sought. By helping to get the city to convert its entire diesel bus fleet to clean diesel, for example, WE ACT, its academic partners, and other allies also helped to pave the way toward the larger goal of conversion to compressed natural gas, and with it the potential for lower asthma rates and a cleaner environment. Finally, WE ACT's leadership role in creating awareness of the need for environmental justice and in fighting for that justice and the consequent reduction in health disparities related to asthma has been widely recognized and cited (Blackwell et al., 2005; Brown et al., 2003; Corburn, 2005).

SUMMARY

As the WE ACT partnership demonstrates, carefully designed community-based participatory research that is committed to strong science, high-level community involvement, engagement in policy steps and activities, and the strategic use of study findings to influence and change policy can be an important part of the broader struggle for environmental justice. The chances for success in such efforts are improved when there is a strong, autonomous community partner with an established track record for effective action on behalf of the community it represents. WE ACT's long history of activism with and for the local community on key community-identified concerns positioned it well to serve as an equal in the partnership with the Columbia Center for Children's Environmental

Health. Yet as this case study has demonstrated, the university partner also had to enter this partnership with an openness to colearning and genuine collaboration. Although influencing policy was not a central goal of the academic partner, appreciation of and commitment to helping the community partner address its policy objectives was critical to partnership success.

Even with the strong and continued collaboration between WE ACT and its academic partners, however, and the powerful and well-publicized findings of its initial Earth Crew study, policy change takes time. And it also takes considerable strategic planning, coalition building, and negotiation along the way. The WE ACT partnership has yet to achieve its most ambitious policy goals, for example, obtaining three hundred new buses powered by compressed natural gas. At the same time, critical incremental changes, new CBPR collaborations with its academic partners, and policy makers' demonstrated recognition of WE ACT as a major player in the struggle for environmental justice locally and statewide all remain important outcomes of this long and fruitful partnership.

QUESTIONS FOR DISCUSSION

1. The collaboration between WE ACT and its epidemiological research partners at Columbia University's Center for Children's Environmental Health seems in many ways an ideal example of a CBPR partnership in which partners share a deep respect for one another and the talents they bring. Yet even in this case study, tensions are evident and the partners display very different levels of interest in working on policy-related goals. Review the principles and guidelines presented in Chapter Three (describing CBPR as an empowering, participatory, and colearning process; fostering community capacity and systems change; balancing research and action; and so forth). Please also look at the guidelines presented in Appendixes A and C. Which of these guidelines might be particularly useful for helping partnerships deal with the different commitments and objectives of diverse partnership members?

2. This case study describes how WE ACT and some of its collaborators used several strategies to achieve their policy goals, including the filing of an administrative complaint. As noted in this chapter and the preceding one, legal strategies like this one can be risky and time consuming yet can also be an important step forward—in this case, more to increase political visibility than out of a strong conviction that the filers could win the legal battle. Do you feel that this legal filing was an appropriate course of action for WE ACT (note that the public health academic partners did not participate in this strategy)? What other strategies, if any, might you have attempted in this situation? Can you think of other real or hypothetical examples of policy-oriented CBPR projects in which a legal approach might be warranted?

KEY TERMS

Environmental justice	Epidemiology	Youth
Legal strategies in CBPR	Diesel bus pollution	

REFERENCES

Blackwell, A. G., Minkler, M., & Thompson, M. (2005). Using community organizing and community building to influence policy. In M. Minkler (Ed.), *Community organizing and community building for health* (2nd ed., pp. 405–418). New Brunswick, NJ.: Rutgers University Press.

Breckwich Vásquez, V., Minkler, M., & Shepard, P. (2006). Promoting environmental health policy through community-based participatory research: A case study from Harlem, New York. *Journal of Urban Health, 83*(1), 101–110.

Brown, P., Mayer, B., Zavestoski, S., Luebke, T., Mandelbaum, J., & McCormick, S. (2003). The health politics of asthma: Environmental justice and collective illness experience in the United States. *Social Science & Medicine, 57*, 453–464.

Brugge, D., & Hynes, H. P. (Eds.). (2005). *Community research in environmental health: Studies in science, advocacy and ethics.* Burlington, VT: Ashgate.

Corburn, J. (2005). *Street science: Community knowledge and environmental health justice.* Cambridge, MA: MIT Press.

Diaz-Sanchez, D. (1997). The role of diesel exhaust particles and their associated polyaromatic hydrocarbons in the induction of allergic airway disease. *Allergy, 52*, 52–56.

Israel, B. A., Schulz, A. J., Parker, E. A., & Becker, A. B. (1998). Review of community-based research: Assessing partnership approaches to improve public health. *Annual Review of Public Health, 19*, 173–202.

Kingdon, J. W. (1995). *Agendas, alternatives, and public policies* (2nd ed.). Reading, MA: Addison-Wesley.

Kinney, P. L., Aggarwal, M., Northridge, M. E., Janssen, N.A.H., & Shepard, P. (2000). Airborne concentrations of $PM_{2.5}$ and diesel exhaust particles on Harlem sidewalks: A community-based pilot study. *Environmental Health Perspectives, 108*, 213–218.

McClellan, R. (1987). Health effects of exposures to diesel exhaust particles. *Annual Review of Pharmaceutical Toxicology, 27*, 279–300.

Milio, N. (1998). Priorities and strategies for promoting community-based prevention policies. *Journal of Public Health Management and Practice, 4*(3), 14–28.

Minkler, M. (2004). Ethical challenges for the "outside" researcher in community-based participatory research. *Health Education & Behavior, 31*(6), 684–697.

Minkler, M., Breckwich Vásquez, V., Tajik, M., & Petersen, D. (2008). Promoting environmental justice through community-based participatory research: The role of community and partnership capacity. *Health Education & Behavior, 35*(1), 119–137.

Morello-Frosch, R., Pastor, M., Sadd, J., Porras, C., & Prichard, M. (2005). Citizens, science, and data judo: Leveraging secondary data analysis to build a community-academic collaborative for environmental justice in southern California. In B. A. Israel, E. Eng, A. J. Schulz, & E. A. Parker (Eds.), *Methods in community-based participatory research for health* (pp. 371–392). San Francisco: Jossey-Bass.

Nicholas, S., Jean-Louis, B., Ortiz, B., Northridge, M., Shoemaker, K., Vaughan, R., et al. (2005). Addressing the childhood asthma crisis in Harlem: The Harlem Children's Zone Asthma Initiative. *American Journal of Public Health, 95*(2), 245–249.

Northridge, M. E., Meyer, I. H., & Dunn, L. (2002). Overlooked and underserved in Harlem: A population-based survey of adults with asthma. *Environmental Health Perspectives, 110*, 217–220.

O'Fallon, L. R., & Dearry, A. (2002). Community-based participatory research as a tool to advance environmental health sciences. *Environmental Health Perspectives, 110*(Suppl. 2), 155–159.

Perera, F., Illman, S., Kinney, P., Whyatt, R. M., Kelvin, E. A., Shepard, P., et al. (2002). The challenge of preventing environmentally related disease in young children: Community-based research in New York City. *Environmental Health Perspectives, 110*, 197–204.

Petersen, D., Minkler, M., Breckwich Vásquez, V., & Baden, A. C. (2006). Community-based participatory research as a tool for policy change: A case study of the Southern California Environmental Justice Collaborative. *Review of Policy Research, 23*(2), 339–353.

Price, R. H., & Behrens, T. (2003). Working Pasteur's quadrant: Harnessing science and action for community change. *American Journal of Community Psychology, 31*(3–4), 219–223.

Shepard, P., Northridge, M., Prakash, S., & Stover, G. (2002). Preface: Advancing environmental justice through community-based participatory research. *Environmental Health Perspectives, 110*(Suppl. 2), 139–140.

Wallerstein, N., Duran, B., Minkler, M., & Foley, K. (2005). Developing and maintaining partnerships with communities. In B. A. Israel, E. Eng, A. J. Schulz, & E. A. Parker (Eds.), *Methods in community-based participatory research for health* (pp. 31–51). San Francisco: Jossey-Bass.

WE ACT for Environmental Justice. (2008). [Home page.] Retrieved May 6, 2008, from www.weact.org.

Yin, R. (2003). *Case study research: Design and methods* (3rd. ed.). Thousand Oaks, CA: Sage.

CHAPTER

19

PARTICIPATORY ACTION RESEARCH WITH HOTEL ROOM CLEANERS IN SAN FRANCISCO AND LAS VEGAS

FROM COLLABORATIVE STUDY TO THE BARGAINING TABLE

PAM TAU LEE, NIKLAS KRAUSE, CHARLES GOETCHIUS, JO MARIE ARGRIESTI, & ROBIN BAKER

THE HOSPITALITY INDUSTRY, with close to 48,000 tourist hotels and a payroll of over 1.8 million, is a major employer of low-wage service workers in metropolitan areas of the United States (American Hotel and Lodging Association, 2006; U.S. Bureau of

Labor Statistics, 2006). Yet despite high rates of injury and disability experienced by these workers, very little health research has been conducted on this population.

The studies described in this chapter grew out of the concerns of low-wage hotel room cleaners and their union, UNITE HERE, in San Francisco and Las Vegas. For many years these workers, up to 99 percent of whom are female and 95 percent of whom are immigrants, had complained of high rates of injuries and musculoskeletal disorders. The union was aware that many had undergone surgery and several had become permanently disabled. Believing that these injuries could be job related, the San Francisco union leadership contacted the University of California, Berkeley (UC-Berkeley) Labor Occupational Health Program (LOHP) to assess its interest in helping to research this issue. The union envisioned a study that would involve participatory action research (PAR), with hotel room cleaners themselves in the role of study collaborators. LOHP would serve as an intermediary with university-based researchers at UC's School of Public Health in conducting original research that would look at workload, health, and employee-employer relationship issues. The results of this San Francisco study later inspired the UNITE HERE Local 226 in Las Vegas to initiate a similar project to study the health of room attendants working in casinos. Activities and insights from both studies are discussed in this chapter.

As Randy Stoecker (in Chapter Six) and others (Reason, 1994) have suggested, collaborations between universities and community organizations such as unions often arise from the interests and priorities of the academic partners rather than from the community organizations or groups themselves. Similarly, the selection of research methods and the design of the study are usually considered to be within the domain of the academics. The studies described in this chapter took a nontraditional path, with the union initiating the partnership and defining the research priorities and methods, which included having hotel room cleaners play an active role in many aspects of the research. Because of LOHP's strong track record in facilitating joint labor-management initiatives around issues of health and safety, both the San Francisco and Las Vegas union locals—which had no prior experience in working with academic researchers—were comfortable having this organization direct the project.

THEORETICAL FRAMEWORK

For the purposes of this study, *participatory action research* (a term used here interchangeably with *community-based participatory research*) was defined as "systematic investigation, with the collaboration of those affected by the issue being studied, for the purpose of education and taking action or effecting social change" (Green et al., 1995, p. 4). As discussed in earlier chapters, this community-driven approach to research begins with the goals and questions of the community, is participatory at every level, is culturally sensitive, and uses a diversity of communication tools and languages. It involves sharing of power and resources with the community and attempts to build a common language among partners (Northridge et al., 2000). In Hagey's (1997) words, "Participatory research is a means of putting research capabilities in the hands of deprived and disenfranchised people so that they can transform their lives for themselves" (p. 1).

A participatory study assembles an appropriate team of research partners, which in this case included health educators and medical researchers, to work in genuine collaboration with the community. It ensures that ownership of data and methods of dissemination are considered collaboratively, and it includes a participatory evaluation process that examines the potential and actual impact of the intervention (National Institute of Environmental Health Sciences, 1997; see also Chapter Twelve). Other objectives include education and empowerment of the community by making resources available for the study of community-defined issues, facilitation of activism, and involvement of both the researchers and the community in improving conditions and quality of life (Hagey, 1997; Israel, Eng, Schulz, & Parker, 2005). Although a participatory research approach is particularly appealing to institutions such as labor unions, applying its principles can be challenging. As Hagey (1997) has pointed out, "Participatory action research, accepting the politics of research, requires a good emotional quotient (EQ), a high tolerance for conflict and excellent group process skills. By definition [it] employs group process to generate and utilize research" (p. 4). Willingness to share power and build trust is key (Northridge et al., 2000; Israel et al., 2005; Jones & Wells, 2007). In this chapter we describe the partners involved in this participatory research effort, examine the challenges and dilemmas faced at different stages of the research, and give a brief overview of the study findings. We then examine how the findings were used to influence policy and practice, and the role of the room cleaners and their academic partners at the bargaining table.

RESEARCH PARTNERS' ROLES AND CONCERNS

UNITE HERE Local 2, which represents approximately 75 percent of all nonmanagerial hotel employees in San Francisco and almost 90 percent of those in large tourist hotels, was the lead community organization in this research. Local 2's membership consists of more than 8,500 workers, the majority of whom are employed in the twenty-three major hotels that have contracts with the union. UNITE HERE Local 226 represents 90 percent of casino workers on "the strip" in Las Vegas and has a total of 55,000 casino workers in thirty-nine casinos as members (Ian Lewis, UNITE HERE, personal communication, January 14, 2007).

In addition to donating considerable amounts of their own time to this project, the union leaders allocated staff and substantial funding. An award of $30,000 from the Rockefeller Foundation helped launch the San Francisco study, and this was augmented with an additional $100,000 from the union to see the project through to completion.

The maids and housekeepers who make up over 20 percent of the workforce in the hotel industry (U.S. Department of Labor, 2001) were another key partner in the study. Through Local 2 and Local 226, union members frequently participate in activities such as picket actions, organizing drives, and workplace committees. Although the workers in San Francisco and Las Vegas had not previously been involved as research partners, these earlier activities may have contributed to individual and community capacity building and laid important groundwork for the women's active participation in the present study.

As noted, LOHP was responsible for direction of the project, coordination between the union and the UC Berkeley School of Public Health researchers, and facilitation and training of room cleaner groups involved in the project. Established in 1974, LOHP is a public service arm of the Center for Occupational and Environmental Health at the School of Public Health. Its primary purpose is to serve working people and their unions, particularly in Northern California, and to assist them in taking an active role in identifying and controlling occupational hazards. Known for its innovative, action-oriented training methods, LOHP is also recognized for its work at the policy level to advance prevention strategies and its strong record of successful collaborations with community-based organizations.

To facilitate a true community-based participatory research (CBPR) study, LOHP identified as potential collaborators public health researchers who were knowledgeable about and comfortable with the use of this approach. Physician and epidemiologist Niklas Krause, a faculty member in occupational and environmental medicine at the University of California, San Francisco, with extensive experience in collaborating with both unions and management, was suggested by LOHP for the role of lead public health researcher. He joined the project after a meeting with union representatives. Pam Tau Lee, LOHP's labor services program coordinator, served as codirector and brought with her her professional background her own experience years earlier as a room cleaner.

By agreeing to collaborate on the original project in San Francisco, both UNITE HERE and the academic researchers were entering uncharted waters. The union believed that workers were getting hurt and sick from the job, but would the survey data support this hunch? How could UNITE HERE mobilize members for action without compromising the scientific protocols? And for the academic partners, how could the needs of the union be respected while the methodological rigor and scientific integrity of the study was also maintained? The union puts it this way: "This was like a marriage with no chance of getting a divorce in case things didn't work out." The academic partners realized they could collaborate with the union when, after a series of exploratory discussions, UNITE HERE made it known that they felt comfortable with the process and would abide by the findings, even if they turned out to be negative for the union. This set a tone of mutual trust.

In both San Francisco and Las Vegas, LOHP's work to facilitate the relationship helped build a foundation for the sharing of power. Assuming a third-party role, LOHP helped to build bridges between the union and the academic researchers. According to one union spokesperson, "We needed a third party to keep us [the union] in line. We had to be disciplined and learn how to participate but not taint the process. A third party helped us sort through our concerns and helped us present these in a way the researchers could understand. We didn't know anything about the world of the academics, and we wouldn't have been able to figure out what to do without the help of people who understood us and understood the researchers as well."

LOHP sometimes held separate discussions with the union and the researchers to hear concerns and brief each party on the interests, needs, constraints, and culture of the other. LOHP also played an important role in keeping the project on track in both its locations, keeping the parties informed, and arranging check-in conference calls before moving the project to the next phase.

As Barbara Israel and her colleagues discuss in Chapter Three, partners in a CBPR project may be differentially involved in different stages of the research. In these studies, for example, the academic partners took primary responsibility for study design. Consistent with CBPR principles, however, they were respectful of and attentive to community partner concerns. So even though these researchers would have preferred a joint labor-management setting for the study, they understood the union's expressed need to focus its limited resources on researching specific room cleaner health and workload issues. These topics were unlikely to generate interest or involvement from the employers during a period just prior to contract negotiations (in both cities, five-year labor contracts were set to expire in about eighteen months after the union first contacted the researchers). The union's preference for a study design that was more limited in scope was accommodated by the academic partners and guided their development of the research design.

DEFINING TOPICS AND ENHANCING PARTICIPATION

Over the years room cleaners in both cities had complained that their workload had increased. Here were two opportunities to cut through the rumors to find out if a significant number of new duties had been added and, if so, with what, if any, impacts on worker health.

In both San Francisco and Las Vegas the study teams agreed to an approach that would combine the knowledge of the workers and the best available science. In each city a core group was identified of twenty-five room cleaners whose racial and ethnic composition reflected that of the overall workforce. Latinas were a high percentage of the team in both cities, followed by African Americans in Las Vegas, and Asians, whites, and African Americans in San Francisco. All core group members were women, and they were chosen on the basis of the high regard in which they were held by peers and the fact that they had frequently sought out union representatives about job-related concerns. An effort also was made to include women with varying years of experience in this work: new hires (under two years), midterm employees (seven to ten years), and senior employees (fifteen to twenty years).

The core group members attended six focus group sessions, held every two weeks for three hours after work. LOHP facilitated these group discussions to look at workload, physical strain, relationship with management, and worker disability. The information that emerged in these discussions provided the study team with several specific issues that could then form the basis of in-depth collaborative research.

Several steps were taken to enhance participation in the focus groups. Since English was not the first language of the great majority of the participants, simultaneous interpretation in Spanish and Chinese was provided in San Francisco and in Spanish in Las Vegas. Translated written materials were made available at each session. Each participant received dinner and a stipend of $15 per hour to communicate appreciation for her expertise and recognition of the hardship of meeting for three hours after work. Finally, because many of the women lived a distance from the meeting locations and had to miss their car pool rides or other commuter hour arrangements in order to participate, the union also provided some travel accommodations.

In keeping with CBPR's emphasis on local capacity building and empowerment (Hagey, 1997; Israel et al., 2005; Jones & Wells, 2007; see also Chapter Three) and to inform the focus group discussions, LOHP integrated training on ergonomics and control measures into the sessions. Each session employed adult education techniques and interactive activities such as compiling illness and injury reports, body charting for workplace pain, brainstorming, and risk mapping. As part of this last activity, participants drew visual maps of their workplaces on which they then identified the various physical, chemical, ergonomic, and other stressors to which they were routinely exposed (Brown, 1995; see also Appendix J). These maps were then used as a basis for subsequent discussion.

Using as a prop a mock hotel room with two beds, a bathtub, a sink, other furniture, and equipment, the San Francisco participants were given a short introduction to ergonomic risk factors. The focus group facilitator then asked for volunteers to go through the motions of cleaning the room while the rest of the participants called out "freeze" when they spotted a cleaner facing a risk factor for injury. Through this process the study team found that factors like the weight and awkwardness of linen carts and vacuum cleaners and ineffective cleaning products that required repeated scrubbing were sources of ergonomic and other forms of stress. In Las Vegas, room attendants held a focus group session at the union's housekeeping training center, where mock hotel rooms were available for their use. Armed with pads of Post-it sticky notes, room attendants were instructed to go into the mock hotel rooms and put Post-its where potential health and safety hazards might be found. After flagging the rooms in this way, the room attendants were divided into small groups and each group was assigned a different part of the room and interviewed there by union staff. The interviews captured in words the reasons for each flag. This information helped the researchers to better understand the risk factors present in each potentially hazardous job task.

To facilitate the academic partners' understanding of the workload and task questions that needed to be posed, the room cleaners listed on index cards every task required to get their job done. The LOHP facilitator then asked the group to identify the tasks that generated time pressures or other stresses for the room cleaner. Finally, these participants were asked to identify when these particular duties had been introduced as part of a room cleaner's job. Participants explained, for example, that linen carts used to be fully stocked during the evening by utility personnel but that over time, that crew had been gradually eliminated and its duties turned over to the room cleaners. Las Vegas room attendants remembered that ten years earlier they had been assigned fewer rooms and suites to clean. The room assignments increased when the employers instituted incentive programs to encourage room attendants to take on more rooms. In exchange, some were given a silver dollar that they could use to try their luck at the dollar slot machine. Others were paid $4 per extra room. Over time, as the room cleaners continued to take on more rooms, their employers simply increased the number of rooms assigned and the incentive programs were dropped.

DESIGNING AND PILOT-TESTING THE SURVEY

In both San Francisco and Las Vegas, once the outside researchers and the core group members had identified the specific data needed, a questionnaire was developed to be distributed to larger numbers of room cleaners. This stage began with the academic partners combing through standardized questionnaires in order to select potentially appropriate psychosocial questions. They also selected and developed other items that would capture accurate information about workload, job pressure, and employer relations. For example, in Las Vegas, information learned from the focus groups generated two new questions addressing incentives to clean extra rooms, questions not included in the San Francisco survey, which was conducted before the Las Vegas survey:

- During your last workweek did you skip breaks, or take shorter breaks in order to clean additional rooms?
- Why did you do the extra rooms: additional pay, overtime pay, gifts, pressure from coworkers, pressure from supervisors, fear of discipline, points, or other penalties?

Additionally, new questions regarding communication were included in the Las Vegas study:

- I am required to speak and understand English when I talk with my superiors at work.
- I received information about changes to personnel policies and rules in writing and in a language I can read or understand.

In San Francisco once the draft questionnaire was produced and shared with the union, union representatives expressed concern that a long and difficult questionnaire could discourage the room cleaners from completing the entire survey. The researchers in turn explained their view that completeness was necessary to maintain the scientific integrity of standardized scales and to provide valid points of comparison. They further suggested that this completeness was important for meeting the union's objective of being able to compare the health conditions of room cleaners with those of other working populations. The core group of room cleaners played a key role at this point. After pilot-testing the draft questionnaire, they shared their perception that the instrument was indeed too long and that some questions were difficult to understand, as a result of having been written in English and then translated into Spanish and Chinese. They helped to reword a number of items, recommended that others be deleted, and further suggested that survey "helpers," fluent in the relevant languages, be available at each survey site to assist the room cleaners in understanding the intent of the questions and the complex directions for filling out the form. A similar process later took place in Las Vegas.

Through this collaborative process, the academic partners were helped to refine the questionnaire, and LOHP and the union came away with concrete ideas for designing the implementation phase, including the training and use of survey helpers.

SELECTING THE SAMPLE POPULATIONS

In selecting the sample populations, the academic partners asked the union to select hotels that differed by business category, by type of customer, or by quality of labor-management relations. Variation in such hotel characteristics, they explained, would allow statistical comparisons that would identify the effects of the different work environments on the health and well-being of room cleaners. Only if differences in working conditions were related to differences in health status could changes in working conditions be proposed to improve the health of hotel workers.

The union explained that San Francisco hotels fall generally into one of four categories: luxury/business, convention/business, tour group/business, and family/tour group. In Las Vegas, hotels fell into several categories: downtown (older, previously family-owned hotels), and medium-sized to very large tourist, luxury, and business hotels located along the Vegas "strip." The unions selected hotels that best represented the diversity of hotel business in the respective sites. In San Francisco two of the four hotels chosen were selected in part because they had relatively positive labor-management relationships and the other two were selected in part because they represented workplaces with more adversarial relationships. The union provided seniority lists from the four selected hotels, and LOHP and the academic partners then worked with a subcommittee of workers from these hotels to update the lists to add new workers and delete those who had retired or left.

PLANNING OUTREACH AND LOGISTICS

To ensure a high response rate in the survey component of the study, an outreach effort was developed in each city that was in effect a mini-campaign waged by the union with its rank and file. The union appointed and trained leaders from each of the targeted hotels to be active members of an outreach team, with one leader selected for approximately each twelve workers, on the basis of commonality of language and other sociocultural factors. Armed with copies of the updated seniority lists, outreach team members followed up with individual workers, explaining the importance of their involvement.

The union supplemented this activity with letters sent to each worker's home, and union staff and workers also distributed leaflets at the various worksites. Announcements were made by union staff at union committee meetings, stressing the importance of this study and encouraging members to contact their friends at these hotels and ask them to participate.

In San Francisco, survey sites—two at churches and one in a union hall—were set up within walking distance of the hotels and staffed by five to twelve people who were available at times convenient for the workers. To maintain confidentiality, each of the rooms selected had a separate entrance and was also strictly off limits to union staff and to employers.

In addition to the room cleaners who had agreed to serve as survey helpers, in San Francisco LOHP hired several UC graduate students and community social service workers who spoke and understood Spanish, Chinese, or Tagalog and thus could serve in this role as well. In Las Vegas the research helpers were students from the University of Nevada, Las Vegas, most majoring in the field of hotels and hospitality, and Las Vegas community members who spoke Croatian. LOHP conducted a special training session for these helpers, covering the protocol for survey administration, the helpers' role as interpreters and explainers, and the importance of not influencing participants' answers.

On the day of each city's survey, the outreach leaders stationed themselves at the time clocks at the selected hotels, where hotel workers punched out at the end of the day, or just outside the employee entrances. In San Francisco, those workers who had agreed to participate walked to their survey site together. In Las Vegas, where many room attendants drive, car pools were arranged to transport the women to the survey site.

To further ensure the neutrality and confidentiality of the process, completed questionnaires were collected only by the university partners, not union members. Finally, and because many of the room cleaners lived in areas that had poor evening transportation, arrangements were made to take these workers home, thus making it less burdensome for them to participate.

The detailed planning that went into the outreach and logistics of survey administration proved very successful. In San Francisco a total of 258 women took part in the survey, resulting in a participation rate of 69.2 percent of all eligible room attendants. In Las Vegas a total of 941 room attendants completed the survey, a participation rate of 74 percent.

Only one adjustment had to be made in the planning. The Las Vegas survey implementation was to have begun in 2001 during the week that brought the tragic events of September 11. The hospitality industry and UNITE HERE Local 226 were both deeply affected by the aftermath of curtailed travel. The hotel industry conducted massive layoffs. Over the next quarter the union had to put the survey on hold and turn its attention to helping its members meet their pressing financial needs. Union members were mobilized and set up food banks and other much needed services. By February 2002, the hotels slowly began to call back their workers, though business was rebounding at a quicker pace than these recalls were.

As workers began to return to the hotels, the union got word that recalled workers were being expected to do the work of two people and that many were getting hurt. UNITE HERE Local 226 again made the survey a priority, and the hotel committees were reinstituted to mobilize room attendants to take the survey and also to get people back to work.

ANALYZING THE DATA

Once the questionnaires were collected, the information was entered into a database program by a graduate student researcher. The academic partners then prepared and provided simple frequency tables for all answers to the questions, stratified by hotel. In keeping with the CBPR principle stressing community ownership of data (Brown & Vega, 1996; Israel et al., 2005; see also Appendix A), the LOHP focus group facilitator then brought together the original core group of room cleaners and UC researchers to review the findings. The room cleaners, academic partners, and union staff broke into several small groups to discuss the data. Each small group was assigned a different set of data, asked to review this information, and then come back to the whole group with an initial analysis. Although this discussion was originally scheduled for three hours, it proved so fruitful that participants voluntarily met for an additional hour.

Because the academic partners did not have firsthand knowledge of how rooms are cleaned, they had many questions and looked to the room cleaners for clarification. For example, when the academic partners questioned why "lots of garbage in the room" surfaced as a big workload problem, core group members explained that there is now far more garbage than there was five years ago because convention and meeting participants collect bags of brochures and trinkets. Convention catalogues and brochures left in a room can weigh ten pounds or more. Guests eat on the run and bring in takeout food, leaving paper containers, cans, and bags on tables or in wastebaskets. More garbage translates into more trips to pick up trash and heavier wastebaskets.

Core group members also explained that "linen" had emerged as a major problem in the study because many hotels now use three sheets per bed and more pillows. A king-size bed can be topped with up to six pillows, requiring more travel to and from the linen closet.

In Las Vegas, heavily trashed and damaged rooms and suites posed a big problem for workers, as did the special-attention task of cleaning up vomit and other biological hazards.

Informed by insights like these, the academic partners in each city spent another four months doing further analysis and cross-checking the data before writing their final report and submitting it to the union.

STUDY FINDINGS

In San Francisco the preliminary study report prepared for the union suggested that the overall health status of room cleaners appeared to be substantially worse than that of the general U.S. population (see Table 19.1). More than three-quarters of the room cleaners reported work-related pain or discomfort. In 73 percent of cases this was severe enough to result in a visit to a doctor, and in 53 percent of cases it required taking time off from work. Yet only 50 percent of workers had reported this pain to their supervisors or management, and just 23 percent had had a formally reported work-related injury during the last year. The relatively high frequency of work-related musculoskeletal symptoms could not be explained by the aging of the workforce, as was suggested by management in discussions with the union. The study found equally high rates of musculoskeletal symptoms among younger and older employees.

Significant differences in health status and workdays lost due to work-related pain were found among the four types of hotels, with employees of one hotel reporting consistently better than average health on nearly all health measures. Further analyses were planned to determine the extent to which these differences were caused by variations in physical workload and psychosocial working conditions, both of which appeared to be more favorable at the hotel showing better health status (Krause, Lee, Thompson, Rugulies, & Baker, 1999; Lee & Krause, 2002).

In Las Vegas, similarly troubling findings emerged. Overall health status was even worse than among San Francisco hotel workers, despite the fact that the Las Vegas workforce was on average six years younger. Almost 80 percent reported pain, with 90 percent reporting that pain had interfered with their work during the last four weeks. Fully 83 percent reported having taken medication for their pain during the last month, yet as in San Francisco, less than a quarter of the workers who experienced work-related pain had reported it to their employer's workers' compensation insurance carrier (see Table 19.1).

TABLE 19.1 **Key Findings from Hotel Room Cleaner Studies, by City**

Article I.	San Francisco 1999 ($n = 258$)	Las Vegas 2002 ($n = 941$)
Survey response rate	69%	74%
Demographics		
Age (average in years) (SD)	47.7 (11.3)	41.7 (9.6)
Female gender	99%	99%
Born outside U.S.	96%	85%
Race or ethnicity		
African American	3%	6%
Latino	28%	76%
Filipino	31%	5%
Other Asian	35%	5%
Other	3%	8%
Employment		
Full time	92%	92%
Years worked as hotel room cleaner (SD)	13.4 (7.6)	7.7 (5.6)
Health status		
General health short form (SF-36) on scale from 1–100, where 1 = poorest (U.S. female population average = 72)[a]	56	39
Took pain medication for pain I had at work during last 4 weeks	Not asked	83%

(Continued)

(Table 19.1, continued)

Severe or very severe low back pain during last 4 weeks[b]	24%	63%
Work-related pain[b]		
Had pain believed to be caused or made worse by work during last 12 months	77%	75%
Visited doctor because of this pain	73%	61%
Reported this pain to supervisor or management	50%	31%
Filed workers' compensation claim during last 12 months	23%	20%
Association between severe bodily pain and physical workload (adj. odds ratio comparing high v. low quartile)[c]	Not analyzed	4.60 ($p < 0.001$)
Association between severe bodily pain and ergonomic problems (adj. odds ratio comparing high v. low quartile)[c]	Not analyzed	4.46 ($p < 0.001$)
Workload intensification[c]		
My job has become more and more demanding over the past few years	87%	87%
Workload increased during past 5 years	44% of job tasks	36% of job tasks
Association between severe bodily pain and workload intensification (adj. odds ratio of high v. low quartile)[c]	Not analyzed	2.16 ($p < 0.01$)
I am often pressed to work overtime	24%	23%
Skipped or shortened lunch or breaks to complete assigned rooms in last workweek	Not asked	66%

(Table 19.1, continued)

Psychosocial job stressors[d]		
I do not get the respect I deserve from my supervisors	Not asked	54%
My job security is poor	48%	69%
Effort-reward imbalance (high effort and low reward)	30%	57%
Association between severe bodily pain and effort-reward imbalance (adj. odds ratio comparing high v. low quartile)	Not analyzed	4.53 ($p < 0.001$)

[a]Short-Form-36 Health Survey developed by Ware, Kosinski, & Keller, 1994.
[b]For more detailed information on selected findings see Scherzer, Rugulies, & Krause, 2005.
[c]For more detailed information on selected findings see Krause, Scherzer, & Rugulies, 2005; Krause et al., 2002.
[d]For more detailed information on selected findings see Rugulies & Krause, 2000.

Prior research has documented that heavy manual labor may lead to overuse and injury of the musculoskeletal system (Bernard, 1997; Institute of Medicine, 2001). Although no longitudinal data were available, the results of both the San Francisco and Las Vegas studies suggested that the physical workload of the room cleaners had increased over the last five years. The extent of the increase, the particular tasks involved, and the reasons for the increase differed among the hotels studied.

In addition to physical job demands, 83 percent of room cleaners in San Francisco reported constant time pressure. In Las Vegas, fully two-thirds of the study participants reported that they skipped lunch or took shorter breaks to accommodate their workload (Scherzer, Rugulies, & Krause, 2005).

Poor job security, limited opportunities for mobility, high levels of job strain—measured as the combination of high job demands and little job control (Karasek et al., 1998; Theorell et al., 1988)—and effort-reward imbalance were also frequently reported. About a third of the room cleaners experienced high levels of job stress and effort-reward imbalance. The study team concluded that the effects of these combined stressors on the health, well-being, and productivity of hotel room cleaners merited further study. Yet the research had also clearly demonstrated significant associations between severe bodily pain and physical workload, ergonomic problems, and effort-reward imbalance, with those in the highest quartile of exposure being more than four times as likely to experience severe pain as those in the lowest quartile.

The studies in both San Francisco and Las Vegas suffered from several limitations. In each case, convenience samples were used, limiting the generalizability of findings.

Although a serious effort was made to ensure the collection of unbiased information (for example, through careful instructions to those administering the survey and the strong safeguards placed on confidentiality), workers may have over- or underestimated the severity and frequency of the problems reported. Finally the data represented a cross section and so precluded the gathering of information on potential changes over time. Despite these limitations, the high response rates achieved, the remarkable similarity of findings between the two cities, and the rigorous analytical methods used in data analysis (including the help received from core group members in interpreting study findings) provided confidence in the validity and usefulness of the study findings. In both cities, moreover, the finding of an association between poor working conditions on the one hand and reduced health, high levels of job stress, and work-related pain and disability in hotel room cleaners on the other served as a basis for action.

TRANSLATING FINDINGS INTO ACTION

Study findings in each city were presented first to the union, which used them as a critical, empirical basis for its negotiations at the bargaining table. Prior to getting to the table, however, other actions were taken in which the room cleaners played a key role. The participatory research in which they had been partners had uncovered information that helped them and their union gain a deeper appreciation of their issues and added legitimacy to their fight. That legitimacy, and in some cases the women's excitement over being part of the research process, helped spur their readiness to act.

In San Francisco many of the women took part in lobby actions at their hotels—four of the largest and best-known tourist hotels in the city. The union called meetings in hotel lobbies during work hours to report on the status of their campaign for a contract. Many room cleaners took the bold step of stopping work to come down to take part in these meetings. At several hotels, focus group participants spoke about their involvement in the study, the issues they had personally raised, and what they had learned through their participation, as a means of educating their fellow workers.

Core group members and study participants also took part in the strike vote, which authorized the union and workers to stop work if the contract bargaining was stalled or not progressing well. A focus group participant was one of the primary speakers at the strike vote meeting.

During a picket line action in front of one of the hotels, a focus group member and a union representative invited other room cleaners to have their hands photographed to show to their employers, as a symbol of the toll in terms of wear and tear that the job was taking on room cleaners' bodies. Two dozen women volunteered, and the photographs were later presented, along with the women's names, to their employers at the bargaining table.

On Labor Day a union action and sit-down civil disobedience action took place on the cable car tracks outside one of the hotels. Approximately ten room cleaners participated in the sit-in and were arrested. For most, this was the first time they had taken part in this kind of action.

Finally, and throughout this process, core group members and focus group participants played a leadership role in their hotels, keeping the workforce informed and mobilizing room cleaners for involvement in both preliminary actions and the bargaining session itself.

Thirty bargaining sessions took place, and the focus group and survey results were two of the main vehicles used to influence the desired changes in hotel policy. Approximately twenty room cleaners attended these daylong bargaining sessions, forfeiting their wages to do so.

Both academic partners and room cleaners played a vital role at the bargaining table. At the union's request the lead UC researcher presented the study findings at a joint contract negotiation session between union and management. A forty-five-minute presentation was made to the entire negotiating committee of over one hundred people, including the union leadership along with many rank-and-file negotiators, the twenty-three hotel general managers, their lawyers, and human resource personnel. Well over two hundred room cleaners came to hear the presentation and signify their support.

The presentation was followed by an hour-long, closed-door session with the employer group and three union representatives. The commitment by the academic partner to present the report in person and to undergo questioning by the employer group lent credibility to the research and allowed the employers to ask questions and discuss the findings.

Equally important, however, was the active involvement of the room cleaners themselves at the bargaining table. A panel of six room cleaners spoke in one of these sessions, including several who had been leaders in the focus group and other aspects of the study. Prior to their presentations, the women selected for the panel met at the union and outlined their talks, received help in writing a simple script, and practiced several times.

When the panel began, each woman told her life story, including the kinds of jobs she had held in her native country and in the United States, the injuries she had incurred as a room cleaner, and the results of these injuries, including severe pain, operations on wrists and shoulders, daily medications, and the wearing of braces. The women also talked about the physical and psychological demands of the job and explained the hardship their injuries caused for them and their families (for example, leaving them with no energy for playing with their children or helping them with homework). Each of the speakers added that room cleaning involved by far the most difficult work she had ever done, and two cried openly during their testimony. In part because of their involvement in the research, the women could speak with great passion and clarity about their situation, the increase in workload they had experienced, and the proposals the union was making to protect their health.

Similarly high-level participation in the action phase of CBPR was observed in Las Vegas. Core group members and study participants attended union meetings, presented their findings and their personal experiences at the bargaining table, and voted overwhelmingly to strike (18, 800 for versus 877 against) if their contract negotiations stalled. To create greater understanding of and support for their cause, the Las Vegas women also participated in creating a video, *In Our Hands,* which poignantly told the stories of a number of the room cleaners and the effects of adverse working conditions on their lives. Among other showings, the video was aired on a huge screen in front of one of the hotels, which increased patron awareness of the plight of the guest room workers.

In both cities the powerful data collected and their effective use at the bargaining table and in these preliminary venues substantially contributed to contract changes. In San Francisco a reduced maximum workload was written into the contracts (from fifteen to fourteen rooms, and to thirteen in some hotels with special cleaning requirements) (Lee & Krause, 2002). This lower maximum work assignment set a new standard, which could potentially be used in efforts to protect the health of room cleaners across the country.

The union also won agreements to have the language in all housekeeping meetings interpreted and to have any written materials that were provided translated as needed. It further won approval for future health and safety studies for other categories of hotel workers, including food servers and kitchen workers. One such study was conducted in 2003 in San Francisco (Shinoff & Krauss, 2003).

Health and safety outcomes of the Las Vegas study were similarly impressive. The new contract negotiated contained language that set a quota of rooms to be cleaned, a formula reducing the number of rooms to be cleaned under particular circumstances, and language giving room attendants the option of wearing pants. It also required the use of hazardous-materials teams to clean up biological hazards, such as vomit, blood, and the like.

Although the primary use of study findings was in influencing policy, successful efforts were also made to bring about changes in practice through less formal means. Some of the hotels, for example, agreed to revise their health and safety programs, some of which inadvertently discouraged workers from reporting work-related injuries.

Presentations of the methods and the outcomes were shared with other groups in the hope of encouraging further use of participatory methods in occupational health research. Such presentations, at national and statewide academic meetings, conferences of health and safety educators, and a popular education workshop for UC's Labor Occupational Safety and Health Program (LOSH) personnel, were among the venues in which this research project was shared. In several of these events, room cleaners served as copresenters. Partly as a result, there has been a growing interest in using this study as a template for further participatory research with workers, including the replication study conducted in Las Vegas.

The study also contributed to individual and community capacity building. One of the Latina focus group members was subsequently elected to the union's executive board. Two Chinese women who had been active in the study were hired as staff and are now union organizers working in a campaign involving a large, nonunion hotel. Several other women active in the study and not previously shop stewards took on that role. One of the focus group members spoke at a national convention of the Hotel Employees and Restaurant Employees Union, where she introduced the newly elected secretary-treasurer of the union to employees—a very high honor.

Core group members and others who played leadership roles in the study have also participated in formal presentations about the research, with several flying to other cities (Toronto, Las Vegas, and Los Angeles) to talk about the study and their own roles in the research.

Finally, all the core group members and many of the other study participants now take part in hotel joint labor and management problem-solving committees, and for many, such activity is a direct outgrowth of their active involvement in the study and the sense of empowerment it has engendered.

University partners involved with the San Francisco and Las Vegas studies also continued to participate, volunteering their time to further analyze some of the original survey data and publish the results in peer-reviewed journals (Scherzer et al., 2005; Krause, Scherzer, & Rugulies, 2005; Rugulies, Scherzer, & Krause, 2008). These subsequent analyses were critical in showing, for example, statistically significant associations between physical workload, work intensification, and ergonomic problems identified by room cleaners, with the prevalence of severe bodily pain, especially in the lower back (Krause et al., 2005). The outside researchers also continued to collaborate with the national UNITE HERE union in the analysis of national injury statistics.

Owing to the success of these initial studies, LOHP was selected by the national union to go to nearly a dozen major metropolitan areas in the United States and Canada to train 250 trainers in worker health and safety action research. The union also started a national campaign for improved worker health and safety conditions, an effort based in part on the findings of the San Francisco and Las Vegas studies. Finally, in 2006, hotel workers, researchers, LOHP, and union representatives participated in town hall meetings sponsored by the National Institute for Occupational Safety and Health (NIOSH) to gather research priorities for NIOSH's National Occupational Research Agenda.

SUMMARY

The hotel room cleaner case studies presented in this chapter are potent examples of CBPR projects that succeeded in "balancing research and action" (Israel et al., 1998, 2005), in part by influencing policy. In each city, study findings constituted the primary data used by the union in its contract negotiation sessions, and the active participation of hotel workers at the bargaining table and in many of the steps leading to the table was crucial to the negotiations' success.

Each case study also demonstrated the effectiveness of a unique partnership among a major union, its university research collaborators, and women from an often invisible sector of the economy for the purposes of community-based participatory research. The vital role of the university-based Labor Occupational Health Program as an organization that could serve as a bridge between the various partners and facilitate the research process was also demonstrated.

Although a hoped-for goal of each participatory research project was to provide data that could be used in subsequent contract negotiations, an emphasis on maintaining high research standards and ensuring that the study findings were not influenced by the union's agenda was adhered to throughout. As noted earlier, it was indeed the union's openness to supporting the studies regardless of the findings they might produce that enabled a relationship based on trust between the academic and union partners to blossom. Reflected throughout the project was its commitment to living up to CBPR's emphasis on community capacity building and empowerment. As illustrated in both case studies, a heavy accent was placed throughout on building on the strengths of the room cleaner partners, increasing their problem-solving abilities, and providing opportunities for them to articulate their own concerns and issues in their own voices.

Finally, it is hoped that these successful CBPR projects with hotel room cleaners in San Francisco and Las Vegas will illuminate the potential for new collaborations among unions, workers, and academic partners as a major new vista for community-based participatory research. In this way, the studies can serve as potent examples of how the application of research findings can be used to promote policy change—in this case, to improve working conditions for low-wage, largely immigrant workers.

QUESTIONS FOR DISCUSSION

1. Hotel management could argue that involving room cleaners (and having union funding) would automatically bias results in a study like the two described in this chapter. What steps were taken to ensure that the data collected were not biased by a union agenda or by community participation in data collection?

2. In Chapter Seventeen Themba-Nixon and her colleagues describe one goal of policy-directed CBPR as helping to lay the groundwork for more good policy. Beyond their contributions to current contract negotiations, how might the hotel room cleaner studies in San Francisco and Las Vegas have helped lay such groundwork for future good policy?

KEY TERMS

Occupational health

Workers

Unions

Participatory action research

REFERENCES

American Hotel and Lodging Association. (2006). *2006 lodging industry profile.* Retrieved June 17, 2007, from www.ahla.com/products info center lip 2006.asp.

Bernard, B. P. (Ed.). (1997). *Musculoskeletal disorders and workplace factors* (DHHS [NIOSH] Pub. No. 97–141). Cincinnati, OH: U.S. Department of Health and Human Services, National Institute for Occupational Safety and Health.

Brown, L., & Vega, W. (1996). A protocol for community-based research. *American Journal of Preventive Medicine, 12*(4), 4–5.

Brown, M. P. (1995). Worker risk mapping: An education-for-action approach. *New Solutions, 5*(2), 22–30.

Green, L. W., George, M. A., Daniel, M., Frankish, C. J., Herbert, C. P., Bowie, W. R., et al. (1995). *Study of participatory research in health promotion: Review and recommendations for the development of participatory research in health promotion in Canada.* Vancouver, BC: Royal Society of Canada.

Hagey, R. (1997). Guest editorial: The use and abuse of participatory action research. *Chronic Diseases in Canada, 18*(1), 1–4.

Institute of Medicine. (2001). *Musculoskeletal disorders and the workplace: Low back and upper extremities.* Washington, DC: National Academies Press.

Israel, B. A., Eng, E., Schulz, A. J., & Parker, E. A. (Eds.). (2005). *Methods in community-based participatory research for health.* San Francisco: Jossey-Bass.

Israel, B. A., Schulz, A. J., Parker, E. A., & Becker, A. B. (1998). Review of community-based research: Assessing partnership approaches to improve public health. *Annual Review of Public Health, 19,* 173–202.

Jones, L., & Wells, K. (2007). Strategies for academic and clinician engagement in community-partnered participatory research. *Journal of the American Medical Association, 297,* 407–410.

Karasek, R., Brisson, C., Kawakami, N., Houtman, I., Bongers, P., & Amick, B. (1998). The Job Content Questionnaire (JCQ): An instrument for internationally comparative assessments of psychosocial job characteristics. *Journal of Occupational Health Psychology, 3*(4), 322–355.

Krause, N., Lee, P. T., Thompson, P. J., Rugulies, R., & Baker, R. L. (1999, Aug.) Working conditions and health of San Francisco hotel room cleaners. Report to the Hotel Employees and Restaurant Employees International Union, Berkeley, CA.

Krause, N., Lee, P. T., Scherzer, T., Rugulies, R, Sinnott, P., & Baker, R. L. (2002). *Health and working conditions of hotel guest room attendants in Las Vegas.* Report to the Culinary Workers' Union, Local 226, Las Vegas.

Krause, N., Scherzer, T., & Rugulies, R. (2005). Physical workload, work intensification, and prevalence of pain in low wage workers: Results from a participatory research project with hotel room cleaners in Las Vegas. *American Journal of Industrial Medicine, 48,* 326–337.

Lee, P. T., & Krause, N. (2002). The impact of a worker health study on working conditions. *Journal of Public Health Policy, 23*(3), 268–285.

National Institute of Environmental Health Sciences. (1997). *Advancing the community-driven research agenda: Conference report.* Research Triangle Park: University of North Carolina.

Northridge, M. E., Vallone, D., Merzel, C., Greene, D., Shepard, P., Cohall, A. T., et al. (2000). The adolescent years: An academic-community partnership in Harlem comes of age. *Journal of Public Health Management and Practice, 6*(1), 53–60.

Reason, P. (1994). Three approaches to participative inquiry. In N. K. Denzin & Y. S. Lincoln (Eds.), *Handbook of qualitative research* (pp. 324–339). Thousand Oaks, CA: Sage.

Rugulies, R., & Krause, N. (2000, Nov. 15–18). The impact of job stress on musculoskeletal disorders, psychological symptoms and general health in hotel room cleaners. In *Proceedings of the 6th International Congress of the International Society of Behavioral Medicine,* Brisbane, Aust.

Rugulies, R., Scherzer, T., & Krause, N. (2008). Associations between psychological demands, decision latitude and job strain with smoking in female hotel room cleaners in Las Vegas. *International Journal of Behavioral Medicine, 15*(1), 34–43.

Scherzer, T., Rugulies, R., & Krause, N. (2005). Work-related pain, injury, and barriers to workers' compensation among Las Vegas hotel room cleaners. *American Journal of Public Health, 95*(3), 478–488.

Shinoff, C. W., & Krause, N. (2003, May 22). *Working conditions and health of hotel kitchen workers in San Francisco.* Report to UNITE HERE, Local 2, San Francisco.

Theorell, T. A., Perski, T., Akerstedt, F., Sigala, G., Ahlberg-Hulten, A., Svensson, J., et al. (1988). Changes in job strain in relation to changes in physiological state. *Scandinavian Journal of Work, Environment, and Health, 14,* 189–196.

U.S. Bureau of Labor Statistics. (2006). *Hotels and other accommodations.* Retrieved Jan. 5, 2008, from www.bls.gov/oco/cg/cgs036.htm.

U.S. Department of Labor. (2001). 1999 national industry-specific occupational employment and wage estimates: SIC 701—hotels and motels: Building and grounds cleaning and maintenance occupations [Table]. Retrieved Jan. 14, 2008, from http://www.bls.gov/oes/1999/oesi3_701.htm#b37–0000.

Ware, J. E., Kosinski, M., & Keller, S. (1994). SF-36 physical and mental health summary scales: A user's manual. Boston: The Health Institute, New England Medical Center.

CHAPTER

ADDRESSING FOOD SECURITY THROUGH POLICY PROMOTING STORE CONVERSIONS

THE ROLE OF A CBPR PARTNERSHIP

VICTORIA BRECKWICH VÁSQUEZ, DANA LANZA,
SUSANA HENNESSEY LAVERY, SHELLEY FACENTE,
HELEN ANN HALPIN, & MEREDITH MINKLER

Note: This chapter is adapted from "Addressing Food Security Through Public Policy Action in a Community-Based Participatory Research Partnership," by V. Breckwich Vásquez, D. Lanza, S. Hennessey Lavery, S. Facente, H. A. Halpin, and M. Minkler, 2007. *Health Promotion Practice, 8*(4), pp. 342–349. Copyright 2007 by Society for Public Health Education. Adapted by permission of Sage Publications. The authors gratefully acknowledge the community, academic, and health department partners and the policymakers whose willingness to share their knowledge and insights made this study possible. We also gratefully acknowledge consultant Angela Blackwell and her team at PolicyLink, and members of the study's national community advisory board for their many contributions. This research was made possible by a grant from the W. K. Kellogg Foundation, with additional financial assistance provided by a dissertation fellowship (Breckwich Vásquez) from the University of California Office of the President.

COMMUNITY-BASED participatory research (CBPR) has achieved growing legitimacy as a useful approach to studying and finding solutions to numerous health and social problems in areas ranging from asthma prevention (Parker et al., 2003) to mental health (Ochocka, Janzen, & Nelson, 2002). As noted in preceding chapters, a distinguishing feature of CBPR is its commitment to action as part of the research endeavor. In particular, by understanding policy change as a potential action component, CBPR has the potential for improving the health of large numbers of people beyond the partners involved or the target populations they serve (see Chapter Seventeen).

This chapter uses a policy engagement framework to describe the specific local food security policy efforts of a CBPR partnership in the Bayview Hunters Point community of San Francisco. The partnership involved a local community-based organization, a local health department, and an external evaluator. Its perceived effectiveness in using a CBPR approach to promote healthy public policy led to its selection in 2003 as one of ten such CBPR partnerships in the United States included in a multisite case study analysis funded by the W. K. Kellogg Foundation (Minkler, Breckwich Vásquez, Chang, Blackwell, et al., 2008a; Minkler, Breckwich Vásquez, Tajik, & Petersen, 2008b).

Following a brief review of food insecurity and background on the CBPR partnership, we briefly describe the methods through which this partnership effort was explored. We then present findings concerning the partnership's food security policy efforts, using relevant steps in the public policymaking process as an organizing framework, and offer implications for practice.

FOOD INSECURITY

Food insecurity is defined as the "limited or uncertain availability of nutritionally adequate and safe foods, or limited or uncertain access to food" (Anderson, 1990, p. 1558). Measured at the community level, food security concerns the underlying social, economic, and institutional factors in a community that affect the quantity and quality of available food and that food's affordability or price relative to the financial resources available to acquire it (Cohen, 2002). Nationwide, poverty-related food insecurity has grown and is associated in part with changes in social safety net programs. In the United States, 35.5 million people were without food for part of 2006, with more than 11 million of those described as having "very low food security," or major disruptions in the amount of food typically eaten. Almost 11 percent of American families were food insecure in 2006 (Nord, Andrews, & Carlson, 2007). Food insecurity is especially prevalent in inner cities, in households with children, in female-headed households, and among African Americans and Latinos. Moreover, individuals who are food insecure have poorer-quality diets, making them vulnerable to a wide variety of adverse conditions and diseases. Health risks and other consequences are also related to the anxiety and trade-offs necessary in food insecure households (Nord et al., 2007).

Dietary choices are influenced by such factors in the local food environment as accessibility and availability of foods (Morland, Wing, & Diez-Roux, 2002; Swinburn, Caterson, Seidell, & James, 2004). Among the documented causes of food insecurity in poor, inner-city neighborhoods are supermarket flight to the suburbs, transportation barriers, the growth of fast-food chains, and a lack of healthy foods at corner stores, which sell foods high in salt, sugar, and fat instead (Bolen & Hecht, 2003; K. Morland, Wing, Diez-Roux, & Poole, 2002; Wang et al., in press). In the Bayview Hunters Point community (hereafter referred to as *Bayview*), the few large grocery stores had all moved out of the area by 1994, making it difficult for local residents to access nutritious foods such as fruits and vegetables (Duggan, 2004; Soltau, 2004). Intake of healthy foods decreases by one-third and fat consumption increases among residents in poor and segregated neighborhoods without supermarkets when compared with residents in a neighborhood with supermarkets (Morland, Wing, Diez-Roux, & Poole, 2002).

THE CBPR PARTNERSHIP

Literacy for Environmental Justice (LEJ) is a nonprofit youth empowerment and environmental justice education organization based in Bayview that was funded by and worked with the San Francisco Department of Public Health's Tobacco Free Project (TFP) to form a CBPR partnership (hereafter referred to as the *LEJ partnership*), which began in 2002. In addition to providing funding, TFP facilitated access to an outside research evaluator for consultation and technical assistance. The LEJ partnership worked collaboratively with youths in assessing food insecurity-related problems and resources in the community and developed a local campaign (the Good Neighbor Program) to reduce the numbers of tobacco company subsidiary food products and tobacco advertisements and to replace them with healthier food alternatives at select commercial businesses. The LEJ partnership then worked with local policymakers to have the Good Neighbor Program adopted by the city, with four city departments contributing staff, resources, and incentives to manage and sustain the program. Efforts are currently under way to evaluate the Good Neighbor Program, explore ways to expand it throughout the city, and develop state policy to support similar efforts throughout California.

Like the WE ACT partnership described in Chapter Eighteen, the LEJ partnership was one of ten CBPR collaborations included in a Kellogg Foundation–funded effort to study and document the impacts of CBPR on health-promoting public policy through a multisite case study analysis (Yin, 2003; see Minkler et al., 2008a, for a discussion of the methods involved in this case study).

LEJ PARTNERSHIP'S POLICY STEPS

The stages of a CBPR partnership generally begin with the identification of a problem and then progress toward deciding on a research question, conducting the study, developing and implementing action plans, and evaluating the outcomes. During the action phase of CBPR, there are few guideposts to provide direction for interventions that undertake policy-related action. Therefore the better-defined field of policymaking can guide the development of a clear pathway through which CBPR can leverage its research findings and translate them into policy change. As discussed in Chapter Seventeen, a number of relevant frameworks for stepwise public policymaking have been developed (cf. Bardach,

2000; Kingdon, 1995). Although policymaking proceeds nonlinearly and is embedded within changing sociohistorical contexts (Milio, 1998), policy steps nonetheless shape the content, course, pace, and development of policy and may contribute to the relative success of some policies over others. The LEJ partnership's engagement in policy steps (problem identification and definition, setting the agenda, constructing policy alternatives, deciding on the policy to pursue, and implementing the policy) is described in the following sections.

Problem Identification and Definition

CBPR partnerships typically come together to research and solve a health or social problem identified by the community, so they commonly begin by identifying and defining the problem. To identify a problem for serious policy consideration, a foundation of research is needed that may dictate policy action (Kingdon, 1995; Richan, 1996). CBPR partnerships necessarily participate in some type of research as part of their endeavor, contributing needed data to identify new problems or issues and then propose solutions to address them.

The TFP was influential in developing the focus of the LEJ partnership and in defining the food security problem. An important focus of TFP is to educate youth and communities about the impact of tobacco globalization and tobacco food subsidiary globalization on people and communities locally and in other countries. Thus the relationship between people's health and the corporate dominance of the food system became an integral part of the LEJ partnership's problem definition and later policy intervention. TFP leveraged state tobacco funds and funded youth-involved organizations that identified issues of concern to their communities and implemented the five steps of the TFP research-to-action model, the *community action model* (Hennessey Lavery, Smith, Esparza et al., 2005; Hennessey Lavery, Smith, & Moore, 2005), to achieve policy-related change (for more information about TFP, see San Francisco Tobacco Free Project, 2008).

Many preliminary developments helped lay the foundation for the LEJ partnership's Good Neighbor Program, among them community organizing around toxics issues, participatory research and forums conducted by local environmental organizations (Bhatia, Calandra, Brainin-Rodríguez, & Jones, 2001), municipal efforts that prioritized food insecurity through environmental justice programs, and health impact assessments. Two important local developments also took place early on and were *foundation builders*—a term used by the TFP staff and the San Francisco Department of Public Health—for the Good Neighbor Program. A group of community elders met regularly in the early 1990s to discuss the problem of the *corner stores* (small, local businesses selling disproportionate amounts of alcohol and cigarettes on Bayview's main thoroughfare), which were attracting loitering and vandalism. It was this group's initial idea to have these stores become "good neighbors" and to deter crime while also improving the quality of food they offered. Together with other local efforts, and with the strong support of a charismatic community leader who later became a city supervisor (Sophie Maxwell), these early stakeholders helped identify food insecurity as a key community concern.

To understand the extent of the food insecurity problem in Bayview from the perspective of various local constituencies, the LEJ partnership undertook several types of research. With training and ongoing technical assistance from their health department and evaluator partners, LEJ youths and project staff designed and conducted a brief (four-question) survey with a convenience sample of 130 residents on a Bayview thoroughfare. The survey covered needs and desires relating to local markets, health behaviors and daily nutrition habits, and what incentives or changes it would take to get people to shop locally.

The LEJ youths also conducted store-mapping research in all eleven central Bayview corner stores to determine how much shelf space was devoted to fast foods, tobacco, liquor, meat, and fresh produce. Youths estimated shelf space with an innovative diagramming method that used Quadrille graph paper and different colors for the various products measured (see Cheadle et al., 1991, for other ways of measuring shelf space). Building on what they had learned from TFP about the relationship between tobacco and food companies, the youths also counted the number of Kraft Foods and Nabisco products as a percentage of the total number of products sold. Using these methods the youths learned that on average, only 2 percent of shelf space in the eleven corner stores was devoted to fresh produce, but 39 percent was allocated to packaged goods and 26 percent to alcohol and cigarettes (see Figure 20.1). Because measures of shelf space commonly approximate sales, in order to minimize restocking costs, what a store offers should closely resemble how much of each major item category is sold at the store.

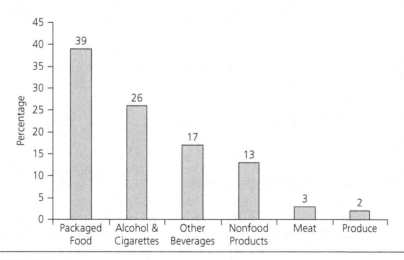

FIGURE 20.1 *Products Sold in Eleven Corner Stores in Bayview Hunters Point in June 2002*
Sources: Adapted from Hennessey Lavery, Smith, & Moore et al., 2005; and Breckwich Vásquez et al., 2007.

The LEJ youths further found that the top three non-tobacco-related and non-alcohol-related products available at these stores were cookies, cereals, and crackers, and that Kraft and Nabisco made 90 percent of the cookies and nearly 80 percent of the cereals and crackers, many of which had a high sugar, fat, and salt content. Finally, the youths learned that 47 percent of the tobacco products and 41 percent of the alcoholic beer products were owned by Philip Morris.

The partnership felt strongly about building relationships with merchants, so during this initial problem identification phase of the project in-depth interviews were conducted with local merchants at five of the corner stores. Merchants were often reluctant to speak with youths who, in the words of an LEJ staff person, "did not look any different than the youth who hang around in front of the store and are often associated with stealing or causing a nuisance." But the store owners who agreed to participate stressed the hardships of owning businesses that attract violent behavior, and the struggles they experienced in keeping their businesses afloat. These merchants also pointed out that alcohol and cigarettes were the most profitable products they sold, due to the cheap bulk price at which distributors offered these items.

To gain additional information for better defining the problem of food insecurity in Bayview, LEJ youths were trained to conduct geographic information system (GIS) mapping and produced maps highlighting locations of corner stores, supermarkets and other grocery stores, transportation routes, and relevant demographic characteristics of the community.

Findings from the GIS mapping showed that census tracts where the majority of the Bayview population lives are primarily hillside areas, whereas the local grocery stores are in the flats over half a mile away. When transportation routes were overlaid on the maps, they revealed that existing public transportation requires about one hour of time and an average of three bus transfers to get from Hunters Point hills to the closest supermarket.

The problem identification phase of the project, in short, included a multipronged approach to data collection and provided a wealth of relevant information about diverse dimensions of the problem of food insecurity in the Bayview neighborhood.

Setting the Agenda

Agenda setting is an important component of public policymaking (Kingdon, 1995; Rochefort & Cobbs, 1994). The LEJ partnership focused on agenda setting by strategically fitting and timing the food insecurity issue within larger, historically based concerns about the community's redevelopment following data collection and analysis. The partnership also focused on building relationships with local policymakers to determine their interest in the issue and garner their support to strengthen their visibility for agenda setting. Disseminating their research findings to key local partners helped the LEJ partnership set a local policy agenda that prioritized food insecurity. LEJ's long relationship with Supervisor Maxwell was credited by the community partners, TFP partners, and policymakers interviewed with opening the door to city agencies and spearheading the Good Neighbor Program. The city-based priorities of redevelopment and reduced community violence may also have served as windows of opportunity to produce an ideal environment for opening the discussion about food insecurity and its connection to community improvement. Revitalizing the area and decreasing the violent crime focused mutual attention on corner stores, which became their primary policy target.

Constructing Policy Alternatives

Developing a policy action plan in a CBPR partnership involves community participation in the interpretation and translation of research findings into concrete policy actions. Partnerships may consider many alternative actions, evaluating their feasibility against political or community pressures and deciding on actions that have the fewest negative consequences for powerful and politically strong allies and constituents. The LEJ partnership considered policy-related strategies that fit with its goal of addressing the link between tobacco and food security and finding a solution to expand access to healthy foods in Bayview. These did not involve a predetermined set of alternatives considered in turn but instead were made part of a larger, ongoing partnership decision-making process that was constantly evolving over time. For all policy options they considered, the partners went through a deliberate process to determine who the key players were and whether the partnership had an appropriate contact or policy connection. After getting to know the merchants and their circumstances, the LEJ partnership considered the foremost policy alternative one that involved working with merchants instead of penalizing them.

Deciding on a Policy to Pursue

Kingdon (1995) describes the separate streams of problems, policies, and politics that may come together at a moment in time to influence how policy decisions are made. Those policies judged politically and analytically feasible present an enormous opportunity for CBPR partnerships to push through policy solutions. The partnership's early focus on trying to craft a city resolution to support a Good Neighbor ordinance was soon abandoned after Supervisor Maxwell reminded the LEJ partnership that "hundreds of resolutions are passed annually," but they are usually ineffective because "they have no teeth."

The LEJ partnership therefore considered trying to get legislation for a *restricted use district* for incoming merchants, which would include making better food available to Bayview residents and requiring that tobacco subsidiary products be removed and that there be restrictions on tobacco and alcohol advertising. However, the partners quickly realized that this might be legally impossible. At the same time, as their understanding of the economic and social complexity of low-income community food distribution increased, they began to see the merchants as another vulnerable constituency, and they developed a focus on working closely with small businesses rather than alienating or challenging them.

Supervisor Maxwell's support seemed clearly behind a third policy option, a voluntary policy targeted at corner stores and involving working with merchants to improve community food security rather than beginning with strong-arm regulatory strategies. As the project evaluator noted: "[The LEJ partnership] decided on a voluntary policy because there are a lot of economic issues involved. They didn't want to go into the neighborhood and say 'we're another group telling you what you should be doing.'" Named the Good

Neighbor Program, this option gathered solid support from other potential partners, including four city departments as well as other city entities, such as the San Francisco Redevelopment Agency (MacLaughlin, 2003). Such a policy was also consistent with sound health promotion theory and practice: incentives-based policy strategies like this one have been used in promoting health, and they work through the building of alliances instead of the threat of penalties (Schauffler, Faer, Faulkner, & Shore, 1994).

To decide on appropriate incentives for the Good Neighbor Program, the LEJ partnership worked with the Good Neighbor Advisory Committee, which brought together LEJ staff and youths, community organizations and residents, city representatives, and other stakeholders. They discussed appropriate merchant incentives in order to devise a plan to partner with incentive-providing entities. The incentives they prioritized included access to low-interest loans and energy efficient appliances, which would help corner stores properly store produce and other healthy foods. An economic feasibility study was conducted to explore existing city-sponsored economic incentive mechanisms for small merchants in San Francisco (MacLaughlin, 2003).

The health-promoting changes corner stores were to make in exchange for incentives were to stock a minimum amount (10 percent of their total items) of fresh produce (encouraging organic and locally grown products); stock an additional minimum (10 percent) of healthy foods (for example, not Kraft or Nabisco products); stock products at affordable prices; participate in food stamp and other related programs; adhere to environmental standards and codes that address loitering, cleanliness, and safety; limit tobacco and alcohol advertising, promotion, and sales (with indoor height requirements for displays and elimination of outdoor tobacco and alcohol advertising); and adhere to laws restricting the sale of tobacco and alcohol to minors. Corner store incentives and health-promoting changes are secured through a memorandum of understanding that the LEJ partnership helped to develop under the direction of its advisory committee.

Implementing the Policy

To see how this voluntary policy might work with merchant criteria and incentives in place to improve access to healthy food products, the LEJ partnership decided on an intervention at one pilot corner store in Bayview, Super Save. Together with the support of the Good Neighbor Advisory Committee and TFP's grant, LEJ launched a six-month Good Neighbor Store pilot in December 2003, with incentives provided by several city agencies (see Table 20.1).

Education and information dissemination are important tools for policymaking that can serve both to change undesirable behaviors and to engage community members in protecting their own health. During this time, LEJ youths promoted products in the pilot store by conducting in-store press events, taste testing, and promotional giveaways of canvas shopping bags and fresh produce. Youths worked with a local graphic artist to develop and implement an award-winning media campaign to raise awareness about the Good Neighbor Program in Bayview (Reed, 2004). The artwork was subsequently featured in a peer-reviewed journal article (Baker, Metzler, & Galea, 2005). The LEJ partnership sent out several press advisories to local media sources, and the pilot store intervention was covered by several local media sources, including KPFA (FM), local

TABLE 20.1 **Good Neighbor Program Incentives for Corner Store Merchants**

Responsible Party	Incentives
Literacy for Environmental Justice	Store branding, external and internal product promotions, healthy food tastings at participating stores, and community outreach and education
San Francisco Community Power Cooperative (SF Coop)	Grants for energy efficient upgrades (lighting and refrigeration), indoor and outdoor motion detector lighting, energy audits, education, and outreach to the business community
San Francisco Department of the Environment	Funds the SF Coop, networking, outreach
San Francisco Department of Public Health	In-kind training, technical assistance, and resources on health promotion, the San Francisco Green Business Program, and food systems
San Francisco Redevelopment Agency	Facade improvements to existing buildings permit expediting
Neighborhood economic development organizations	Free business development training
Mayor's Office on Economic Development	.25 FTE for Good Neighbor Program; consulting with grocers on store layout
Rainbow Grocery	Collective buying of whole foods for participating merchants
San Francisco Produce Market	Facilitate purchase and instruct on care of organic produce; refrigeration units
Veritable Vegetable	Delivers organic produce from warehouse twice per week; collective bulk purchasing of organic produce

ABC news, and the *San Francisco Chronicle.* This coverage also helped to promote the Good Neighbor Program within the nonprofit funding community and city government.

LOCAL POLICY-RELATED OUTCOMES

The LEJ partnership, together with a high level of commitment among influential partners, including a city supervisor, has realized policy outcomes at the local, municipal and state levels. According to those interviewed and the multiple documents reviewed, the partnership's research and policy actions have contributed to these outcomes. The partnership's impact on the involved youths is currently being examined, but initial findings are promising (Breckwich Vásquez, Lanza, Hennessey Lavery, Facente, Halpin, & Minkler, 2007).

The pilot store intervention was seen as a local success, producing broad interest in replication and expansion. Community and TFP partners told us that the *combination* of research and media coverage both raised awareness of the issues and influenced policymakers to address them in this preliminary way. Super Save's manager reported in July 2004 that these efforts had led to an increase in fresh produce sales from 5 percent to 15 percent in the first seven months of Good Neighbor involvement, with similarly dramatic declines in alcohol sales (from 25 percent to 15 percent). By early 2008, fresh produce made up 15 to 17 percent of total sales, with alcohol sales making up 14 percent and cigarettes about 10 percent (Sam Aloude, Super Save manager, personal communication, January 14, 2008). The decline in alcohol sales was believed to reflect the fact that fewer individuals were coming into the store solely to buy alcohol now that the store had a more family-friendly ambience and decreased alcohol advertising. Although the increased sale of cheap cigarettes through other outlets in the neighborhood was believed to be a factor in the declining tobacco sales, decreased tobacco advertising and, again, the family-friendly ambience were also seen as contributors to this trend. Finally, and of equal importance for sustainability, the store's gross sales have remained up by 10 to 12 percent since the beginning of the Good Neighbor Program (Sam Aloude, personal communication, January 14, 2008). Although changes in actual consumption patterns are more difficult to document (Wang et al., in press), efforts are under way to determine whether the greater availability of fresh produce through the local stores is having an impact on the dietary habits of residents.

Building on its initial success, the LEJ partnership secured additional funding through The California Endowment and the TFP to expand the Good Neighbor Program to a goal of eight corner stores in Bayview and to evaluate the partnership's efforts. LEJ is the lead partner on these expansion plans and has four city agency partners. As of this writing, six additional stores have agreed to become good neighbors.

Policymakers in the city government have credited the LEJ partnership with producing credible research evidence of food insecurity in Bayview and for playing a key role in persuading policymakers of the importance of the problem and an appropriate policy solution. A local policymaker commented that the partnership's research findings and LEJ's youth involvement "shed a lot of light" on the nature and urgency of the food insecurity problem among city policymakers and decision makers.

At the level of state policy the LEJ partnership is currently working with Assembly-man Mark Leno and the California Food Policy Advocates on legislation (Assembly Bill 2384) to support Good Neighbor efforts throughout the state. The legislation would create a demonstration project to (1) improve the supply of healthy choices (fresh fruit and vegetables) in small corner stores; (2) provide grocers with technical assistance to procure, store, display, and market healthy choices; and (3) increase the demand in underserved communities by providing food stamp recipients with "bonus" dollars toward the purchase of fruits and vegetables.

SUMMARY

The LEJ partnership is a community-driven CBPR partnership that stands firmly in the environmental justice movement, with youths at its center. Undergoing strategic efforts to frame food insecurity as an environmental justice issue, the LEJ partnership proceeded with funding from a local health department to advance a policy agenda in collaboration with a local legislator and several city agencies. This partnership has helped to bring about an impressive series of policy-related victories in just a few years. These include youth-led research on the understudied problem of food insecurity, a successful pilot Good Neighbor store intervention, community outreach and education to influence community knowledge and behavioral change, the development of a city- and foundation-sponsored initiative to expand the Good Neighbor Program, and state legislation that, if passed, would support similar efforts throughout California. The success of this effort demonstrates the potential for involving youths in a policy-focused process to promote healthy environments in some of this nation's most challenged urban communities.

QUESTIONS FOR DISCUSSION

1. As discussed in Chapters One and Two, participatory research ideally engages participants in a discussion of some of the root causes of problems they have collectively identified. In what ways were the LEJ youths in this case study helped to consider some of the problems behind the problem of food insecurity in low-income neighborhoods like theirs?

2. The partners in this case study did a good job of doing their homework in order to better decide on the courses of action that might be most feasible and realistic to pursue. What examples of such background reconnaissance can you point to? If you were a member of this partnership, what other kinds of information or data, if any, might you have wanted to collect to help inform your decision making?

3. The LEJ partnership ended up deciding to pursue a policy promoting what is in essence a voluntary agreement by store owners in the neighborhood to offer healthier food choices and to decrease the availability and advertising of alcohol and tobacco. Was a voluntary policy the best way to go in this case, or can you think of other alternatives that would have been preferable? Can you think of other examples of cases in which a voluntary agreement might be the most expedient policy goal to pursue?

KEY TERMS

Food insecurity

Tobacco

Good Neighbor Program

Policy

REFERENCES

Anderson, S. (1990). Core indicators of nutritional state for difficult-to-sample populations. *Journal of Nutrition, 120*(11, Suppl.), 1557–1600.

Baker, E. A., Metzler, M. M., & Galea, S. (2005). Addressing social determinants of health inequities: Learning from doing. *American Journal of Public Health, 95*(4), 553–555.

Bardach, E. (2000). *A practical guide for policy analysis: The eightfold path to more effective problem solving.* New York: Chatham House.

Bhatia, R., Calandra, C., Brainin-Rodríguez, L., & Jones, P. (2001). *Food access study of the Bayview Hunters Point.* San Francisco: San Francisco Department of Public Health and San Francisco League of Urban Gardeners.

Bolen, E., & Hecht, K. (2003). *Neighborhood groceries: New access to healthy food in low-income communities.* San Francisco: California Food Policy Advocates.

Breckwich Vásquez, V., Lanza, D., Hennessey Lavery, S., Facente, S., Halpin, H. A., & Minkler, M. (2007). Addressing food security through public policy action in a community-based participatory research partnership. *Health Promotion Practice, 8*(4), 342–349.

Cheadle, A., Psaty, B. M., Curry, S., Wagner, E., Diehr, P., Koepsell, T., et al. (1991). Community-level comparisons between the grocery store environment and individual dietary practices. *Preventive Medicine, 20,* 250–261.

Cohen, B. (2002). *United States Department of Agriculture community food security assessment toolkit.* Washington, DC: U.S. Department of Agriculture.

Duggan, T. (2004, July 16). Bringing healthy produce to poor neighborhoods: Food activists, small farmers lead project. *San Francisco Chronicle.*

Hennessey Lavery, S., Smith, M. L., Esparza, A. A., Hrushow, A., Moore, M., & Reed, D. F. (2005). The community action model: A community-driven model designed to address disparities in health. *American Journal of Public Health, 95*(4), 611–616.

Hennessey Lavery, S., Smith, M. L., & Moore, M., (2005). The community action model: Organizing for change in San Francisco's Tobacco Free Project. *Health Education and Behavior, 32(3),* 293–297.

Kingdon, J. W. (1995). *Agendas, alternatives, and public policies* (2nd ed). Reading, MA: Addison-Wesley.

MacLaughlin, K. (2003). *Making good neighbors: Creating food security with small food retailers in Bayview/ Hunters Point.* Berkeley: University of California, Berkeley, Department of City and Regional Planning.

Milio, N. (1998). Priorities and strategies for promoting community-based prevention policies. *Journal of Public Health Management and Practice, 4*(3), 14–28.

Minkler, M., Breckwich Vásquez, V., Chang, C., Blackwell, A. G., Thompson, M., and Rubin, V. (2008a). *Promoting healthy public policy through community-based participatory research.* Oakland, CA: PolicyLink.

Minkler, M., Breckwich Vásquez, V., Tajik, M., & Petersen, D. (2008b). Promoting environmental justice through community-based participatory research: The role of community and partnership capacity. *Health Education & Behavior, 35*(1), 119–137.

Morland, K., Wing, S., & Diez-Roux, A. (2002). The contextual effect of the local food environment on residents' diets: The Atherosclerosis Risk in Communities Study. *American Journal of Public Health, 92*(11), 1761–1768.

Morland, K., Wing, S., Diez-Roux, A., & Poole, C. (2002). Neighborhood characteristics associated with the location of food stores and food service places. *American Journal of Preventive Medicine, 22*(1), 23–29.

Nord, M., Andrews, M., & Carlson, S. (2007). *Household food security in the United States, 2006* (Economic Report No. 49). Washington, DC: U.S. Department of Agriculture.

Ochocka, J., Janzen, R., & Nelson, G. (2002). Sharing power and knowledge: Professional and mental health consumer/survivor researchers working together in a participatory action research project. *Psychiatric Rehabilitation Journal, 25*(4), 379–387.

Parker, E. A., Israel, B. A., Williams, M., Brakefield-Caldwell, W., Lewis, T. C., Robins, T., et al. (2003). Community action against asthma: Examining the partnership process of a community-based participatory research project. *Journal of General Internal Medicine, 18*(7), 558–567.

Reed, D. (2004). *Literacy for Environmental Justice—Youth Envision's Good Neighbor Program in Bayview Hunters Point: A case study.* San Francisco: San Francisco Department of Public Health & Tobacco Free Project.

Richan, W. C. (1996). *Lobbying for social change* (2nd ed.). Binghamton, NY: Haworth Press.

Rochefort, D. A., & Cobbs, R. W. (1994). *The politics of problem definition: Shaping the policy agenda.* Lawrence: University of Kansas Press.

San Francisco Tobacco Free Project. (2008). [Home page.] Retrieved May 7, 2008, from http://sftfc.globalink.org.

Schauffler, H., Faer, M., Faulkner, L., & Shore, K. (1994). Health promotion and disease prevention in health care reform. *American Journal of Preventive Medicine, 10*(Suppl. 5) 1–31.

Soltau, A. (2004, Jan. 6). Fresh look for the Bayview. *San Francisco Independent.*

Swinburn, B. A., Caterson, I., Seidell, J. C., & James, W.P.T. (2004). Diet, nutrition and the prevention of excess weight gain and obesity. *Public Health Nutrition, 7*(1A), 123–146.

Wang, M. C., MacLeod, K., Steadman, C., Williams, L., Bowie, S. L., Herd, D., et al. (in press). Is the opening of a neighborhood full-service grocery store accompanied by a change in the food behavior of residents? *Journal of Hunger and Environmental Nutrition.*

Yin, R. (2003). *Case study research: Design and methods.* Thousand Oaks, CA: Sage.

PART

6

NEXT STEPS AND STRATEGIES FOR THE FUTURE OF CBPR

The primary goal of this book has been to stimulate and enhance CBPR practice as a collaborative approach to knowledge creation and application to eliminate health disparities. Our central aim is to support students, scholars, community members, and allies in becoming comfortable with applying CBPR approaches in their community-based research, and beyond that to inspire them with CBPR's potential.

We began this new edition by providing a historical and conceptual grounding in core issues such as cross-cultural and power dynamics, the role of race and racism, and self- and community reflection, embedded in the processes of CBPR partnerships. The book then further explored methods for identifying community strengths and concerns and the special considerations in undertaking CBPR with hidden populations, youths, and other diverse groups.

In addition to addressing continuing concerns in CBPR processes and practices, this new edition has given greater attention to the issues of evidence and outcomes, more description of methodologies, and more discussions of rigor and internal and external validity. It has also recognized that CBPR's reach in the health field goes well beyond public health to include such partners as clinical medicine, nursing, and, increasingly, policymakers. We have included updated chapters from the first edition in order to document longer-term outcomes, and we have offered new case studies, selected in part because the projects they discuss have demonstrated effectiveness in getting to outcomes, including policy changes.

The final chapter now turns to several questions that are central to the future of CBPR research as the field moves beyond its earlier focus on processes to the study of linkages between processes and outcomes. The latter may be systems or capacity outcomes, such as more culturally attuned interventions, or outcomes related to health and the reduction of health disparities. In this chapter, Nina Wallerstein and her colleagues present findings from a pilot research project that identified a conceptual model and hypothesized potential pathways between contexts, characteristics of participation and partnership, and outcomes. These authors urge that further research be focused on assessing the added value of CBPR and on identifying those best practices that might be most salient in various contexts, conditions, and models to enhancing health and reducing health disparities.

CHAPTER

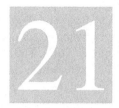

WHAT PREDICTS
OUTCOMES
IN CBPR?

NINA WALLERSTEIN, JOHN OETZEL, BONNIE DURAN,
GREG TAFOYA, LORENDA BELONE, & REBECCA RAE

WITH THE INCREASING recognition over the last decade that communities need to be partners in order to reduce disparities and improve health status, community-based participatory research (CBPR) has moved to center stage in intervention research (Israel, Eng, Schulz, & Parker, 2005; Viswanathan et al., 2004; Minkler & Wallerstein, 2003; Wallerstein

Note: Funding for this pilot CBPR study (U26IHS300009A Supplement, N. Wallerstein, PI; B. Duran, co-PI) came from the National Center on Minority Health and Health Disparities (NCMHD, 2006–2008) in partnership with the Native American Research Centers for Health (NARCH). To incorporate a community-based participatory research (CBPR) approach within this funded research, a national advisory committee was formed that included principal investigators from the NCMHD and NARCH partnerships, other CBPR national experts, community members involved in selected CBPR projects, and representatives of the Navajo Nation.

& Duran, 2006). Nonetheless, the actual study of the science of CBPR, that is, the *effects of participation and partnerships* on public health interventions and health outcomes, remains insufficient. The majority of CBPR intervention literature has employed case studies to describe partnerships, research designs, and interventions. Articles to date primarily report strategies for creating and maintaining research partnerships, methods of data collection and analysis that have been adapted and adopted by partners, and facilitators and challenges to building trust among stakeholders. Far fewer papers have documented outcomes that can be attributed to CBPR partnerships and interventions (Viswanathan et al., 2004; Cargo & Mercer, 2008; see also Chapters Fourteen and Eighteen).

As CBPR has received greater attention from the National Institutes of Health (NIH) and other agencies, foundations, and training programs (discussed in Chapter One), however, academic and community investigators have become increasingly interested in documenting the outcomes and impacts of CBPR research. A number of recent studies, including some explored in this second edition, report policy and capacity changes that have resulted from CBPR (Minkler, Breckwich Vásquez, Tajik, & Petersen, 2008). Nevertheless, documenting the health outcomes of CBPR remains a challenge (Viswanathan et al., 2004; Cargo & Mercer, 2008).

This chapter seeks to further advance the study of how CBPR processes influence or predict outcomes. To this end, we report results of a two-year pilot study to identify the core processes and pathways to CBPR outcomes. This study focused on two central questions: What is the added value of CBPR to the research itself and to producing outcomes? and, What are the potential pathways to intermediate system and capacity change outcomes, and to more distal health outcomes?

In this final chapter, we provide a brief rationale for the study, and we discuss the results of our CBPR literature review, our Internet survey, and the consensus process of a national CBPR advisory committee[1] formed to synthesize a unifying, conceptual logic model of CBPR processes leading to outcomes. We present the conceptual model and the list of characteristics for each dimension in the model as a framework for future research into the identified gaps in CBPR knowledge. We further offer examples of testable hypotheses regarding the pathways and relationships between different dimensions of CBPR. Although the focus of this chapter is intervention research, the conceptual logic model can also be used to inform research about partnership processes in CBPR epidemiologic or other assessment studies.

STUDY BACKGROUND

Gaps in the CBPR and related scientific literatures motivated this pilot study that addressed three major challenges: (1) translating evidence-based interventions to widespread implementation and sustainability in diverse settings with populations that face health disparities; (2) evaluating *community-supported* interventions—those founded on cultural normative beliefs and practices rather than on evidence-based practice per se—and (3) gaps in the scientific knowledge base of CBPR itself, that is, lack of knowledge about what constitutes effective participatory processes and practices, about the ways these processes and practices may manifest differently in different contexts; and about what constitutes systems-level and capacity changes, such as new policies or culturally centered interventions that have an impact on health outcomes in CBPR. Each of these challenges is discussed in the following paragraphs.

1. *Translation of research to multiple settings.* The NIH roadmap has recently heightened the importance of translational research (which moves science into practical applications), with issues of context and external validity assuming greater importance (National Institutes of Health, Office of Portfolio Analysis and Strategic Initiatives, 2008). As noted in Chapter One, efficacy studies and randomized controlled trials, which focus on internal validity, do not provide the knowledge necessary for translating and disseminating interventions to real-world settings with high variability in culture, context, and levels of acceptance (Wallerstein, 2007; Glasgow et al., 2006; Fixsen, Naoom, Blasé, Friedman, & Wallace, 2005; Miller & Shinn, 2005). In a comprehensive review of the implementation literature, Fixsen and colleagues (2005) articulate that although evidence-based interventions have core elements, that is, underlying principles or best practices, they need to be flexible in applying these elements to the "noise" (the organizational, cultural, and policy differences) of different settings (Hohmann & Shear, 2002). Green, Glasgow, and colleagues argue for greater practitioner [and community] engagement. They advocate for the use of practice-based evidence or frameworks, such as RE-AIM, to enhance external validity; increase the use of research findings; and enable greater implementation, adaptation, and dissemination to new settings, with higher potential for sustainability (Green & Glasgow, 2006; Glasgow & Emmons, 2007; Green & Ottoson, 2004; Bull, Gillette, Glasgow, & Estabrooks, 2003). A recent systematic review of diffusion of innovations supports a better understanding of the range of intervention adoption methods, from passive diffusion through active dissemination (Greenhalgh, Robert, Macfarlane, Bate, & Kyriakidou, 2004).

2. *Empirically supported interventions (ESIs) in the dominant culture do not necessarily translate to minority cultures,* especially when culturally supported interventions (CSIs), including their theories and contexts, are excluded from the research (terms adapted from Hall, 2001; Persaud & Mamdani, 2006). Culturally supported interventions, although rarely circulated in the academic literature or tested with Western scientific methods, fit within the values and social service systems of local communities, support cultural revitalization, and remain highly used and sustained over time (see Chapter Five; Duran & Walters, 2004; Smith, 1999). CBPR offers a valuable means of creating an integrated, or a hybrid, approach to knowledge and to codeveloped interventions by (a) translating and testing the core components of empirically supported interventions with communities while also (b) integrating culturally supported interventions to enhance translation and sustainability within the local context.

3. The challenge persists of identifying the specific CBPR practices and processes needed to improve community capacity building or other system changes and health outcomes; and of specifying the conditions under which participation is effective

in contributing to these outcomes. There are limitations (Buchanan, Miller, & Wallerstein, 2007) as well as potential for using randomized controlled trials (see Chapter Four) to study participation as an independent variable, and other innovative methodologies will be needed to assess variability of participation and potential outcomes from this variability across CBPR sites. With the reality of CBPR falling across a continuum of participatory characteristics (such as being more university driven or more community driven), the starting place remains the identification of effective CBPR partnership processes and practices (Wallerstein, Duran, Minkler, & Foley, 2005; see also Chapter Two).

LITERATURE SEARCH

The purpose of our literature review was to summarize the state of the knowledge about existing partnering characteristics as preparation for creating a new model with hypothesized pathways of the ways in which CBPR processes predict outcomes. (See Table 21.1; the model and the description of characteristics are discussed later in this chapter.) We examined two earlier reviews: the CBPR study by Green and colleagues (1995) and the systematic literature review commissioned by the Agency for Healthcare Research and Quality (AHRQ) (Viswanathan et al., 2004). From the earlier literature, we created an initial list of CBPR characteristics, paying particular attention to the comprehensive dimensions generated by Schulz, Israel, and Lantz (2003), who adapted a nationally used, validated, coalition instrument (Sofaer, 2000), including group dynamics variables (Johnson & Johnson, 1999). We used search terms that paralleled the AHRQ study terms and expanded our literature review to the year 2007 and to several new databases. Table 21.1 displays the databases, search terms, inclusion criteria, and number of articles reviewed.

Articles were coded in an iterative process to generate a larger inclusive list of characteristics within six categories. For PubMed, SciSearch and SocioFile, and "colleague-recommended" articles, the largest number of mentions was in the dimension of group dynamics (236), followed by context/environmental characteristics (141), structural dynamics of the partnership (126), CBPR capacity and systems outcomes (95), and individual characteristics of the principal investigator or community investigators (46). Linkages to health had the fewest mentions (27).

We also sought new literatures to deepen our understanding of participation from the perspective of the macro- and micro-forces of power and relationships. To identify these new literatures we examined (1) the Business Source Premier database, which covers organizational and international development, highlighting historical and power relations within CBPR; (2) the indigenous CBPR articles from the United States, Canada, New Zealand, and Australia that centered on historical contexts of colonization, trust or mistrust, and race relations; and (3) the mass communication literature (including that indexed in PsycInfo) that highlighted organizational and micro-team dynamics in workforce and community partnerships.

The Business Source Premier database contributed literatures on the positive contributions to participatory research by consumer and advocate researchers (Drew, Nyerges,

TABLE 21.1 **Literature Review Databases and Inclusion Criteria**

Database & search terms	Search limits	Inclusion criteria	Articles reviewed
PubMed (10 exact terms used by AHRQ) "Community-based Participatory Research," "CBPR," "participatory research," "action research," "Participatory Action Research," "participatory evaluation," "community driven research," "action science," "collaborative inquiry," "empowerment evaluation"	English; 2002 to 2007; Male; Female; Humans	If yes to these questions, include the article: **a.** Dimensions between collaborators discussed? **b.** Participation characteristics mentioned? **c.** Dimensions of the participatory process measured? **d.** Are the CBPR processes linked to outcomes?	45
SciSearch; SocioFile Same search terms as PubMed	English; published in the last 6 years		85
Business Source Premier "Community-based Participatory Research," "Participatory Action Research"	2003–2007; English; removal of PubMed duplicates		21
Communication & Mass Media Complete; PsycINFO Under each category, Group, Organization, or Team: "effectiveness," "process," "structure," "communication," "participation," "satisfaction," "roles," "leadership," "outcomes," "climate," "voice"	English; Adulthood; Human; Original Journal Article	**a.** Not therapy groups **b.** Not computer-mediated communication **c.** Not educational groups (research on teaching group dynamics)	87
Colleague-recommended articles	N/A	N/A	20

& Leschine, 2004; Resnik, Zeldin, & Sharp, 2005; Russell, 2006) and on the importance of interdisciplinary collaborations and political analysis for CBPR policy success (Spielman et al., 2006). Of equal importance from the international development literature were the methodological and theoretical critiques of power issues in participatory processes. Among these issues are the challenge of governance and conflict of interest in interdisciplinary groups (Special section on urban planning & public health, 2006), the conflation of methods and politics by politically activist researchers (Danieli & Woodhams, 2005), and the obscuring of systematic oppression even in the arguments related to power dimensions in participation (Williams, 2004). These literatures supported CBPR processes of political education and analysis as necessary for both practice and research in public health.

The CBPR literature from American Indian and Alaska Native communities has helped to set the standard for community voice, ownership, and control, in opposition to the historical acculturative force of medicine and public health research (Smith-Morris, 2007; Manson, Garroutte, Goins, & Henderson, 2004). With sovereign nation status, Native communities involved in CBPR and tribal participatory research have pioneered the joint interpretation and application of research results and cultural revitalization (Fisher & Ball, 2002, 2003, 2005; see also Appendix H) and have stressed indigenous theories such as historical trauma, lateral oppression, and other tribally specific determinants of disease and wellness (DeJong & Holder, 2006; English, Fairbanks, et al., 2004; English, Wallerstein, et al, 2006; Jumper Thurman, Allen, & Deters, 2004; Strickland, 2006; Denzin, Lincoln, & Smith, 2008). Many tribal health workers have challenged the use of evidence-based practices and research, seeing it as a veiled attempt to repackage acculturative public health instead of promoting a partnership based on power sharing and collaborative knowledge creation.

Although CBPR researchers stress the importance of participation, very few have discussed how or why the group interaction plays out (two exceptions are Schulz et al., 2003; Israel, Lantz, McGranaghan, Kerr, & Guzman, 2005). In contrast, the Communication and Mass Media Complete and PsycInfo databases included research on the micro-processes, or the "black box," of group dynamics (Pelled, Eisenhardt, & Xin, 1999; Wheelan, 1999). This research addresses the individual, cultural, and structural factors that influence and shape group communication; the patterns of group dynamics over time; and the correlations of these patterns with positive and negative group outcomes (for example, productivity, quality decision making, and so forth). These micro-processes demonstrate why certain patterns might occur in CBPR partnerships and how to craft and sustain the most effective partnership.

In summary, our literature review gave depth and breadth to the previously identified barriers and promoters of CBPR practice and also provided new characteristics for the next stage of model development. For CBPR that has an emancipatory purpose of co-creating knowledge for democratizing society (see Chapter Two), these characteristics involved, most prominently, the role of context (historical, governance, and power differences) and its influence on group dynamics; cultural issues (that is, cultural humility, the ability to bridge across cultures in group settings, culturally centered interventions, and outcomes of cultural revitalization); and recognition of the importance of CBPR intermediate system and capacity change outcomes in producing health outcomes.

ASSESSING DIMENSIONS OF PARTICIPATION AND PARTNERSHIP

Internet Survey

As noted previously and as graphically illustrated later in Figure 21.1, we identified characteristics under each of four dimensions of CBPR that are critical to consider if communities and researchers are to achieve a greater understanding of the pathways by which CBPR may lead to outcomes. These characteristics range from historical trust or mistrust to evidence of shared power, and they operate on individual, partnership, and contextual levels (see Figure 21.1). Employing the list of characteristics, our evolving model, and iterative discussions and input from our national advisory committee, we developed an Internet survey instrument to begin to test the saliency of the identified characteristics. The goals of the survey were to elicit community member and researcher opinions about the *importance* of different contexts and participatory characteristics and practices for CBPR projects and to pilot-test questions on the relationship of these participatory processes to outcomes. We sent the survey by e-mail link to the twenty-five CBPR projects funded by the National Center on Minority Health and Health Disparities (NCMHD), to the thirteen Native American Research Centers for Health (NARCH) projects, to our advisory committee members, and to additional CBPR projects. The following lists provide an overview of some of the questions included in this survey. All questions had Likert scale response categories.

Internet Survey Questions About Contexts

How important is

- the issue of historical trust or mistrust between a community and the university's overall research efforts to the eventual success of the CBPR project?
- the level of community strengths or history of organizing?
- the level of the university's support and capacity to engage the community as partners?
- community concern about or perceived severity of the health problem as a stimulus to working together?
- cultural difference between the university and the community?
- openness and respect from the principal investigator or lead researcher?
- the actual distribution of resources?

Internet Survey Questions About Participation Issues Within Group Dynamics:

How important is

- diversity of the partnership to achieving overall CBPR and health outcomes?
- complexity of the partnership (number and kind of partners and issues)?
- formality (for example, memorandums of agreement [MOAs], written principles, or by-laws)?
- ability to bridge across cultural differences?

- ability to accept, manage, and maintain trust through conflicts?
- ability to negotiate and make decisions in a participatory manner?
- ability to communicate and complete tasks?
- ability in a partnership to have a sense of closeness or supportive relationships?

Although this was explicitly *not* a survey created to evaluate any individual partnership, we did ask about respondents' own experiences with their overall participation in CBPR projects. Questions were framed, for example, on how much "cross-cultural bridging by the university members" or "power-sharing" they thought had really been achieved in the partnerships they had worked with.

A final section of the survey adapted the RAND/UCLA appropriateness method[2] to two contexts (Shekelle, 2004; Shekelle & Schriger, 1996): (1) high and low trust between universities and communities and (2) high and low community capacity to organize. Questions in this section asked respondents to think about how each context might affect, first, their group dynamics and, second, their ability to have an impact on the internal outcome of a strengthened partnership or on external outcomes of improved CBPR capacities, policies, practices, and health status. The purpose of adapting this appropriateness method was to demonstrate whether there was a consensus about best practices in CBPR and whether each participatory practice was considered worthwhile or a waste of time. There has been an assumption in the field, for example, that certain group dynamic practices should be implemented, but before this survey, there has been no empirical evidence supporting this assumption.

Findings from the online survey of ninety-six respondents were generated (from sixteen NCMHD and seven NARCH projects) and used as discussion points for a meeting of our national advisory committee. In brief, the importance of *CBPR group dynamics* in creating effective CBPR processes leading to outcomes was ranked high, with little difference among racially and ethnically diverse respondents. Highest among these were the ability within the partnership to

- accept, manage, and maintain trust through conflicts;
- communicate and complete tasks;
- negotiate and make decisions in a participatory manner;
- bridge across cultural differences;
- manage, recognize, and share power and resources.

The *contexts* ranked highest for the success of the CBPR project were the importance or level of

- trust/mistrust between a community and the specific university research team;
- university support and capacity to engage the community as partners;
- openness and respect from the principal investigator;
- community concern or perceived severity about the health problem;
- historic trust/mistrust between a community and the university's overall research effort.

National Advisory Committee Consensus Process

As described earlier, a national advisory committee of CBPR experts has acted as participatory partners to provide consultation and direction throughout our research, offering feedback on the iterations of the list of characteristics and the evolving model, on the survey items, and on the committee members' own experiences in taking the pilot survey. In a face-to-face consensus meeting, committee members interpreted survey results, sharpened the model, and discussed implications for further research. There was much discussion of the adapted RAND appropriateness method section because of findings which suggested differences in community member and university staff responses to low trust and low community capacity conditions, versus similarities in responses in high trust or high capacity conditions. Although there were concerns about the validity of the findings from this adapted RAND appropriateness method section (because of the compressed and abstract language used), important discussion emerged on the salience of *context* for influencing outcomes based on potential pathways in the model. The discussion provoked us to grapple with the challenge of creating methodologies and instruments for assessing contextual differences, whether they are differences in socio-economic inequities, cultural or population context, level of university or community capacity to work in partnership, or the dynamic and nuanced issues of trust and mistrust between the community and the university or university team. In particular, this led us to the inadequacy of current measurement tools to assess contextual and partnership power inequities and to our next steps to develop methodologies and instruments that take into consideration the complex contexts of power and the comparability of these complicated contextual constructs cross-culturally.

Open-ended questions at the end of the survey revealed data that triangulated with the quantitative results. These data identified key barriers to success, such as time conflicts, lack of trust between partners, nonsustainable funding, power differences, and lack of communication. Key facilitators identified in the survey were successful communication, having a respected community member in the partnership, having a PI truly open to the CBPR process, and having long-standing partnerships characterized by commitment, trust, mutual understanding, and power sharing.

The consensus meeting helped generate a final model (discussed later). Additionally, the following CBPR research questions for future research were developed:

1. What is the variability of CBPR projects within different contexts and partnerships, and are there minimal standards for classifying projects as being truly inside or outside the universe of CBPR?

2. How do we better understand dynamic power relations between academic and community partners?

3. How do we better define best or promising practices within varying contexts of CBPR?

4. How can we best research the theoretical pathways between processes and outcome dimensions of the CBPR model?

FINAL MODEL AND RELATIONSHIPS BETWEEN DIMENSIONS

The final model is presented in Figure 21.1, with examples of the characteristics or variables in each dimension (for a detailed outline of characteristics, see our project Web site: http://mycbpr.org). This model identifies four dimensions of CBPR characteristics and suggests relationships between each category. First, *contextual factors* shape the nature of the research and the partnership and can determine whether and how a partnership is initiated. Next, *group dynamics,* consisting of three subdimensions (structural and individual dynamics that influence relational dynamics), interact with contextual factors to produce *the intervention and its research design.* Finally, *intermediate system and capacity changes, and ultimately, health outcomes* result directly from the intervention research. Although CBPR partnership processes and practices are presented linearly in this model, they are in reality dynamic and changing, with embedded paradoxes and tensions that are driven by both external and internal context changes (for example, loss of funding, new leadership, differences in partners' interpretations of events, and so forth). In the remainder of this chapter, we discuss the potential relationships among and within the four general dimensions represented in the model, constructs within each dimension, as well as testable hypotheses for research on CBPR processes leading to outcomes. We hope partnerships will use this model and possibly identify additional constructs meaningful for their situation. For more in-depth descriptions of currently identified constructs within the dimensions, see http://mycbpr.org.

Contexts

Five specific constructs are part of the context that frames any CBPR partnership. First, socio-economic, environmental, and cultural factors provide the backdrop to all of our work, with inequitable structural conditions being a primary risk factor for health disparities, and with cultural dimensions influencing both risk and protective factors. Second, *national and local policies and trends* relevant to CBPR shape its frequency and prestige. Despite increased funding for CBPR in recent years (see Appendix B), skepticism remains among many scientists, and there are far fewer avenues for funding CBPR than there are for traditional research approaches, such as clinical trials (Schulz et al., 2003; Buchanan et al., 2007; see also Chapter Fourteen). *Governance and leadership* are also policy contexts in that questions may be raised, for example, regarding whether CBPR projects in Indian country, grounded in sovereign nation status and formal tribal leadership approval (see Appendix H), would have impacts different from the impacts of other CBPR projects operating under multiple leadership models in more diffuse community settings.

Third, the *historical contexts of collaboration* influence how CBPR partnerships face and address issues of trust or mistrust over time. The multiple contextual challenges to building trust include (1) the congruence or lack of congruence over core values and mission, with communities traditionally focused on services and action and universities focused on new knowledge and scholarship; (2) historical, institutionalized racism in research, health care, and U.S. government–community relations, such that communities of color have less faith in health research than white Americans (Yonas et al., 2006; Aday, 2001; du Pré, 2000; Williams, 2001); and (3) the specific histories (both positive and negative) of university relationships with particular communities.

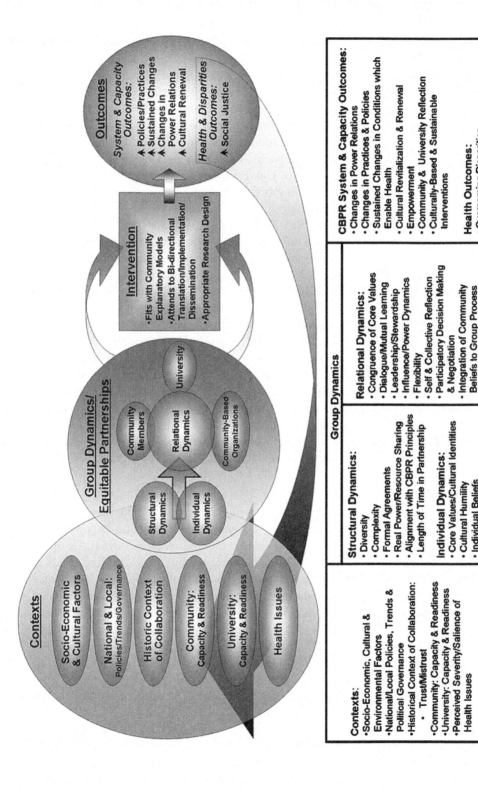

Contexts:
- Socio-Economic, Cultural & Environmental Factors
- National/Local Policies, Trends & Political Governance
- Historical Context of Collaboration:
  • Trust/Mistrust
- Community: Capacity & Readiness
- University: Capacity & Readiness
- Perceived Severity/Salience of Health Issues

Group Dynamics

Structural Dynamics:
- Diversity
- Complexity
- Formal Agreements
- Real Power/Resource Sharing
- Alignment with CBPR Principles
- Length of Time in Partnership

Individual Dynamics:
- Core Values/Cultural Identities
- Cultural Humility
- Individual Beliefs
- Community Reputation of PI

Relational Dynamics:
- Congruence of Core Values
- Dialogue/Mutual Learning
- Leadership/Stewardship
- Influence/Power Dynamics
- Flexibility
- Self & Collective Reflection
- Participatory Decision Making & Negotiation
- Integration of Community Beliefs to Group Process

CBPR System & Capacity Outcomes:
- Changes in Power Relations
- Changes in Practices & Policies
- Sustained Changes in Conditions which Enable Health
- Cultural Revitalization & Renewal
- Empowerment
- Community & University Reflection
- Culturally-Based & Sustainable Interventions

Health Outcomes:
- Overcoming Disparities

FIGURE 21.1 *Conceptual Logic Model of Community-Based Participatory Research: Processes to Outcomes*

The fourth contextual characteristic is the *community's capacity for research,* or more broadly, its *capacity to create change.* These capacities encompass the community's history of successful organizing, its ability to mobilize local cultural strengths and practices, its articulation of a shared identity and vision, and its organizational readiness to embrace changes. The capabilities for handling the time and commitment needed for a CBPR research process may be greater when the community has experience with organizing efforts, whether they were political, social, cultural, economic, or health related.

Fifth, much like the community's capacity, the *university's capacity for CBPR* is critical to the success of the partnership. University practices that promote CBPR— for example, supportive tenure and promotion guidelines or existing CBPR research centers—have been shown to foster greater university capacity (see Appendix E). Formal university agreements to share resources, knowledgeable institutional review boards, and university legal counsel who are supportive of CBPR approaches are essential to avoid undue bureaucracy and time delays. Finally, diversity of the research team matters. Even though historically CBPR researchers have been primarily white, ethnic or minority and bicultural academics are increasingly embracing CBPR research practice. Diverse research teams, built with research assistants and students who identify with the communities with which they are working, are critical for cultural understanding.

The sixth contextual factor that shapes the CBPR process is the *perceived severity and seriousness of the health issues.* Communities and researchers need to tap into health issues that are salient enough to mobilize involvement yet are not perceived as overwhelming. Community organizing and capacity-building strategies, including adequate incentives such as sharing grant funds with communities, also are important in enabling marginalized communities to participate in studying and addressing issues high on their list of concerns. Funding streams often dictate the health conditions to be studied, however, and therefore may limit the opportunity for true negotiation of the health issue of most concern.

Group Dynamics

The second overarching dimension is that of *group dynamics*, or *how* the practice of CBPR takes place with our core values of creating equitable partnerships. Group dynamics has three subdimensions: the *individual, structural,* and *relational* dynamics of the partnership. At the individual level, CBPR team members may have differing levels of motivation and belief about their own self-efficacy to do CBPR, and these levels may also change over time. The principal investigator is a critical team member, and his or her ability to work across cultures with flexibility and grace is critical for the project's success. This spanning ability is equally important for the community coinvestigator or key leaders. Cultural humility and critical self reflection, especially from high-status or otherwise privileged members of the respective teams (including a reflection on white privilege by white researchers) may be critical to high emotional and social capacity, trust, empathy, and a successful partnership (Yonas et al., 2006; Tervalon & Murray-Garcia, 1998; Goleman, 1995, 2006; see also Appendix I).

Structural dynamics refers to the nature of the team, its composition, extent of diversity, and level of complexity of membership or issues addressed and to the rules and resources used to guide the CBPR partnership. Diversity in values influences the way that individuals communicate in teams (Oetzel, 1998), and partnerships may face challenges because of cultural distance in values, ethnic or racial group identities, or even differences in profession and sector among partners (Oetzel, 2005). Higher complexity, such as that found with a health coalition that addresses many issues with multiple organizations as members, may also pose challenges not seen in a more limited partnership that addresses one set of issues, such as immunizations with providers as partners. Partnerships differ in their structural agreements, with tribal partners, for example, requiring formal tribal resolutions or memorandums of agreement whereas other partners may have more informal rules. Other factors, such as the closeness of alignment among partners' principles and expectations and the length of time the partnership has existed, may also influence the need for formal agreements.

Relational dynamics are the core interactive or communicative processes used to negotiate work, relationships, and identities during the partnership. Although group dynamics can be both problematic and positive (Hirokawa, 1988; Hirokawa & Keyton, 1995), effective CBPR dynamics might well include reflection on core values to enhance mutual respect and congruence, dialogue, and mutual learning; recognizing power dynamics; self- and collective reflection (especially about the group's process); participatory decision making; integrating local beliefs into the group's process; and the research team's involvement with the community, for example, holding meetings in community locations and participating in community social and cultural events.

Intervention

The third dimension of the model, the *intervention,* is both a result of the contextual factors and group dynamics and the major independent variable leading to outcomes. While this category focuses on interventions, it includes research designs that also are influenced by contextual factors and group dynamics. Often initiated by university partners who use the evidence-based literature, both CBPR interventions and the research designs used for implementation need to be shaped by the interaction with community partners in order to reflect local culture, community-supported practices, contexts, and program environments. Attention to implementation and translation issues in diverse contexts becomes especially important for sustainability as a system change outcome. The extent of organizational readiness to adopt new interventions, for example, can enhance the likelihood of sustainability of the intervention even after the grant funding ends. As seen in the AHRQ study, CBPR studies enhanced the implementation of the research (producing, for example, greater participation rates and decreased loss to follow-up) and also enhanced outcomes of capacity, without decreasing research rigor, as feared (Viswanathan et al., 2004). For CBPR projects not engaged in intervention research—namely, for epidemiologic or other descriptive studies—implementation and translation research knowledge is equally important for constructing appropriate research designs and collaborating with community members and leaders in research issues of recruitment, data collection, and participatory data analysis, among others.

Outcomes

The final category in the model focuses on *outcomes:* intermediate system and capacity change outcomes, and health outcomes. System and capacity outcomes focus on structural and relationship changes that promote greater equity in power dynamics. These include new institutional practices and policies in the university and community, new policies, new capacities such as community research infrastructures, and cultural revitalization (Wallerstein, Duran, Aguilar, Belone, Loretto, Padilla, et al., 2003; Appendix D). They also include enhanced empowerment for individuals, organizations, and communities and opportunities for sustained changes in conditions that enable health. Sustainability of interventions is key for communities and is more likely with the integration of local culture and attention to organizational readiness to adopt interventions. Although community capacity is mentioned frequently in published articles, equally important are *researcher capacity* in CBPR and supportive institutional practices within universities, factors that are seldom mentioned (Viswanathan et al., 2004).

Health outcomes and the reduction of health disparities toward social justice are the ultimate goals of research interventions designed through a CBPR partnership, though as shown through our literature review, evidence is still limited as to the impact of CBPR processes on health outcomes and disparities. Because of the wide variation in studies, Viswanathan et al. (2004) found insufficient evidence for CBPR effectiveness. Only twelve out of sixty studies had health outcome data: four randomized clinical trials had moderate effects, and the others had mixed or no effects. A recent comprehensive review article on participatory research cited seven other studies with health impacts, and there is a promise of more in the publishing pipeline due to the current infusion of CBPR intervention research dollars (Cargo & Mercer, 2008). Other recent case studies on CBPR efforts aimed in part at health-promoting public policy have demonstrated some success in terms of health outcomes, though in each case the CBPR effort was one among a number of associated factors (see Chapters Eighteen, Nineteen, and Twenty; Minkler et al., 2008; Minkler, Brechwich Vásquez, Chang, Blackwell, et al., 2008).

Relationships Among the Categories

Although the model presented here can serve as a framework for individual partnerships to evaluate selected characteristics and their own practices, its overall purpose is to strengthen the CBPR research agenda on pathways and on relationships that may link CBPR processes and practices to CBPR system and capacity changes and health outcomes. Presented here are potentially testable propositions derived from the model. Although not exhaustive, these propositions serve to illustrate potential starting points for further research.

Context and Group Dynamics   The first propositions consider the relationships between context and group dynamics. The six contextual constructs frame the nature of the interactions between CBPR team members. Although there are multiple bivariate relationships, we made an assumption that relational dynamics have a consistent relationship with the context factors (that is, all relational dynamics will be positive or negative). In fact, it is possible to have differing relational dynamics characteristics (for example, a group may be good with leadership but not necessarily good with dialogue), but the characteristics likely follow one another. The following propositions are offered as concrete testable hypotheses.

> *Proposition One.* Communities that have histories of being exploited and used by universities without attention to community engagement will have more relational dynamic difficulties within the partnership, even over the long term, than will communities that have histories of trust with researchers.

> *Proposition Two.* Formal governance structures in communities promote greater equality in group decision making with university partners early on in the partnership.

CBPR projects have the opportunity to benefit from a structural and environmental scan of these contextual issues, both in terms of assessing their potential influence on the partnership, and also because contexts can be influenced by the success (or failure) of CBPR processes.

Within Group Dynamics Given the primacy of group dynamics within CBPR, it is important to investigate the relationships among structural, individual, and relational dynamics. In fact, prior CBPR researchers have strongly emphasized investigating and evaluating group dynamics as a primary goal for CBPR projects (for example, Schulz et al., 2003).

> *Proposition Three.* The more culturally diverse the CBPR partnership, the more difficulty it will have with relational dynamics.

> *Proposition Four.* The more individuals demonstrate cultural humility or collectivistic identities, or both, the stronger relational dynamics will be.

These propositions are based in the literature on group dynamics from management, intercultural, and group communication; cross-cultural psychology; and social psychology. Although cultural diversity can provide important benefits in terms of insights and innovation, it also raises challenges (McLeod, Lobel, & Cox, 1996; Oetzel, 2005). A consistent finding about organizational processes is that the more cultural diversity there is, the more likely it is that high levels of tension, lack of respect for group members, and inequality in turn-taking will exist (Oetzel, Burtis, Chew Sanchez, & Perez, 2001; Watson, Kumar, & Michaelsen, 1993). Recognizing the potential for these tensions in culturally diverse groups, especially when there are power differences, therefore becomes an important starting place for generating best and promising practices to create positive relational and structural dynamics.

The cultural and individual identities that members bring to the partnership influence their communication styles and the overall climate of the interactions (Bond & Ng, 2004; Earley, 1993; Oetzel et al., 2001). Prior research demonstrates that individuals who bring a sense of collectivistic (as opposed to individualistic) identity and values and a willingness to reflect on their own culture and understand how it influences their behavior are more likely to engage in positive relational dynamics such as collaborative conflict resolution, shared decision making, and collective reflection (Oetzel, 1998; Oetzel et al., 2001; Yonas et al., 2006).

Context, Group Dynamics, and Outcomes Some of the more complex relationships in the model focus on the mediating and moderating role of group dynamics in the CBPR process.

Specifically, group dynamics are the medium through which contexts (for example, health problems and historical factors) are addressed and changed and result in concrete outcomes. Group dynamics can simply mediate or enable the work to be done but also can moderate or change the contexts to produce positive (or negative) outcomes. The potential negative outcome is important to consider, because poorly done CBPR (or research done under the guise of CBPR) can do more harm than good. One exemplar proposition is offered.

> *Proposition Five.* In CBPR partnerships that begin in a context of historical mistrust or low community capacity, increased use of formal structures for the partnership (for example, memorandums of agreement detailing the roles of partners), relate positively to relational dynamics and CBPR outcomes.

The fifth proposition recognizes the need to explore the relationship between structural and personal relationships. Contextual historical mistrust, based on egregious university or government action, is sufficiently prevalent in communities of color facing health disparities that strategies need to be supported to enable research partnerships to be successful. As indicated in the Internet survey, in low-trust conditions, community members may question the value of structural agreements, though for CBPR within tribes, official tribal approvals are mandated. The empirical questions remain, however: Do structural agreements facilitate the growth of trust through setting mutual expectations and guidelines for action, and how do these structural arrangements interact with the importance of personal relationships?

Group Dynamics, Intervention Research, and Outcomes The final complex relationship examines the last three characteristics of the CBPR model and places some emphasis on the mediating and moderating role of intervention and research methods in the CBPR process. The following propositions suggest some of the research possibilities related to these three factors.

> *Proposition Six.* The better group dynamics are, the greater the probability of CBPR system and capacity changes and improved health outcomes.
>
> *Proposition Seven.* The more a CBPR partnership can integrate local beliefs in the research, the more positive the CBPR system and capacity change outcomes will be.
>
> *Proposition Eight.* The better the CBPR system and capacity change outcomes, the better the health outcomes for the community.

These propositions are based on the experience of the research team (coauthors of this chapter) and the advisory board as well as prior research on CBPR interventions, especially in the literature on indigenous CBPR and CBPR with other communities of color. Enhanced use of culturally supported beliefs and practices (Hall, 2001) within relational dynamics that honor shared decision making and community power can create culturally acceptable interventions to address health problems and increase capacities in the community. The additional question is, What else is necessary to create system change within universities? Viswanathan et al.'s (2004) survey of sixty CBPR studies found that forty-seven studies reported strong community involvement, resulting in new community capacities, such as grant funding and job creation as well as better intervention quality. The last proposition is more speculative: it states that health outcomes are a direct result of CBPR system and capacity change outcomes, such as collaboratively produced and more sustainable interventions, transformed policies, and other practices, rather than a result of positive group dynamics per se. The specifics of the health impact, of course, depend on the specifics of the intervention or policy target. The health-enhancing factors of partnership participation may also have an impact on individuals. Yet to have an impact on community health, participation needs to be sustained through systems-level support and infrastructures in order to reach beyond the impact of a single CBPR project.

MEASUREMENT ISSUES

Measurement issues have, intentionally, not been considered in this chapter, although we are currently compiling a comprehensive list of measurement tools for dimensions and characteristics in the model. The majority of existing instruments focus on the group dynamics core of the model. However, study of the *contexts* underlying these dynamics, the relationship among structural conditions, institutional history, and personal participation, the individual characteristics of partners, and the unfolding power dynamics are not addressed by currently available tools. We suggest that measurement be directed toward these issues and toward each end of the model, for example, the contextual factors and system and capacity change outcomes. In particular, measurement efforts should focus on the ability of interventions to reach culturally and deeply into the communities served. Research would benefit from the development of vignette-based instruments that would make the contextual factors more concrete and potentially culturally-centered (King & Wand, 2007; Noe et al., 2007). The compiled list of existing tools and initial vignette-based questions that address contextual variables and others currently without measurement tools are both available on our Web site (http://mycbpr.org). We hope to use these instruments to create the next stage of cross-site research on CBPR projects, assessing variability in core participation dimensions and their relationships to outcomes in order to test the model.

SUMMARY AND IMPLICATIONS FOR FUTURE RESEARCH

The story of a baby hippo and a 130-year-old male tortoise living in an animal facility in Mombassa, Kenya, offers an allegory for the challenges and potentials of CBPR. Swept into the Indian Ocean during the 2004 tsunami, the baby hippo (an animal that typically stays with its mother for four years) latched onto the tortoise after its rescue. Since this time, they have become inseparable, sleeping, swimming, and eating together ("We can all learn from the animals," 2006). Like the hippo in this unexpected partnership, the lumbering and sometimes clumsy university can bond with communities—and the ancient and newer histories communities bring to the table—to find common ground.

In this study we have sought to find the common-ground characteristics of effective research partnerships that allow them to produce system and capacity change outcomes and improve well-being and health status within communities. We have garnered knowledge from our review of "outside" literature, from discussions with and experiences of working with our advisory board, and from the findings of an Internet-based survey in order to develop a new unifying, conceptual model that embodies the next stages for CBPR research. Our review uncovered challenges to this burgeoning research movement and suggested that constructive analysis of social and environmental contexts, political governance, historical institutional dynamics, and evolving power dynamics between partners and also self-reflection among members of research teams and partners should be included in the list of minimal core characteristics of CBPR, aimed at reducing health disparities.

The next steps are clearly indicated. Future research needs to assess variability in CBPR contexts and processes and to identify which processes and practices are most salient in which contexts, to test the various pathways of the model from processes to outcomes, and to develop a better understanding of best and promising practices for successful CBPR efforts. As community-based participatory research achieves greater acceptance within the research community, it becomes essential for the field to engage in the science of discovery and to learn how CBPR pathways work to promote new capacities, system changes, and health outcomes, both to generate stability for the field and to enhance our collective ability to have an impact on health status and health equity.

QUESTIONS FOR DISCUSSION

1. From the core dimensions of the CBPR model presented here (the contexts, group dynamic processes, and interventions), pick one or two and provide examples from your experience or reading of the literature about the ways in which each of the dimensions you picked might influence the ability of CBPR research projects to successfully affect outcomes. What are the core tensions within each dimension as described here or in your experience?

2. Why are power dimensions so central to CBPR processes, and how do you think they have an impact on CBPR system and capacity change outcomes and health outcomes?

3. Of the testable hypotheses discussed here, which two or three would you prioritize as the most important, and why? If you were to construct your own, what hypotheses or propositions would you propose as priorities for CBPR research?

NOTES

1. The national advisory committee members were Margarita Alegria, Beverly Becenti-Pigman, Eugenia Eng, Barbara Israel, Jeffrey Henderson, Michele Kelley, Loretta Jones, Paul Koegel, Marjorie Mau, Meredith Minkler, Lynn Palmanteer-Holder, Amy Schulz, Edison Trickett, Jesus Valles, Kenneth Wells, Earnestine Willis, and Kalvin White. New participating members include: Magdalena Avila, Elizabeth

Baker, Shelley Frazier, Ella Greene-Morton, Lyndon Haviland, Sarah Hicks, Laurie Lachance, Tassy Parker, Cynthia Pearson, Victoria Sanchez, and Lauro Silva.

2. The RAND/UCLA appropriateness method has typically been used to develop a consensus of expert opinion on the appropriateness of clinical procedures or other inputs that do not yet have proven effectiveness (in our case CBPR participatory processes and practices) for different patient conditions (in our case different contexts) in order to produce different outcomes (in our case capacity and system changes and public health outcomes).

REFERENCES

Aday, L. A. (2001). *At risk in America: The health and health care needs of vulnerable populations in the United States* (2nd ed.). San Francisco: Jossey-Bass.

Bond, M. H., & Ng, I. W.-C. (2004). The depth of a group's personality resources: Impacts on group process and group performance. *Asian Journal of Social Psychology, 7,* 285–300.

Buchanan, D. R., Miller, F. G., & Wallerstein, N. (2007). Ethical issues in community-based participatory research: Balancing rigorous research with community participation in community intervention studies. *Progress in Community Health Partnerships: Research, Education, and Action 1*(2), 153–160.

Bull, S. S., Gillette, C., Glasgow, R. E., & Estabrooks, P. (2003). Work site health promotion research: To what extent can we generalize the results and what is needed to translate research to practice? *Health Education & Behavior, 30*(5), 537–549.

Cargo, M., & Mercer, S. L. (2008). The value and challenges of participatory research: Strengthening its practice. *Annual Review of Public Health, 29,* 325–350.

Special section on urban planning and public health 2006. *Journal of the American Planning Association, 72*(1), 119–120.

Danieli, A., & Woodhams, C. (2005). Emancipatory research methodology and disability: A critique. *International Journal of Social Research Methodology, 8*(4), 281–296.

DeJong, J. A., & Holder, S. R. (2006). Indian boarding schools and the therapeutic residential model project. *American Indian and Alaska Native Mental Health Research, 13*(2), 1–16.

Denzin, N. K., Lincoln, Y. S., & Smith, L. T. (2008). *Handbook of critical and indigenous methodologies.* Thousand Oaks: Sage.

Drew, C. H., Nyerges, T. L., & Leschine, T. M. (2004). Promoting transparency of long-term environmental decisions: The Hanford decision mapping system pilot project. *Risk Analysis, 24*(6), 1641–1664.

du Pré, A. (2000). *Communicating about health: Current issues and perspectives.* Mountain View, CA: Mayfield.

Duran, B., & Walters, K. L. (2004). HIV/AIDS prevention in "Indian country": Current practice, indigenist etiology models, and postcolonial approaches to change. *AIDS Education and Prevention, 16*(3), 187–201.

Earley, P. C. (1993). East meets West meets Mideast: Further explorations of collectivistic and individualistic work groups. *Academy of Management Journal, 36,* 319–348.

English, K. C., Fairbanks, J., Finster, C. E., Rafelito, A., Luna, J., & Kennedy, M. (2006). A socioecological approach to improving mammography rates in a tribal community. *Health Education & Behavior, 35*(3), 396–409.

English, K. C., Wallerstein, N., Chino, M., Finster, C. E., Rafelito, A., Adeky, S., et al. (2004). Intermediate outcomes of a tribal community public health infrastructure assessment. *Ethnicity & Disease, 14*(3, Suppl. 1), S61–S69.

Fisher, P. A., & Ball, T. J. (2002). The Indian Family Wellness project: An application of the tribal participatory research model. *Prevention Science, 3*(3), 235–240.

Fisher, P. A., & Ball, T. J. (2003). Tribal participatory research: Mechanisms of a collaborative model. *American Journal of Community Psychology, 32*(3–4), 207–216.

Fisher, P. A., & Ball, T. J. (2005). Balancing empiricism and local cultural knowledge in the design of prevention research. *Journal of Urban Health, 82*(2, Suppl. 3), iii, 44–55.

Fixsen, D. L., Naoom, S. F., Blasé, K. A., Friedman, R. M., & Wallace, F. (2005). *Implementation research: A synthesis of the literature* (FMHI Pub. No. 231). Tampa: University of South-Florida, Louis de la Parte Florida Mental Health Institute, National Implementation Research Network.

Glasgow, R. E., & Emmons, K. M. (2007). How can we increase translation of research into practice? Types of evidence needed. *Annual Review of Public Health. 28,* 413–433.

Glasgow, R. E., Green, L. W., Klesges, L. M., Abrams, D. B., Fisher, E. B., Goldstein, M. G., et al. (2006). External validity: We need to do more. *Annals of Behavioral Medicine, 31,* 105–108.

Goleman, D. (1995). *Emotional intelligence.* NY: Bantam Books.

Goleman, D. (2006). *Social intelligence: The new science of human relations.* NY: Bantam Books.

Green, L. W., George, M. A., Daniel, M., Frankish, C. J., Herbert, C. J., Bowie, W. R., et al. (1995). *Study of participatory research in health promotion: Review and recommendations for the development of participatory research in health promotion in Canada.* Vancouver, BC: Royal Society of Canada.

Green, L. W., & Glasgow, R. E. (2006). Evaluating the relevance, generalization, and applicability of research: Issues in external validation and translation methodology. *Evaluation & the Health Professions, 29*(1), 126–153.

Green, L. W., & Ottoson, J. M. (2004). From efficacy to effectiveness to community and back: Evidence-based practice vs. practice-based evidence. In L. Green et al. (Eds.), *From clinical trials to community: The science of translating diabetes and obesity research.* Bethesda, MD: National Institutes of Health.

Greenhalgh, T., Robert, G., Macfarlane, F., Bate, P., & Kyriakidou, O. (2004), Diffusion of innovations in service organizations: Systematic review and recommendations. *Milbank Quarterly, 82*(4), 581–629.

Hall, G. (2001). Psychotherapy research with ethnic minorities: Empirical, ethical, and conceptual issues. *Journal of Consulting and Clinical Psychology, 69*(3), 502–510.

Hirokawa, R. Y. (1988). Group communication and decision-making performance: A continued test of the functional perspective. *Human Communication Research, 14,* 487–515.

Hirokawa, R. Y., & Keyton, J. (1995). Perceived facilitators and inhibitors of effectiveness in organizational work teams. *Management Communication Quarterly, 8,* 424–446.

Hohmann, A., & Shear, M. (2002). Community-based intervention research: Coping with the noise of real life in study design. *American Journal of Psychiatry, 159,* 201–207.

Israel, B. A., Eng, E., Schulz, A. J., & Parker, E. A. (Eds.). (2005). *Methods in community-based participatory research for health.* San Francisco: Jossey-Bass.

Israel, B. A., Lantz, P. M., McGranaghan, R. J., Kerr, D. L., & Guzman, J. R. (2005). Documentation and evaluation of CBPR partnerships: In-depth interviews and close-ended questions. In B. A. Israel, E. Eng, A. J. Schulz, & E. A. Parker (Eds.), *Methods in community-based participatory research for health* (pp. pp. 255–278). San Francisco: Jossey-Bass.

Johnson, D. W., & Johnson, F. P. (1999). *Joining together: Group theory and group skills* (7th ed.). Englewood Cliffs, NJ: Prentice Hall.

Jumper Thurman, P., Allen, J., & Deters, P. B. (2004). The Circles of Care evaluation: Doing participatory evaluation with American Indian and Alaska Native communities. *American Indian and Alaska Native Mental Health Research, 11*(2), 139–154.

King, G., & Wand, J. (2007). Comparing incomparable survey responses: Evaluating and selecting anchoring vignettes. *Political Analysis, 15,* 46–66.

Manson, S. M., Garroutte, E., Goins, R. T., & Henderson, P. N. (2004). Access, relevance, and control in the research process: Lessons from Indian country. *Journal of Aging and Health, 16*(5, Suppl.), 58S–77S.

McLeod, P. L., Lobel, S. A., & Cox, T. H. (1996). Ethnic diversity and creativity in small groups. *Small Group Research, 27,* 248–264.

Miller, R. L., & Shinn, M. (2005). Learning from communities: Overcoming difficulties in dissemination of prevention and promotion efforts. *American Journal of Community Psychology, 35*(3–4), 169–183.

Minkler, M., Breckwich Vásquez, V., Chang, C., Blackwell, A. G., Thompson, M., & Rubin, V. (in press). *Promoting healthy public policy through community-based participatory research.* Oakland, CA: PolicyLink.

Minkler, M., Breckwich Vásquez, V., Tajik, M., & Petersen, D. (2008). Promoting environmental justice through community-based participatory research: The role of community and partnership capacity. *Health Education & Behavior, 35*(1), 119–137.

Minkler, M., & Wallerstein, N. (Eds.). (2003). *Community-based participatory research for health.* San Francisco: Jossey Bass.

National Institutes of Health, Office of Portfolio Analysis and Strategic Initiatives. (2008). NIH Roadmap for Medical Research. Retrieved May 12, 2008, from nihroadmap.nih.gov.

Noe, T., Manson, S., Croy, C., McGough, H., Henderson, J., & Buchwald, D. (2007). The influence of community-based participatory research principles on the likelihood of participation in health research in American Indian communities. *Ethnicity & Disease, 17*(Suppl. 1), S6–S14.

Oetzel, J. G. (1998). Explaining individual communication processes in homogeneous and heterogeneous groups through individualism-collectivism and self-construal. *Human Communication Research, 25,* 202–224.

Oetzel, J. G. (2005). Intercultural work group communication theory. In W. B. Gudykunst (Ed.), *Theorizing about intercultural communication* (pp. 351–371). Thousand Oaks, CA: Sage.

Oetzel, J. G., Burtis, T. E., Chew Sanchez, M. I., & Perez, F. G. (2001). Investigating the role of communication in culturally diverse work groups: A review and synthesis. In W. B. Gudykunst (Ed.), *Communication Yearbook 25* (pp. 237–269). Mahwah, NJ: Erlbaum.

Pelled, L. H., Eisenhardt, K. M., & Xin, K. R. (1999). Exploring the black box: An analysis of work group diversity, conflict, and performance. *Administrative Science Quarterly, 44,* 1–28.

Persaud, N., & Mamdani, M. (2006). External validity: The neglected dimension in evidence ranking. *Journal of Evaluation in Clinical Practice, 12*(4), 450–453.

Resnik, D. B., Zeldin, D. C., & Sharp, R. R. (2005). Research on environmental health interventions: Ethical problems and solutions. *Accountability in Research: Policies & Quality Assurance, 12*(2), 69–102.

Russell, C. A. (2006). Consumer researchers for public health: Insights from three government-funded programs. *Advances in Consumer Research, 33*(1), 59–62.

Schulz, A. J., Israel, B. A., & Lantz, P. M. (2003). Instrument for evaluating dimensions of group dynamics within community-based participatory research partnerships. *Evaluation and Program Planning, 26,* 249–262.

Shekelle, P. (2004). The appropriateness method [Editorial]. *Medical Decision Making, 24*(2), 228–231.

Shekelle, P., & Schriger, D. L. (1996). Evaluating the use of the appropriateness method in the Agency for Health Care Policy and Research clinical practice guidelines development process. *Health Services Research, 31*(4), 453–468.

Smith, L. T. (1999). *Decolonizing methodologies: Research and indigenous peoples.* New York: Zed Books.

Smith-Morris, C. (2007). Autonomous individuals or self-determined communities? The changing ethics of research among Native Americans. *Human Organization, 66*(3), 327–337.

Sofaer, S. (2000). *Working together, moving ahead: A manual to support effective community health coalitions.* City University of New York, Baruch College, School of Public Affairs.

Spielman, S. E., Golembeski, C. A., Northridge, M. E., Vaughan, R. D., Swaner, R., Jean-Louis, B., et al. (2006). Interdisciplinary planning for healthier communities. *Journal of the American Planning Association, 72*(1), 100–108.

Strickland, C. J. (2006). Challenges in community-based participatory research implementation: Experiences in cancer prevention with Pacific Northwest American Indian tribes. *Cancer Control, 13*(3), 230–236.

Tervalon, M., & Murray-Garcia, J. (1998). Cultural humility versus cultural competence: A critical distinction in defining physician training outcomes in multicultural education. *Journal of Health Care for the Poor and Underserved, 9*(2), 117–125.

Viswanathan, M., Ammerman, A., Eng, E., Gartlehner, G., Lohr, K. N., Griffith, D., et al. (2004). *Community-based participatory research: Assessing the evidence* (Evidence Report/Technology Assessment No. 99; prepared by RTI, University of North Carolina). Rockville, MD: Agency for Healthcare Research and Quality.

Wallerstein, N. (2007). Making traces: Evidence for practice and evaluation. In J. Green & R. Labonté (Eds.), *Critical perspectives in public health* (pp. 80–92). New York: Routledge.

Wallerstein, N., & Duran, B. (2006). Using community-based participatory research to address health disparities. *Health Promotion Practice, 7*(3), 312–323.

Wallerstein, N., Duran, B., Aguilar, J., Belone, J. L., Loretto, F., Padilla, R., Shendo, K., Toya, A., & Yepa-Waquie, H. (2003). Jemez Pueblo: Built and social-cultural environments and health within a rural American Indian community in the Southwest. *American Journal of Public Health, 93*(9), 1517–1518.

Wallerstein, N., Duran, B., Minkler, M., & Foley, K. (2005). Developing and maintaining partnerships with communities. In B. A. Israel, E. Eng, A. J. Schulz, & E. A. Parker (Eds.), *Methods in community-based participatory research for health* (pp. 31–51). San Francisco: Jossey-Bass.

Watson, W. E., Kumar, K., & Michaelsen, L. K. (1993). Cultural diversity's impact on interaction process and performance: Comparing homogeneous and diverse task groups. *Academy of Management Journal, 36,* 590–602.

"We can all learn from the animals." (2006). Retrieved May 12, 2008, from www.criticalconcern.com/hiipo-and-turtle.htm.

Wheelan, S. (1999). *Creating effective teams: A guide for members and leaders.* Thousand Oaks, CA: Sage.

Williams, D. R. (2001). Race and health: Trends and policy implications. In. J. A. Auerbach & B. K. Krimgold (Eds.), *Income, socioeconomic status, and health: Exploring the relationships* (pp. 67–85). Washington, DC: National Policy Association.

Williams, G. (2004). Evaluating participatory development: Tyranny, power and (re)politicisation. *Third World Quarterly, 25*(3), 557–578.

Yonas, M. A., Jones, N., Eng, E., Vines, A. I., Aronson, R., Griffith, D. M., et al. (2006). The art and science of integrating undoing racism with CBPR: Challenges of pursuing NIH funding to investigate cancer care and racial equity. *Journal of Urban Health, 83*(6), 1004–1012.

APPENDIXES

APPENDIX

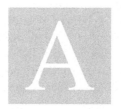

A PROTOCOL FOR COMMUNITY-BASED RESEARCH

LELAND BROWN & WILLIAM A. VEGA

This protocol is a starting point for a wider dialogue around the nature of academic research—specifically, whom it serves, whom it benefits, and who reports it. In essence, the question is, How relevant is academic research to the specific health needs of our community?

The protocol was developed in 1994 by a committee of the Oakland Community-Based Public Health Initiative (CBPHI), a collaboration among community-based organizations, the University of California, Berkeley School of Public Health, and the Alameda County Department of Public Health. The CBPHI in turn was part of the nation-wide W. K. Kellogg Foundation–funded Community-Based Public Health Initiative (CBPHI) designed to promote long-term change in institutions of public health research and public health practice. As Thomas Bruce (1995, p. 11), formerly of the W. K. Kellogg Foundation, has pointed out, "If an informed and involved community works in active

Note: Adapted from "A Protocol for Community Based Research," by L. Brown and W. A. Vega, 1996. *American Journal of Preventive* Medicine, *12*(4), pp. 4–5. Copyright 1996 by American Journal of Preventive Medicine. Adapted with permission of Elsevier Science.

collaboration with a responsive and knowledgeable health agency, enormous progress can be made against many resistant health problems." The aim of this protocol was to establish ground rules about the ways in which research institutions and communities in Oakland might best work together. Of special concern was moving from models focusing on community deficits and professional-client relationships to models that empower communities by building on local assets and professional-community partnerships (Kretzmann & McKnight, 1993). The CBPHI community-based research protocol reinforces the type of dialogue that must occur between communities and research institutions in order for legitimate community-based solutions to local public health problems to emerge. The protocol ensures that rigorous, academically sound community-based research can and should involve communities at every step.

The protocol was developed as a series of questions around which the community-researcher dialogue can take place. It is by no means exhaustive. The questions can be viewed from at least two perspectives: (1) questions that communities should ask every researcher and (2) questions every researcher should ask himself or herself.

1.   How will research processes and outcomes serve the community?

      Will community people be hired?

      Will community people be trained?

      Will the research build on community assets and enhance them?

      Will there be continuity over time?

2.   How will the community be involved in defining the objectives of the research?

3.   Are researchers committed to doing the follow-up necessary to implement larger applications?

4.   How will the community be involved in the analysis of the data?

      What are the hypotheses?

      What are the biases?

5.   What perceptions about the community are likely to be created or persist as a result of analysis and publication of the results? Will the spirit of confidentiality be violated as a result of making public the research findings?

6.   How, when, and by whom should findings be released?

7.   What is the focus of the research vis-à-vis addressing long-term community needs?

8.   Are the research methods sufficiently rigorous yet true to community-based principles that incorporate perspectives and beliefs of community residents?

Perhaps one of the most germane and elusive questions for university-based researchers is who really represents their partner community. This question is not static, as time and circumstances create new landscapes and landscape architects within the community. It is sometimes impossible to know who can represent the true spirit of the community. Nevertheless, the questions on our list cannot be answered without the benefit of community participation involving those who will be the subjects of research and the potential beneficiaries of that research. If answers to the questions can be mutually agreed on, the results and the effects of collaborative research will be worth far more than time and money invested in the conduct of this research. This should be a lesson for federal, state, and private funding sources as well. Such research takes time, enormous goodwill, and infinite patience.

REFERENCES

Bruce, T. A. (1995). Community health science: A discipline whose time has already come; Research linkages between academia and public health practice. *American Journal of Preventive Medicine, 11*(Suppl.), 1–7.

Kretzman, J. P., & McKnight, J. L. (1993). *Building communities from the inside out: A path toward finding and mobilizing a community's assets.* Evanston, IL: Northwestern University, Center for Urban Affairs and Policy Research.

APPENDIX

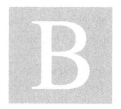

FEDERAL FUNDING AND SUPPORT FOR PARTICIPATORY RESEARCH IN PUBLIC HEALTH AND HEALTH CARE

SHAWNA L. MERCER & LAWRENCE W. GREEN

Much has been made of the need for people's participation in public health and health education. Health promotion has emerged as a field spanning health education and other aspects of public health and social policy development, with participation—expressed as enabling people to control the determinants of their health—written into the very definition of this emerging field (World Health Organization, 1986).

Note: The findings and conclusions in this appendix are those of the authors and do not necessarily represent the views of the Centers for Disease Control and Prevention.

At first, the emphasis on participation in the health field was directed toward people's participation in the adoption or endorsement of scientifically validated programs or services delivered by experts to their localities. Later, the emphasis shifted to the need for people's cooperation in the implementation of such programs; later still, it focused on participation in advocating and planning programs and policies; and most recently, it has sought participation in translating research to local circumstances and in the research itself. These gradual shifts from downstream to upstream involvement of people in the continuum from research to policy and practice have resulted from various converging strands of theory, practice, politics, and policy (Green, 1986). Many of these strands are reflected in the chapters of this volume. Appendix B of the first edition of this book discussed how these strands influenced federal interest in public participation in health research over the course of the twentieth century and how they led to the recent increases in federal funding for participatory research (Minkler & Wallerstein, 2003). The purpose of the present appendix is to represent and reflect on recent and current U.S. federal support for participatory research (PR).

RECENT EFFORTS OF FEDERAL HEALTH AGENCIES

In the 1980s, research and evaluation funding programs that were at least partially aligned with the ideals of PR were introduced by the Health Resources and Services Administration (HRSA), the Indian Health Service (IHS), the Substance Abuse and Mental Health Services Administration (SAMHSA), and the Centers for Disease Control and Prevention (CDC). Some of these programs aligned themselves more closely with PR in the 1990s and were joined by new National Institutes of Health (NIH) and CDC funding streams expressly dedicated to PR or requiring grantees to incorporate a PR component. More recent years have seen a mixture of research funding dedicated specifically to community-based participatory research (CBPR), funding for PR more broadly (for a discussion of CBPR as a type of PR, see Cargo & Mercer, 2008; Green et al., 1995), and funding calls open to receiving PR applications among others. Determining whether the total amount of federal funding available for PR is increasing is complicated by fluctuations in the amount of federal funding available for all research and also by changes in the openness of non-PR funding calls to PR approaches. Given recent reductions in overall federal research funding, the number of funding calls specific to or accepting of PR is particularly noteworthy.

Early Efforts

HRSA and the IHS pursued a model of *community-oriented primary care* in the 1980s that had many of the markings of CBPR. Staff of migrant health centers, community health centers, and Indian Health facilities were trained to engage the community collaboratively in conducting community assessments of the population served by the practice (Nutting, 1987). The growing insistence by Congress and federal agencies in the 1980s on accountability by state and local grantees for their expenditure of federal funds required partnered evaluation between the agencies receiving federal funds and the local stakeholders. This was reflected in partnerships funded by SAMHSA and the CDC. The Anti-Drug Abuse Act of 1988 authorized SAMHSA's Community Partnership Demonstration Grant Program, whose initial 251 grantees were required to plan and conduct process and outcome evaluations of their projects using local evaluators. Systematic efforts to study these and other local evaluation partnerships led to the formulation of the PR approach known as *empowerment evaluation* (Dugan, 1996; Fetterman, 1994; Yin, Kaftarian, & Jacobs, 1996).

CDC-Based Efforts

At the CDC, a long tradition of "bootstrap epidemiology" and strong ties to state and local health departments have provided a sympathetic environment for promoting participatory concepts in the development and fielding of surveillance systems, planning, training, evaluation, and research. The university-based Centers for Health Promotion and Disease Prevention Research (also known as Prevention Research Centers, or PRCs), funded through the CDC by Congress in 1984, have had a clear mandate for greater collaboration between academic researchers and state or community public health practitioners and citizen groups (CDC, 2006). Three centers were funded in 1986, and the thirty-three currently funded PRCs—housed in schools of public health or medicine—compete for approximately $40 million per year by submitting proposals for peer-reviewed cooperative agreements. The PRCs represent a nationwide network of academic, public health, and community partners linking science and practice.

A committee of the Institute of Medicine (IOM), National Academy of Sciences, commissioned by the CDC to assess the PRCs in the mid-1990s, concluded that they needed to "adopt a community-based approach to their research and demonstration efforts" (Stoto, Green, & Bailey, 1997). Responding to the IOM recommendation, the CDC placed considerably more emphasis on building collaborative community partnerships through the PRCs (Green, 2007). Since 1998, community-based advisory boards have been required for all PRCs, representing community members, volunteers, health and education professionals, and representatives of local and state service organizations. The current policy statement for core research projects of the PRCs states that they "conduct participatory, community-based research" and that the researchers and community advisory groups "design, test and disseminate effective strategies to improve community and personal health" (CDC, 2006). The PRC national program evaluation is assessing how CBPR is implemented across the PRCs (Faridi, Grunbaum, Gray, Franks, & Simoes, 2007).

In 1994, the Epidemiology Program Office (EPO) at the CDC solicited applications for Urban Research Centers (URCs) in public health that would place emphasis on PR (Metzler et al., 2003). Three URCs were funded in 1995, as extensions of the PRC program, with a mandate to establish community partnerships to govern the selection and execution of research projects and participate in all phases of the research. The three URCs leveraged core federal funds of $705,000 to $1.6 million per year, and received additional grants of $26 million from other federal agencies and philanthropic foundations. Several URCs forged new infrastructures and have competed successfully for federal PR funding after the end of their initial round of CDC funding.

Even though not specifically required to use PR approaches, about one-third of the projects funded in the first round of the Extramural Prevention Research Program (EPRP;

known then as the Prevention Research Initiative) in 1999 involved participatory research. In 2002, the CDC's Public Health Practice Program Office (PHPPO) announced $12 million in funding through the EPRP for twenty-five investigator-initiated, peer-reviewed grants (with a twenty-sixth grant added in 2003) of approximately $450,000 each per year for three years for community-based participatory prevention research. This grant program solicited multidisciplinary, multilevel (including community residents and groups, practitioners, and policymakers) PR aimed at enhancing the capacity of communities and population groups to address health promotion and the prevention of disease, disability, and injury (CDC, 2002; Green & Mercer, 2001).

NIH-Based Efforts

In 1995, the National Institute of Environmental Health Sciences (NIEHS) became the first of the National Institutes of Health to support CBPR (by that name) when it funded fifteen CBPR projects at about $6.1 million per year (NIH, NIEHS, 2007; O'Fallon, Tyson, & Dearry, 2000). Among the NIH Institutes, NIEHS had been under the greatest pressure to undertake PR, owing to public skepticism about the reliability of environmental research—a skepticism brought on by Love Canal and other pollution disasters in which residents perceived government scientists as protecting industry or failing to represent community knowledge, concerns, and perspectives in their environmental research.

From 2002 through 2005, NIEHS sponsored a federal Interagency Working Group (IWG) on CBPR (NIH, Office of Extramural Research, 2007), with active ongoing participation from eleven federal agencies. The purpose of this IWG was to strengthen communication among federal agencies with an interest in supporting CBPR methodologies in the conduct of biomedical research, education, health care delivery, or policy. One of the IWG's most important products was the development and release in December 2004 of a funding announcement titled "Community Participation in Research," cosponsored by the NIH, AHRQ (Agency for Healthcare Research and Quality), and CDC. The goal was to support research on health promotion, disease prevention, and health disparities that was jointly conducted by communities and researchers. The funding announcement was active until January 2008 and was then replaced with two announcements calling for "community participation in research targeting the medically underserved" and sponsored by NIH, and one "community participation in research" announcement cosponsored by NIH and CDC. Although the only CDC entity initially identified on the latter announcement is the National Institute for Occupational Safety and Health (NIOSH), the inclusion of NIOSH enables other parts of the CDC to consider cosponsorship in future years when funding becomes available.

In the years between the 2004 release of the initial funding announcement and its replacements in 2008, a number of individual NIH institutes have also provided funding for PR. Of particular note is CBPR-specific funding awarded by the National Institute of Nursing Research, National Center on Minority Health and Health Disparities, National Institute of Mental Health, and National Cancer Institute. An extensive list of NIH and other federal (and nonfederal) funding sources for CBPR was developed by Community-Campus Partnerships for Health in association with the Northwest Health Foundation

(Seifer, Kauper-Brown, & Robbins, 2004). Although some of the funding calls are now obsolete and other calls have arisen since its publication, the directory includes valuable Web sites, reports, and other resources that researchers can access to learn about funding priorities and identify ongoing and future research calls.

Another recent NIH initiative with implications for increasing PR funding is the Clinical and Translational Science Awards program (CTSA). The first twelve awards were offered in 2006, twelve more were added in 2007, and a total of sixty will be offered when the program is fully implemented in 2012. The CTSA aims to transform "how clinical and translational work is conducted at academic health centers across the country" and "will enable researchers to provide new treatments more efficiently and quickly to patients" (NIH, National Center for Research Resources, 2007). One of the key components of CTSA is community engagement, with the intent to "foster collaborative partnerships and enhance public trust in clinical and translational research" with approaches engaging "both the public and community providers" (NIH, National Center for Research Resources, 2007).

AHRQ-Based Efforts

The AHRQ has funded a systematic review of the effectiveness of CBPR, as part of its influential series of evidence reports (Viswanathan et al., 2004). The AHRQ also provides support for primary care practice-based research networks (PBRNs) to undertake research on questions encountered by primary care clinicians in their practices "in community settings" and to "produce scientific information that is externally valid, and, in theory, assimilated more easily into everyday practice" (AHRQ, 2006). A number of PBRNs engage clinicians, their patients, and academic researchers in research. A recent article suggests that several PBRNs have active involvement by community members in generating research ideas, reviewing research protocols, interpreting results, and disseminating findings (Westfall, VanVorst, Main, & Herbert, 2006).

Other Recent Federal Initiatives

The NIH has established a CBPR Scientific Interest Group to build on the earlier work of the IWG on CBPR by strengthening communication among federal agencies with an interest in supporting CBPR (NIH, Office of Extramural Research, 2007). Federal agencies have also funded special issues dedicated to PR in important journals such as the *Journal of General Internal Medicine* (with an AHRQ-funded special issue in 2003), and the *American Journal of Preventive Medicine* (with a special issue about the CDC's PRC program in 2007). PR conferences for federal staff, researchers, and nonacademic partners have been sponsored by the NIH (NIEHS in 2000), AHRQ in 2001, CDC (PRC program in 2006), and others.

The CDC's Racial and Ethnic Approaches to Community Health (REACH) program uses participatory approaches in establishing and evaluating community-based programs and culturally appropriate interventions to eliminate health disparities (CDC, 2007). The Office of the Director of both the NIH and CDC have sponsored large meetings exploring community engagement. Additionally, several parts of the CDC have issued recommendations for increased federal support for PR (for example, CDC,

Agency for Toxic Substances and Disease Registry, 2006; Navarro, Voetsch, Liburd, Giles, & Collins, 2007). Finally, the Guide to Community Preventive Services (Community Guide) is using PR approaches to reinvigorate and extend its network of official liaisons and partners—to ensure that research questions; data collection, analysis, and interpretation; and dissemination reflect the needs of practitioners, policymakers, and communities, and that the Task Force on Community Preventive Services receives broad input from intended users when formulating its recommendations for policy, practice, and research.

FEDERAL QUANDARIES IN FURTHERING PARTICIPATORY RESEARCH

The first and most paradoxical of the issues confronting federal agencies in trying to support CBPR is the apparent contradiction of a centralized agency of government controlling the funds and selection of applicants for grants to support local initiative, autonomy, self-determination, and self-sufficiency. Federal agencies struggle to find the optimal level of restraint of their own hegemony and that of research scientists in their collaborations with health professionals and with nonscientifically trained policymakers, local lay residents, and citizens (for example, Mercer, MacDonald, & Green, 2004).

A related problem is that most of the federal funds for research are allotted to congressionally restricted vertical silos as categorical disease earmarks or line items in agency budgets. The principle of local autonomy in selecting local needs to define research priorities may seem somewhat hollow if the research funds can be used only in relation to specific diseases, age groups, risk factors, or other categories. Some relief has been provided by nondedicated funding available through the CDC's URC and EPRP programs, the NIH's CTSA, and AHRQ's PBRNs.

A third issue on which federal agencies and many PR scholars and practitioners may disagree is how much involvement of the non-scientifically trained collaborators is needed in each research phase and type of research (Cargo & Mercer, 2008). Although equal, or at least equitable, participation of researchers and community participants in every phase of the research process may be the ideal for many PR approaches, recent reviews found that only four of sixty CBPR studies and no PBRNs demonstrated full participation by communities (for CBPR) or patients (for PBRNs) (Viswanathan et al., 2004; Westfall et al., 2006). Federal expectations of participation by all partners in all phases may therefore often be unrealistic. There is broad agreement that maximal involvement of both parties in the first and last stages—in specifying the research questions or otherwise contributing to the study direction and in interpreting and applying the findings—is key to ensuring that community interests are being represented in the research, its publication, and its use. However, community partners are usually volunteers in the research partnership, so their devotion of time and effort to the technical phases of design and data collection could become exploitive, particularly if their preference is not to participate (Green & Mercer, 2001). Although nonacademic partners should at least be given the opportunity to participate in all phases, the involvement of academic and nonacademic partners in these technical research phases may therefore depend on: their interests, expertise, and time; what is negotiated; and how much support is available for participation by the various partners (Cargo & Mercer, 2008). Additional consideration of trade-offs, advantages, and disadvantages of involvement in different stages and across study types requires further study.

Finally, the logic and apparent advantages to a better fit between research and local or practitioner needs makes a strong but not compelling case for PR. The only systematic review of PR approaches in intervention research concluded that there was insufficient evidence in 2004 to determine its effectiveness in leading to better health outcomes (Viswanathan et al., 2004). Federal needs for accountability—for evidence that PR projects are progressing adequately toward health outcomes—will continue to grow, requiring more definitive evidence of effectiveness, greater conceptual clarity, and more consistent measurement of core PR elements such as capacity building, empowerment, ownership, and sustainability (Cargo & Mercer, 2008). Encouragingly, studies published since the AHRQ review and new publications expected from the recent federal PR funding calls described earlier will likely add to the growing evidence base.

REFERENCES

Agency for Healthcare Research and Quality. (2006). AHRQ support for primary care practice-based research networks (PBRNs). Retrieved Feb. 3, 2008, from http://www.ahrq.gov/research/pbrn/pbrnfact.htm.

Cargo, M., & Mercer, S. L. (2008). The value and challenges of participatory research: Strengthening its practice. *Annual Review of Public Health, 29,* 325–350.

Centers for Disease Control and Prevention. (2002). *Science Coordination & Innovation: Community-based participatory prevention research grants.* Retrieved Feb. 3, 2008, from http://www.cdc.gov/od/science/PHResearch/grants/community/index.htm.

Centers for Disease Control and Prevention. (2006). *Prevention Research Centers: Policy statement for core research projects.* Retrieved Feb. 3, 2008, from http://www.cdc.gov/prc/about-prc-program/program-policy.htm.

Centers for Disease Control and Prevention. (2007). *Racial and ethnic approaches to community health: REACH U.S.* Retrieved Feb. 3, 2008, from http://www.cdc.gov/reach/index.htm.

Centers for Disease Control and Prevention, Agency for Toxic Substances and Disease Registry. (2006). *Advancing the nation's health: A guide to public health research needs, 2006–2015.* Retrieved Feb. 5, 2008, from http://www.cdc.gov/od/science/PHResearch/cdcra/Guide_to_Public_Health_Research_Needs.pdf.

Dugan, M. A. (1996). Participatory and empowerment evaluation: Lessons learned in training and technical assistance. In D. M. Fetterman, S. J. Kaftarian, & A. Wandersman (Eds.), *Empowerment evaluation: Knowledge and tools for self-assessment and accountability* (pp. 277–303). Thousand Oaks, CA: Sage.

Faridi, Z., Grunbaum, J. A., Gray, B. S., Franks, A., & Simoes, E. (2007). Community-based participatory research: Necessary next steps. *Preventing Chronic Disease, 4,* A70.

Fetterman, D. M. (1994). Empowerment evaluation. *Evaluation Practice, 15,* 1–15.

Green, L. W. (1986). The theory of participation: A qualitative analysis of its expression in national and international health policies. In W. B. Ward (Ed.), *Advances in health education and promotion* (Vol. 1, Part A, pp. 211–236). Greenwich, CT: JAI Press.

Green, L. W. (2007). The prevention research centers as models of practice-based evidence: Two decades on. *American Journal of Preventive Medicine, 33*(1, Suppl.), S6–S8.

Green, L. W., George, M. A., Daniel, M., Frankish, C. J., Herbert, C. P., Bowie, W. R., et al. (1995). *Study of participatory research in health promotion: Review and recommendations for the development of participatory research in health promotion in Canada.* Vancouver, BC: Royal Society of Canada.

Green, L. W., & Mercer, S. L. (2001). Can public health researchers and agencies reconcile the push from funding bodies and the pull from communities? *American Journal of Public Health, 91*, 1926–1929.

Mercer, S. L., MacDonald, G., & Green, L. W. (2004). Participatory research and evaluation: From best practices for all states to achievable practices within each state in the context of the Master Settlement Agreement. *Health Promotion Practice, 5*(3, Suppl.), 167S–178S.

Metzler, M. M., Higgins, D. L., Beeker, C. G., Freudenberg, N., Lantz, P. M., Senturia, K. D., et al. (2003). Addressing urban health in Detroit, New York City, and Seattle through community-based participatory research partnerships. *American Journal of Public Health, 93*, 803–811.

Minkler, M., & Wallerstein, N. (Eds.). (2003). *Community-based participatory research for health.* San Francisco: Jossey-Bass.

National Institutes of Health, National Center for Research Resources. (2007). *Clinical and translational science awards.* Retrieved Feb. 3, 2008, from http://www.ctsaweb.org/Docs/CTSA_FactSheet.pdf.

National Institutes of Health, National Institute of Environmental Health Sciences. (2007). *Environmental justice & community-based participatory research.* Retrieved Feb. 3, 2008, from http://www.niehs.nih.gov/research/supported/programs/justice/index.cfm.

National Institutes of Health, Office of Extramural Research. (2007). *Community-Based Participatory Research Scientific Interest Group.* Retrieved Feb. 3, 2008, from http://grants.nih.gov/grants/training/esaig/cbpr_sig.htm.

Navarro, A. M., Voetsch, K. P., Liburd, L. C., Giles, W., & Collins, J. L. (2007). Charting the future of community health promotion: Recommendations from the National Expert Panel on Community Health Promotion. *Preventing Chronic Disease, 4*, 1.

Nutting, P. A. (Ed.). (1987). *Community-oriented primary care: From principle to practice.* Washington, DC: U.S. Department of Health and Human Services, Health Resources and Services Administration.

O'Fallon, L. R., Tyson, F. L., & Dearry, A. (Eds.). (2000). *Successful models of community-based participatory research: Final report.* Research Triangle Park, NC: National Institute of Environmental Health Sciences.

Seifer, S. D., Kauper-Brown, J., & Robbins, A. (2004). *Directory of funding sources for community-based participatory research.* Retrieved Feb. 3, 2008, from http://depts.washington.edu/ccph/pdf_files/directory-062704f.pdf.

Stoto, M. A., Green, L. W., & Bailey, L. A. (Eds.). (1997). *Linking research and public health practice: A review of CDC's program of centers for research and demonstration of health promotion and disease prevention.* Washington, DC: National Academies Press.

Viswanathan, M., Ammerman, A., Eng, E., Gartlehner, G., Lohr, K. N., Griffith, D., et al. (2004). *Community-based participatory research: Assessing the evidence* (Evidence Report/Technology Assessment No. 99; Prepared by RTI International-University of North Carolina). Rockville, MD: Agency for Healthcare Research and Quality.

Westfall, J. M., VanVorst, R. F., Main, D. S., & Herbert, C. (2006). Community-based participatory research in practice-based research networks. *Annals of Family Medicine, 4*(1), 8–14.

World Health Organization. (1986). *Ottawa Charter for health promotion.* Copenhagen: Author.

Yin, R. K., Kaftarian, S. J., & Jacobs, N. F. (1996). Empowerment evaluation at federal and local levels: Dealing with quality. In D. M. Fetterman, S. J. Kaftarian, & A. Wandersman (Eds.), *Empowerment evaluation: Knowledge and tools for self-assessment and accountability* (pp. 188–207). Thousand Oaks, CA: Sage.

APPENDIX

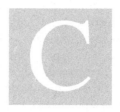

RELIABILITY-TESTED GUIDELINES FOR ASSESSING PARTICIPATORY RESEARCH PROJECTS

SHAWNA L. MERCER, LAWRENCE W. GREEN, MARGARET CARGO,

MARGARET A. POTTER, MARK DANIEL,

R. SCOTT OLDS, & ERIKA REED-GROSS

This appendix presents a revised set of guidelines (criteria and rating scales) for assessing participatory research. It discusses the purposes of the original guidelines and key differences between the original and new reliability-tested guidelines. It then presents the reliability-tested guidelines in their entirety and concludes with considerations for their use.

Note: The findings and conclusions in this appendix are those of the authors and do not necessarily represent the views of the Centers for Disease Control and Prevention. We acknowledge with thanks the authors of the original guidelines (Green et al., in Minkler & Wallerstein, 2003). In addition to current coauthors Lawrence W. Green and Mark Daniel, they are M. Anne George, C. James Frankish, Carol P. Herbert, William R. Bowie, and Michel O'Neill.

The purposes of the guidelines are (1) to help funding agencies and peer reviewers assess the participatory nature of proposals submitted for funding as participatory research, (2) to aid evaluators in assessing the extent to which projects meet participatory research criteria, and (3) to assist researchers and intended users of the research who partner with researchers (that is, nonacademic partners) in strengthening the participatory nature of their project proposals and funding applications.

The original version of the guidelines appeared in the first edition of this book (Green et al., 2003). Those guidelines were developed through a comprehensive, data-driven process that involved locating and reviewing more than 400 participatory research (PR) articles, distilling key PR concepts and processes into a definition of PR and PR guidelines, and subjecting the resulting definition and guidelines to multiple rounds of review and validity testing by several expert panels (for a detailed discussion of this comprehensive development process, see Green et al., 1995; George, Daniel, & Green, 1998–1999). The guidelines have since undergone extensive reliability testing (manuscripts detailing the multiple rounds of reliability testing are currently in preparation), and the revised set of guidelines is presented here. These guidelines can be used with both community-based participatory research (CBPR) and other forms of PR (for a discussion of CBPR as a type of PR, see Cargo & Mercer, 2008; Green et al., 1995).

Several factors converged in the early 1990s to signal the need for such a set of guidelines—and each of these factors remains equally important today. First, although there is a growing interest in PR, many health researchers, research funding agencies, and intended users of research are unaware of the complexities and challenges inherent in designing and conducting research that is truly participatory. Second, with the increasing interest among federal agencies and others in funding PR (see Appendix B in this volume) comes the funders' need to assess and compare PR proposals using consistent standards so they can award funding to the projects that are the most meritorious not only in terms of their significance and methods but also in terms of their participatory aspects. More recently, a number of reports have called for the development of standards and tools to facilitate evaluation of PR projects (O'Toole, Aaron, Chin, Horowitz, & Tyson, 2003; Viswanathan et al., 2004). Although addressing this third need was implicit in the initial guidelines, the purpose statement for the revised reliability-tested guidelines now explicitly states that the guidelines can be used to assist in evaluating PR projects.

KEY DIFFERENCES BETWEEN THE OLD AND NEW GUIDELINES

Since the initial publication of the guidelines in 1995, interest in PR approaches has continued to grow in policy- and practice-based public health and health care arenas, especially among those interested in translating the knowledge gained through research into action (Cargo & Mercer, 2008). One barrier for some of these potential PR users has been the use of the word *community* in the original guidelines to describe many of those involved in PR. Despite attempts to broaden the definition of *community* beyond geographical, geopolitical, or racial and ethnic units to include people sharing common characteristics or interests (Green et al., 1995; Green & Mercer, 2001), many of those interested in using PR approaches do not see their work as dealing with a community or fitting under the label of CBPR (Glasgow & Emmons, 2007; Graham et al., 2006; Jones & Wells, 2007; Potter & Quill, 2006). To address the needs of all groups engaged in PR, the word *community* used in the original version of the guidelines has now been replaced with the terms *intended users* (defined in the guidelines instrument as being users, beneficiaries, or stakeholders of the research findings, as discussed further later) and *nonacademic partners*. For most CBPR projects, the intended users or nonacademic partners participating in the research are community participants. Although in reality researchers can also be seen as intended users, and although all are co-collaborators in the research process, distinguishing *researchers* and *intended users* in the guidelines enables clear examination not only of the roles of traditional academic researchers but also of those who need to be engaged in the research in order for the findings to be applicable to and applied in policy, practice, advocacy, or everyday living.

In the decade between the initial development of the guidelines and their reliability testing, the roles of capacity building and sustainability have taken on increasing importance. Although these concepts were included in the original guidelines, the revised guidelines use these specific terms.

The ordering of response categories varied from guideline to guideline in the original set. The intent was to provide flexibility in case different response options might be preferred by different individuals or groups. For example, it was believed that some people might consider it more valuable to have community participants who were able to fully contribute their physical and intellectual resources, with researchers acting only as facilitators, or to have research benefiting the community only, while other people might place higher value on having researchers and community participants contributing resources equitably or on having the research benefit both researchers and community participants. This variable ordering of response categories became a formidable challenge when rating grant proposals, however, because raters could not stop feeling that the final response option should be the one most aligned with PR ideals, and they worried that projects would appear less participatory if given a middle rating. Moreover, recent research has underscored that providing benefits to all partners is essential for sustaining partnerships and research products (Israel et al., 2006). The revised guidelines therefore consider benefits for both nonacademic partners and researchers as being most aligned with the ideals of PR and consistently order the response categories from least to most participatory.

Finally, the first round of reliability testing revealed that raters did not consistently use all five available response categories. The second round of reliability testing revealed that three response categories provided sufficient discriminability.

GUIDELINES FOR ASSESSING PR PROJECTS

Key Terms
Participatory research is defined as systematic inquiry, with the collaboration of those affected by the issue being studied, for the purposes of education and of taking action or effecting change.

Intended users are the users, beneficiaries, and stakeholders of the research findings. Depending on the purposes of the project, the intended users may include any or all of the following:

- *Beneficiaries or ultimate users:* Individuals or organizations who are expected to apply the research findings to improve their own health or that of their family members, friends, or community (geographical, ethnic, indigenous, religious, cultural, or other grouping), or on whose behalf the research findings are to be used by professional intermediaries.
- *Immediate users:* Health, service, and other professionals and organizations who are expected to use the research results in their planning, policymaking, or practice.
- *Stakeholders:* Other stakeholders whose involvement or obstruction might have a substantial impact on completion of the research or ultimate use of the research findings.

Intended users (nonacademic partners) participating in the research process are those users, beneficiaries, or stakeholders who engage with researchers in the research activities. Projects that engage ultimate beneficiaries and users in the research process are typically more aligned than other projects are with the ideals of participatory research.

Researchers (academic partners) are those individuals who are generally located in academic, health, or related institutions and whose job descriptions usually include conducting research.

Instructions for Use

The guidelines can be used to

1. Help funding agencies and peer reviewers assess the participatory nature of proposals submitted for funding as participatory research.
2. Aid evaluators in assessing the extent to which projects meet participatory research criteria.
3. Assist researchers and intended users of the research who partner with researchers (that is, nonacademic partners) in strengthening the participatory nature of their project proposals and funding applications.

Response categories for each guideline increase in their alignment with participatory research as the list progresses from top to bottom. For each guideline, check only one box.

If there is insufficient information to know whether a guideline has been addressed *at all,* select the lowest rating on the response scale. If information is insufficient to know whether a guideline has been addressed *adequately,* select the middle rating. Ratings of *not applicable* or *insufficient information* should not usually be required. If either is believed to be required in a particular instance, then write in the appropriate term and provide a brief explanation.

The guidelines are intended to be used both qualitatively and quantitatively. Detail on how each of funding agencies, evaluators, researchers, and nonacademic partners can tailor the guidelines to their specific needs is found in the section on considerations following these guidelines.

Guidelines

1. Participants and the Nature of Their Involvement

1a. Are the intended users (may include users, beneficiaries, and/or stakeholders)[1] of the research described adequately enough to assess their representation in the project?

❑ No description or description provides minimal help in assessing representation [or there are no plans to include intended users in the research process].

❑ Description provides partial but not adequate help in assessing representation.

❑ Description is adequate for assessing representation.

1b. Is the mix of participants included in the research process sufficient to consider the needs of the project's intended users?

❑ The mix suggests that the research will not consider or will minimally consider the needs of the intended users [or there are no plans to include intended users in the research process].

❑ The mix suggests that the research will partially but not sufficiently consider the needs of the intended users.

❑ The mix suggests that the research will sufficiently consider the needs of the intended users.

1c. Is effort made to address barriers to participation in the research process by intended users who might otherwise tend to be underrepresented?

❑ No or minimal effort to address barriers that might limit their participation [or there are no plans to include intended users in the research process].

❑ Partial but not substantial effort to address barriers that might limit their participation.

❑ Substantial effort to address barriers that might limit their participation.

1d. Has provision been made to build trust between researchers and intended users participating in the research process?

❑ No or minimal provision has been made [or there are no plans to include intended users in the research process].

❑ Moderate provision has been made.

❑ Substantial provision has been made.

---

[1]Please refer to the *Key Terms* for an explanation of how intended users is defined and used in this and all subsequent guidelines.

1e. Do the researchers and intended users participating in the research process have a formal or informal agreement (verbal or written) regarding management of the project?

☐ There is no mention of a formal or informal agreement or of plans to develop a formal or informal agreement [or there are no plans to include intended users in the research process].

☐ There are plans to develop a formal or informal agreement.

☐ A formal or informal agreement has been developed.

2. **Shaping the Purpose and Scope of the Research**

2a. Was (were) the research question(s) developed (or refined) through a collaborative process between researchers and intended users?

☐ Research question(s) was (were) developed (or refined) mostly or entirely by the researchers with no or minimal contributions from the intended users [or development of the research question(s) is not discussed].

☐ Research question(s) was (were) developed (or refined) mostly or entirely by the intended users with no or minimal contributions from the researchers.

☐ Both intended users and researchers made relatively substantial contributions to development (or refinement) of the research question(s).

2b. Has the proposed research project applied the knowledge and experience of intended users in conceptualizing and/or designing the research?

☐ Knowledge and experience of intended users has not been applied or has been minimally applied.

☐ Knowledge and experience of intended users has been partially but not sufficiently applied.

☐ Knowledge and experience of intended users has been sufficiently applied.

2c. Does the proposed research project provide for mutual learning among intended users and researchers?

☐ No or minimal provision for mutual learning.

☐ Moderate provision for mutual learning.

☐ Substantial provision for mutual learning.

2d. Does the proposed research project consider multiple levels of determinants of health (for example, individual, familial, organizational, political, social, and/or economic)?

☐ Consideration of determinants at only one level.

☐ Consideration of determinants at two levels.

☐ Consideration of determinants at three or more levels.

2e.   Does the proposed research project plan to build the capacity of intended users to address individual or broader determinants of health?

- ❑   No or minimal plans to build capacity.

- ❑   Moderate plans to build capacity.

- ❑   Substantial plans to build capacity.

3. Research Implementation and Context

3a.   Does the proposed research project apply the knowledge and experience of intended users in the implementation of the research?

- ❑   No or minimal application of knowledge and experience of intended users.

- ❑   Moderate application of knowledge and experience of intended users.

- ❑   Substantial application of knowledge and experience of intended users.

3b.   Does the proposed research project provide intended users participating in the research process with *opportunity* to learn about research (whether or not the intended users choose to take that opportunity)?

- ❑   No or minimal opportunity to learn about research methods [or there are no plans to include intended users in the research process].

- ❑   Moderate opportunity to learn about research methods.

- ❑   Substantial opportunity to learn about research methods.

3c.   Does the proposed research project provide researchers with *opportunity* to learn about user perspectives on the issue(s) being studied?

- ❑   No or minimal opportunity to learn about user perspectives.

- ❑   Moderate opportunity to learn about user perspectives.

- ❑   Substantial opportunity to learn about user perspectives.

3d.   Do the researchers and intended users participating in the research process have a formal or informal agreement (verbal or written) regarding mutual decision making about potential changes in research methods or focus?

- ❑   There is no mention of a formal or informal agreement or of plans to develop a formal or informal agreement [or there are no plans to include intended users in the research process].

- ❑   There are plans to develop a formal or informal agreement.

- ❑   A formal or informal agreement has been developed.

3e.   Does the proposed research project provide intended users with *opportunity* to participate in planning and executing the data collection (whether or not the intended users choose to take that opportunity)?

❑   No or minimal opportunity to participate.

❑   Moderate opportunity to participate.

❑   Substantial opportunity to participate.

3f.   Does the proposed research project provide intended users with *opportunity* to participate in planning and/or executing the analysis (whether or not the intended users choose to take that opportunity)?

❑   No or minimal opportunity to participate.

❑   Moderate opportunity to participate.

❑   Substantial opportunity to participate.

3g.   Are plans to involve intended users in interpreting the research findings sufficient to reflect knowledge of the particular context and circumstances in the interpretation?

❑   Plans to involve intended users suggest that knowledge of the particular culture and circumstances will not be reflected or will be minimally reflected in the interpretation [or there are no plans to involve intended users in interpretation of the research findings].

❑   Plans to involve intended users suggest that knowledge of the particular culture and circumstances will be partially but not sufficiently reflected in the interpretation.

❑   Plans to involve intended users suggest that knowledge of the particular culture and circumstances will be sufficiently reflected in the interpretation.

4.   Nature of the Research Outcomes

4a.   Does the proposed research project reflect sufficient commitment by researchers and intended users participating in the research process to action (for example, social, individual, and/or cultural) following the (learning acquired through) research?

❑   Proposed project reflects no or minimal commitment to action by both researchers and intended users, or partial commitment by one and no or minimal commitment by the other [or there are no plans to include intended users in the research process].

❑   Proposed project reflects partial but not sufficient commitment to action by both researchers and intended users, or sufficient commitment to action by one and partial, minimal, or no commitment by the other.

❑   Proposed project reflects sufficient commitment to action by both researchers and intended users.

4b.   Do the researchers and intended users engaged in the research process have a formal or informal agreement (verbal or written) for acknowledging and resolving in a fair and open way any differences in the interpretation of research results?

❑   There is no mention of a formal or informal agreement or of plans to develop a formal or informal agreement [or there are no plans to include intended users in the research process].

❑   There are plans to develop a formal or informal agreement.

❑   A formal or informal agreement has been developed.

4c.   Do the researchers and intended users engaged in the research process have a formal or informal agreement (verbal or written) regarding ownership and sharing of the research data?

❑   There is no mention of a formal or informal agreement or of plans to develop a formal or informal agreement [or there are no plans to include intended users in the research process].

❑   There are plans to develop a formal or informal agreement.

❑   A formal or informal agreement has been developed.

4d.   Do the researchers and intended users engaged in the research process have a formal or informal agreement (verbal or written) regarding feedback of research results to intended users?

❑   There is no mention of a formal or informal agreement or of plans to develop a formal or informal agreement [or there are no plans to include intended users in the research process].

❑   There are plans to develop a formal or informal agreement.

❑   A formal or informal agreement has been developed.

4e.   Do the researchers and intended users engaged in the research process have a formal or informal agreement (verbal or written) regarding the dissemination (and/or translation or transfer) of research findings?

❑   There is no mention of a formal or informal agreement or of plans to develop a formal or informal agreement [or there are no plans to include intended users in the research process].

❑   There are plans to develop a formal or informal agreement.

❑   A formal or informal agreement has been developed.

4f.   Does the proposed research project provide intended users with *opportunity* to participate in dissemination of project findings to other intended users and researchers (whether or not the intended users choose to take that opportunity)?

❑   No or minimal opportunity to participate in dissemination to other intended users and researchers, or moderate opportunity to participate in dissemination to either intended users or researchers and no or minimal opportunity to participate in dissemination to the other.

❑ Moderate opportunity to participate in dissemination to other intended users and researchers, or substantial opportunity to participate in dissemination to either intended users or researchers and moderate, minimal, or no opportunity to participate in dissemination to the other.

❑ Substantial opportunity to participate in dissemination to other intended users and researchers.

4g. Is there sufficient provision for assistance to intended users to indicate a high probability of research results being applied?

❑ No or minimal provision for assistance has been made.

❑ Partial but not sufficient provision for assistance has been made.

❑ Sufficient provision for assistance has been made.

4h. Does the proposed research project plan for sustainability in relation to the purpose of the research (for example, by fostering collaboration between intended users and resource providers, funding sources, policymakers, holders of community assets, and the like)?

❑ No or minimal plans for sustainability.

❑ Moderate plans for sustainability.

❑ Substantial plans for sustainability.

CONSIDERATIONS IN USING THE GUIDELINES

A tension existed between a desire to enable research funders, evaluators, researchers, and nonacademic partners to exhibit flexibility in using the guidelines so that the issues of most importance to them can receive the greatest weight (Green et al., 2003), and a desire to ensure that the guidelines will enable consistent and equitable ratings of PR project proposals submitted in response to the same funding call.

Resolution of this tension has been achieved. Funding agencies, evaluators, researchers, and nonacademic partners have flexibility in deciding (a) whether to use all twenty-five guidelines (the default) or to exclude one or more guidelines that are less important to them or that do not fit their particular situation (for example, a funder could drop guideline 2a if it has established firm research questions), and (b) whether to weight all guidelines equally (the default) or to weight some more heavily (that is, as more important than others). At the same time, research funders, evaluators, researchers, and nonacademic partners can have confidence that different PR proposals or projects will be rated consistently on the guidelines they choose to retain because all of the guidelines use the same ordering of response categories and because the guidelines have been found to be reliable.

Researchers and their nonacademic partners developing PR projects may gain the most benefit from using the guidelines primarily in a qualitative fashion and considering what they would need to do to receive the rating most aligned with the tenets of PR (the final response category for each guideline). Evaluators of an individual PR project may also want to consider which response category the project is most aligned with for each guideline, and why.

In contrast, for simultaneously evaluating multiple PR projects and for peer review of PR funding proposals, the guidelines will be most valuable when they are used both quantitatively and qualitatively. The quantitative ratings can identify a general picture of the participatory nature of a project—by identifying how many guidelines overall and within each domain (or guidelines of most importance to a funder or evaluator) a particular project scored as most participatory. This information should then be interpreted in light of an accompanying qualitative write-up that highlights weaknesses and strengths of specific PR aspects of the proposal, identified by applying the guidelines. This could address such things as why a particular project received ratings of "less participatory" on certain guidelines while it was consistently high on others and whether these ratings reflect realities of the particular situation or a lack of attention to particular PR components that should have been addressed. This approach is consistent with peer review practices of federal funding agencies, which request narrative descriptions for each of the aspects (for example, significance, approach, innovation, and so forth) considered during peer review, with the guidelines identifying key PR criteria to be considered by peer reviewers who may vary in the extent of their PR knowledge and experience.

A link to the guidelines should be provided in the original funding announcement every time that project proposals are to be rated against them. This will increase the likelihood that the proposals will explicitly address all the areas covered by the guidelines.

Finally, the developers of the guidelines all continue to be interested in their further refinement. The first two authors would very much like to hear from those who intend to use the guidelines in order to engage their assistance in further refinement and in evaluating the guidelines' usefulness for different types of projects and participants (please see the Web site www.lwgreen.net/guidelines.html).

REFERENCES

Cargo, M., & Mercer, S. L. (2008). The value and challenges of participatory research: Strengthening its practice. *Annual Review of Public Health, 29,* 325–350.

George, M. A., Daniel, M., & Green, L. W. (1998–1999). Appraising and funding participatory research in health promotion. *International Quarterly of Community Health Education, 18,* 181–197. (Reprinted in 2006–2007, *26,* 171–187.)

Glasgow, R. E., & Emmons, K. M. (2007). How can we increase translation of research into practice? Types of evidence needed. *Annual Review of Public Health, 28,* 413–433.

Graham, I. D., Logan, J., Harrison, M. B., Straus, W. E., Tetroe, J., Caswell, W., et al. (2006). Lost in knowledge translation: Time for a map? *Journal of Continuing Education in the Health Professions, 26*(1), 13–24.

Green, L. W., George, M. A., Daniel, M., Frankish, C. J., Herbert, C. P., Bowie, W. R., et al. (1995). *Study of participatory research in health promotion: Review and recommendations for the development of participatory research in health promotion in Canada.* Vancouver, BC: Royal Society of Canada.

Green, L. W., George, M. A., Daniel M., Frankish, C. J., Herbert, C. P., Bowie, W. R. et al. (2003). Guidelines for participatory research in health promotion. In M. Minkler & N. Wallerstein (Eds.), *Community-based participatory research for health* (pp. 419–428). San Francisco: Jossey-Bass.

Green, L. W., & Mercer, S. L. (2001). Can public health researchers and agencies reconcile the push from funding bodies and the pull from communities? *American Journal of Public Health, 91,* 1926–1929.

Israel, B. A., Krieger, J. W., Vlahov, D., Ciske, S., Foley, M., Fortin, P., et al. (2006). Challenges and facilitating factors in sustaining community-based participatory research partnerships: Lessons learned from the Detroit, New York City, and Seattle urban research centers. *Journal of Urban Health, 83,* 1022–1040.

Jones, L., & Wells, K. (2007). Strategies for academic and clinician engagement in community-partnered participatory research. *Journal of the American Medical Association, 297,* 407–410.

Minkler, M., & Wallerstein, N. (Eds.). (2003). *Community-based participatory research for health.* San Francisco: Jossey-Bass.

O'Toole, T. P., Aaron, K. F., Chin, M. H., Horowitz, C., & Tyson, F. (2003). Community-based participatory research: Opportunities, challenges and the need for a common language. *Journal of General Internal Medicine, 18,* 592–594.

Potter, M. A., & Quill, B. E. (Eds.). (2006). Demonstrating excellence in practice-based research for public health. *Public Health Reports, 121,* 1–16.

Viswanathan, M., Ammerman, A., Eng, E., Gartlehner, G., Lohr, K. N., Griffith, D., et al. (2004). *Community-based participatory research: Assessing the evidence* (Evidence Report/Technology Assessment No. 99; Prepared by RTI International-University of North Carolina). Rockville, MD: Agency for Healthcare Research and Quality.

APPENDIX

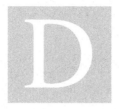

D

SUPPORTING PARTICIPATORY EVALUATION USING THE COMMUNITY TOOL BOX ONLINE DOCUMENTATION SYSTEM

STEPHEN FAWCETT & JERRY SCHULTZ

A key challenge in evaluating comprehensive community health initiatives is documenting the unfolding of the intervention, that is, the multiple changes in the environment that can lead to widespread behavior change and improvement in population-level outcomes. Using principles of community-based participatory research (CBPR), partners can document changes in the community and system (for example, a new program or policy), analyze how the changing environment contributes to more distant health outcomes, and make adjustments along the way.

BACKGROUND AND FRAMEWORK FOR THE ONLINE SUPPORT SYSTEM

The Work Group for Community Health and Development (2008a) at the University of Kansas (KU) has developed an Internet-based support for participatory evaluation, known as the Online Documentation and Support System (ODSS), which has been used with various community health initiatives (for example, Collie-Akers et al., 2007; Fawcett et al., 1997, 2003; Fawcett, Schultz, Carson, Renault, & Francisco, 2003; Paine-Andrews et al., 2002). Each customized workstation integrates tools for participatory evaluation, such as online graphing and reporting, with capacity-building resources in the Community Tool Box (CTB) (Work Group for Community Health and Development, 2008b). The CTB contains over 7,000 pages of free resources for learning skills (for example, conducting listening sessions), doing the work (for example, assessing needs and resources), solving problems (such as not enough participation), and exploring best approaches for change.

The Institute of Medicine's (2003, pp. 178–211) framework for collaborative public health action in communities suggests a general model for promoting community health. As shown in adapted form in Figure D.1, the KU work group's online documentation system focuses attention on four participatory evaluation questions related to the framework. In using this or other frameworks, CBPR partners collaboratively select and interpret measures of process and intended outcomes based on an agreed-upon logic model.

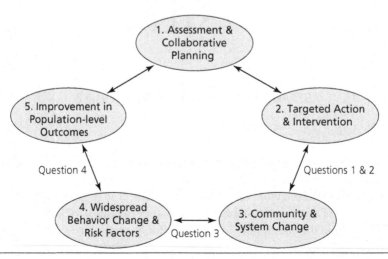

FIGURE D.1 *Framework for Collaborative Public Health Action in Communities*

CORE QUESTIONS AND RELATED MEASURES

1. *Is the community health initiative serving as a catalyst for community and system change related to its mission?* To capture the unfolding of changes in the environment, the online system supports documentation of key events such as community and system change: that is, new or modified programs, policies, and practices facilitated by the effort and related to its aims (for example, to prevent substance abuse or injuries). Using online graphs, community and research partners can examine the rate of community and system changes over time (see Figure D.2). We recommend that partners regularly document discrete instances of community and system change (for example, a new after-school program or a modified road safety policy) and review the time series graphs to look for discontinuities (marked increases or decreases) in rates of change.

2. *What factors or processes are associated with the rate of community and system change?* We recommend engaging CBPR partners in obtaining qualitative information on critical events in the initiative (for example, a completed action plan or implementation of intervention components). Updated annually, identified critical events can be overlaid on the time series graph(s) of community and system changes (see the boxes in Figure D.2). When particular events (for example, completion of action plan or change

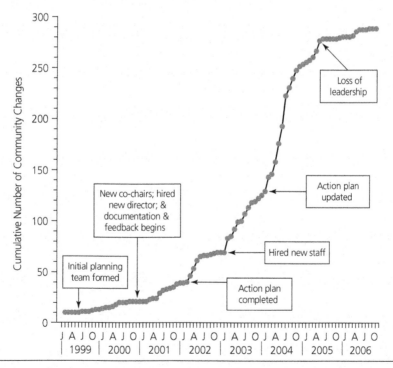

FIGURE D.2 *Cumulative Community and System Changes (Such as New Programs or Policies) Facilitated by a Hypothetical Coalition, and Associated Critical Events and Processes*

in leadership) are associated with marked discontinuities (increases or decreases) in the rate of community change—and where these associations are replicated across contexts—they may suggest key processes that can advance or inhibit efforts to reach outcomes.

3. *How are community and system changes contributing to efforts to promote community health?* We recommend that CBPR partners conduct regular analyses of contribution by reviewing how the community and system changes are distributed along several dimensions related to the logic model or intervention plan. Secondary scoring of documented changes and online graphs (such as pie charts of the proportion of changes occurring in different sectors) can aid systematic reflection. We recommend examining the distribution of community and system changes by (a) primary goal or aim (for example, to promote healthy nutrition or physical activity); (b) primary strategy of intervention used (for example, providing information or bringing about policy change); (c) expected duration of change (for example, a one-time event or an ongoing process); (d) primary population to benefit (for example, children or adults); (e) primary sector addressed (for example, schools or health organizations); (f) primary ecological level addressed (for example, individual, relationship, or community); and (g) place (for example, a particular city or county).

4. *Are community and system changes associated with improvements in population-level outcomes related to the objectives?* Annually, the CBPR partners examine whether the cumulative unfolding of community and system changes is sufficient to "tip," or improve, indicators of population-level improvement (for example, the prevalence of violence or reported cases of HIV/AIDS) (see the sample graph in Figure D.3). We recommend using the analysis of contribution to discover the "dose" or conditions under which associated population-level improvements are noted. For instance, we might expect population-level

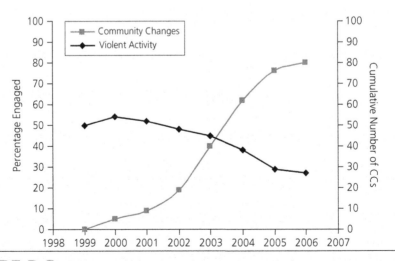

FIGURE D.3 *Possible Association of the Unfolding of Community and System Changes and Improvement in Population-Level Outcomes.*

improvement when there are larger numbers of environmental changes that are focused on the goal, and when these changes are of longer duration, with a greater intensity of change strategy, and delivered through multiple sectors in places where people experience the problem. Multiple case studies can help researchers establish the generality of observed associations across contexts and conditions.

SUMMARY AND ADVANTAGES

There are several advantages to this and similar systems for supporting CBPR and related efforts to promote community health. First, such a support system can help partners to systematically document the unfolding of comprehensive community interventions in dynamic and diverse contexts. Second, it focuses attention on core evaluation questions, such as whether an initiative is serving as a catalyst for environmental change and whether the changes are associated with population-level improvement. Third, all required online capabilities for documenting and analyzing the contribution of community health efforts (for example, for online data entry, graphing, participatory sense making, reporting, and making adjustments) have been field-tested using the CTB Online Documentation and Support System.

Fourth, it provides integrated supports for targeted action and related participatory evaluation. For instance, when viewing online graphs, community and research partners can use tailored reflection questions to consider what the results mean. If the results show a low level of change or improvement, for example, guiding questions may be asked (for example, Is this what we expected to see? What affects progress? What might lead to improvement?). For identified problems, the participants are referred to relevant how-to sections in the Community Tool Box (for example, how to respond to opposition). Fifth, the community and system changes documented by collaborating partners can suggest promising approaches for intervention in other communities. Each initiative's postings of accomplishments are readily viewable by other CBPR partners, thus contributing to empowerment and co-learning within and across initiatives. When coupled with other technical assistance, this online support system can help make easier the collaborative work of creating conditions that promote health and health equity.

REFERENCES

Collie-Akers, V., Fawcett, S. B., Schultz, J. A., Carson, V., Cyprus, J., & Pierle, J. (2007, July). Analyzing a community-based coalition's efforts to reduce health disparities and the risk for chronic disease in Kansas City, Missouri. *Preventing Chronic Disease.* Retrieved May 12, 2008, from http://www.cdc.gov/pcd/issues/2007/jul/06_0101.htm.

Fawcett, S. B., Boothroyd, R., Schultz, J. A., Francisco, V., Carson, V., & Bremby, R. (2003). Building capacity for participatory evaluation within community initiatives. *Journal of Prevention and Intervention in the Community, 26*(2), 21–36.

Fawcett, S. B., Lewis, R. K., Paine-Andrews, A., Francisco, V. T., Richter, K. P., Williams, E. L., et al. (1997). Evaluating community coalitions for prevention of substance abuse: The case of Project Freedom. *Health Education & Behavior, 24*(6), 812–828.

Fawcett, S. B., Schultz, J. A., Carson, V. L., Renault, V. A., & Francisco, V. T. (2003). Using Internet-based tools to build capacity for community-based participatory research and other efforts to promote community health and development. In M. Minkler & N. Wallerstein (Eds.), *Community-based participatory research for health* (pp. 155–178). San Francisco: Jossey-Bass.

Institute of Medicine. (2003). *The future of the public's health in the 21st century.* Washington, DC: National Academies Press.

Paine-Andrews, A., Fisher, J. L., Berkley-Patton, J., Fawcett, S. B., Williams, E. L., Lewis, R. K., et al. (2002). Analyzing the contribution of community change to population health outcomes in an adolescent pregnancy prevention initiative. *Health Education & Behavior, 29*(2), 183–193.

Work Group for Community Health and Development. (2008a). *Services.* Retrieved Apr. 24, 2008, from http://communityhealth.ku.edu.

Work Group for Community Health and Development. (2008b). *The community tool box.* Retrieved Apr. 24, 2008, from http://ctb.ku.edu.

APPENDIX

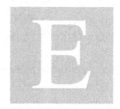

MAKING THE BEST CASE FOR COMMUNITY-ENGAGED SCHOLARSHIP IN PROMOTION AND TENURE REVIEW

SARENA D. SEIFER

Our experience suggests that even those faculty with the belief that a participatory community based approach to research is appropriate and relevant to their work may find the process daunting, given the pressures of academic institutions on faculty to publish and obtain grant money.

ISRAEL, SCHULZ, PARKER, & BECKER (1998)

A frequently cited barrier to faculty conducting community-based participatory research (CBPR) is the risk associated with trying to achieve promotion and tenure (Israel, Schulz, Parker, & Becker, 1998; Maurana, Wolff, Beck, & Simpson, 2001; Gelmon & Agre-Kippenhan, 2002; Calleson, Jordan, & Seifer, 2005). This appendix is intended primarily to serve as a resource for faculty who are engaged in CBPR and concerned about successfully preparing for and navigating their institution's review, promotion, and tenure (RPT) process.

A good place to start is to become familiar with three influential reports on scholarship that help to "make the case" for community-engaged scholarship (CES): *Scholarship Reconsidered* (Boyer, 1990), *Scholarship Assessed: Evaluation of the Professoriate* (Glassick, Huber, & Maeroff, 1997), and *Linking Scholarship and Communities,* the report of the Commission on Community-Engaged Scholarship in the Health Professions (2005).

Numerous initiatives are underway to apply the definitions, frameworks, and recommendations in these reports in the health professions and in higher education as a whole. A growing number of higher education institutions are rewriting their RPT policies to recognize and reward CES. Links to these initiatives and policies are included in the online CES Toolkit (Calleson, Kauper-Brown, & Seifer, 2005). Community-engaged faculty might share these with department chairs and RPT committee members as evidence of the growing legitimacy of CES in higher education and to educate these colleagues about this approach.

DOCUMENTING AND ASSESSING CES

Community-engaged scholarship requires the scholar to be engaged with the community in a mutually beneficial partnership. The role of expert is shared, the relationship with the community must be reciprocal and dynamic, and community-defined concerns direct the scholarly activities. A challenge for faculty engaged in CBPR is to describe clearly how accepted standards of scholarship are implemented in the context of community. The Peer Review Work Group of the Community-Engaged Scholarship for Health Collaborative (Jordan, 2007) elaborated on Glassick's work to articulate eight characteristics of quality CES. Excerpts from these guidelines, particularly as they pertain to research, are highlighted in the following section. They may be useful both to community-engaged faculty to guide the documentation needed for their review, promotion, and tenure portfolio, and to RPT committees as a tool for assessing cases that emphasize community-engaged scholarship.

CHARACTERISTICS OF QUALITY CES

1. **Clear Academic and Community Change Goals**

    A scholar should clearly define objectives of scholarly work and clearly state basic questions of inquiry. Clarity of purpose provides a critical context for evaluating scholarly work.

    Possible evidence includes:

    - Clearly stating the basic purpose of the work and its value for the public good
    - Identifying intellectual and significant questions in the discipline and in the community

2. **Adequate Preparation in Content Area and Grounding in the Community**

A scholar must be well prepared and knowledgeable about developments in his or her field. The ability to educate others and conduct meaningful research depends upon mastering existing knowledge.

Possible evidence includes:

- Investing time and effort in developing community partnerships
- Participating in training and professional development that builds skills and competencies in CES

3. **Appropriate Methods: Rigor *and* Community Engagement**

Meaningful scholarly work must always be conducted with appropriate rigor. In the case of research, rigor facilitates methodologically sound research design, data collection and interpretation and reporting of results, so that valid conclusions can be drawn from the findings. In many instances, the engagement of communities can enhance rigor and facilitate the study of issues and research questions (e.g., research related to health disparities).

Possible evidence includes:

- Refining a research question, or confirming its validity, through co-generation with community partner

4. **Substantive and Important Results: Impact on the Field and the Community**

Scholars should evaluate whether or not they achieve their goals, and whether this achievement had an important impact on others, and whether the work is used by others. A primary goal of CES is to beneficially impact the communities in which such scholarship is conducted. The assessment of CES impact must go beyond just the reporting of positive, neutral, or negative project outcomes: The scholar should explicitly state what knowledge was created or applied and what impact it has had or may likely have in the future.

Possible evidence includes:

- The community contributing to as well as benefiting from the research
- Disseminating geographically limited work with clear discussion of issues concerning generalizability and the project's potential role as a model that can be further investigated in other settings.

5. **Effective Presentation/Dissemination to Academic and Community Audiences**

Central to scholarly pursuits is the effective presentation and dissemination of results. Scholars should possess effective oral and written communication skills that enable them to convert knowledge into language that a lay audience can understand. Scholars should communicate with appropriate audiences and subject their ideas to critical inquiry and independent review.

Possible evidence includes:

- Publishing research results in peer-reviewed journals, practitioner journals and professional journals, with community partner co-authors

- Disseminating information through media that reaches community members, practitioners or policy makers (e.g., radio, newsletters, podcasts)

6. Reflective Critique: Lessons Learned to Improve the Scholarship and Community Engagement

Community-engaged scholars should demonstrate an ability to critically reflect on their work, their community partnerships, the issues and challenges that arise, and how they are able to address them. Scholars further should demonstrate an ability to consider such questions as: Why did this project succeed or fail to achieve its intended outcomes? What could be done differently in succeeding projects to improve outcomes? Does this project involve an idea that is deserving of further time and effort?

Possible evidence includes:

- Changing project based on stakeholder feedback and lessons learned
- Engaging in personal reflection concerning, for example, issues of privilege or racism

7. Leadership and Personal Contribution

One of the most consistent criteria for promotion or tenure in the academy is evidence of a national or international reputation. Community-engaged scholars should demonstrate, within their discipline, within the arena of CES, or both, that their work has earned them a reputation for rigor, impact and the capacity to move the discipline or community change work forward. In addition, community-engaged scholars should demonstrate an ability to serve in leadership roles.

Possible evidence includes:

- Receiving invitations to serve on advisory or policy-making committees at national, regional, state and/or community levels
- Receiving awards or letters of appreciation from community-based organizations

8. Consistently Ethical Behavior: Socially Responsible Conduct of Research and Teaching

Scholarly work must be conducted with honesty, integrity, perseverance and courage. Ethical behavior considers that scholars will foster a respectful relationship with students, community participants, peers, and others who participate in or benefit from their work. Ethical behavior must consider cultural or community implications as well as university policies.

Possible evidence includes:

- Focusing scholarly work on community assets, and allowing community members to take active, meaningful roles in research rather than simply serving as research subjects
- Appropriately involving community partners in writing and reviewing products of the scholarship before they are published or otherwise disseminated

For additional ideas, including excerpts of actual portfolios, see the CES Toolkit (Calleson, Kauper-Brown, & Seifer, 2005).

IDEAS FOR DOCUMENTING QUALITY CES IN A DOSSIER

The following are examples of documents that could be included in a faculty member's RPT portfolio and ways they can help to "make the case" for promotion or tenure. These ideas, of course, should be implemented in the context of one's institutional culture and requirements. For additional ideas, including excerpts of actual portfolios, consult the CES Toolkit (Calleson, Kauper-Brown and Seifer, 2005). [*Note:* faculty members who have been promoted or tenured based on CES are asked to consider submitting excerpts of their portfolios for posting on the CES Toolkit so that junior colleagues may learn from their experience.]

- *Career statement.* As a part of their career statement, scholars can discuss the role of CES in their career and academic development. Some institutions require scholars to specifically address research and teaching accomplishments in either subsections of the Career Statement or in separate essays. The scholar should take this opportunity to illustrate how CES enhances the rigor of their research or teaching, the reach of their work, community impact, and student outcomes.
- *Curriculum vita.* Scholars can use their vita to highlight the importance of community-engagement to their scholarly work. For example, sections of the vita could be developed to highlight community activities, consultative and advisory positions, and articles or reports co-authored with community partners. It is particularly important that the role of community partners be highlighted and that the work undertaken is scholarly, in that it creates, advances, or extends knowledge. Mere provision of community service, while a form of community engagement, cannot be considered to be CES.
- *Statement of assigned responsibilities/work assignment.* Scholars can also document the importance of community engagement as it relates to their assigned responsibilities. Sadly, in many academic settings, faculty members are evaluated based on criteria that are out of alignment with the responsibilities they are asked to assume on a daily basis. Inclusion of a statement of assigned responsibilities or work assignment may call attention to the importance of community engagement as it relates to a scholar's work.
- *Teaching portfolios.* Teaching portfolios are ideal vehicles for documenting the value of community engagement as it relates to teaching as well as scholarship related to community-engaged teaching activities.
- *Letters of support & appreciation from community members/partners.* Such letters can be used to help document the value of the scholarly work as perceived by community leaders, and to illustrate community impact and breadth of dissemination.
- *Peer review letters from community leaders.* To be valuable, such letters must provide an analytical critique of the scholar's work from the community's perspective. Letters of a general nature that lack critical analysis may be counterproductive to the scholar's promotion or tenure application.

As CES is increasingly being recognized and rewarded as a legitimate form of scholarship, the future appears bright for faculty who seek community-engaged careers in the academy.

REFERENCES

Boyer, E. L. (1990). *Scholarship reconsidered: Priorities of the professoriate.* Princeton, NJ: Carnegie Foundation for the Advancement of Teaching.

Calleson, D. C., Jordan, C., & Seifer, S. D. (2005). Community-engaged scholarship: Is faculty work in communities a true academic enterprise? *Academic Medicine, 80*(4), 317–321.

Calleson, D. C., Kauper-Brown, J., & Seifer, S. D. (2005). *Community-engaged scholarship toolkit.* Community-Campus Partnerships for Health. Retrieved May 12, 2008, from http://www.communityengagedscholarship.info.

Commission on Community-Engaged Scholarship in the Health Professions. (2005). *Linking scholarship and communities.* Seattle, WA: Community-Campus Partnerships for Health.

Jordan, C. (Ed.). (2007). *Community-engaged scholarship review, promotion and tenure package.* Seattle, WA: Community-Campus Partnerships for Health, Community-Engaged Scholarship for Health Collaborative, Peer Review Workgroup.

Gelmon, S., & Agre-Kippenhan, S. (2002, Jan.). Promotion, tenure, and the engaged scholar: Keeping the scholarship of engagement in the review process. *AAHE Bulletin,* pp. 7–11.

Glassick, C. E., Huber, M. T., & Maeroff, G. I. (1997). *Scholarship assessed: Evaluation of the professoriate.* San Francisco: Jossey-Bass.

Israel, B. A., Schulz, A. J., Parker, E. A., & Becker, A. B. (1998). Review of community-based research: Assessing partnership approaches to improve public health. *Annual Review of Public Health, 19,* 173–202.

Maurana, C., Wolff, M., Beck, B. J., & Simpson, D. E. (2001). Working with our communities: Moving from service to scholarship in the health professions. *Education for Health, 14*(2), 207–220.

APPENDIX

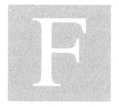

COMMUNITY PARTNERSHIP THROUGH A NURSING LENS

JENNIFER AVERILL

The domain of professional nursing has a rich history of partnership with communities and affinity for the principles of community-based participatory research (CBPR). Collaborations are long-standing in care settings, educational arenas, and research efforts aimed at expanding the knowledge base of the discipline. Care settings such as clinics, hospitals, homes, rural communities, refugee and labor camps, schools, and organizations have always been sites where nurses developed meaningful, trusting relationships with people who were suffering, partnerships with patients and their families, and linkages with resources available to aid in the restoration of health (such as places to rest and heal, medications and treatment, adequate nutrition and hydration, cleanliness and hygiene, and access to available providers) (Nightingale, 1859/1992; Stanhope & Lancaster, 2008; Anderson & McFarlane, 2004).

Nursing education has long promoted and depended on partnerships with the communities integral to the learning process, among them students, educators, clinical preceptors, and managers of hospitals, clinics, community-based agencies, senior centers, and health and human service departments. Nursing knowledge development and nursing research have also embraced the fundamental principles of CBPR. The National Institute of Nursing Research (NINR) was established within the National Institutes of Health (NIH) in 1986 (NINR, 2007), and the American Nurses Association (ANA) has produced a set of research priorities aimed at demonstrating social responsibility and engaging communities in the analysis and resolution of health disparities (ANA, 2003).

In addition to funding research addressing physiological issues, end-of-life care, symptom management, health behavior and minority health, HIV/AIDS and oncology, neuroscience, and reproductive health, NINR funds *community-partnered interventions to reduce health disparities.* In all these priority areas, but especially in community-partnered interventions, NINR emphasizes building collaborative, culturally reflective alliances with populations accustomed to marginalization and deprivation (NINR, 2007).

Consistent with this emphasis on community partnership, several examples of CBPR applications offer evidence of CBPR's value to the discipline of nursing. In 1996, Anderson and McFarlane (2004) developed the community-as-partner model for practice and education. Blending public health science with nursing process, the model systematically guides phases of community assessment, analysis, planning, intervention, analysis, and evaluation. Key to this model is the collaborative work of negotiating the substance of each phase, from start to finish. This model has been used in improving the health status of many groups, including homeless people, immigrants and refugees, chronically ill elders, and the members of various schools, organizations, and rural communities. Partnerships are forged among the nurses, gatekeepers, and representatives of particular groups, representatives of resource units or agencies, and local politicians whose voices affect legislation and policy. Educationally, the model has been used in preparing several generations of public health nurses to identify and engage holistically with as many key stakeholders as possible in both urban and rural settings for the purposes of improving health care access and health status.

Falk-Rafael (2001) has spent a decade working to build awareness and capacity in both nurses and the communities they serve, toward the end of changing health care environments and reducing major health disparities. Using the qualitative techniques of community meetings, focus groups, journaling, and recorded narratives, she has undertaken several projects aimed at enhancing the awareness, active participation, knowledge, survival skills, and change-making ability of both clients and nurses in primary care and public health practice. Central to her CBPR work are relationship building and nurturance, political advocacy and voice, knowledge and skill development, and capacity building so that resources can be identified and applied to the process of making change while barriers are reduced or eliminated. Finally, and consistent with CBPR's emphasis on action to effect broader social change, Falk-Rafael (2005) has called for nurses to add political advocacy to the list of essential skills they use in practice and research activities.

Holkup Tripp-Reimer, Salois, and Weinert (2004) have conducted an innovative CBPR project with a Native American community aimed at helping Native families resolve internal problems while maintaining self-determination. The core CBPR tenets and practices incorporated in this work have included an emphasis on the community's defined problem, partnering with respected members of the community for guidance, holding regular meetings to dialogue and keep the relationships strong, sharing all information from the project with the community, and devising strategies for long-term commitments from all partners in the process. Respecting the culture was essential, and this pilot project was successful in winning the endorsement of the community so that a larger investigation, still under way, could move forward. The CBPR team created a conference and model built on the *family*, with participation by numerous local residents, who retain primary ownership for the ongoing project.

More recently, Chen et al. (2007) employed CBPR principles to open and cultivate trusting relationships with patients in China who have HIV and are caught in the tensions surrounding Confucian ideals of collectivism and familial authority, severe stigmatization of HIV, and Western ideas about autonomy and privileged personal information. Chen and her team proposed that health care providers (HCPs) could be pivotal in an effort to stop the escalation of HIV in the Chinese population by providing health-related, financial, and emotional support to HIV-positive individuals. Working in the context of these factors, a team of nurses, social workers, and educators interviewed twenty-nine Chinese HIV-positive patients to learn their perceptions and experiences with the HCPs involved in their HIV care. The results of the team's work suggested ways in which capacity building in both HIV patients and their HCPs could be instituted to reduce discrimination and stigma; provide education, care, and support; and intervene with families sensitively, in ways that respected traditions and culture.

As these examples illustrate, many diverse opportunities exist in the field of nursing for CBPR involving collaborations with patients and their families and communities and also with educational, administrative, research, and interdisciplinary partners and stakeholders. The long-standing covenant between professional nursing and CBPR remains vibrant, dynamic, and progressive in a variety of settings and applications.

REFERENCES

American Nurses Association. (2003). *Nursing's social policy statement* (2nd ed.). Silver Spring, MD: Author.

Anderson, E. T., & McFarlane, J. M. (2004). *Community as partner: Theory and practice in nursing* (4th ed.). Philadelphia: Lippincott Williams & Wilkins.

Chen, W., Starks, H., Shiu, C., Fredriksen-Goldsen, K., Simoni, J., Pearson, C., et al. (2007). Chinese HIV-positive patients and their health care providers: Contrasting Confucian versus Western notions of secrecy and support. *Advances in Nursing Science, 30*(4), 329–342.

Falk-Rafael, A. R. (2001). Empowerment as a process of evolving consciousness: A model of empowered caring. *Advances in Nursing Science, 24*(1), 1–16.

Falk-Rafael, A. (2005). Advancing nursing theory through theory-guided practice: The emergence of a critical caring perspective. *Advances in Nursing Science, 28*(1), 38–49.

Holkup, P. A., Tripp-Reimer, T., Salois, E. M., & Weinert, C. (2004). Community-based participatory research: An approach to intervention research with a Native American community. *Advances in Nursing Science, 27*(3), 162–175.

National Institute of Nursing Research. (2007). [Home page]. Retrieved Oct. 28, 2007, from http://www.ninr.nih.gov.

Nightingale, F. (1992). *Notes on nursing: What it is and what it is not* (commemorative ed.). Philadelphia: Lippincott Williams & Wilkins (Original work published 1859).

Stanhope, M., & Lancaster, J. (2008). *Public health nursing* (7th ed.). St. Louis: Mosby.

APPENDIX

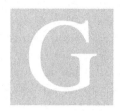

ETHICAL REVIEW OF COMMUNITY-BASED PARTICIPATORY RESEARCH

CONSIDERATIONS FOR INSTITUTIONAL REVIEW BOARDS

SARAH FLICKER, ROBB TRAVERS, ADRIAN GUTA, SEAN McDONALD, & AILEEN MEAGHER

Ethical guidelines generally use autonomy, nonmaleficence, beneficence, and justice as touchstone principles for conducting an *ethical review* (Office of the Secretary, National Commission for the Protection of Human Subjects, 1979). Despite increasingly rigorous review procedures, however, ethical problems continue to arise in health research. Community-based participatory research (CBPR) strives to address many of the problems associated with more traditional enquiry. Nevertheless, though sensitivity to the vulnerability of participants is implicit in CBPR, a different and often unanticipated set of ethical issues may emerge.

The guidelines typically used by institutional review boards (IRBs) or ethics review boards (ERBs) to evaluate protocols reflect biomedical ethical frameworks used to assess risk to *individuals* and not necessarily to *communities*. Consequently, they may not be as appropriate in the case of alternative approaches to research, including CBPR. After carefully reviewing IRB and ERB assessment forms at a sample of thirty schools of public health, we sought to assist in the development of new guidelines that might benefit communities in the long run and the field of CBPR in the present. To begin with, we offer three overarching recommendations for enhancing the quality of CBPR ethical review:

1. IRBs and ERBs engaged in reviewing CBPR and other community-based intervention grants should be provided with basic training in the principles of CBPR.

2. IRBs and ERBs should mandate that CBPR projects seeking ethical review must provide signed *terms of reference* or *memorandums of understanding*. These should clearly outline the goals of the project, the partnership principles to be followed, the decision-making processes to be used, the partners' roles and responsibilities, and the partnership's guidelines for handling and disseminating data.

3. IRBs/ and ERBs should require CBPR projects to document the processes through which key research design decisions were made and the processes through which the communities most affected were consulted.

Ultimately, we propose that there is a need for protocol forms that ground the potential ethical problems inherent in CBPR studies in a framework that includes assessment of risk to communities and attention to other CBPR principles. IRBs/ and ERBs have an important role to play in assessing the ethical challenges posed by CBPR. But if they are to prevent an ethical splintering—with CBPR researchers and communities looking for outside means of ethical review—they must work closely with CBPR researchers and communities toward better integrating research and community needs. In Table G.1, we provide some ways of addressing the issues already found in current protocol forms with increased sensitivity to community interests.

The questions suggested do not negate the importance of individual ethical concerns, but they do broaden the scope of risk assessment. They can serve two purposes: (1) they can inform future research design, helping research teams to clarify their conceptualization of new projects, and (2) they can guide the development of improved and more holistic ethics protocol review forms. Although the role of designing and conducting ethical research is ultimately in the hands of investigators, IRBs and ERBs constitute an important framework that supports ethical practices. The questions in Table G.1 may help both these boards and the researchers themselves as they think through and address the special, community-level ethical issues and challenges that may arise in CBPR.

TABLE G.1   **Alternate Ways of Addressing the Issues Covered by Current Protocol Forms**

Traditional questions	Potential new questions
Background, purpose, objectives	
Provide a description of the background, purpose, objectives, and hypothesis for the research.	How was the community involved or consulted in defining the need? Who came up with the research objectives and how? Is this research *really* justified? Are there concrete action outcomes? Who benefits? How?
Research methodology	
Describe exactly *how* the research will be carried out. Answer the who's, what's, when's, where's, and why's. Describe the procedures to be used in the conduct of the research (for example, interviews, questionnaires, chart reviews). State the period during which the procedures will be carried out and how long each will last, and be specific about the number and frequency of the procedures.	How will the community be involved in the research? At what levels? What training or capacity-building opportunities will be built in? Will the methods used be sensitive and appropriate to various communities (consider literacy issues, language barriers, cultural sensitivities, and so forth)? How will the project balance scientific rigor and accessibility?
Participants	
Describe who the participants are and why they were selected. State the proposed *sample size*: that is, the number of people who will be involved. Provide relevant inclusion and exclusion criteria. Describe any special issues with the proposed population: that is, incompetent patients or minors.	Are you talking to the "right" people to get the research questions answered appropriately (for example, service providers, community members, leaders, and the like)? How will the research team protect vulnerable groups? Will the research process include or engage marginalized or disenfranchised community members? How? Is there a reason to exclude some people? Why?

(Table G.1, continued)

Recruitment

Describe how and by whom participants will be approached and recruited; include copies of any recruiting materials (for example, letters, advertisements, flyers, telephone scripts). State where participants will be recruited from (for example, a hospital, clinic, or school).

Provide a statement of the investigator's relationship, if any, to the participants (for example, treating physician or teacher).

What provisions have been put in place to ensure culturally relevant and appropriate recruitment strategies and materials?

Has the research team considered *power* relationships in its recruitment strategies? (No coercion!)

Who approaches people about the study and how?

Risks and benefits

List the anticipated risks and benefits to participants.

Describe how the risks and benefits are balanced, and explain what strategies are in place to minimize and manage any risks.

What are the risks and benefits of the research for communities? For individuals?

Be honest about risks—and consider how the project will minimize them.

Are there built-in mechanisms for dealing appropriately with unflattering results?

Privacy and confidentiality

Describe how privacy and confidentiality will be protected. Include descriptions of data maintenance, data storage, processes for release of information and access to information, use of names or codes, and destruction of data at the conclusion of the research; include information on the use of audio- or videotapes.

Where will the research team store data? Who will have access to the data? How?

What processes will the team put in place to be inclusive about data analysis and yet maintain the privacy of participants?

What rules will the team have for working with transcripts or surveys with identifying information?

How will team members maintain boundaries between multiple roles (for example, researcher, counselor, peer)?

Compensation

Describe any reimbursement, remuneration, or other compensation that will be provided to the participants, and the terms of this compensation.

It is important to reimburse people for their time and to honor their efforts; however, economic incentives should never become coercive. How will the research team approach compensation?

What provisions has the team made for minimizing barriers to participation (for example, providing for food, travel, child care)?

Who is managing the budget? How are these decisions negotiated?

Conflicts of interest

Provide information relevant to actual or potential conflicts of interest (to allow the review committee to assess whether participants require information for informed consent).

What happens when the researcher's job depends on the results?

What happens when a person is both the researcher *and* the friend, peer, service provider, doctor, nurse, social worker, educator, or funder, or the like?

How will the research team appropriately acknowledge and negotiate power differentials?

Informed consent process

Describe the procedures that will be followed to obtain informed consent.

Include a copy of the information letter(s) and consent form(s).

Where written informed consent is not being obtained, explain why.

Where minors are to be included as participants, provide a copy of the assent script to be used.

What does informed consent mean for *vulnerable* populations (for example, children or people who have mental illnesses or are developmentally challenged)?

What processes does the research team have in place for gathering individual consent?

What processes does the team have in place for gathering community consent?

Are the consent processes culturally sensitive and appropriate for the populations that the team is working with?

Outcomes and results

How will the research be disseminated to academic audiences?

How will the research be disseminated to community audiences?

What are the new ways in which this research will be acted on to ensure community, policy, or social change?

(Table G.1, continued)

Ongoing reflection and partnership development	
	Please attach a copy of this partnership's agreement or memorandum of understanding, signed by all partners and describing how all partners will work together.
	What internal process evaluation mechanisms does the research team have in place?
	When the team's plans change to accommodate community concerns (as they invariably do in CBPR), how will the team communicate this to the IRB or ERB?

Source: This table and portions of the explanatory text were adapted from Flicker, Travers, Guta, McDonald, & Meagher, 2007. Adapted with the permission of Springer Publishing Company.

REFERENCES

Flicker, S., Travers, R., Guta, A., McDonald, S., and & Meagher, A. (2007). "Ethical dilemmas in community-based participatory research: Recommendations for institutional review boards. *Journal of Urban Health, 84*(4), 478–493.

Office of the Secretary, National Commission for the Protection of Human Subjects (1979). *The Belmont Report: Ethical principles and guidelines for the protection of human subjects of biomedical and behavioral research.* Retrieved May 14, 2008, from www.hhs.gov/ohrp/humansubjects/guidance/belmont.htm.

APPENDIX

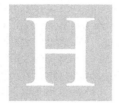

RESEARCH POLICIES, PROCESSES, AND PROTOCOL

THE NAVAJO NATION HUMAN RESEARCH REVIEW BOARD

BEVERLY BECENTI-PIGMAN, KALVIN WHITE, BEA BOWMAN, NANCY "LYNN" PALMANTEER-HOLDER, & BONNIE DURAN

This appendix presents a description of the Navajo Nation Human Research Review Board policies and procedures, which were developed in 1996 and revised in 2004 in response to an increase in requests for approval for research on the people of the Navajo Nation. Although this protocol is specific to the Navajo Nation, it illustrates the level of circumspection needed when conducting research with indigenous populations. (See Navajo Nation Human Research Review Board, 2008, for related additional documents.)

Tribal research policies and protocols are derived from the ethical principles and legal protections inherent in the rights of indigenous nations (Assembly of First Nations, 2007; Sahota, 2007). The Navajo Nation (NN) has exercised its sovereignty by vesting a tribal board with the authority to review, approve or deny, and oversee human research involving tribal members.

HISTORY AND DEVELOPMENT OF THE REVIEW BOARD

Although Navajo people have had indigenous knowledge and science for millennia (Mann, 2006), most researchers in Western academic institutions are non-Indian. The earliest health research on the Navajos was published in 1862. Most of the historical health research about Indian Country has been exploitive and unethical (Smith, 1999), has produced biased representations (Waldram, 2004), has denied Native people self-definition (Kelm, 1998), and has been a force for acculturation (Crazy Bull, 2004; Deloria, 1991). Even culturally sensitive research results often failed to improve, the health status of American Indians, though such research routinely furthered the careers of academic researchers (Jones, 2002).

In 1987, the Belmont Report on federal research regulations prompted the Indian Health Service (IHS) to establish an institutional review board (IRB) committee to implement the new regulations (Sahota, 2007). However, it was not until the 1992 to 1993 period that the IHS formed the Navajo Area Indian Health Service (NAIHS) Human Research Review Board (HRRB), comprising IHS medical professionals and staff and Navajo representatives. In 1995, Navajo community members recognized the need to transfer decision making from the NAIHS to the Navajo Nation Council and created the Navajo Nation Human Research Review Board (NNHRRB). Legislative amendments in 2002 expanded the authority of the NNHRRB to review, approve, and monitor all human research, and to ensure that the research is beneficial to the tribe and consistent with NN values.

RESEARCH PROTOCOL APPLICATION PROCESS

The principal investigator (PI) must submit a research protocol application to the HRRB two months prior to an in-person presentation. The application must include at least two *approving resolutions* from *agency councils* or *chapters* of the NN or IHS service unit health boards; support letters from CEOs of relevant NAIHS service units and NN program directors; permission from affected NN offices or agencies; other study-specific documents; and a detailed budget.

NN STANDARDS OF APPROVAL

The NN Standards of Approval go beyond typical research protections, and so we will explain them in detail before proceeding to the next step.

> *Community involvement.* How will local chapters, tribal programs, and community members be active participants in the research?
>
> *Benefits to the NN.* How will the study improve the overall health of the Navajo people?
>
> *NN authority.* Does the researcher recognize the civil jurisdiction of the NN over the research and agree to submit study results for NN approval prior to publication?
>
> *Research project description.* What are the rationale, objectives, targeted populations, methods, study design, data gathering and analysis methods, and publication plans?

Informed consent form. Researchers must attach informed consent forms and must list their institutional affiliations and list IRB and NN HRRB offices as contacts for inquiries. All adverse events must be reported to the NN HRRB office.

Certification by the principal investigator (PI). The PI must certify agreement to adhere to tribal laws and protocols when conducting research.

Once a research application is submitted, the project is scheduled for presentation and review at a monthly HRRB meeting. Upon approval, the PI provides quarterly updates on the project at HRRB meetings. When the research is completed, findings are provided to Navajo offices and programs.

REVIEW AND APPROVAL STAGES

The NNHRRB uses a twelve-phase review and approval process for all research protocols (see Table H.1). Phases I to III require researchers to verify community involvement and tribal participation in the research or approval process. In phase IV, research decisions are made. Phases V through VII provide input and support for researchers to ensure the accuracy and relevance of their work to the target population and to their respective professions. The dissemination phases, VII to XI, guarantee that the Navajo Nation will be adequately apprised of the research outcomes and findings. Finally, phase XII ensures that the NN will take possession of its own data (Assembly of First Nations, 2007; National Congress of American Indians, 2005). The Navajo Nation Office of Research holds a biennial health research conference that investigators are strongly encouraged to attend.

This is a rigorous process intended to ensure that culturally competent, ethical research is conducted. Such research is more likely than other studies to have a positive effect on both the Navajo Nation and the research scientists and institutions.

TABLE H.1 **Twelve-Phase Navajo Nation Human Research Review Board Review and Approval Processes**

Phase	NN research protocol	Description of processes
Phase I	Community partnership	PI formalizes partnerships with NN chapters, boards, health and community organizations, securing resolutions supporting the study.
Phase II	Tribal program partnership	PI partners with tribal programs, providing them with a benefits analysis of the study, and secures a support letter—for example, from the program manager of the NN Division of Health.
Phase III	Screening of research application	PI submits NNHRRB application to NN Division of Health staff for review. Application is placed on NNHRRB agenda for the next meeting. The NNHRRB has a 2-week review period.

(Table H.1, continued)

Phase IV	NNHRRB meeting and presentation	PI gives a 10-minute summary of study. After completion of inquiry, the NNHRRB meets in executive session to (1) approve, (2) request amendments, or (3) disapprove. If amendments are requested, PI can resubmit proposal for the next meeting.
Phase V	Study implementation	Within 30 days of research approval, PI will receive a 1-year, annually renewable, research permit. Quarterly and annual progress reports are required. NNHRRB vetting is requested prior to national and international presentations. This stipulation is in effect for 1 year after end of study.
Phase VI	Data analysis & preliminary findings	Upon completion of data collection, PI conducts preliminary data analysis and presents findings to NNHRRB.
Phase VII	Data work session	PI schedules a work session with partnering tribal programs, staff of the NN Division of Health, and others. A modified research report presented back to NNHRRB will include unique interpretations offered by NN partners and staff.
Phase VIII	Final report & submission for dissemination plan	PI compiles a final comprehensive report and submits all research products (materials, videos, photographs, and the like). Final report also includes a dissemination plan containing dates, times, and sites for NNHRRB approval.
Phase IX	Transfer of data to NN	PI and NNHRRB determine the NN program that will receive the data. PI then submits data to that program and trains program staff.
Phase X	Manuscript publications (optional)	PI as first author will submit a completed manuscript in an approved, publishable format. Upon its publication, PI submits three copies to the NN Division of Health.
Phase XI	Community feedback & presentations	PI will present research results to chapters, schools, health boards and facilities, tribal programs, and so forth, discussing the research findings and implications for practice.
Phase XII	Final transfer of data	All data are given to the NN Data Resource Center.

REFERENCES

Assembly of First Nations. (2007). *Ownership, control, access and possession: First Nations' inherent right to govern First Nations data.* Ottawa, ON: Author.

Crazy Bull, C. (2004). Decolonizing research: Indigenous scholars can take over the research process. *Tribal College, 16*(2), 14.

Deloria, V. (1991). Research, redskins, and reality. *American Indian Quarterly, 15*(4), 457–468.

Jones, D. S. (2002). The health care experiments at Many Farms: The Navajo, tuberculosis, and the limits of modern medicine, 1952–1962. *Bulletin of the History of Medicine, 76*(4), 749–790.

Kelm, M.-E. (1998). *Colonizing bodies: Aboriginal health and healing in British Columbia, 1900–50.* Vancouver, BC: UBC Press.

Mann, C. C. (2006). *1491: New revelations of the Americas before Columbus.* New York: Vintage Books.

National Congress of American Indians. (2005). *Tribal ownership of health-related data* (Resolution TUL-05–059). Washington, DC: Author.

Navajo Nation Human Research Review Board. (2008). [Home page]. Retrieved May 14, 2008, from http://www.nnhrrb.navajo.org.

Sahota, P. C. (2007). *Research regulation in American Indian/Alaska Native communities: Policy and practice considerations.* Washington, DC: National Congress of American Indians, Policy Research Center.

Smith, L. T. (1999). *Decolonizing methodologies: Research and indigenous peoples.* New York: Zed Books.

Waldram, J. B. (2004). *Revenge of the Windigo: The construction of the mind and mental health of North American aboriginal peoples.* Toronto: University of Toronto Press.

APPENDIX

UNDOING RACISM TRAINING AS A FOUNDATION FOR TEAM BUILDING IN CBPR

ROBERT E. ARONSON, MICHAEL A. YONAS, NORA JONES,
NETTIE COAD, & EUGENIA ENG

Community-based participatory research (CBPR) is increasingly used to study and address racial and ethnic disparities in health and health care. The threats to partnering effectively in investigations of the health effects arising from inequities are numerous, however, because the genesis and the legacy of racism in the United States have generated conditions antagonistic to forming partnerships between academic institutions and many communities. Partnerships may break down because issues of trust, communication, and culture make it difficult to develop a shared vision and action plans as well as to mobilize and sustain broad community involvement over time in the research enterprise.

Note: Portions of this appendix are adapted from "The Art and Science of Integrating Undoing Racism with CBPR: Challenges of Pursuing NIH Funding to Investigate Cancer Care and Racial Equity," by M.A. Yonas, N. Jones, E. Eng, A. I. Vines, R. E. Aronson, D. M. Griffith, et al., 2006. *Journal of Urban Health, 83*(6), pp. 1004–1012. Adapted with the permission of the New York Academy of Medicine.

Given these historical and contemporary realities, openly addressing racism is an essential first step in the development of partnerships for CBPR that can be effective in seeking to understand and eliminate racial disparities in health and health care. In this appendix we briefly describe the importance of integrating the principles and skills of *undoing racism training,* or *antiracism training,* with those of CBPR, and then highlight our experience with the training and its utility in our North Carolina CBPR partnership's successful efforts to prepare a proposal for the National Institutes of Health (NIH) to study and address race-based disparities in breast cancer care (Yonas et al., 2006). We conclude by offering recommendations for other partnerships interested in exploring how training in undoing racism can be combined with CBPR to build and maintain strong CBPR collaborations focused on eliminating racial and ethnic health disparities.

WHAT IS UNDOING RACISM TRAINING?

Anti-racism training engages people in a process of understanding the origins of the concept of race in the United States, the current experience and effects of ongoing racism, and how power is used to the advantage of some and the disadvantage of others based on race. Such training efforts seek to develop a cadre of leaders, and also organizations and partnerships, who can be effective organizers for social justice and social change in their communities. This training can also benefit academically trained researchers and their community partners as they work to address racism head on in developing respectful and authentic partnerships.

The People's Institute for Survival and Beyond (2006), an organization "dedicated to training and organizing with intelligence and integrity—with values and vision" offers what is arguably the best known antiracism training. The institute's Undoing Racism™/ Community Organizing workshops with follow up technical assistance begin with a two-and-one-half-day workshop that challenges participants to analyze the social forces that create disparities and hinder racial equity. The multiple learning outcomes established by the institute address abilities particularly important to building and maintaining CBPR partnerships:

- Develop a common definition of racism and an understanding of its different forms: individual, institutional, linguistic, and cultural;
- Develop a common language and analysis for examining racism in the United States;
- Understand one's own connection to institutional racism and its impact on his/her work;
- Understand the historical context for how racial classifications in the United States came to be and how and why they are maintained;
- Understand why people are poor and the role of institutions in exacerbating institutional racism, particularly for people and communities of color;
- Understand the historical context for how U.S. institutions came to be and who they have been designed to serve;
- Develop awareness and understanding about ways to begin Undoing Racism [People's Institute for Survival and Beyond, 2006].

THE NEED FOR ANTIRACISM TRAINING IN CBPR

CBPR efforts that seek to eliminate racial and ethnic disparities in health may find Undoing Racism workshops useful for at least two reasons. They provide a framework for understanding racism that is often missing in health disparities research and at the same time help to create conditions that make effective cross cultural partnerships possible.

Although there is growing recognition that racism in its various forms has contributed to unequal health care treatment across races (Smedley, Stith, & Nelson, Institute of Medicine, 2003) and to inequalities in health status (Williams, Neighbors, & Jackson, 2003; Krieger, 2003), few frameworks for understanding how racism contributes to health disparities appear in the literature (Krieger, 2003; Harrell, Hall, & Taliaferro, 2003). Personal beliefs and prejudices as well as negative experiences and discomfort with the topic itself have made the discussion of race and racism exceedingly difficult. Such dialogue, however, is critical to moving forward, and particularly in CBPR, in which partnership makeup often inadvertently reflects the patterns of race, power, and privilege in the larger society (see Chapter Five).

Facilitated by trained antiracism community organizers, Undoing Racism workshops facilitate such critical dialogue and are offered to ten to fifteen groups across the country each month. Before planning a workshop, a CBPR partnership must first recognize that a need exists, and that the training will help partners move forward on addressing their concerns. The partnership must also consider whom to invite to the training, being sure to reflect the diversity of the community and the partnership and to include key gatekeepers of institutions and organizations that serve the community.

INSIDE AN UNDOING RACISM WORKSHOP

The workshop training seeks to create an environment in which openness, self-reflection, and healing can occur. Given participants' diversity of background and experience, this environment is both essential and difficult to achieve. Throughout the training, participants sit in a circle, and all attendees are urged to actively participate in every aspect of the training. At the beginning of the two-and-one-half-day experience, participants create and commit to a set of guidelines and principles for the interactions within the group, focusing on such issues as respect, honesty and openness, and making a commitment to listen and maintain confidentiality. Appreciating the importance of conflict in relationship building and facilitating understanding is also highlighted and embraced.

The workshop includes large-group discussions and small-group working sessions. One crucial component is the *power analysis,* which explains how institutions such as banks, insurance companies, schools, public housing agencies, police departments, and so forth can disempower people who live in low-income communities by denying them the power to control their own lives. Although these institutions function within a community, they are primarily accountable to interests outside the community and not to the people they serve. Residents rarely share in the decision-making policies, and therefore programs and services often fail to address community needs. Undoing Racism training teaches that people, regardless of race, cannot solve a problem as long as they have the same consciousness that created that problem in the first place.

The training also presents fundamental definitions of race, prejudice, racism, and internalized racial oppression (the latter occurs when members of a stigmatized group devalue and accept the stereotypes about their race). Participants hold in-depth discussions about racial classifications and the different types of racism and culture, with the aim of fostering a common language as a basis for learning and change. Following the workshop, participants engage in *cultural sharing,* an activity in which they share stories about their families or another aspect of their personal histories over several weeks. Because cultural sharing comes at the conclusion of this two-and-one-half-day workshop, participants tend to be reflective at this point, and have come to realize how deeply racism has affected everyone. Finally, because a goal of the training is to equip a cadre of social justice leaders, the trainers help the participants to generate a list of the qualities of a good organizer.

OUR EXPERIENCE

Our experience, as the Greensboro Health Disparities Collaborative (GHDC), in combining CBPR with an Undoing Racism workshop has been described by Yonas et al. (2006). Briefly, thirty-five members of our community-academic partnership (twelve medical or academic professionals and twenty-three community members) undertook the training in conjunction with the partnership's efforts to write an NIH grant proposal for a breast cancer disparities research project. After completing the full training, these participants were then engaged in four educational and five discussion sessions over the following six months.

While the initial Undoing Racism/Community Organizing workshop provided an essential primary step, it is naive to believe that participation in a single workshop could be sufficient to set the stage for an effective partnership. The doubts and distrust that communities have about research institutions are so deep and pervasive that constant monitoring, dialogue, and renewal are needed if ongoing collaboration is to be sustained. By combining antiracism training with the principles of CBPR (Israel et al., 1998; see also Chapter Three), however, the GHDC partners were able to establish shared principles that anticipated and even embraced conflict.

Following the workshop the GHDC continued the collaborative learning process through exploring the dynamics of institutional culture, power, and collaboration. A system of accountability and trust was established within the GHDC by developing a *full value contract,* using a consensus process. The contract defines ownership of the research findings, protects the integrity of the collaborative process, and delineates a process for negotiating conflict and continued cultivation of the interpersonal relationships within the group.

With this foundation the GHDC partners established expectations for working together to develop an NIH research proposal. Interdisciplinary subgroups were formed to work on key sections of the proposal (research question, methodology, data analysis, budget, and so forth). On average, in each subgroup two-thirds of the members were from the community and one-third of the members were from an academic or other outside institution. This process involved sixteen meetings over a four-month period and used consensus building as the sole means of decision making. Consistent with the earlier Undoing Racism workshop training, this process accommodated and negotiated conflict, which was intense, emotional, passionate, and warranted.

The GHDC's work in combining antiracism training with CBPR greatly contributed to its efforts to prepare a successful grant application to NIH's National Cancer Institute that in turn enabled GHDC to begin a CBPR study of racial disparities in breast cancer care. The GHDC remains committed to the principles of undoing racism training and CBPR and to constructive responses to conflict and has reflected these in its subsequent work in creating by-laws, electing officers to guide the work of the GHDC, and other activities. As the GHDC grows and changes, it continues to incorporate new members. Part of the process of joining includes an orientation to CBPR and the completion of an Undoing Racism/Community Organizing workshop.

Our experience strongly suggests that the Undoing Racism workshop training may benefit other CBPR partnerships committed to studying and addressing race-based health disparities. To take best advantage of such a training experience, we recommend that it be incorporated at the very beginning of partnership formation and that a diversity of key stakeholders be invited, with the majority being community members involved in the partnership. It is important that partnerships do not enter this process naively or without a steadfast commitment to seeing it through. The terrain is rough, but trust and real change will be achieved only when the parties are committed to working through the conflicts that will occur.

REFERENCES

Harrell, J. P., Hall, S., & Taliaferro, J. (2003). Physiological responses to racism and discrimination: An assessment of the evidence. *American Journal of Public Health, 93*(2), 243–248.

Israel, B. A,. Shultz, A. J., Parker, E. A., & Becker, A. B. (1998). Review of community-based research: Assessing partnership approaches to improve public health. *Annual Review of Public Health, 19,* 173–202.

Krieger, N. (2003). Does racism harm health? Did child abuse exist before 1962? On explicit questions, critical science, and current controversies: An ecosocial perspective. *American Journal of Public Health, 93*(2), 194–199.

People's Institute for Survival and Beyond. (2006). [Home page]. Retrieved June 28, 2007, from http://www.pisab.org.

Smedley, B. D., Stith, A. Y., & Nelson, A. R. (Eds.), Institute of Medicine. (2003). *Unequal treatment: Confronting racial and ethnic disparities in health care.* Washington, DC: National Academies Press.

Williams, D. R., Neighbors, H. W., & Jackson, J. S. (2003). Racial/ethnic discrimination and health: Findings from community studies. *American Journal of Public Health, 93*(2), 200–208.

Yonas, M. A., Jones, N., Eng, E., Vines, A. I., Aronson, R. E., Griffith, D. M., et al. (2006). The art and science of integrating undoing racism with CBPR: Challenges of pursuing NIH funding to investigate cancer care and racial equity. *Journal of Urban Health, 83*(6), 1004–1012.

APPENDIX

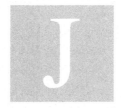

RISK MAPPING AS A TOOL FOR CBPR AND ORGANIZING

MARIANNE P. BROWN

The community members, all from the same neighborhood, gather around a large sheet of paper taped to the wall. One of them is creating a map of the neighborhood and marking where certain heath and safety hazards are. The others are giving guidance—"Don't forget the diesel exhaust from the idling trucks outside the frozen food plant." "Remember the broken concrete on the sidewalk in front of the corner store." "There's noise from the freeway that goes right by the elementary school."

This is what happens when people get together to develop a *risk map*—a visual representation of areas where there are hazards that could result in injury, illness, or even

Note: Adapted from "Worker Risk Mapping: An Education-for-Action Approach," by M. P. Brown, 1995. *New Solutions,* 5(2), 1995, pp. 22–30. Copyright 1995. Adapted with the permission of Marianne P. Brown.

death. This appendix summarizes the risk map method, an approach to action-oriented research and organizing that is increasingly being used to improve health and safety conditions in communities and workplaces around the United States.

WHY MAKE RISK MAPS?

The risk map method lends itself to community-based participatory research (CBPR) for several reasons:

- It draws on people's knowledge and insights about their community.
- It helps people become active investigators.
- It incorporates experiential learning principles and offers a new method for involvement of study subjects.
- It is effective in a variety of settings.

Draw on Community Knowledge and Insight

In the United States the people who assess community environmental hazards, recommend control measures, and see that they are implemented are typically health professionals—safety engineers, industrial hygienists, epidemiologists, physicians, nurses. These professionals use terms and concepts not commonly understood by laypersons, such as *dose-response, parts per million, ambient air levels, relative risk, particulates,* and *microns.* Consequently, their inspection reports, studies, and presentations are often written in a scientific jargon that is unclear to many who could benefit from the information provided. The risk map method breaks from this traditional approach by acknowledging the vital contributions that people who might potentially be exposed to environmental hazards can make and by drawing on their knowledge when they develop risk maps based on their everyday experiences.

Health professionals use a "scientific approach" when they look at environmental hazards, relying heavily on quantitative measures to establish possible risks to humans. For example, industrial hygienists measure the levels of formaldehyde vapor in the air and then compare the results with what are considered acceptable levels previously established by a governmental agency through a process that is both scientific and political. Although such quantitative approaches are important, they need to be supplemented by the perceptions of community groups who can share vital information concerning when and where they experience irritation, smell odors, see dust. In this way the worst exposure periods can be pinpointed. By systematically combining the knowledge of community members with the expertise of outside professionals, a more complete picture of the hazards can be visualized.

Help People Become Active Investigators

In the risk map method, the people doing the mapping are both the investigators and the subjects of the investigation. The standard approach used in a work setting is described by Jorge Mujica (1992): "The participatory method draws on the established organization of workers in the workplace. For management purposes, workers are classified by the duties they perform, such as maintenance workers in a plant, assembly workers on an assembly line, and word processors in an office. By virtue of their shared work, these employees also share work hazards. This participatory method utilizes these existing groupings by bringing together these subgroups to both actively assess specific hazards and take action to correct them" (p. 767).

Incorporate Experiential Learning and Involve Study Subjects

The risk map method is visual. People are asked to picture their neighborhood and then fill out a questionnaire or report on the hazards they know about. They are then asked to draw the hazards so that their neighbors can also see them. This method can be a particularly effective tool for those who have limited literacy or English reading or speaking skills.

The risk map method can also help people learn to function effectively in a task-based group. This in turn builds their confidence and shows them they can directly control aspects of their lives—and that environmental conditions in their community that could affect their health are not solely the purview of health and safety professionals. Such realizations can create a sense of ownership over such problems while also helping people see the collective, rather than individual, nature of the problems. Finally, in the process of prioritizing the problems to work on, participants gain perspective so that the small concerns of a few do not dominate.

Be Effective in a Variety of Settings

The risk map method evolved out of the experiences of workers in an auto plant in Italy in the early 1960s, who identified workplace hazards by drawing on a blueprint of the factory circles of different colors and sizes indicating where the hazards were located. A group of scientists then verified the practical evidence. Since that time, versions of this approach have been used in a variety of settings around the world. In the United States, these settings have included state health departments, companies, labor unions, university labor centers, and community-based organizations (see Chapter Nine).

LESSONS FOR CBPR RESEARCHERS AND ORGANIZERS

Researchers who have used risk mapping as part of a CBPR project or with community-organizing efforts have found it effective for a variety of reasons. First and foremost, it is an approach people immediately respond to in a positive way. Risk mapping can be a confidence-building exercise and can also function as an immediate needs assessment tool. The outside researcher in a CBPR effort can see what the community members perceive the hazards to be and can use this information in subsequent work with the community to determine the specific health issue or issues to be studied. The risk map method also provides participants with a good way to learn about a neighborhood without asking a lot of questions.

HOW TO MAKE A RISK MAP

Risk mapping is a technique to obtain information about hazards in the community or workplace. It can be useful in identifying hazards and developing priority issues and long-range goals. Risk mapping can be used as a way to visually portray the results of a previously conducted survey. Members of a group can engage in it at a group meeting.

To make a risk map, follow these steps:

1. On a very large piece of paper, draw a picture of your neighborhood or community. Be sure to draw everything—streets and alleys; buildings such as homes, businesses, schools, and factories; parks; and all the other features of your neighborhood. For the workplace, draw a picture of the area where you spend most of your time. Be sure to draw everything—furniture, machinery, equipment, and tools.

2. Label everything on your drawing.

3. With other community members or workers, draw any vehicular activity in your neighborhood and other mobile sources of hazards; draw stick figures where people live, work, go to school, or play. If it's a workplace, draw the flow of production and put stick figures where people work.

4. Mark the locations of the hazards, using colored circles:

   Use green for physical safety hazards such as noise, heat or cold, leaks, slippery floors, unguarded equipment, radiation, and electrical hazards.

   Use red for chemical hazards such as dust, vapors, fumes, gases, and mists.

   Use blue for hazards related to physical exertion or bad ergonomics, which can cause musculoskeletal injuries.

   Use purple for hazards associated with work-related stress, such as lack of training, inadequate supervision, or too much overtime.

5. List hazards that would be simple to correct.

6. List items that require more information and investigation.

7. List priorities for research or change.

On the downside, however, risk mapping takes a considerable amount of time. It takes about fifteen minutes for the map to be drawn and about twenty minutes for each individual or small group to explain its map. The outside researcher or organizer describes the exercise, provides the writing materials, and most important, asks probing questions about the maps. The answers to these questions can then assist the outside researcher or group in working with the community to further identify hazards and prioritize problems to form the basis of further action-oriented research.

Finally, and consistent with CBPR's emphasis on balancing research and action (Hall, 1981; Israel, Schulz, Parker, & Becker, 1998; Israel, Eng, Schulz, & Parker, 2005), there must be a commitment to follow through on the risk mapping effort. As noted, in CBPR this follow-up typically consists of a collaborative effort to identify specific problem areas for further study, conduct the research, and use the results as the basis of determining and implementing concrete action strategies to bring about change. For both organizers and partners in a CBPR project, the risk map serves as a powerful and evolving record of the hazards on which the group wants to work. When subsequent research and action take place and improvements in living or working conditions result, the risk map can further stand as a visual testimony of the participants' success.

REFERENCES

Hall, B. L. (1981). Participatory research, popular knowledge, and power: A personal reflection. *Convergence, 14*(3), 6–19.

Israel, B. A., Eng, E., Schulz, A. J., & Parker, E. A. (2005). Introduction to methods in community-based participatory research. In B. A. Israel, E. Eng, A. J. Schulz, & E. A. Parker (Eds.), *Methods in community-based participatory research for health* (pp. 3–26). San Francisco: Jossey-Bass.

Israel, B. A., Schulz, A. J., Parker, E. A., & Becker, A. B. (1998). Review of community-based research: Assessing partnership approaches to improve public health. *Annual Review of Public Health, 19,* 173–202.

Mujica, J. (1992). Coloring the hazards: Risk maps, research, and education to fight health hazards. *American Journal of Industrial Medicine, 22,* 767–770.

APPENDIX

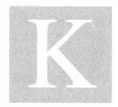

USING CBPR TO PROMOTE POLICY CHANGE

EXERCISES AND ONLINE RESOURCES

**CASSANDRA RITAS, MEREDITH MINKLER,
ANGELA NI, & HELEN ANN HALPIN**

This set of exercises is designed for small groups. It is divided into five parts, and each part may be used independently of the others, depending on the emphasis of the course, community partnership, or other group participating in the exercise. However, to do exercises 2 through 4 in part 1, you will need to decide in advance on the real or hypothetical issue or problem area and on the policy objective on which the group will be working.

Each part of the set is designed to take from thirty to forty minutes. At the conclusion of each of the first three parts, additional time can fruitfully be spent having participants

Note: The authors are grateful to the Policy Project (www.policyproject.org) and PolicyLink (www.policylink.org) for their excellent work in this area, which in turn stimulated our thinking in the development of these exercises.

reflect on and share some of the insights they gained from the exercises so far. Sample questions to aid in this process are provided. The final exercise is intended to be staged in front of the whole group and requires the completion of one of the small-group projects in advance.

For all parts of this set of exercises, begin by breaking into small groups around common issue areas (for example, reproductive rights, HIV/AIDS, environmental justice, affordable housing). Then have participants follow the instructions given here.

Part 1: Defining the Policy Objective (30 minutes)

1. Brainstorm the problems involved in your issue area.

2. From this list choose *the single problem* you want to address. Consider the magnitude of each problem (that is, how many are affected and how adversely?) in making your choice.

3. Brainstorm possible *solutions* to the identified problem.

4. Decide on a *policy objective*. (Note that this can be getting a new or existing policy implemented or repealed.) This objective is framed as the *solution* (or partial solution) to your problem, so before making a final decision be sure to discuss briefly the political viability and potential unintended consequences of the top two to three policy objectives you are considering.

Questions for reflection: What was the most difficult part of this exercise? Why? What criteria were most helpful in coming up with your policy objective? If unintended consequences were identified, how did they influence your thinking?

Part 2: Power Mapping: Defining Policymakers and Other Key Players (40 minutes)

Before beginning, select the *specific change* you want to bring about (it must be one amenable to a policy solution) and select one *policy objective* you hope to achieve in order to help effect this change.

1. Identify the policy *target* or *targets:* the individuals and organizations with the power to make a particular change happen.

2. Identify the other *key players* in this situation: the individuals, organizations, or in some cases communities that may be affected by the problem or policy or that have the potential to influence the situation. Keep in mind that as change becomes imminent, many people will be drawn into the issue who did not know or care about it before. Try to anticipate who might be in this category.

3. On a sheet of paper with your policy objective stated at the top, label the left side *supporters,* the middle undecided, and the right side *opposition*. Onto this page place your *targets* (depicted as circles) and *key players* (squares), according to where they fall along the spectrum. As illustrated in Figure K.1, for visual reference use larger squares and circles to indicate more powerful targets and players and smaller squares and circles to indicate weaker ones.

Remember that many considerations go into decisions about relative power (depicted in the size of the squares or circles), among them the target's or player's scope (size), resources (staff, money, lobbyists), skills, and access, and also how

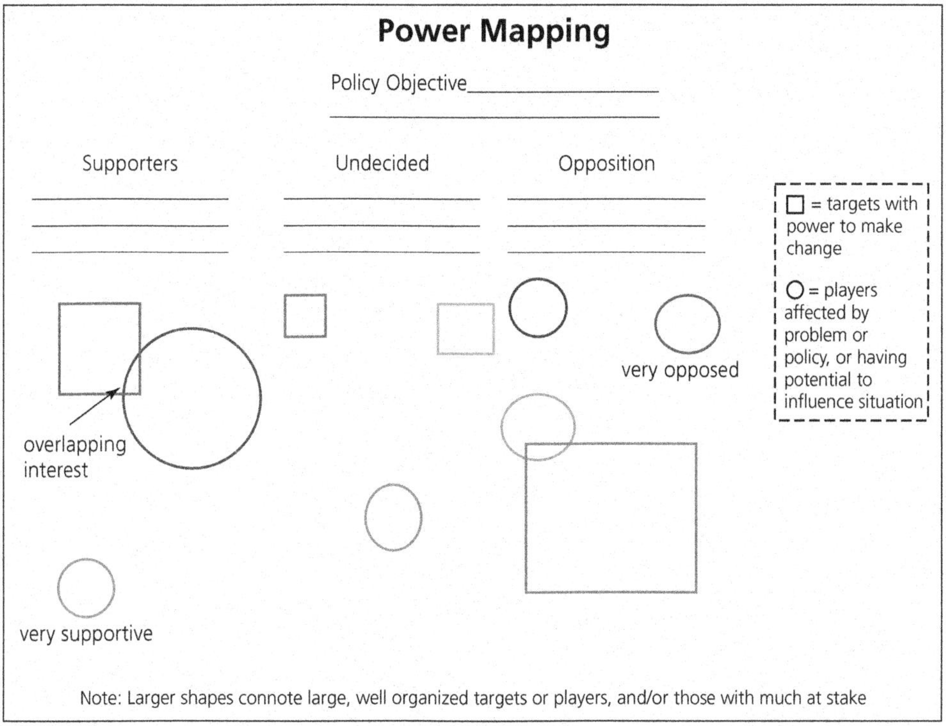

Power Mapping

Policy Objective_____

_____

| Supporters | Undecided | Opposition |

□ = targets with power to make change

○ = players affected by problem or policy, or having potential to influence situation

very opposed

overlapping interest

very supportive

Note: Larger shapes connote large, well organized targets or players, and/or those with much at stake

FIGURE K.1 *Power Mapping*

intensely the issue affects each target or player (is it seen, for example, as a burning issue or as a tangential concern?). A small group that cares deeply about an issue and has great resources and organization may be more effective as a player than a larger group that has few resources at its disposal, is poorly organized, or experiences the issue less intensely. Where possible, allow the circles and squares to overlap where interests overlap (this is not always feasible, however, because some supporters may share interests with the opposition).

4. Choose the three most important individuals and organizations to influence. Consider the following when making your choices:

▪ Is it more important now to strengthen your allies, persuade those who are neutral, or to weaken the opposition?

▪ Is it time to approach a target, or to work with key players?

Questions for reflection: For the issue you have chosen to examine, was it easier to identify potential supporters or sources of opposition? Why? Were there any surprises when you considered potential overlapping interests among targets and players? If your group decided that the time was right to approach a key target or a key player, what *next steps* might this approach usefully entail?

Part 3: Force-Field Analysis: Defining Points of Persuasion (30 minutes)

1. At the top center of a sheet of paper write the name of the *first policy target* (individual, organization, or community) you want to influence. Underneath, draw three columns and label them "Forces/Individuals/Factors in Our Favor," "Forces/Individuals/Factors Against Us," and "Strategies to Promote Change."

2. Fill in the first two columns, using one or more plus signs (+) to indicate the relative strength of each supporting or resisting force, individual, or factor you list.

3. Considering the list of forces, individuals, and factors against you and in your favor, come up with a list of five or more potential *strategies* for influencing the targeted group or individual.

4. Choose the two to three best strategies to move your issue forward. Consider the following questions when making your strategy choice:

    ■ Which strategies seem the most productive across multiple targets and key players?
    ■ Will these strategies anger potential or existing allies?
    ■ Will these strategies weaken the position of existing allies?
    ■ Could these strategies increase the opposition of a player who was once neutral?

Part 4: Group Homework

Write a one- to two-page policy brief that includes your concrete recommendations for change. This will require researching the topic outside of your meetings or your class to come up with the best solution. The group will need to meet to brainstorm the most effective and persuasive way to present the information.

The brief should include

■ The policy goal
■ A definition of the problem and the scope of the problem
■ Current policies affecting the problem
■ Past policies and their effects
■ A short but specific presentation of potential solutions
■ An argument for the solution(s) that the group is advocating

Part 5: Mock-Legislative Visit (30 minutes per group, including feedback)

One group presents its policy brief and proposed changes to another group, whose members take the roles of a legislator and her aides. This exercise can be modified if necessary, depending on the audience chosen by the group for its brief. (For example, group members could pretend they are going door to door in the community or meeting with hospital administrators or health department officials.) The larger group or full class serves as the audience and at the end offers reflections on the small group's performance. The objective of this exercise is for people to get experience in dealing with the kind of commonsense, and occasionally adversarial, questions that would likely be encountered if this were an actual change campaign. *The group should be prepared to discuss the implementation of its plan and that plan's potential unintended consequences and to answer questions about the fiscal implications and political viability of any proposal(s) presented.*

SELECTED ONLINE TOOLS FOR WORKING TO EFFECT POLICY CHANGE

Networking for Policy Change: An Advocacy Training Manual, produced by POLICY Project, 1999, www.policyproject.com.

Advocating for Change, an online manual produced by PolicyLink, n.d., http://www. policylink.org/AdvocatingForChange.

Speaking Truth, Creating Power: A Guide to Policy Work for Community Based Participatory Research Practitioners, by C. Ritas, 2003, http://futurehealth.ucsf.edu/pdf_files/ Ritas.pdf.

The Community Tool Box, an Internet-based support for participatory evaluation produced by Work Group for Community Health and Development, at the University of Kansas, 2008, http://ctb.ku.edu. (See also Appendix D.)

The Praxis Project, offers an information resource center and other support, www. thepraxisproject.org.

APPENDIX

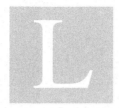

SELECTED CENTERS AND OTHER RESOURCES FOR PARTICIPATORY RESEARCH IN NORTH AMERICA

MEREDITH MINKLER, NINA WALLERSTEIN,
ANGELA NI, & ROSANNA TRAN

The dramatic increase in community-based participatory research is reflected in part in the rapidly growing number of networks and centers engaged in or supporting those who engage in such work. What follows is a partial list of local, regional, national, and international resources in the United States and Canada. Many other excellent centers and networks exist, and the reader is encouraged to use this list as a jumping-off point for a fuller exploration.

NATIONAL AND INTERNATIONAL CENTERS AND NETWORKS HEADQUARTERED IN THE UNITED STATES AND CANADA

Catalyst Centre
720 Bathurst Street
Toronto, ON M5S 2R4
Phone: (416) 516–9546
E-mail: catalystcentre@web.ca
Web: http://www.catalystcentre.ca
Contact: Matt Adams

Community-Based Public Health Caucus
American Public Health Association
c/o School of Public Health
University of Michigan
2649B Crossroads Building
109 South Observatory
Ann Arbor, MI 48109
Phone: (734) 936–0936
E-mail: cbphcaucus@umich.edu
Web: http://www.sph.umich.edu/cbph/caucus/index.html
Contact: Toby Citrin
tcitrin@umich.edu

Community-Campus Partnerships for Health
8701 Watertown Plank Road
Milwaukee, WI 53226–0509
E-mail: maurana@mcw.edu
Web: www.ccph.info
Contact: Cheryl Maurana, Executive Director

Community Research Project
The Bonner Foundation
10 Mercer Street
Princeton, NJ 08540
Phone: (609) 924–6663
E-mail: rhackett@bonner.org
Web: http://www.bonner.org/campus/cbr/home.htm
Contact: Robert Hackett, Vice President

Highlander Research and Education Center
1959 Highlander Way
New Market, TN 37820
Phone: (865) 933–3443
E-mail: hrec@highlandercenter.org
Web: http://www.highlandercenter.org
Contact: Kristi Coleman, Office Manager

International Council for Adult Education
720 Bathurst Street, Suite 500
Toronto, ON M5S 2R4
Phone: (416) 588–1211
E-mail: icae@icae.ca
Web: http://www.unesco.org/education/aladin/members/49.htm
Contact: Eva Kupidura, Information and Communications Coordinator

Institute for People's Education and Action
c/o Cobscook Community Learning Center
10 Commissary Point Road
Lubec, ME 04652
Contact: Alan Furth, Executive Director
Phone: (207) 733–2233
E-mail: alan@thecclc.org
Web: www.thecclc.org

Kellogg Health Scholars Program, Community Track
National Program Office
School of Public Health
University of Michigan
2657 Crossroads Building
109 Observatory Street
Ann Arbor, MI 48109
Phone: (734) 647–3065
E-mail: chsp@umich.edu
Web: http://www.sph.umich.edu/chsp
Contact: Saundra Bailey, Program Administrator

National Network for Aboriginal Mental Health Researchers
Institute of Community and Family Psychiatry
Sir Mortimer B Davis-Jewish General Hospital
4333 Cote Ste Catherine Road
Montreal, QB H3T 1E4
Phone: (514) 340–8222 x5244
E-mail: laurence.kirmayer@mcgill.ca
Web: http://www.mcgill.ca/namhr
Contact: Lawrence Kirmayer

National Network on Environments and Women's Health
c/o Centre for Health Studies
York University
4700 Keele Street
Toronto, ON M3J 1P3
Phone: (416) 736–5941
E-mail: nnewh1@yorku.ca
Web: http://www.yorku.ca/nnewh

Participatory Development Forum
207 Bank Street, Suite 202
Ottawa, ON K2P 2N2
Phone: (613) 792–1006
E-mail: pdforum@pdforum.org
Web: http://www.pdforum.org

Society for Community Research and Action
Division 27 of the American Psychological Association
16 Sconticut Neck Road, #290
Fairhaven, MA 02719
Phone: (508) 441–2471
E-mail: SCRA@telepath.com
Web: office@scra27.org
Contact: Janet Singer

U.S. LOCAL AND REGIONAL CENTERS

Action Research Center
University of Cincinnati
Edwards One
45–51 Corry Road
Cincinnati, OH 45221
E-mail: mary.brydon-miller@uc.edu
Web: http://www.uc.edu/arc

Applied Research Center
900 Alice Street, Suite 400
Oakland, CA 94607
Phone: (510) 653–3415
E-mail: arc@arc.org
Web: http://www.arc.org
Contact: Sonia Peña, Associate Director

Center for AIDS Prevention Studies (CAPS)
University of California, San Francisco
50 Beale Street, Suite 1300
San Francisco, CA 94105
Phone: (415) 597–9100
E-mail: skegeles@psg.ucsf.edu
Web: http://www.caps.ucsf.edu
Contact: Susan Kegeles, Co-Director

Center for Community Partnerships
University of Pennsylvania
133 South 36th Street, Room 519
Philadelphia, PA 19104
Phone: (215) 898–5351
Fax: (215) 573–2799
E-mail: weeks@pobox.upenn.edu or harkavy@pobox.upenn.edu
Web: http://www.upenn.edu/ccp
Contact: Ian Harkavy, Associate Vice President and Founding Director

Center for Community and Urban Health
Hunter College, City University of New York
425 East 25th Street, 8th Floor
New York, NY 10010
Phone: (212) 481–4284
E-mail: Meredith.halpern@hunter.cuny.edu
Web: http://www.hunter.cuny.edu/schoolhp/centers/comm_urb/index.htm
Contact: Shawn McGinniss, Research Assistant, Trainer, and Administrative Coordinator
shawn.mcginniss@hunter.cuny.edu

Center for Health, Environment and Justice
PO Box 6806
Falls Church, VA 22040
Phone: (703) 237–2249
E-mail: chej@chej.org
Web: http://www.chej.org
Contact: Barbara Sullivan

Center for Research on Women
University of Memphis
337 Clement Hall
Memphis, TN 38512
Phone: (901) 678–2770
Fax: (901) 678–3652
E-mail: CROW@memphis.edu
Web: http://cas.memphis.edu/isc/crow
Contact: Phyllis Betts, Steering Committee Member

Center for Urban Epidemiological Studies
New York Academy of Medicine
1216 Fifth Avenue
New York, NY 10029
Phone: (212) 822–7382
E-mail: dvlahov@nyam.org
Web site: http://www.nyam.org/initiatives/cues.shtml
Contact: Dr. David Vlahov, Director

Center for Urban and Regional Affairs
330 HHH Center
301 19th Avenue S
Minneapolis, MN 55455
Phone: (612) 625–1551
Web: www.cura.umn.edu

Center for Urban Research and Learning
Loyola University Chicago
820 North Michigan Avenue, 10th Floor
Chicago, IL 60611
Phone: (312) 915–7760
E-mail: curlweb@luc.edu
Web: http://www.luc.edu/curl
Contact: Philip Nyden, Director
pnyden@luc.edu

College of Public and Community Service
University of Massachusetts, Boston
Wheatley, 4th Floor
100 Morissey Boulevard
Boston, MA 02124
Phone: (617) 287–5000
E-mail: marie.kennedy@umb.edu
Web: http://www.umb.edu/academics/cpcs
Contact: Marie Kennedy

Datacenter
1904 Franklin Street, Suite 900
Oakland, CA 94612
Phone: (510) 835–4692, x305
E-mail: datacenter@datacenter.org
Web: http://www.datacenter.org
Contact: Celia Davis

Detroit Community-Academic Urban Research Center
School of Public Health and Medical Sciences
University of Michigan
1420 Washington Heights
Ann Arbor, MI 48109
Phone: (734) 764–5171
E-mail: rojomcg@umich.edu
Web: http://www.sph.umich.edu/urc
Contact: Robert J. McGranaghan, Project Manager

Harlem Health Promotion Center
Mailman School of Public Health
Columbia University
215 West 125th Street, Ground Floor
New York, NY 10027
Phone: (646) 284–9777
E-mail: staff@healthyharlem.org
Web: http://www.healthyharlem.org
Contact: Nydia Rodriguez, Administrative Assistant

Health Research for Action Center
2140 Shattuck Avenue, 10th Floor
Berkeley, CA 94704
Phone: (510) 643–9543
www.uchealthaction.org
E-mail: healthaction@berkeley.edu
Contacts: Linda Neuhauser, Co-Principal Investigator and Susan Ivey, Director of
Research

Institute for Community Research
2 Hartford Square West, Suite 100
146 Wyllys Street
Hartford, CT 06106
Phone: (860) 278–2044
Fax: (860) 278–2141
E-mail: info@icrweb.org
Web: http://www.incommunityresearch.org
Contact: Jean J. Schensul, Senior Scientist and Founding Director

Poverty and Race Research Action Council
1015 15th Street NW, Suite 400
Washington, DC 20005
Phone: (202) 906–8023
Fax: (202) 842–2885
E-mail: info@prrac.org
Web: http://www.prrac.org
Contact: Chester Hartman, Director of Research

Project South
Institute for the Elimination of Poverty and Genocide
9 Gammon Avenue SW
Atlanta, GA 30315
Phone: (404) 622–0602
Fax: (404) 622–6618
E-mail: emery@projectsouth.org
Web: http://www.projectsouth.org
Contact: Emery Wright, Program Director

Southern Regional Council
1201 W. Peachtree Street NE, Suite 2000
Atlanta, GA 30309
Phone: (404) 522–8764
Fax: (404) 522–8791
E-mail: hsenghor@southerncouncil.org
Web: http://www.southerncouncil.org
Contact: Hiewet Senghor, Executive Director

Sustainable Urban Neighborhoods
Urban Studies Institute
University of Louisville
426 West Bloom Street
Louisville, KY 40208
Phone: (502) 852–8557
Fax: (502) 852–4558
E-mail: a0mulu01@gwise.louisville.edu
Web: http://www.louisville.edu/org/sun
Contact: John Gilderbloom

CANADIAN LOCAL AND REGIONAL CENTERS

Aboriginal Capacity and Developmental Research Environments
University of British Columbia
College of Health Disciplines
Institute for Aboriginal Health Instructional Resources Centre
429–2194 Health Sciences Mall
Vancouver, BC V6T 1Z3
Phone: (613) 827–5464
E-mail: lindaday@interchange.ubc.ca
Web: http://www.health-disciplines.ubc.ca/iah/acadre
Contact: Linda Day, Program Director

The Alberta ACADRE Network
1059 Research Transition Facility
University of Alberta
Edmonton, AB T6G 2V2
Phone: (780) 492–1827
E-mail: acadre@ualberta.ca
Web: http://www.acadre.ualberta.ca
Contact: Malcolm King, Principal Investigator

Anisnwabe Kenendazone Network Environment for Aboriginal Health Research
1 Stewart Street, Room 319
Ottawa, ON K1N 6N5
Telephone: 1 (613) 562–5393
Fax: 1 (613) 562–5392
E-mail: cietcanada@ciet.org
Web: http://www.ciet.org/en/documents/projects/200629171753.asp

Atlantic Centre of Excellence for Women's Health
502–1465 Brenton Street
Halifax, NS B3J 3T4
Phone: (902) 494–7850
E-mail: barbara.clow@dal.ca
Web: http://www.acewh.dal.ca
Contact: Barbara Clow, Executive Director

Atlantic Health Promotion Research Centre
Dalhousie University
City Centre Atlantic, Suite 209
1535 Dresden Row
Halifax, NS B3J 3T1
Phone: (902) 494–2240
E-mail: renee.lyons@dal.ca
Web: http://www.ahprc.dal.ca/welcome/default.asp
Contact: Renee Lyons, Senior Scientist

BC Centre of Excellence for Women's Health
E311–4500 Oak Street, Box 48
Vancouver, BC V6H 3N1
Phone: (604) 875–2633
Fax: (604) 875–3716
E-mail: lgreaves@cw.bc.ca
Web: http://www.bccewh.bc.ca
Contact: Dr. Lorraine Greaves, Executive Director

Centre for Aboriginal Health Research
Department of Community Health Sciences
Suite 715, 7th Floor
J. Buhler Research Centre
The University of Manitoba
715 McDermot Avenue
Winnipeg, MB R3E 3P4
Phone: (204) 789–3250
E-mail: oneilj@ms.umanitoba.ca
Web: http://www.umanitoba.ca/centres/cahr
Contact: John O'Neil, Professor

Centre for Community Health Promotion Research
University of Victoria, UH3
PO Box 3060
Victoria, BC V8W 3R4
Phone: (250) 472–4102
E-mail: mhills@uvic.ca
Web: http://web.uvic.ca/~chpc
Contact: Marcia Hills, Director

Centre for Health Promotion
155 College Street, Suite 400
Health Sciences Building
Toronto, ON M5T 3M7
Phone: (416) 978–2182
E-mail: suzanne.jackson@utoronto.ca
Web: http://www.utoronto.ca/chp
Contact: Suzanne Jackson, Director

Centre for Health Promotion Studies
5–10 University Terrace
8303 112th Street
Edmonton, AB T6G 2T4
Phone: (780) 492–9415
Fax: (780) 492–9579
E-mail: kim.raine@ualberta.ca
Web: http://www.chps.ualberta.ca
Contact: Kim Raine, Professor and Director

Centre for Human Settlements
University of British Columbia
1933 West Mall, 2nd Floor
Vancouver, BC V6T 1Z2
Phone: (604) 822–5254
E-mail: peterb@interchange.ubc.ca or angeles@interchange.ubc.ca
Web: http://www.chs.ubc.ca
Contact: Peter Boothroyd, Professor Emeritus or Leonora Angeles, Associate Professor

Centre for Population Health Promotion Research/Partnering in Community Health
Research
426–2206 East Mall, LPC Building
Vancouver, BC V6R 1Z3
Phone: (604) 822–6515
E-mail: faye.pedersen@ubc.ca
Web: www.pchr.net
Contact: Faye Pedersen, Training Program Manager

Groupe de recherche et d'intervention en promotion de la santé de l'Université
Laval
École des sciences infirmiégres
Université Laval
Pavillon Paul-Comtois
2425, rue de l'Agriculture, local 4106
Québec, QB G1K 7P4
Phone: (418) 656–3356
Web: http://www.ulaval.ca/fsi/gripsul.html
Contact: Michel O'Neill

Health Promotion Research Group
University of Calgary
Community Health Sciences
3330 Hospital Drive NW
Calgary, AB T2N 4N1
Phone: (403) 220–8242
Web: http://www.hprg.ucalgary.ca/notice.php
Contact: Dr. Penny Hawe

Indigenous Health Research Development Program
Six Nations Polytechnic
2160 Fourth Line Road
Ohsweken, ON N0A 1M0
Phone: (519) 445–0023, ext. 236
E-mail: vobrien@mcmaster.ca
Web: http://www.ihrdp.ca
Contact: Valerie O'Brien, Research and Training Coordinator

Indigenous Peoples' Health Research Centre
CK 115, University of Regina
3737 Wascana Parkway
Regina, SK S4S 0A2
Phone: (306) 337–2461
E-mail: marlene.lerat@uregina.ca
Web: http://www.iphrc.ca
Contact: Marlene Lerat-Stetner, Research Coordinator

Institute of Health Promotion Research
University of British Columbia
2206 East Mall, Room 324
Vancouver, BC V6T 1Z4
Phone: (604) 822–2258
E-mail: frankish@interchange.ubc.ca
Web: http://www.ihpr.ubc.ca
Contact: C. James Frankish

Kahnawake Schools Diabetes Prevention Project
Kahnawake Education Center
PO Box 989
Kahnawake Territory, Mohawk Nation
via QB, Canada J0L 1B0
Phone: (450) 635–4374
E-mail: ann.macaulay@mcgill.ca
Web: http://www.ksdpp.org
Contact: Ann Macaulay, MD, Co-Investigator

Nasivvik NEAHR Centre for Inuit Health and Changing Environments
Unité de recherche en santé publique
Université Laval,
Centre de recherche du CHUL-CHUQ
Édifice Delta 2, Bureau 600
2875, boulevard Laurier, 6e étage
Sainte-Foy, QC, G1V 2M2
Phone: (418) 656–4141, ext. 46516
E-mail: susie.bernier@crchul.ulaval.ca
Web: http://www.nasivvik.ulaval.ca
Contact: Susie Bernier, Executive Director

Participatory Research at McGill
McGill University
Department of Family Medicine
517 Pine Avenue West
Montreal, QC H2W 1S4
Phone: (514) 398–1357
E-mail: pram.med@mcgill.ca
Web: http://pram.mcgill.ca
Contact: Ann Macaulay, Director

Prairie Region Health Promotion Research Centre
University of Saskatchewan
Health Sciences Building
107 Wiggins Road
Saskatoon, SK S7N 5E5
Phone: (306) 966–7842
Web: http://prhprc.usask.ca
Contact: Lewis Williams, Director

Prairie Women's Health Centre of Excellence
56 The Promenade
Winnipeg, MB R3B 3H9
Phone: (204) 982–6630
Fax: (204) 982–6637
E-mail: pwhce@uwinnipeg.ca
Web: http://www.pwhce.ca
Contact: Margaret Haworth-Brockman, Executive Director

Rural Development Institute
Brandon University
270 18th Street
Brandon, MB R7A 6A9
Phone: (204) 571–8518
Web: http://www.brandonu.ca/rdi
Contact: Robert Annis, Director

Saskatchewan Indian Federated College
1 First Nations Way, Room 0127
Regina, SK S4S 7K2
Phone: (306) 790–5950, x2600
E-mail: tpelletier@firstnationsuniversity.ca
Web: http://www.firstnationsuniversity.ca
Contact: Tina Pelletier

Wellesley Institute
45 Charles Street E, Suite 101
Toronto, ON M4Y 1S2
Phone: (416) 972–1010
E-mail: contact@wellesleyinstitute.com
Web: http://wellesleyinstitute.com
Contact: Brenda Roche, Director, Community-Based Research

NAME INDEX

SUBJECT INDEX

CPSIA information can be obtained at www.ICGtesting.com
Printed in the USA
BVOW04n0829280816

459798BV00003B/1/P